Motor Control and Human Movement

Motor Control and Human Movement

Editor: Lael Dickson

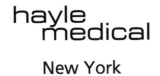

New York

Hayle Medical,
750 Third Avenue, 9th Floor,
New York, NY 10017, USA

Visit us on the World Wide Web at:
www.haylemedical.com

ISBN 978-1-64647-583-4 (Hardback)

Cataloging-in-Publication Data

Motor control and human movement / edited by Lael Dickson.
    p. cm.
Includes bibliographical references and index.
ISBN 978-1-64647-583-4
1. Motor ability. 2. Human mechanics. 3. Kinesiology. 4. Human locomotion. 5. Musculoskeletal system.
6. Human physiology. I. Dickson, Lael.
QP301 .M68 2023
612.044--dc23

Contents

Preface

The regulation of movement in the organisms which have a nervous system is known as motor control. It consists of both reflexes as well as deliberate movement. Biomechanics refers to the study of movements in a living body, which involves the manner in which bones, ligaments, muscles and tendons collaborate for producing movement. It encompasses not only the structure and movement of muscles and bones but also the mechanics of renal function, blood circulation and other body functions. The human body comprises many joints and muscles that work in tandem. The nervous system needs to combine multimodal sensory input in order to regulate movement. Furthermore, it must elicit the required signals for recruiting muscles to complete a task. Motor control then initiates, directs and grades deliberate voluntary movement while also regulating movement related mechanisms. This book includes some of the vital pieces of work being conducted across the world, on various topics related to motor control and human movement. The topics included herein are of utmost significance and bound to provide incredible insights to readers.

Significant researches are present in this book. Intensive efforts have been employed by authors to make this book an outstanding discourse. This book contains the enlightening chapters which have been written on the basis of significant researches done by the experts.

Finally, I would also like to thank all the members involved in this book for being a team and meeting all the deadlines for the submission of their respective works. I would also like to thank my friends and family for being supportive in my efforts.

Editor

Guidelines for Assessment of Gait and Reference Values for Spatiotemporal Gait Parameters in Older Adults: The Biomathics and Canadian Gait Consortiums Initiative

Olivier Beauchet [1,2,3*], Gilles Allali [4,5], Harmehr Sekhon [1], Joe Verghese [5], Sylvie Guilain [6,7], Jean-Paul Steinmetz [8], Reto W. Kressig [9], John M. Barden [10], Tony Szturm [11], Cyrille P. Launay [12], Sébastien Grenier [13], Louis Bherer [13,14], Teresa Liu-Ambrose [15], Vicky L. Chester [16], Michele L. Callisaya [17,18], Velandai Srikanth [18], Guillaume Léonard [19], Anne-Marie De Cock [20], Ryuichi Sawa [21], Gustavo Duque [22], Richard Camicioli [23] and Jorunn L. Helbostad [24,25]

[1] Department of Medicine, Division of Geriatric Medicine, Sir Mortimer B. Davis—Jewish General Hospital and Lady Davis Institute for Medical Research, McGill University, Montreal, QC, Canada, [2] Dr. Joseph Kaufmann Chair in Geriatric Medicine, Faculty of Medicine, McGill University, Montreal, QC, Canada, [3] Centre of Excellence on Aging and Chronic Diseases of McGill Integrated University Health Network, QC, Canada, [4] Department of Neurology, Geneva University Hospital and University of Geneva, Geneva, Switzerland, [5] Division of Cognitive & Motor Aging, Department of Neurology, Albert Einstein College of Medicine, Yeshiva University, Bronx, NY, United States, [6] Geriatric Department, Liège University Hospital, Liege, Belgium, [7] Laboratory of Human Motion Analysis, Liège University, Liege, Belgium, [8] Centre for Memory and Mobility, Luxembourg City, Luxembourg, [9] Basel University Center for Medicine of Aging, Felix Platter Hospital and University of Basel, Basel, Switzerland, [10] Faculty of Kinesiology and Health Studies, Neuromechanical Research Centre, University of Regina, Regina, SK, Canada, [11] Department of Physical Therapy, College of Rehabilitation Sciences, University of Manitoba, Winnipeg, MB, Canada, [12] Division of Geriatrics, Angers University Hospital, Angers, France, [13] Centre de Recherche, Institut Universitaire de Gériatrie de Montréal, Montreal, QC, Canada, [14] Department of Medicine and Montreal Heart Institute, University of Montreal, Montreal, Canada, [15] Aging, Mobility and Cognitive Neuroscience Laboratory, University of British Columbia, Vancouver, BC, Canada, [16] Andrew and Marjorie McCain Human Performance Laboratory, Richard J. Currie Center, Faculty of Kinesiology, University of New Brunswick, Fredericton, NB, Canada, [17] Menzies Institute of Medical Research, University of Tasmania, Hobart, TAS, Australia, [18] Stroke and Ageing Research Group, Department of Medicine, Southern Clinical School, Monash University, Melbourne, VIC, Australia, [19] Research Center on Aging, CIUSSS de l'Estrie-CHUS, Sherbrooke, QC, Canada, [20] Department of Geriatrics and Department of Primary and Interdisciplinary Care (ELIZA), University of Antwerp and AZ St. Maarten Mechelen, Antwerp, Belgium, [21] Department of Physical Therapy, School of Health Sciences at Narita, International University of Health and Welfare, Narita, Japan, [22] Australian Institute for Musculoskeletal Science, University of Melbourne and Western Health, St. Albans, VIC, Australia, [23] Division of Neurology, Department of Medicine, University of Alberta, Edmonton, AB, Canada, [24] Department of Neuro-Medicine and Movement Science, Faculty of Medicine and Health Sciences, Norwegian University of Science and Technology, Trondheim, Norway, [25] Clinic for Clinical Services, St. Olav University Hospital, Trondheim, Norway

*Correspondence:
Olivier Beauchet
Olivier.beauchet@mcgill.ca

Background: Gait disorders, a highly prevalent condition in older adults, are associated with several adverse health consequences. Gait analysis allows qualitative and quantitative assessments of gait that improves the understanding of mechanisms of gait disorders and the choice of interventions. This manuscript aims (1) to give consensus guidance for clinical and spatiotemporal gait analysis based on the recorded footfalls in older adults aged 65 years and over, and (2) to provide reference values for spatiotemporal gait parameters based on the recorded footfalls in healthy older adults free of cognitive impairment and multi-morbidities.

Methods: International experts working in a network of two different consortiums (i.e., Biomathics and Canadian Gait Consortium) participated in this initiative. First, they identified items of standardized information following the usual procedure of formulation of consensus findings. Second, they merged databases including spatiotemporal gait assessments with GAITRite® system and clinical information from the "Gait, cOgnitiOn & Decline" (GOOD) initiative and the Generation 100 (Gen 100) study. Only healthy—free of cognitive impairment and multi-morbidities (i.e., ≤ 3 therapeutics taken daily)—participants aged 65 and older were selected. Age, sex, body mass index, mean values, and coefficients of variation (CoV) of gait parameters were used for the analyses.

Results: Standardized systematic assessment of three categories of items, which were demographics and clinical information, and gait characteristics (clinical and spatiotemporal gait analysis based on the recorded footfalls), were selected for the proposed guidelines. Two complementary sets of items were distinguished: a minimal data set and a full data set. In addition, a total of 954 participants (mean age 72.8 ± 4.8 years, 45.8% women) were recruited to establish the reference values. Performance of spatiotemporal gait parameters based on the recorded footfalls declined with increasing age (mean values and CoV) and demonstrated sex differences (mean values).

Conclusions: Based on an international multicenter collaboration, we propose consensus guidelines for gait assessment and spatiotemporal gait analysis based on the recorded footfalls, and reference values for healthy older adults.

Keywords: gait, aged, guidelines, reference values

INTRODUCTION

Gait—the medical term used to describe the human locomotor movement of walking in healthy adults—is simple in terms of execution, but complex in terms of biomechanics and motor control (Nutt et al., 1993; Zajac et al., 2002; McCann and Higginson, 2008; Dicharry, 2010; Kuo and Donelan, 2010). Gait is usually considered as a dynamic balance condition in which the body's center of gravity is maintained within a slight base of support while moving (Farley and Ferris, 1998; Dicharry, 2010; Kuo and Donelan, 2010). During the past decade, it has been highlighted that even the simplest walking condition, such as straight-line walking at a comfortable steady-state pace without any disturbance, involves important cortical networks and cognitive functions (Alexander and Crutcher, 1990; Seidler et al., 2010; Zwergal et al., 2012; Beauchet et al., 2015b, 2016).

Numerous studies show that gait changes over an individual's lifetime (Nutt et al., 1993; Hausdorff et al., 1996; Nutt, 2001; Verghese et al., 2006; Montero-Odasso et al., 2012). Although, gait disorders are common in older (i.e., >65 years) adults, they are not unavoidable. With aging, there are physiological changes in the sensorimotor systems, which when combined with adverse effects of chronic diseases, may cause gait disorders (i.e., a deviation of normal gait performance leading to gait instability and related adverse health consequences; American Geriatrics Society and British Geriatrics Society and American Academy of Orthopedic Surgeons Panel on Falls Prevention, 2001; Nutt, 2001). Gait disorders in old age are a risk factor for

falls and are associated with increased morbidity, mortality, loss of independent living, disability, altered quality of life, and as such can lead to increased health care expenditures (Panel on Prevention of Falls in Older Persons and American Geriatrics Society and British Geriatrics Society, 2011). The prevalence of gait disorders can be as high as 80% in the oldest-old (i.e., >85 years) age category and gait disorders represent a major worldwide concern based on their expanding prevalence (American Geriatrics Society and British Geriatrics Society and American Academy of Orthopedic Surgeons Panel on Falls Prevention, 2001; Verghese et al., 2006; Panel on Prevention of Falls in Older Persons and American Geriatrics Society and British Geriatrics Society, 2011).

The assessment of gait characteristics in older adults has enhanced our understanding of the mechanisms of gait disorders, which have been helpful in developing preventive and curative interventions (Nutt, 2001; Panel on Prevention of Falls in Older Persons and American Geriatrics Society and British Geriatrics Society, 2011). Clinical gait assessment has typically been based on visual observation (Nutt, 2001). However, this approach has two main limitations. First, visual observation depends on the background and experience of the clinician who performs the gait assessment, which explains the poor inter-rater reliability of this approach (Eastlack et al., 1991; Kressig et al., 2006). Second, a limited amount of information is collected, which limits the possibility of detecting gait impairments at an early stage as well as understanding the disorganization of gait control (Kressig et al., 2006; Montero-Odasso et al., 2012). The use of quantitative and standardized clinical tests, such as the Timed Up & Go (TUG) test has been shown to be useful as a complement to visual gait observation (Podsiadlo and Richardson, 1991). Indeed, it improves the inter-rater reliability of gait assessment and provides a common objective language that facilitates exchanges between clinicians and researchers. However, it is insufficient in detecting relevant subtle gait abnormalities like changes in gait variability (Kressig et al., 2006; Beauchet et al., 2014a). For instance, an increase in stride time variability (STV) has been identified as the best motor phenotype of cognitive decline in older adults, suggesting that increases in STV could be used to improve the prediction of dementia such as Alzheimer Disease (AD; Montero-Odasso et al., 2012; Beauchet et al., 2014a). It has been proposed that subclinical gait changes may be used as a surrogate marker of development of future diseases or adverse clinical outcomes, such as falls or disability (Verghese et al., 2009; Rao et al., 2011; Ayers et al., 2014; Beauchet et al., 2014a; Artaud et al., 2015).

Currently, advanced technology has changed the practice of gait analysis because it surpasses the limits of clinical observation (i.e., visual observation and standardized test) of gait and is easily accessible and feasible (Webster et al., 2005; Beauchet et al., 2008). The initial trade-off between the accuracy of gait measuring systems and their clinical use due to cost, labor-intensity, and time consumption has disappeared. There are numerous validated and user-friendly portable gait analysis systems, like electronic gait mats, insole footswitch systems and body worn inertial sensor systems that allow objective gait parameters to be easily obtained at low cost (Kressig et al., 2006; Beauchet et al., 2008). Gait analysis systems may be separated into three categories: the first includes non-wearable sensors and consists of devices based on image processing and pressure-sensitive floor sensors, such as the GAITRite® system, which provided all spatiotemporal parameters based on the recorded footfalls. The second category includes wearable sensors such as pressure-sensitive insoles and body worn accelerometers/inertial measurement units (IMUs), with this last category providing the opportunity to analyse gait outside the laboratory and obtain information about gait during the individual's everyday activities. The third category of devices includes a combination of both previous systems. Though promising, the research on gait characteristics derived from wearable sensors in free living situations is still in its infancy. It is therefore too early to give strong recommendations on gait assessment and on the protocols that should be used to derive reliable and valid information about gait from these systems.

While this is an important advancement for researchers, as well as for patients and clinicians, it presents a new challenge based on a combination of different issues: (1) the lack of consensus on which gait parameters to assess and their clinical relevance; (2) the lack of a consensus concerning data acquisition; (3) the lack of standardized data from a large number of people to correctly define reference values related to healthy aging; (4) the excessive fragmentation, dispersion and confinement of data, skills, and knowledge of teams of researchers and/or clinicians; (5) and finally the lack of sufficient research funding in science and medicine. The successful future of scientific and medical research in the field of gait disorders mainly depends on sharing and/or pooling of resources, research and databases between teams. Hence, there is an emergence of networks with a common interest to provide mutual assistance and useful information. Recently, two networks have been formalized, with the aim of helping clinicians and researchers to increase their knowledge and improve the field of age-related gait disorders by sharing knowledge and data sets: these are (1) the Biomathics (Beauchet et al., 2014c) and (2) the Canadian Gait Consortium. Both consortiums connect academic research teams working on age-related gait changes, and share their databases in order to compound a larger, more comprehensive and representative database. This provides fast and comprehensive answers to research questions with minimal additional financial resources and large population-based samples. Furthermore, it is likely that some objectives identified in a specific study may be relevant to other teams, and at the very least the initial investigators can respond to queries of a secondary team. In such cases, the requesting team launches an initiative within the consortium and contacts all team members who may be able to help. Willing researchers are included in the initiative to participate in the research, contribute to the collaborative publication and be included in the list of co-authors depending on their contribution to the study and the number of included participants. For instance, the Biomathics consortium recently focused on gait disorders in older individuals with cognitive decline: the objective was to compare spatiotemporal gait parameters based on the recorded footfalls in cognitively healthy individuals (CHIs), individuals with amnestic (aMCI) and non-amnestic mild cognitive impairment (naMCI), and individuals with mild and moderate stages AD and non-Alzheimer's disease (non-AD; Allali et al., 2016). They merged databases for a first initiative called "Gait, cOgnitiOn & Decline" (GOOD), which involved 2717 participants and represented the largest database in this field of research. The GOOD study demonstrated that spatiotemporal gait parameters are more disturbed in the advanced stages of dementia with worse performance in the non-AD dementias than in AD. These results suggest that quantitative gait parameters may be used for improving the accuracy of classifying dementia (Allali et al., 2016), as well as supporting clinical follow-ups that try to prevent adverse events such as falls or disability.

This first initiative underscored the requirement of utilizing standardized assessment when performing spatiotemporal gait analysis. Although, some reference values for gait parameters in older adults already exist (Oberg et al., 1993; Oh-Park et al., 2010; Bohannon and Williams Andrews, 2011; Hollman et al., 2011; Hass et al., 2012), this first initiative demonstrated that there is a need for quantitative reference values of spatiotemporal gait parameters for large numbers of healthy older adults. Importantly, older adults are considered to be healthy when they are free of cognitive deficits and comorbidities. Combining and integrating evaluations performed in populations from different countries is crucial for the development of future research on gait disorders. Indeed, the definition of gait disorders requires comparisons with quantitative reference values for spatiotemporal gait parameters in healthy older adults with diverse social, cultural, ethnic, and demographic backgrounds. Based on this first experience of the GOOD initiative, the Biomathics and Canadian Gait Consortiums decided to launch an initiative with the following aims: (1) to give consensus guidance for clinical and spatiotemporal gait analysis based on the recorded footfalls in older adults aged 65 years and over, and (2) to provide reference values for spatiotemporal gait parameters based on the recorded footfalls in healthy older (i.e., >65 years) adults free of cognitive impairment and multi-morbidities.

METHODS

Guidelines for Clinical and Spatiotemporal Gait Analysis Based on the Recorded Footfalls in Older Adults Aged 65 Years and Over

The guidelines for clinical and spatiotemporal gait analysis based on the recorded footfalls in older adults followed the usual procedure of formulation of a consensus finding, consisting of a three-step process (Annweiler et al., 2015). In the first step, between May and October 2015, the lead author (OB) invited members of the Biomathics and Canadian Gait Consortiums composed with experts of gait disorders in aging, to form a group. The members of both consortiums are experts in gait and/or movement and are presented in **Table 1**. In a second step from July 2015 to May 2016, all experts communicated by email, phone calls or videoconferencing with the first author to identify items required for spatiotemporal gait analysis in older adults. The first author, as the leader of both consortiums, contacted each member to explain the initiative, obtain their agreement to the consensus procedures, and propose an initial version of the guidelines. Each member of the consortium formulated changes and/or proposed additional information. The first author merged all changes and wrote the second version of the guidelines. All experts reviewed this version and finally a consensual

TABLE 1 | Composition of Biomathics and Canadian Gait Consortiums.

Country/Canadian province	Town	University	Centre	Reference person
BIOMATHICS CONSORTIUM				
Australia	Hobart	University of Tasmania	Menzies Institute of Medical Research	Michele L Callisaya; PhD
	Melbourne	University of Melbourne & Western Health	Australian Institute for Musculoskeletal Science	Gustavo Duque; MD, PhD
	Victoria	Monash University	Department of Medicine	Velandai Srikanth; PhD
Belgium	Antwerp	University of Antwerp	Department of geriatrics and department of primary and interdisciplinary care (ELIZA)	Anne-Marie De Cock; MD
	Liege	University of Liege	Department of Geriatrics	Sylvie Gilain; MD
France	Angers	University of Angers	Department of Neuroscience, Geriatrics division	Cyrille P Launay; MD, PhD
Japan	Chiba-ken	University of Health and Welfare	Department of Physical Therapy, School of Health Sciences at Narita International	Ryuichi Sawa; PhD
Luxembourg	Luxembourg-city	Zitha Senior	Centre for Memory and Mobility	Jean-Paul Steinmetz; PhD
Norway	Trondheim	Norwegian University of Science and Technology	Department of Neuromedicine and Movement Science	Jorunn L. Helbostad; PT, PhD
USA	New York	Yeshiva University	Department of Neurology, Division of Cognitive & Motor Aging	Joe Verghese; MD, MBBS
Switzerland	Basel	University of Basel	Basel University Center for Medicine of Aging	Reto W. Kressig; MD
	Geneva	University of Geneva	Department of Neurology	Gilles Allali; MD, PhD
CANADIAN GAIT CONSORTIUM				
Alberta	Edmonton	University of Alberta	Department of Medicine, Division of Neurology	Richard Camicioli; MD, PhD
British Columbia	Vancouver	University of British Columbia	Aging, Mobility, and Cognitive Neuroscience Lab Djavad Mowafaghian Centre for Brain Health	Teresa Liu-Ambrose; PT, PhD
Manitoba	Winnipeg	University of Manitoba	College of Rehabilitation Sciences	Tony Szturm; PT, PhD
Quebec	Montreal	University of Concordia	Perform institute	Louis Bherer; PhD
		University of McGill	Department of Medicine, Division of Geriatrics, Jewish General Hospital	Olivier Beauchet; MD, PhD
		University of Montreal	Institut universitaire de gériatrie Montreal Heart Institute Research Center and Departement of Medicine	Sébastien Grenier; PhD Louis Bherer; PhD
	Sherbrooke	University of Sherbrooke	Research Centre on Aging	Léonard Guillaume; PhD
New Brunswick	Fredericton	University of New Brunswick	Richard J. Currie Center	Victoria L. Chester; PhD
Saskatchewan	Regina	University of Regina	Neuromechanical Research Centre, Faculty of Kinesiology and Health Studies	John M. Barden; PhD

agreement was obtained. A dataset of common items divided into three categories was selected: demographic characteristics, clinical characteristics, and gait characteristics. Furthermore, a standardized procedure for spatiotemporal gait analysis based on the recorded footfalls was defined and two types of datasets were individualized: a minimum dataset corresponding to items required for all gait analysis in older individuals, and a full dataset corresponding to items of the minimum dataset plus additional items recorded when possible and for specific purposes. All selected items are shown in **Table 2.**

Quantitative Reference Values for Spatiotemporal Gait Parameters Based on the Recorded Footfalls
Participant Selection
Data were extracted from two databases: the GOOD initiative (Clinical trials registration number: NCT02350270) (Allali et al., 2016) and the Generation 100 (Clinical trials registration number: NCT01666340) (Stensvold et al., 2015). The GOOD initiative was based on a cross-sectional design such that the main objective was to compare spatiotemporal gait characteristics based on the recorded footfalls of CHIs, and participants with MCI or dementia. Data collection, study procedures and criteria for categorization of participants have been described in detail elsewhere (Allali et al., 2016). In brief, data from seven countries (Australia, Belgium, France, India, Luxembourg, Switzerland, and the United States) were merged. Data sources were the "Tasmanian Study of Cognition and Gait" (TASCOG) (Tasmanian), the Mechelen memory clinic database (Belgium), the "Gait and Alzheimer Interactions Tracking" (GAIT) study (France), the "Kerala-Einstein Study" (KES) (India), the Center for Memory and Mobility (Luxembourg), the "Central Control of Mobility in Aging" (US), and the Basel mobility center (Switzerland).

The Generation 100 study is a population-based large randomized controlled clinical trial (Stensvold et al., 2015). The primary aim of this study is to examine the effects of 5 years of exercise training on mortality in the elderly (Stensvold et al., 2015). The data collection and study procedures have been described in detail elsewhere (Stensvold et al., 2015). In summary, it is an ongoing phase IIb clinical trial. The participants are stratified by sex and marital status and randomized 1:1 into an exercise training group or a control group. They are assessed at baseline and at follow-up after 1, 3, and 5 years. For this analysis, we used the data collected at baseline.

Exclusion criteria for the present study were age <65 years, non-Caucasian, cognitive decline (i.e., MCI and dementia), walking with personal assistance, polypharmacy defined as more than 3 therapeutic drug classes taken daily, history of falls in the past 12-month period, the presence of depressive and/or anxiety symptoms, moderate or severe distance vision impairment (when information was accessible), and absence of spatiotemporal gait data. From the 2,717 participants initially recruited in the GOOD initiative, 548 (20.2%) healthy older adults met the inclusion criteria. A total of 457 (29.7%) participants from the

1,541 participants who had a gait assessment at baseline in the Generation 100 study met the inclusion criteria. Fifty-one of the 1005 (19.7%) identified participants were excluded because of incomplete gait data. Finally, 954 participants were included in the analysis.

Assessment
Age, sex, and anthropometric measures (i.e., height in metres and weight in kilograms) were recorded. Body mass index (BMI, in kg/m^2) was also calculated. Spatiotemporal gait parameters based on the recorded footfalls were measured during steady-state walking using the GAITRite®-system. This gait system is an electronic walkway with an integrated pressure-sensitive electronic surface connected to a portable computer via an interface cable. The GAITRite®-system is a well-established method of quantifying gait and provides reliable and accurate measures of spatiotemporal gait parameters. Spatiotemporal gait parameters have shown excellent test-retest reliability in clinical and research settings in community-dwelling older people when using the GAITRite®-system (Brach et al., 2008). During the past decade over 100 manuscripts have been published using data collected and processed with the GAITRite® system.

The active recording area of the gait mats ranged from 4.6 m (TASCOG study) to 7.9 m (GAIT study). Participants completed one (GAIT, CCMA, and KES studies; the Mechelen memory clinic, the Centre for Memory and Mobility of Luxembourg-city, The Basel mobility center), two (Generation 100 study) or six (TASCOG study) trials at their usual self-selected walking speed in a quiet, well-lit environment, wearing their own footwear. The mean of the 2 (the Generation 100) or 6 trials (the TASCOG studies) was used to calculate the gait variables. The mean value and coefficient of variation [CoV = (standard deviation/mean) × 100] of the spatiotemporal gait parameters were used as outcomes. For a list of the included spatiotemporal variables, see **Table 2.**

Standard Protocol Approvals and Registrations
Each site involved in this study obtained approval from their local ethics committee to conduct site-specific assessments: the Southern Tasmanian Health and Medical Human Research Ethics Committee for the TASCOG study (Australia), the ethics committee of Angers University hospital for the GAIT study (France), the ethics committee of Emmaus—St Maarten General Hospital Mechelen for the Mechelen memory clinic database (Belgium), the institutional ethics committee of Baby Memorial Hospital for KES study (India), the ethics committee of Luxembourg for the Center for Memory and Mobility database (Luxembourg), the ethics committee of Albert Einstein College of Medicine for the "Central Control of Mobility in Aging" (US) study, and the ethics committee of Basel for the Basel mobility center database (Switzerland). The ethics committee of Angers (France) University hospital approved the GOOD initiative (2014/17). The regional committee of Mid Norway for Medical and Health Research Ethics approved the transfer and the merging (number 2015/1797) of the Generation 100 database with the GOOD database.

TABLE 2 | Selected items for gait analysis in the elderly.

Items for the minimum dataset	Additional items for the full dataset
DEMOGRAPHIC CHARACTERISTICS	
Age (year)	
Sex	
Ethnicity coded as follows: 1, Black; 2, Caucasian; 3, Asian; 4, Other	
CLINICAL CHARACTERISTICS	
Height (m)	
Weight (kg)	
Medication; Number of therapeutic classes used per day >3 (coded yes vs. no)	
	Number of therapeutic classes taken daily
	Use of psychoactive drugs (i.e., benzodiazepines, antidepressants, neuroleptics) (coded yes vs. no)
History of falls (i.e., defined as an event resulting in a person coming to rest unintentionally on the ground or at another lower level, not as the result of a major intrinsic event or an overwhelming hazard) in the previous 12-month period (coded yes vs. no)	Recurrent falls (i.e., ≥ 2) (coded yes vs. no)
	Severe falls (i.e., fractures, cranial trauma, large and/or deep skin lesions, post-fall syndrome; inability to get up; time on ground ≥ 1 h; hospitalization) (coded yes vs. no).
	Fear of falling (Are you afraid of falling? Never, almost never, sometimes, often, and very often)
Neurological diseases:	
• Dementia (coded yes vs. no)	• Cognitive complaint (coded yes vs. no)
	• Mild cognitive impairment (coded yes vs. no)
	• Dementia (coded yes vs. no), if yes stage (i.e., mild, moderate, severe) and etiology (i.e., AD, non-AD neurodegenerative, non-AD vascular, mixed)
	• Global cognitive performance: MoCA score (Nasreddine et al., 2005)
• Other (coded yes vs. no)	• Parkinson's disease or parkinsonian syndromes (coded yes vs. no)
	• Idiopathic normal pressure hydrocephalus (coded yes vs. no)
	• Cerebellar disease (coded yes vs. no)
	• Myelopathy (coded yes vs. no)
	• Peripheral neuropathy (coded yes vs. no)
Depressive symptoms (coded yes vs. no)	4-item Geriatric Depression Scale score (Shah et al., 1997)
Anxiety symptoms (coded yes vs. no)	5-item Geriatric Anxiety Inventory (Byrne and Pachana, 2011)
Major orthopedic diagnoses (e.g., osteoarthritis) involving the lumbar vertebrae, pelvis or lower extremities (coded yes vs. no)	
Vision disorders (coded yes vs. no)	Distance binocular vision measured at 5 m with a standard scale, vision assessed with corrective lenses if needed
Lower limb proprioception disorders (coded yes vs. no)	Lower limb proprioception evaluated with a graduated tuning fork placed on the tibial tuberosity: The mean value obtained for the left and right sides (/8)
Muscle strength impairment (coded yes vs. no)	Hand grip strength: mean value of the highest value of maximal isometric voluntary contractions (3 trials) measured with computerized dynamometers expressed in Newtons per square meter
Use of walking aid (coded yes vs. no)	
GAIT CHARACTERISTICS	
Clinical analysis	
Subjective self-reported difficulties (coded never, almost never, sometimes, often, and very often)	
Clinical gait abnormalities (coded yes vs. no)	
Timed Up & Go score (s) (Podsiadlo and Richardson, 1991)	Timed Up & Go imagined form score (s) (Beauchet et al., 2010)
Walking speed: time to walk 4 m at steady-state walking	

(Continued)

TABLE 2 | Continued

Items for the minimum dataset	Additional items for the full dataset
Spatiotemporal analysis	
• Conditions	
✓ In a quiet, well-lit environment	
✓ Steady state walking (acceleration and deceleration phase of 1 m each)	
✓ Wearing participant's own footwear	
✓ Usual self-selected walking speed	
	• Fast walking speed
	• Dual tasking:
	✓ Backward counting by ones from 50
	✓ Verbal fluency task (animal names)
• Parameters	
✓ Walking speed [mean value (cm/s)]	
✓ Stride time [mean value (ms) and coefficient of variation (%)]	
✓ Swing time [mean value (ms) and coefficient of variation (%)]	
✓ Stride width [mean value (cm) and coefficient of variation (%)]	
	• Stride length [mean value (cm) and coefficient of variation (%)]
	• Stance time [mean value (ms) and coefficient of variation (%)]
	• Single support time [mean value (ms) and coefficient of variation (%)]
	• Double support time [mean value (ms) and coefficient of variation (%)]
	• Stride velocity [mean value (cm/s) and coefficient of variation (%)]

m, meter; kg, kilogram; s, second; cm, centimeter.

Statistics

Participants' baseline characteristics were summarized using means and standard deviations or frequencies and percentages. Participants were separated into three age groups (65–74 years, 75–84 years, and ≥85 years), and each group was dichotomized by sex. First, between-group comparisons were performed using unpaired t-test or Mann–Whitney tests, as appropriate. $P < 0.0006$ were considered as statistically significant after adjustments for multiple comparisons ($n = 79$). Second, multiple linear regressions showing the association of each spatiotemporal gait parameter (dependent variable) with age and sex (independent variable), adjusted for BMI and test center were performed. $P < 0.05$ were considered as statistically significant. All statistics were performed using SPSS (version 15.0; SPSS, Inc., Chicago, IL).

RESULTS

Guidelines for Clinical and Spatiotemporal Gait Analysis Based on the Recorded Footfalls

Two complementary sets of standardized information were identified: a minimal data set and a full data set. All items of both sets are shown in **Table 2**. They have been separated into three categories: demographic, clinical, and gait characteristics. This last category has been divided into clinical and spatiotemporal gait analysis based on the recorded footfalls.

Demographic and Clinical Characteristics

Demographic (i.e., age in years, sex and ethnicity) and anthropometric items [height in meters (m), weight in kilograms (kg), body mass index (BMI) in kg/m^2], are required because each may influence spatiotemporal gait parameters (American Geriatrics Society and British Geriatrics Society and American Academy of Orthopedic Surgeons Panel on Falls Prevention, 2001; Kressig et al., 2006; Verghese et al., 2006; Beauchet et al., 2008; Dicharry, 2010; Panel on Prevention of Falls in Older Persons and American Geriatrics Society and British Geriatrics Society, 2011). Given that the burden of disease can influence gait performance, it was decided to record this information as well (American Geriatrics Society and British Geriatrics Society and American Academy of Orthopedic Surgeons Panel on Falls Prevention, 2001; Panel on Prevention of Falls in Older Persons and American Geriatrics Society and British Geriatrics Society, 2011). Different scales have been developed to score the burden of morbidity, but they remain difficult to use in older adults, especially because of possible recall bias when reporting chronic disease among individuals with cognitive disorders, and lack of feasibility in clinical practice (due to their complexity and value for physicians, physiotherapists, or other health care professionals; Linn et al., 1968; Parmelee et al., 1995; Salvi et al., 2008; de Decker et al., 2013). Recently, an independent association was found between the Cumulative Illness Rating Scale Geriatric form (CIRS-G), which provides a morbidity score, and the number of drug classes taken daily (de Decker et al., 2013). The results showed that an increase of three drug classes corresponds to a one-point increase on the CIRS-G (de Decker et al., 2013). This result is consistent with previous studies in the general population, which reported that pharmacy data using the Anatomical Therapeutic Chemical Classification (ATCC) system might be used to provide reliable prevalence estimates of several common comorbid conditions (Von Korff et al., 1992;

Maio et al., 2005; Chini et al., 2011). In addition, it has been demonstrated that pharmacy data provide a stable measure of morbidity status, and are associated with physician-rated disease severity as well as with individual-rated health status (Von Korff et al., 1992). Hence, the decision was made to record the use of drugs in the clinical assessment. Polypharmacy is defined as the use of more than three drugs per day, which was used as the item for the minimum data set, and was combined with the exact number of therapeutic drug classes taken daily and the use of psychoactive drugs (i.e., benzodiazepines, antidepressants, neuroleptics), which was coded as yes or no in the full dataset.

Information about falls, with a fall being defined as an event resulting in a person coming to rest unintentionally on the ground or at another lower level, not as the result of a major intrinsic event or an overwhelming hazard, in the previous 12 month-period before the assessment, is also proposed (American Geriatrics Society and British Geriatrics Society and American Academy of Orthopedic Surgeons Panel on Falls Prevention, 2001; Panel on Prevention of Falls in Older Persons and American Geriatrics Society and British Geriatrics Society, 2011). For the minimum data set, only the existence (or not) of a fall(s) history is required, while for the full data set information on recurrence (i.e., ≥ 2 falls) and severity (defined as fractures, cranial trauma, large, and/or deep skin lesions, post-fall syndrome including an association of fear of falling (FOF), postural instability with absence of postural reflexes, inability to get up, time on ground ≥ 1 h, and hospitalization) are proposed for the data collection. Recently, a systematic review and meta-analysis reported that FOF might increase gait instability (Ayoubi et al., 2015). Thus, it was determined to measure FOF using the single question: "Are you afraid of falling?" with a graded answer (i.e., never, almost never, sometimes, often, and very often) for the full dataset.

In addition to FOF, collecting information on disorders or diseases that directly influence gait performance is also advised. First, information on neurological diseases (limited to the existence or non-existence of dementia) and other diseases (coded as yes or no) are collected for the minimal data set. Information on memory complaints, MCI, nature of dementia (i.e., AD, non-AD neurodegenerative, non-AD vascular, mixed), Parkinson disease, idiopathic normal pressure hydrocephalus, cerebellar disease, stroke, myelopathy, and peripheral neuropathy are also proposed for the full dataset (Alexander and Crutcher, 1990; Nutt et al., 1993; Nutt, 2001; Verghese et al., 2006; Montero-Odasso et al., 2012). A quantification of global cognitive functioning is also recommended, using for example the Montreal Cognitive Assessment (MoCA) (Nasreddine et al., 2005). In addition, among the neuropsychiatric disorders, it is important to collect information about depression symptoms because they can lead to gait instability and falls. This is limited to a simple binary question in the minimum data set and the score for the 4-item geriatric depression scale in the full data set (Shah et al., 1997). A measure of anxiety is also proposed using the 5-item Geriatric Anxiety Inventory (Byrne and Pachana, 2011).

Information on major orthopedic diagnoses (e.g., osteoarthritis) involving the lumbar vertebrae, pelvis, or lower extremities, coded yes vs. no, as well as the use of a walking aid, should also be recorded (American Geriatrics Society and British Geriatrics Society and American Academy of Orthopedic Surgeons Panel on Falls Prevention, 2001; Panel on Prevention of Falls in Older Persons and American Geriatrics Society and British Geriatrics Society, 2011).

Information on sensory and motor subsystems such as muscle strength, lower-limb proprioception and vision are required because the age-related impairment in the performance of these subsystems may affect gait performance (Beauchet et al., 2014a). For the minimal data set, impairments were coded as binary (i.e., yes or no), while in the full dataset standardized measures are required. First, the Maximum isometric Voluntary Contraction (MVC) of handgrip strength must be measured with a computerized hydraulic dynamometer. The test should be performed three times with the dominant hand. The mean value of MVC over the three trials should be used as the outcome measure. Second, distance binocular vision should be measured at a distance of 5 m with a standard scale (Lord et al., 1994). Vision needs to be assessed with corrective lenses, if used regularly. Third, lower extremity vibration sense should be measured, using a graded tuning fork placed on a bony area, such as the tibial tuberosity, medial malleolus or big toe. This is correlated with proprioception, which is critical to balance (Beauchet et al., 2014a).

Gait Characteristics

Before conducting a spatiotemporal gait analysis based on the recorded footfalls, a standardized clinical evaluation is advised. First, the individual's subjective perception of gait difficulties is registered using a single question: "Do you have any difficulty walking?" with a graduated answer (i.e., never, almost never, sometimes, often, and very often). Second, a visual observation of gait during habitual walking is proposed with a binary answer (yes vs. no) to the question "are there gait abnormalities during physical examination?"

Third, the TUG test score and gait speed (distance divided by ambulation time) when walking a distance of 4 m at a steady-state pace is suggested (Podsiadlo and Richardson, 1991; Goldberg and Schepens, 2011). These measures are proposed for the minimal dataset, while for the full data set an additional measure is proposed; that being the time to achieve the imagined TUG (iTUG) (Beauchet et al., 2015a). Exploring the higher levels of gait control may be more difficult in clinical practice. There are two alternatives: using a dual-task paradigm (i.e., walking while simultaneously executing an attention-demanding task), or using motor imagery of gait (i.e., the mental simulation of gait without its actual execution; Beauchet et al., 2015a). Recently, interest in the latter alternative has been underscored using the mental chronometry approach applied to the TUG, a well-known motor test used in clinical practice (Beauchet et al., 2010, 2014b, 2015a). The TUG is a standardized assessment of a basic functional mobility task of relevance to daily living and records the time needed to stand up, to walk 3 m, to turn back and sit down (Podsiadlo and Richardson, 1991). It has been reported that cognitive performance, and in particular executive functioning, contributes to the temporal correspondence between executing and imaging gait in individuals with neuropsychiatric conditions like dementia, schizophrenia or multiple sclerosis (Linn et al., 1968; Von Korff et al., 1992; Oberg et al., 1993; Lord et al., 1994; Parmelee et al., 1995; Shah et al., 1997; Maio et al., 2005; Nasreddine et al., 2005; Brach et al., 2008; Salvi et al., 2008; Beauchet et al., 2010, 2014a,b, 2015a; Bohannon and Williams Andrews, 2011; Byrne and Pachana, 2011; Chini et al., 2011; Goldberg and Schepens, 2011; Allali et al., 2012; Hass et al., 2012; Lallart et al., 2012; de Decker et al., 2013; Annweiler et al., 2015; Ayoubi et al., 2015; Stensvold et al., 2015). It has also been shown that older individuals with cognitive impairment executed the iTUG more rapidly than they performed it (Allali et al., 2012; Beauchet et al., 2015a). On the contrary, there has been no significant difference between the two conditions in healthy younger adults (Lallart et al., 2012). This difference in terms of performance between pTUG and iTUG, called "delta TUG," can be interpreted as the awareness of movement and physical performance, and thus may be used as a biomarker of the disorders of higher levels of gait control (Beauchet et al., 2010, 2014b, 2015a; Allali et al., 2012; Lallart et al., 2012).

It is necessary to underscore that the spatiotemporal gait analysis based on the recorded footfalls should be performed in a reproducible, quiet, well-lit environment, with patients wearing their own footwear (walking shoes, no slippers) with heel height not exceeding 3 cm and comfortable and non-restrictive clothing. Depending on the participant's fall risk, the use of safety support systems is recommended, such as a safety belt around the participant's waist. We recommend assessing the normal walking condition for the minimal data set, and for the full dataset we recommend three additional walking conditions; a fast walk at a maximum speed, and two dual-task conditions, in which the patient is instructed to walk normally while (a) counting backwards by ones starting from 50 and (b) to enumerate animal names (Kressig et al., 2006; Beauchet et al., 2012; Montero-Odasso et al., 2012). For the dual task condition, no prioritization should be given to a single task and the trial should be performed to the best of the participant's ability. Steady-state gait and gait trials in the same walking direction are required for all conditions and may be achieved by instructing participants to start walking at least 1 m prior to the data recording zone and stopping at least 1 m beyond it. It is also advisable to use simple, clear and standardized walking instructions to explain the various tasks to the participants.

Regardless of the type of category of devices used to assess gait, we recommend using a validated system that provides reliable measures. For the minimum data set, four gait parameters during normal walking including the mean value of walking speed, and mean values and coefficient of variation of stride time, swing time and stride width need to be reported. We suggest adding more stressful walking conditions (i.e., fast speed and dual tasking conditions) and reporting mean values and coefficients of variation of stride length, stance time, single and double support, and stride velocity for the full dataset. This choice is based on the fact that in terms of control of gait, gait variability has been identified as a biomarker for cortical control of gait in normal aging individuals and in individuals with dementia (Beauchet et al., 2010, 2012, 2014b, 2015a; Allali et al., 2012; Lallart et al., 2012). In addition, higher (i.e., worse) STV during normal walking has been associated with lower cognitive performance in non-demented older community-dwellers (Beauchet et al., 2012). This result has been confirmed by a meta-analysis underscoring that higher STV during normal walking was related to both MCI and dementia (Beauchet et al., 2014a). In terms of gait variability, a certain level of "healthy" variability of the motor control system is necessary to adapt to unexpected instability. Indeed, both high and low gait variability during habitual walking have been reported in younger and older CHIs with safe gait, depending on the type of gait parameters being examined (Beauchet et al., 2009). In particular, safe gait has been characterized by a low STV, an intermediate swing time variability and a high stride width variability in CHIs (Beauchet et al., 2009). These results can be explained by the fact that temporal and spatial gait parameters appear to reflect different constructs of gait control (Gabell and Nayak, 1984; Newell and Corcos, 1993; Nutt et al., 1993; Nutt, 2001; Launay et al., 2013). Stride time and stride width variability provide an indication of control of the rhythmic stepping mechanism and dynamic postural control, respectively, while swing time is indicative of both mechanisms (Gabell and Nayak, 1984; Beauchet et al., 2009). Furthermore, it is important to consider the number of steps recorded. Indeed, the accuracy of gait variability measures are highly dependent on obtaining a sufficient number of steps, with a study suggesting that a minimum of 400 steps are needed to obtain valid measures of gait variability during treadmill walking (Faude et al., 2012). However, even if it is recommended to have the highest number of gait cycles possible from a practical standpoint to assess gait variability of spatiotemporal parameters, it has been suggested that a minimum of three consecutive gait cycles should be obtained for both the left and right sides (i.e., a total of six gait cycles; Kressig et al., 2006). Furthermore, including steps from several shorter walks is recommended when obtaining the number of steps over a long walking distance is not possible.

For the collection of gait data, we suggest that gait should be assessed without assistive devices whenever possible. When a device is required it is important to describe the type of device used by the individual. Given that there are no established reference values for assistive devices, the first assessment should be used as the reference point for individuals who repeatedly use the same device.

The operational definitions of spatiotemporal gait parameters, based on GAITRite® software are as follows: (1) Stride length (in cm): anterior-posterior distance between the heel strikes of two successive placements of the same foot; stride width (in cm): lateral distance between the midlines of the right and left heels; stride time (in ms): time elapsed from the first contact of two consecutive footsteps of the same foot; swing time (in ms): time elapsed from the last contact of the current footstep to the first contact of the next footstep on the same foot; stance time (in ms): time elapsed from the initial contact and the last contact of consecutive footstep of the same foot; single support time (in ms): time elapsed from the last contact of the opposite footfall to the initial contact of the next footstep of the same foot; double support time (in ms): time elapsed during which both feet are in ground contact; stride velocity (in cm/s): stride length divided by the stride time; and walking speed (in cm/s): distance walked divided by the ambulation time.

Procedure for Clinical and Spatiotemporal Gait Analysis Based on the Recorded Footfalls

All adults aged 65 and over should be systematically interviewed or examined for gait disorders at least once per year. In addition, those who report a fall or have an acute medical condition should be asked about difficulties with gait and should be examined for gait disorders.

Clinical assessment should be separated into two main parts: global and analytic clinical assessment. The global assessment detecting gait difficulties begins with watching individuals as they walk into the examination room. The use of a walking aid and its nature (i.e., cane, walker, personal assistance, and supervision) should be noticed and the individual should be asked about his/her subjective perception of gait difficulties. This visual observation should be completed with one of the two standardized motor tests to provide an objective measure of gait performance: the TUG score and the gait speed value. After this clinical assessment and if an abnormality is recorded, a spatiotemporal gait analysis based on the recorded footfalls (collection of all information described in **Table 2**) in laboratory setting is suggested. If necessary and based on abnormalities recorded during the clinical and clinical and spatiotemporal gait analysis, an analysis outside the laboratory using wearable sensors may be propose to obtain information about gait during the individual's everyday activities. The role of other laboratory testing and diagnostic evaluation for gait and balance disorders has not been well-studied, and there is no recommended systematic investigation to perform. However, the following complementary investigations are recommended: (1) Bone radiography in the event of acute pain, joint deformation and/or functional disability, (2) Standard 12-lead ECG in case of dizziness, 3) Blood glucose level in patients with diabetes, and (4) Serum 25OHD concentration if there is no vitamin D supplementation. Cerebral imaging in the absence of specific indications based on a clinical examination may not be necessary.

Quantitative Reference Values for Spatiotemporal Gait Parameters

Table 3 shows the group mean values, standard deviations and CoV of spatiotemporal gait parameters separated by age groups and sex. In most cases, men demonstrated greater performance for mean values (i.e., less difference relative to normal values for healthy young adults) than women, but not for CoV. This effect was observed in the total sample as well as for the 65–74 year age category. Interestingly, walking speed and stride velocity were similar in both males and females when considering the total sample and each age strata separately.

The results of multiple linear regression analyses exploring the effects of age and sex on spatiotemporal gait parameters,

adjusted for BMI and test center are shown in **Table 4**. Increasing age was associated with significant lower performance for mean values and CoV for all gait parameters, except for the mean value of stride width ($P = 0.861$) and CoV of double support time ($P = 0.186$). Women demonstrated lower mean values for all temporal gait parameters compared to men, except for the mean value of double support time ($P = 0.059$) CoV of spatial parameters were significantly greater in women compared to men. In addition, both mean and CoV of stride velocity were significantly worst with increasing age in women.

DISCUSSION

Standardized systematic assessment of three categories of information, which included demographics, clinical features and gait characteristics were selected for the development of gait assessment guidelines. Two complementary sets of guidelines have been proposed: a minimal data set and a full data set. Concerning the quantitative reference values, we observed lower values in several spatiotemporal gait parameters with age as well as differences between men and women. Age had a negative effect on mean values and CoV, while sex was mainly associated with mean values. Stride velocity parameters were affected both by age and sex.

Our study provides quantitative normative values for widely used and clinically relevant spatiotemporal gait parameters. Compared to previous studies on this topic, the strategy of recruiting participants through an intercontinental initiative provides access to probably the highest number of participants involved in a study exploring reference values until now. Furthermore, we chose to select "very healthy" older participants to avoid any interaction with morbidities or cognitive impairments that can affect gait performance. Previous studies have controlled for the potential effects of morbidities using statistical analysis (Oberg et al., 1993; Oh-Park et al., 2010; Bohannon and Williams Andrews, 2011; Hollman et al., 2011; Hass et al., 2012). However, it has recently been suggested that the strategy of statistical adjustment may be limited and does not take into consideration the complex interplay and potential effects of morbidities (Kressig et al., 2006; Byrne and Pachana, 2011; Montero-Odasso et al., 2012). For instance, a recent study reported the results of the independent and combined effects of impairments of muscle strength, distance vision, lower-limb proprioception, and cognition on gait performance using pTUG and iTUG (Byrne and Pachana, 2011). It was shown that cognitive impairment, considered either separately or in combination with any other subsystem decline, notably muscle strength, was strongly associated with decreased performance on the pTUG and delta TUG scores. In contrast, lower-limb proprioceptive impairment was associated with worse performance (i.e., lower) on the iTUG. The subsystem's impairment has been associated with worse (i.e., greater) delta TUG scores; the highest impact being reported when combining muscle strength and cognition. In our study, all participants were free of morbidities, and thus

TABLE 3 | Quantitative reference values (i.e., mean ± standard deviation) for spatiotemporal gait parameters by age group (65–74 years, 75–84 years and ≥ 85 years) and sex (n = 954).

	Total population (n = 954)			P-value*	Age 65–74 years (n = 711)			P-value*	Age 75–84 years (n = 207)			P-value*	Age ≥85 years (n = 36)			P-value*
	Total	Female (n = 437)	Male (n = 517)		Total	Female (n = 312)	Male (n = 399)		Total	Female (n = 101)	Male (n = 106)		Total	Female (n = 24)	Male (n = 12)	
Age (years), mean ± SD	72.8 ± 4.8	73.2 ± 5.1	72.4 ± 4.5	0.006	70.6 ± 2.4	70.7 ± 2.4	70.5 ± 2.3	0.649	77.6 ± 2.6	77.8 ± 2.5	77.4 ± 2.6	0.274	87.7 ± 2.8	87.2 ± 2.0	88.6 ± 4.0	0.585
BMI (kg/m²), mean ± SD	26.2 ± 4.1	26.0 ± 4.8	26.4 ± 3.3	0.105	26.0 ± 3.8	25.6 ± 4.4	26.2 ± 3.2	0.094	26.6 ± 4.1	26.2 ± 4.7	27.0 ± 3.4	0.171	28.0 ± 7.2	28.2 ± 8.4	27.6 ± 3.8	0.379
STRIDE TIME																
Mean value (ms)	1123.7 ± 122.4	1095.5 ± 109.8	1147.6 ± 127.4	**<0.001**	1118.5 ± 122.3	1081.5 ± 104.3	1147.3 ± 127.5	**<0.001**	1132.7 ± 117.0	1124.3 ± 109.4	1140.7 ± 123.7	0.314	1176.1 ± 140.9	1155.7 ± 139.2	1216.9 ± 141.1	0.177
CoV (%)	2.2 ± 1.1	2.2 ± 1.1	2.1 ± 1.1	0.244	2.1 ± 1.1	2.1 ± 1.0	2.1 ± 1.0	0.520	2.3 ± 1.1	2.4 ± 1.1	2.2 ± 1.0	0.053	2.8 ± 1.3	3.1 ± 1.3	2.3 ± 1.3	0.067
SWING TIME																
Mean value (ms)	414.1 ± 40.2	402.1 ± 36.5	424.2 ± 40.5	**<0.001**	416.3 ± 40.0	403.4 ± 36.2	426.3 ± 40.0	**<0.001**	409.6 ± 39.6	401.2 ± 36.7	417.5 ± 40.8	0.003	396.7 ± 43.1	388.6 ± 37.5	413.1 ± 50.2	0.188
CoV (%)	4.2 ± 1.8	4.2 ± 2.0	4.2 ± 1.6	0.863	4.0 ± 1.7	3.9 ± 1.9	4.1 ± 1.6	0.063	4.5 ± 1.7	4.7 ± 1.8	4.4 ± 1.6	0.199	6.0 ± 2.7	6.5 ± 2.7	4.9 ± 2.3	0.020
STANCE TIME																
Mean value (ms)	706.6 ± 91.2	689.3 ± 87.3	721.2 ± 92.0	**<0.001**	700.9 ± 88.1	677.6 ± 79.0	719.0 ± 90.6	**<0.001**	713.5 ± 91.6	706.6 ± 90.3	720.1 ± 92.7	0.291	779.4 ± 114.9	767.0 ± 122.6	804.0 ± 97.9	0.212
CoV (%)	3.1 ± 1.4	3.1 ± 1.3	3.1 ± 1.4	0.309	3.1 ± 1.3	3.1 ± 1.3	3.1 ± 1.4	0.743	3.2 ± 1.5	3.3 ± 1.4	3.0 ± 1.5	0.124	3.5 ± 1.7	3.8 ± 1.8	2.9 ± 1.4	0.029
SINGLE SUPPORT TIME																
Mean value (ms)	414.3 ± 39.8	401.5 ± 35.5	425.2 ± 40.0	**<0.001**	417.2 ± 39.5	403.4 ± 36.2	427.4 ± 39.6	**<0.001**	407.8 ± 38.7	396.8 ± 34.3	418.3 ± 39.8	**<0.001**	396.7 ± 43.1	388.6 ± 37.5	413.1 ± 50.2	0.188
CoV (%)	4.0 ± 1.8	4.1 ± 2.0	4.0 ± 1.6	0.453	3.9 ± 1.7	3.9 ± 1.9	3.9 ± 1.5	0.154	4.3 ± 1.7	4.5 ± 1.8	4.2 ± 1.6	0.102	6.0 ± 2.7	6.5 ± 2.8	4.9 ± 2.3	0.062
DOUBLE SUPPORT TIME																
Mean value (ms)	292.6 ± 71.0	288.1 ± 74.1	296.4 ± 68.2	0.072	284.2 ± 64.5	274.5 ± 62.1	291.8 ± 65.4	**<0.001**	305.7 ± 74.2	308.8 ± 77.3	302.9 ± 71.4	0.569	381.4 ± 100.2	376.4 ± 115.3	391.3 ± 63.1	0.398
CoV (%)	6.6 ± 2.8	6.8 ± 2.7	6.5 ± 2.8	0.079	6.8 ± 2.9	7.0 ± 2.8	6.6 ± 2.9	0.117	6.3 ± 2.5	6.5 ± 2.8	6.1 ± 2.2	0.273	6.0 ± 2.1	6.2 ± 2.8	5.5 ± 2.6	0.177
STRIDE LENGTH																
Mean value (cm)	134.1 ± 18.9	126.5 ± 17.1	140.7 ± 18.0	**<0.001**	138.0 ± 16.6	131.1 ± 14.8	143.3 ± 15.9	**<0.001**	126.5 ± 19.7	118.2 ± 15.1	134.4 ± 20.4	**<0.001**	102.9 ± 15.3	100.7 ± 16.2	107.3 ± 13.0	0.166
CoV (%)	2.3 ± 1.2	2.7 ± 1.3	2.2 ± 1.1	0.005	2.2 ± 1.1	2.2 ± 1.2	2.1 ± 1.0	0.087	2.6 ± 1.3	2.7 ± 1.3	2.6 ± 1.3	0.743	3.6 ± 2.1	4.1 ± 2.4	2.7 ± 1.0	0.026
STRIDE WIDTH																
Mean value (cm)	9.9 ± 3.1	9.4 ± 3.1	10.2 ± 3.0	**<0.001**	9.9 ± 3.1	9.5 ± 3.1	10.3 ± 3.0	0.001	9.6 ± 3.2	9.0 ± 3.4	10.1 ± 2.9	0.010	10.0 ± 3.2	9.9 ± 2.5	10.2 ± 4.3	0.804
CoV (%)	26.6 ± 49.0	30.9 ± 69.8	23.0 ± 17.2	0.013	24.6 ± 34.7	27.4 ± 48.5	22.5 ± 17.2	0.057	33.0 ± 82.6	43.4 ± 116.9	23.0 ± 12.8	0.075	28.2 ± 23.4	22.5 ± 9.1	39.5 ± 36.8	0.934
WALKING SPEED (CM/S)																
mean ± SD	121.5 ± 23.4	120.2 ± 23.8	122.7 ± 23.0	0.103	125.4 ± 21.7	126.1 ± 21.7	124.9 ± 21.6	0.488	113.9 ± 23.5	109.7 ± 21.3	118.0 ± 24.9	0.011	88.5 ± 17.8	88.3 ± 19.4	88.9 ± 14.9	0.934
STRIDE VELOCITY																
Mean value (cm/s)	119.9 ± 22.5	118.8 ± 23.2	120.8 ± 21.8	0.175	122.9 ± 21.2	123.6 ± 21.2	122.3 ± 21.0	0.426	114.8 ± 22.8	111.1 ± 22.7	118.5 ± 22.5	0.020	89.0 ± 17.8	88.9 ± 19.4	89.3 ± 15.0	0.251
CoV (%)	3.5 ± 1.7	3.5 ± 1.7	3.4 ± 1.6	0.244	3.4 ± 1.6	3.4 ± 1.7	3.4 ± 1.6	0.244	3.7 ± 1.7	3.8 ± 1.8	3.6 ± 1.6	0.280	4.2 ± 2.0	4.6 ± 2.0	3.5 ± 1.9	0.084

SD, standard deviation; m, meter; s, second; ms, millisecond; CoV, coefficient of variation; *Comparison based on unpaired t-test; P significant (i.e., P < 0.0006) indicated in bold.

TABLE 4 | Multiple linear regression showing the association of spatiotemporal gait parameters (dependent variables) with age and sex (independent variables) adjusted for body mass index and test center among participants ($n = 954$).

Spatiotemporal gait parameters* (Dependent variables)	Independent variables					
	Age			Sex		
	β	[95%CI]	*P*-value	β	[95%CI]	*P*-value
STRIDE TIME						
Mean value (ms)	3.14	[1.55; 4.73]	**<0.001**	−50.62	[−65.85; −35.38]	**<0.001**
CoV (%)	0.04	[0.02; −0.05]	**<0.001**	00.13	[−0.00; 0.25]	0.056
SWING TIME						
Mean value (ms)	−0.52	[−1.03; −0.00]	**0.049**	−21.69	[−26.62; 16.76]	**<0.001**
CoV (%)	0.10	[0.07; 0.12]	**<0.001**	−0.02	[0-0.25; 0.21]	0.880
STANCE TIME						
Mean value (ms)	3.51	[2.34; 4.69]	**<0.001**	−31.11	[−42.38; −19.83]	**<0.001**
CoV (%)	0.03	[0.01; 0.05]	**0.004**	0.14	[−0.04; 0.31]	0.122
SINGLE SUPPORT TIME						
Mean value (ms)	−0.59	[−1.10; −0.09]	**0.021**	−22.66	[−27.50; −17.82]	**<0.001**
CoV (%)	0.10	[0.08; 0.13]	**<0.001**	−0.00	[−0.23; 0.22]	0.992
DOUBLE SUPPORT TIME						
Mean value (ms)	−4.03	[3.14; 4.92]	**<0.001**	−8.22	[−16.73; 0.30]	0.059
CoV (%)	−0.03	[−0.06; 0.01]	0.186	0.34	[−0.01; 0.70]	0.057
STRIDE LENGTH						
Mean value (cm)	−1.49	[−1.68; −1.29]	**<0.001**	−14.48	[−16.34; 12.62]	**<0.001**
CoV (%)	0.07	[0.06; 0.09]	**<0.001**	0.22	[0.08; 0.36]	**0.002**
STRIDE WIDTH						
Mean value (cm)	0.00	[−0.04; −0.04]	0.861	−0.95	[−1.33; −0.57]	**<0.001**
CoV (%)	0.77	[0.11; 1.44]	**0.023**	8.09	[1.71; 14.47]	**0.013**
STRIDE VELOCITY						
Mean value (cm/s)	−1.47	[−1.75; −1.20]	**<0.001**	−2.62	[−5.23; −0.01]	**0.049**
CoV (%)	0.05	[0.03; 0.07]	**<0.001**	0.27	[0.08; 0.46]	**0.005**

*ms, millisecond; s, second; cm, centimeter; CoV, coefficient of variation; CI, confidence interval; β, coefficient of regression corresponding to a decrease or increase in value of gait parameters; *Used as dependent variable in the multiple linear regression. P-value significant (i.e., <0.05) indicated in bold; each linear Model is adjusted for Body mass index and test center.*

provided the opportunity to report real normative quantitative reference values by age category from 65 to 85 years and above. The decline in gait performance with age is consistent with the literature and supports the validity of the reported values.

Some limitations, however, need to be acknowledged. First, the number of participants in the 85 and over age category was low, probably because healthy individuals only represent a low percentage of this age group. More effort needs to be made to explore this population, as they currently represent the fastest growing age group in many countries and have the highest prevalence and incidence of gait disorders (American Geriatrics Society and British Geriatrics Society and American Academy of Orthopedic Surgeons Panel on Falls Prevention, 2001; Panel on Prevention of Falls in Older Persons and American Geriatrics Society and British Geriatrics Society, 2011). Second, because this initiative merged data from clinical and research centers in different countries and different clinical settings, assessment was not strictly uniform even if the same procedures and equipment were used.

CONCLUSIONS

The past decade has been characterized by an acceleration of knowledge in medicine and science, particularly in the area of neuroscience. Considerable efforts have been (and continue to be) made in developing accessible and practical technology-based assessment tools aiming at providing accurate measurements of spatiotemporal gait parameters. These advances challenge researchers and clinicians, pushing them to develop new ways of thinking and working. Currently, new opportunities exist as the result of working as part of an internationally structured consortium. The GOOD initiative (Allali et al., 2016) underscores the fact that there is still a lot of work to do, but significant progress has been made and the future is optimistic with respect to the development of the Biomathics and Canadian Gait Consortiums. This work represents an important first step in the development of guidelines for clinical and spatiotemporal gait analysis based on the recorded footfalls in laboratory setting and the definition of quantitative reference values in healthy older adults. These guidelines facilitate the ability to work together and think broadly and effectively in the field of gait disorders and aging.

AUTHOR CONTRIBUTIONS

Study concept and design: OB, GA and JH; acquisition of data: OB, JV, JS, RK, CL, MC, VS, AD, and JH; analysis and interpretation of data: OB, GA, and JH; drafting of the manuscript: OB, GA, CL, and JH; critical revision of the manuscript for important intellectual content: HS, JV, SGu, JS, RK, JB, TS, CL, SGr, LB, TL, VC, MC, VS, GL, AD, RS, GD, and RC; obtained funding: OB, JV, and JH; statistical expertise: OB; administrative, technical, or material support: OB and JH; study supervision: OB and JH. All the authors have participated in the research reported, have seen and approved the final version of the manuscript, and have agreed to be an author of the paper.

FUNDING

The Kerala-Einstein Study was funded by the National Institutes of Health, USA (R01 AG039330). The CCMA study was funded by the National Institutes of Health, USA (R01AG036921, RO1AGO44007-01A1). TASCOG was funded by the National Health and Medical Research Council (NHMRC grant number 403000 and 491109) and the Royal Hobart Hospital Research Foundation. The study was financially supported by the French Ministry of Health (Projet Hospitalier de Recherche Clinique national n°2009-A00533-54). MC is funded by an NHMRC Early Career Fellowship (1034483); VS is funded by an NHRMC CDF/HF Future Leader fellowship.

REFERENCES

Alexander, G. E., and Crutcher, M. D. (1990). Functional architecture of basal ganglia circuits: neural substrates of parallel processing. *Trends Neurosci.* 13, 266–271. doi: 10.1016/0166-2236(90)90107-L

Allali, G., Annweiler, C., Blumen, H. M., Callisaya, M. L., De Cock, A. M., Kressig, R. W., et al. (2016). Gait phenotype from MCI to moderate dementia: results from the GOOD initiative. *Eur. J. Neurol.* 23, 527–541. doi: 10.1111/ene.12882

Allali, G., Laidet, M., Assal, F., Beauchet, O., Chofflon, M., Armand, S., et al. (2012). Adapted timed up and go: a rapid clinical test to assess gait and cognition in multiple sclerosis. *Eur. Neurol.* 67, 116–120. doi: 10.1159/0003 34394

American Geriatrics Society and British Geriatrics Society and American Academy of Orthopedic Surgeons Panel on Falls Prevention (2001). Guideline for the prevention of falls in older persons. *J. Am. Geriatr. Soc.* 49, 664–772. doi: 10.1046/j.1532-5415.2001.49115.x

Annweiler, C., Dursun, E., Féron, F., Gezen-Ak, D., Kalueff, A. V., Littlejohns, T., et al. (2015). 'Vitamin, D., and cognition in older adults': updated international recommendations. *J. Intern. Med.* 277, 45–57. doi: 10.1111/joim.12279

Artaud, F., Singh-Manoux, A., Dugravot, A., Tzourio, C., and Elbaz, A. (2015). Decline in fast gait speed as a predictor of disability in older adults. *J. Am. Geriatr. Soc.* 63, 1129–1136. doi: 10.1111/jgs.13442

Ayers, E. I., Tow, A. C., Holtzer, R., and Verghese, J. (2014). Walking while talking and falls in aging. *Gerontology* 60, 108–113. doi: 10.1159/000355119

Ayoubi, F., Launay, C. P., Annweiler, C., and Beauchet, O. (2015). Fear of falling and gait variability in older adults: a systematic review and meta-analysis. *J. Am. Med. Dir. Assoc.* 16, 14–19. doi: 10.1016/j.jamda.2014.06.020

Beauchet, O., Allali, G., Annweiler, C., and Verghese, J. (2016). Association of motoric cognitive risk syndrome with brain volumes: results from the GAIT study. *J. Gerontol. A Biol. Sci. Med. Sci.* 71, 1081–1088. doi: 10.1093/gerona/glw012

Beauchet, O., Allali, G., Annweiler, C., Bridenbaugh, S., Assal, F., Kressig, R. W., et al. (2009). Gait variability among healthy adults: low and high stride-to-stride variability are both a reflection of gait stability. *Gerontology* 55, 702–706. doi: 10.1159/000235905

Beauchet, O., Allali, G., Montero-Odasso, M., Sejdiæ, E., Fantino, B., and Annweiler, C. (2014a). Motor phenotype of decline in cognitive performance among community-dwellers without dementia: population-based study and meta-analysis. *PLoS ONE* 9:e99318. doi: 10.1371/journal.pone. 0099318

Beauchet, O., Annweiler, C., Assal, F., Bridenbaugh, S., Herrmann, F. R., Kressig, R. W., et al. (2010). Imagined Timed Up & Go test: a new tool to assess higher-level gait and balance disorders in older adults? *J. Neurol. Sci.* 294, 102–106. doi: 10.1016/j.jns.2010.03.021

Beauchet, O., Annweiler, C., Montero-Odasso, M., Fantino, B., Herrmann, F. R., and Allali, G. (2012). Gait control: a specific subdomain of executive function? *J. Neuroeng. Rehabil.* 9:12. doi: 10.1186/1743-0003-9-12

Beauchet, O., Herrmann, F. R., Grandjean, R., Dubost, V., and Allali, G. (2008). Concurrent validity of SMTEC footswitches system for the measurement of temporal gait parameters. *Gait Posture* 27, 156–159. doi: 10.1016/j.gaitpost.2006.12.017

Beauchet, O., Launay, C. P., Fantino, B., Allali, G., and Annweiler, C. (2015a). Respective and combined effects of impairments in sensorimotor systems and cognition on gait performance: a population-based cross-sectional study. *PLoS ONE* 10:e0125102. doi: 10.1371/journal.pone.0125102

Beauchet, O., Launay, C. P., Fantino, B., Annweiler, C., and Allali, G. (2015b). Episodic memory and executive function impairments in non-demented older adults: which are the respective and combined effects on gait performances? *Age* 37:9812. doi: 10.1007/s11357-015-9812-y

Beauchet, O., Launay, C. P., Sejdiæ, E., Allali, G., and Annweiler, C. (2014b). Motor imagery of gait: a new way to detect mild cognitive impairment? *J. Neuroeng. Rehabil.* 11:66. doi: 10.1186/1743-0003-11-66

Beauchet, O., Merjagnan-Vilcoq, C., and Annweiler, C. (2014c). From industrial research to academic discoveries, toward a new concept of partnership: the Biomathics model. *Front. Pharmacol.* 5:166. doi: 10.3389/fphar.2014. 00166

Bohannon, R. W., and Williams Andrews, A. (2011). Normal walking speed: a descriptive meta-analysis. *Physiotherapy* 97, 182–189. doi: 10.1016/j.physio.2010.12.004

Brach, J. S., Perera, S., Studenski, S., and Newman, A. B. (2008). The reliability and validity of measures of gait variability in community-dwelling older adults. *Arch. Phys. Med. Rehabil.* 89, 2293–2296. doi: 10.1016/j.apmr.2008.06.010

Byrne, G. J., and Pachana, N. A. (2011). Development and validation of a short form of the Geriatric Anxiety Inventory–the GAI-SF. *Int. Psychogeriatr.* 23, 125–131. doi: 10.1017/S1041610210001237

Chini, F., Pezzotti, P., Orzella, L., Borgia, P., and Guasticchi, G. (2011). Can we use the pharmacy data to estimate the prevalence of chronic conditions? a comparison of multiple data sources. *BMC Public Health* 11:688. doi: 10.1186/1471-2458-11-688

de Decker, L., Launay, C., Annweiler, C., Kabeshova, A., and Beauchet, O. (2013). Number of drug classes taken per day may be used to assess morbidity burden in older inpatients: a pilot cross-sectional study. *J. Am. Geriatr. Soc.* 61, 1224–1225. doi: 10.1111/jgs.12345

Dicharry, J. (2010). Kinematics and kinetics of gait: from lab to clinic. *Clin. Sports Med.* 29, 347–364. doi: 10.1016/j.csm.2010.03.013

Eastlack, M. E., Arvidson, J., Snyder-Mackler, L., Danoff, J. V., and McGarvey, C. L. (1991). Interrater reliability of videotaped observational gait-analysis assessments. *Phys. Ther.* 71, 465–472. doi: 10.1093/ptj/71.6.465

Farley, C. T., and Ferris, D. P. (1998). Biomechanics of walking and running: center of mass movements to muscle action. *Exerc. Sport Sci. Rev.* 26, 253–285. doi: 10.1249/00003677-199800260-00012

Faude, O., Donath, L., Roth, R., Fricker, L., and Zahner, L. (2012). Reliability of gait parameters during treadmill walking in community-dwelling healthy seniors. *Gait Posture* 36, 444–448. doi: 10.1016/j.gaitpost.2012.04.003

Gabell, A., and Nayak, U. S. (1984). The effect of age on variability in gait. *J. Gerontol.* 39, 662–666. doi: 10.1093/geronj/39.6.662

Goldberg, A., and Schepens, S. (2011). Measurement error and minimum detectable change in 4-meter gait speed in older adults. *Aging Clin. Exp. Res.* 23, 406–412. doi: 10.1007/BF03325236

Hass, C. J., Malczak, P., Nocera, J., Stegemöller, E. L., Wagle Shukla, A., Malaty, I., et al. (2012). Quantitative normative gait data in a large cohort of ambulatory persons with Parkinson's disease. *PLoS ONE* 7:e42337. doi: 10.1371/journal.pone.0042337

Hausdorff, J. M., Purdon, P. L., Peng, C. K., Ladin, Z., Wei, J. Y., and Goldberger, A. L. (1996). Fractal dynamics of human gait: stability of long-range correlations in stride interval fluctuations. *J. Appl. Physiol.* 80, 1448–1457.

Hollman, J. H., McDade, E. M., and Petersen, R. C. (2011). Normative spatiotemporal gait parameters in older adults. *Gait Posture* 34, 111–118. doi: 10.1016/j.gaitpost.2011.03.024

Kressig, R. W., Beauchet, O., and European GAITRite Network Group (2006). Guidelines for clinical applications of spatio-temporal gait analysis in older adults. *Aging Clin. Exp. Res.* 18, 174–176. doi: 10.1007/BF03327437

Kuo, A. D., and Donelan, J. M. (2010). Dynamic principles of gait and their clinical implications. *Phys. Ther.* 90, 157–174. doi: 10.2522/ptj.20090125

Lallart, E., Jouvent, R., Herrmann, F. R., Beauchet, O., and Allali, G. (2012). Gait and motor imagery of gait in early schizophrenia. *Psychiatry Res.* 198, 366–370. doi: 10.1016/j.psychres.2011.12.013

Launay, C., De Decker, L., Annweiler, C., Kabeshova, A., Fantino, B., and Beauchet, O. (2013). Association of depressive symptoms with recurrent falls: a cross-sectional elderly population based study and a systematic review. *J. Nutr. Health Aging* 17, 152–157. doi: 10.1007/s12603-012-0370-z

Linn, B. S., Linn, M. W., and Gurel, L. (1968). Cumulative illness rating scale. *J. Am. Geriatr. Soc.* 16, 622–626. doi: 10.1111/j.1532-5415.1968.tb02103.x

Lord, S. R., Ward, J. A., Williams, P., and Anstey, K. J. (1994). Physiological factors associated with falls in older community-dwelling women. *J. Am. Geriatr. Soc.* 42, 1110–1117. doi: 10.1111/j.1532-5415.1994.tb06218.x

Maio, V., Yuen, E., Rabinowitz, C., Louis, D., Jimbo, M., Donatini, A., et al. (2005). Using pharmacy data to identify those with chronic conditions in Emilia Romagna, Italy. *J. Health Serv. Res. Policy* 10, 232–238. doi: 10.1258/135581905774414259

McCann, D. J., and Higginson, B. K. (2008). Training to maximize economy of motion in running gait. *Curr. Sports Med. Rep.* 7, 158–162. doi: 10.1097/01.CSMR.0000319711.63793.84

Montero-Odasso, M., Verghese, J., Beauchet, O., and Hausdorff, J. M. (2012). Gait and cognition: a complementary approach to understanding brain function and the risk of falling. *J. Am. Geriatr. Soc.* 60, 2127–2136. doi: 10.1111/j.1532-5415.2012.04209.x

Nasreddine, Z. S., Phillips, N. A., Bédirian, V., Charbonneau, S., Whitehead, V., Collin, I., et al. (2005). The montreal cognitive assessment (MoCA): a brief screening tool for mild cognitive impairment. *J. Am. Geriatr. Soc.* 53, 695–699. doi: 10.1111/j.1532-5415.2005.53221.x

Newell, K. M., and Corcos, D. M. (1993). "Issues in variability and motor control," in *Variability and Motor Control*, eds K. M. Newell and D. M. Corcos (Champaign, IL: Human Kinetics), 1–12.

Nutt, J. G. (2001). Classification of gait and balance disorders. *Adv. Neurol.* 87, 135–141.

Nutt, J. G., Marsden, C. D., and Thompson, P. D. (1993). Human walking and higher-level gait disorders, particularly in the elderly. *Neurology* 43, 268–279. doi: 10.1212/WNL.43.2.268

Oberg, T., Karsznia, A., and Oberg, K. (1993). Basic gait parameters: reference data for normal subjects, 10–79 years of age. *J. Rehabil. Res. Dev.* 30, 210–323.

Oh-Park, M., Holtzer, R., Xue, X., and Verghese, J. (2010). Conventional and robust quantitative gait norms in community-dwelling older adults. *J. Am. Geriatr. Soc.* 58, 1512–1518. doi: 10.1111/j.1532-5415.2010.02962.x

Panel on Prevention of Falls in Older Persons and American Geriatrics Society and British Geriatrics Society (2011). Summary of the Updated American Geriatrics Society/British Geriatrics Society clinical practice guideline for prevention of falls in older persons. *J. Am. Geriatr. Soc.* 59, 148–157. doi: 10.1111/j.1532-5415.2010.03234.x

Parmelee, P. A., Thuras, P. D., Katz, I. R., and Lawton, M. P. (1995). Validation of the Cumulative Illness Rating Scale in a geriatric residential population. *J. Am. Geriatr. Soc.* 43, 130–137. doi: 10.1111/j.1532-5415.1995.tb06377.x

Podsiadlo, D., and Richardson, S. (1991). The timed "Up & Go": a test of basic functional mobility for frail elderly persons. *J. Am. Geriatr. Soc.* 39, 142–148. doi: 10.1111/j.1532-5415.1991.tb01616.x

Rao, A. K., Mazzoni, P., Wasserman, P., and Marder, K. (2011). Longitudinal change in gait and motor function in pre-manifest Huntington's Disease. *PLoS Curr.* 3:RRN1268. doi: 10.1371/currents.RRN1268

Salvi, F., Miller, M. D., Grilli, A., Giorgi, R., Towers, A. L., Morichi, V., et al. (2008). A manual of guidelines to score the modified cumulative illness rating scale and its validation in acute hospitalized elderly patients. *J. Am. Geriatr. Soc.* 56, 1926–1931. doi: 10.1111/j.1532-5415.2008.01935.x

Seidler, R. D., Bernard, J. A., Burutolu, T. B., Fling, B. W., Gordon, M. T., Gwin, J. T., et al. (2010). Motor control and aging: links to age-related brain structural, functional, and biochemical effects. *Neurosci. Biobehav. Rev.* 34, 721–733. doi: 10.1016/j.neubiorev.2009.10.005

Shah, A., Herbert, R., Lewis, S., Mahendran, R., Platt, J., and Bhattacharyya, B. (1997). Screening for depression among acutely ill geriatric inpatients with a short Geriatric Depression Scale. *Age Ageing* 26, 217–221. doi: 10.1093/ageing/26.3.217

Stensvold, D., Viken, H., Rognmo, Ø., Skogvoll, E., Steinshamn, S., Vatten, L. J., et al. (2015). A randomised controlled study of the long-term effects of exercise training on mortality in elderly people: study protocol for the Generation 100 study. *BMJ Open* 5:e007519. doi: 10.1136/bmjopen-2014-007519

Verghese, J., Holtzer, R., Lipton, R. B., and Wang, C. (2009). Quantitative gait markers and incident fall risk in older adults. *J. Gerontol. A Biol. Sci. Med. Sci.* 64, 896–901. doi: 10.1093/gerona/glp033

Verghese, J., LeValley, A., Hall, C. B., Katz, M. J., Ambrose, A. F., and Lipton, R. B. (2006). Epidemiology of gait disorders in community-residing older adults. *J. Am. Geriatr. Soc.* 54, 255–261. doi: 10.1111/j.1532-5415.2005.00580.x

Von Korff, M., Wagner, E. H., and Saunders, K. (1992). A chronic disease score from automated pharmacy data. *J. Clin. Epidemiol.* 45, 197–203. doi: 10.1016/0895-4356(92)90016-G

Webster, K. E., Wittwer, J. E., and Feller, J. A. (2005). Validity of the GAITRite® walkway system for the measurement of averaged and individual step parameters of gait. *Gait Posture* 22, 317–321. doi: 10.1016/j.gaitpost.2004.10.005

Zajac, F. E., Neptune, R. R., and Kautz, S. A. (2002). Biomechanics and muscle coordination of human walking. Part I: introduction to concepts, power transfer, dynamics and simulations. *Gait Posture* 16, 215–232. doi: 10.1016/s0966-6362(02)00068-1

Zwergal, A., Linn, J., Xiong, G., Brandt, T., Strupp, M., Jahn, K., et al. (2012). Aging of human supraspinal locomotor and postural control in fMRI. *Neurobiol. Aging* 33, 1073–1084. doi: 10.1016/j.neurobiolaging.2010.09.022

2

Effects of Age-Related Macular Degeneration on Postural Sway

Hortense Chatard[1,2,3]*, Laure Tepenier*[4]*, Olivier Jankowski*[3]*, Antoine Aussems*[3]*,*
Alain Allieta[3]*, Talal Beydoun*[4]*, Sawsen Salah*[4]* and Maria P. Bucci*[1,2]

[1] UMR 1141, Institut National de la Santé et de la Recherche Médicale—Université Paris 7, Robert Debré University Hospital,
Paris, France, [2] Vestibular and Oculomotor Evaluation Unit, ENT Department, Robert Debré University Hospital, Paris, France,
[3] Centre Ophtalmologique du Val-d'Oise (OPH95), Osny, France, [4] Groupe Hospitalier Cochin-Hôtel-Dieu, Department of
Ophthalmology, Assistance Publique-Hôpitaux de Paris, Paris Descartes University, Paris, France

*Correspondence:
Hortense Chatard
chatardhortense@gmail.com

Purpose: To compare the impact of unilateral vs. bilateral age-related macular degeneration (AMD) on postural sway, and the influence of different visual conditions. The hypothesis of our study was that the impact of AMD will be different between unilateral and bilateral AMD subjects compared to age-matched healthy elderly.

Methods: Postural stability was measured with a platform (TechnoConcept®) in 10 elderly unilateral AMD subjects (mean age: 71.1 ± 4.6 years), 10 elderly bilateral AMD subjects (mean age: 70.8 ± 6.1 years), and 10 healthy age-matched control subjects (mean age: 69.8 ± 6.3 years). Four visual conditions were tested: both eyes viewing condition (BEV), dominant eye viewing (DEV), non-dominant eye viewing (NDEV), and eyes closed (EC). We analyzed the surface area, the length, the mean speed, the anteroposterior (AP), and mediolateral (ML) displacement of the center of pressure (CoP).

Results: Bilateral AMD subjects had a surface area ($p < 0.05$) and AP displacement of the CoP ($p < 0.01$) higher than healthy elderly. Unilateral AMD subjects had more AP displacement of the CoP ($p < 0.05$) than healthy elderly.

Conclusions: We suggest that ADM subjects could have poor postural adaptive mechanisms leading to increase their postural instability. Further studies will aim to improve knowledge on such issue and to develop reeducation techniques in these patients.

Keywords: age-related macular degeneration, postural sway, elderly, visual condition, balance

INTRODUCTION

Age-Related Macular Degeneration (AMD) is the first cause of blindness after fifty years old in developed countries (Kocur and Resnikoff, 2002; Augood et al., 2006). This pathology is characterized by uni- or bi-lateral photoreceptor degeneration, which generates a large scotoma including central vision (Leveziel et al., 2009). Peripheral vision is conserved. AMD is a multifactorial and polygenic pathology with three main risk factors: age, environment and genetics (Chakravarthy et al., 2007; Wang et al., 2008, 2009). AMD represents a true public health issue because of the prevalence (1.6% before 64 years old and 27.9% after 85 years old; Ferris, 1983; Hyman and Neborsky, 2002; Friedman et al., 2004), the cost of care (which increases with disease severity; Bandello et al., 2008), psychological impact and functional disability (difficulty reading, driving restriction, difficulty of stereoscopic vision, difficulty recognizing faces, etc.; Augustin et al., 2007; Christoforidis et al., 2011; Hochberg et al., 2012; Sengupta et al., 2014; McCloud and Lake, 2015). This pathology affects more than one million people in France.

According to HAS (*Haute Autorité de Santé*) and other authors, 33% of subjects older than 65 years have experienced at least one fall per year (Tinetti et al., 1988; Campbell et al., 1989; Wood et al., 2011). It is a real public health problem because of autonomy loss and of the medical cost ($6–8 billion by year in the United States alone; Carroll et al., 2005).

Postural control is an elaborated process which allows a coordinated relationship of body segments (static and dynamic positions; Paillard, 1971; Gurfinkel and Shik, 1973). It is controlled by vestibular, proprioceptive, and visual information (Nashner, 1979; Horak and Shupert, 1994; Fetter and Dichgans, 1996). The vestibular system contributes to postural stability with eyes open (Fitzpatrick and McCloskey, 1994). Vision and proprioception participate to the detection of slow movements in the visual environment. When the visual or the vestibular system is affected, subjects need to compensate with other sensorial inputs (Brandt, 2003).

Some studies examined the impact of AMD on postural control (Elliott et al., 1995; Wood et al., 2009; Kotecha et al., 2013). Elliott et al. (1995) explored balance control (anterior-posterior sways of CoP) in AMD subjects compared to age-matched control subjects on a stable/unstable platform. They showed that postural stability in AMD subjects was poor when the inputs of kinesthetic sensory system were disrupted. The authors suggested that in normal standing condition, the vestibular and kinesthetic systems compensated for the lack of visual information in AMD subjects. Wood et al. (2009) studied postural stability in older adults with age-related maculopathy in order to identify the visual factors associated with postural control and falls. They proved that diminution of contrast sensitivity and visual field loss lead to postural instability and mobility difficulties. Kotecha et al. (2013) examined the effect of a secondary task on standing balance in elderly subjects with central visual field loss (AMD) or peripheral visual field loss (glaucoma) compared with age-matched healthy subjects. They compared two standing conditions: eyes open on a firm or a foam surface. These authors found that during the secondary task, AMD subjects were more unstable than healthy elderly on a firm and foam surface, while glaucoma subjects were more unstable on the foam surface only. Authors suggested that when subjects have visual impairment, they have to increase somatosensory contribution to obtain a good postural stability, and that peripheral vision is important when somatosensory inputs are disturbed.

The role of central vs. peripheral vision information in control of movements and posture was examined in numerous studies (i.e., Berencsi et al., 2005; Marigold and Patla, 2007). These authors suggested that peripheral vision is used for postural control and most particularly for stabilization of fore-aft sways; central vision is more used for foot trajectory planning, targeting, obstacle avoidance, and for stabilization of lateral sways.

Taken together all these findings showed poor postural stability in patients with AMD, particularly under eyes open condition; the novelty of the present study was to explore further AMD pathology (i) unilateral vs. bilateral AMD (ii) and the effect of different visual condition (both eyes open, and one eye alternatively open, dominant and non-dominant).

The hypothesis of our study was that the impact of AMD could be different between unilateral and bilateral AMD subjects compared with age-matched healthy elderly, and that postural sways could be different for different eye viewing conditions.

MATERIALS AND METHODS

Subjects

A total of 10 unilateral AMD patients between 62.8 and 76.7 years old (mean age: 71.1 ± 4.6 years) and 10 bilateral AMD patients between 57.1 and 78.5 years old (mean age: 70.8 ± 6.1 years) participated in the study. We also tested 10 age-matched healthy controls (mean age: 69.8 ± 6.3 years). All participants were recruited from the Department of Ophthalmology, Hôtel-Dieu Hospital in Paris and from the *Centre Ophtalmologique du Val-d'Oise* (France). Their participation was voluntary.

All participants had to fulfill criteria: ametropia inferior to five dioptries (spherical equivalent), no ocular surgery background, no retina laser treatment, no other ophthalmology pathologies, no diabetes, no known cognitive loss, no known vestibular abnormality, and no known orthopedic surgeries and abnormalities.

The investigation adhered to the principles of the Declaration of Helsinki and was approved by our Institutional Human Experimentation Committee (*Comité de Protection des Personnes CPP, Ile de France V*). Written informed consent was obtained from each participant after an explanation of the experimental procedure.

Ophthalmologic and Orthoptic Evaluation

All AMD subjects underwent ophthalmologic and orthoptic examination to evaluate their visual function. Clinical data of each AMD patients are shown in **Tables 1, 2**. Clinical data of healthy elderly subjects are shown in **Table 3**.

Visual acuity was measured separately for each eye at far distance (5 m) with the Monoyer chart. Next we have translated to ETDRS with an adapted scale. Stereoscopic acuity was measured by TNO test (Test of Netherlands Organization for Applied Scientific Research; Walraven, 1975). Unilateral AMD patients have a corrected monocular visual acuity between 20/125 and 20/20, and bilateral AMD patients a corrected monocular acuity between 20/800 and 20/25. Only eight of the ten AMD participants have a stereoscopic acuity <480 s of arc. Visual functions are also evaluated for control subjects. They have a monocular corrected visual acuity of 20/20 and stereoscopic acuity for 120 s of arc.

Age-related macular degeneration severity scale of AREDS was used for each eye (AREDS, 2001). SD-OCT (Spectralis®, Heidelberg Engineering) for each eye allows identifying AMD level by locating geographic atrophies (deterioration of the photoreceptors) and choroidal neovascularization (growth of

TABLE 1 | Clinical characteristics of unilateral AMD subjects.

Patient (Age, years)	ETDRS		Glasses correction		AMD level		Type of AMD	Scotoma		Stereoacuity (TNO)	Eye dominant
S1 (62.8)	RE:	20/40	RE:	+1.75 (−0.75) 100°	RE:	3	CNV	RE:	Perimacular	200″	LE
	LE:	20/20	LE:	+1.5 (−1.75) 85°	LE:	1	/	LE:	/		
S2 (63.8)	RE:	20/125	RE:	+2.25 (−0.25) 130°	RE:	4	GA	RE:	Perimacular	/	LE
	LE:	20/20	LE:	+2 (−0.5) 60°	LE:	1	/	LE:	/		
S3 (63.5)	RE:	20/20	RE:	+1.25 (−0.25) 80°	RE:	2	/	RE:	/	/	RE
	LE:	20/32	LE:	+1.5 (−0.25) 85°	LE:	4	CNV	LE:	/		
S4 (70.5)	RE:	20/40	RE:	+0.75 (−0.75) 40°	RE:	4	CNV	RE:	Perimacular	/	LE
	LE:	20/25	LE:	+2.5 (−0.75) 160°	LE:	2	/	LE:	/		
S5 (72.4)	RE:	20/20	RE:	−0.5 (−0.5) 105°	RE:	1	/	RE:	/	/	RE
	LE:	20/32	LE:	+0.5 (−0.75) 80°	LE:	4	CNV		Paramacular		
S6 (72.5)	RE:	20/25	RE:	+4.75	RE:	3	GA	RE:	/	480″	LE
	LE:	20/20	LE:	+4.75 (−0.75) 130°	LE:	2	/	LE:	/		
S7 (72.7)	RE:	20/20	RE:	+2.5 (−1) 90°	RE:	1	/	RE:	/	/	RE
	LE:	20/50	LE:	+2.75 (−1.5) 100°	LE:	4	CNV		Perimacular		
S8 (73.4)	RE:	20/40	RE:	+1.75 (−0.75) 80°	RE:	4	CNV	RE:	Perimacular	480″	LE
	LE:	20/40	LE:	+2 (−1)110°	LE:	3	/	LE:	/		
S9 (76.3)	RE:	20/32	RE:	+3 (−0.75) 95°	RE:	3	CNV	RE:	/	480″	LE
	LE:	20/20	LE:	+3.25 (−0.75) 125°	LE:	1	/	LE:	/		
S10 (76.7)	RE:	20/20	RE:	+0.75 (−0.75) 115°	RE:	1	/	RE:	/	480″	RE
	LE:	20/40	LE:	+0.75 (−0.75) 60°	LE:	4	CNV		Paramacular		

Data are reported for each participant with unilateral AMD. Their corrected visual acuity (ETDRS), glasses correction, AMD level, type of AMD (GA, geographic atrophy; CNV, choroidal neovascularization), stereoscopic acuity (seconds of arc, TNO test) and dominant eye are reported (LE, left eye; RE, right eye).

pathologic blood vessels from the choroid into the subretinal space).

Among participants, 60% of bilateral AMD and 80% of unilateral AMD are choroidal neovascularization. Other studies have reported that there is two AMD with choroidal neovascularization for one AMD with geographic atrophy (Chakravarthy et al., 2007).

The eye with the better corrected visual acuity is considered as the dominant eye.

Posturography

A force platform (AFP40/16 Stabilotest, principle of strain gauge) consisting of two dynamometric clogs was used to measure and quantify postural stability (Standards by *Association Française de Posturologie*, produced by TechnoConcept®, Céreste, France; **Figure 1**). Foot position is standardized with footprints. This platform included a 16-bit analog-digital and acquisition frequency was 40 Hz. The excursion of center of pressure was measured during 25.6 s. Postural parameters were calculated following Gagey's standards (Gagey et al., 1993; Gagey and Weber, 1999).

Postural Recording Procedure

In a dark room, participants stood on the platform and fixed a target (3 × 3 cm; identically for all subjects) in front of their eye level (150 cm). Four visual conditions were tested: binocular eye viewing (BEV), dominant eye viewing (DEV), non-dominant eye viewing (NDEV), and eyes closed (EC). We choose to test postural control separately for each eye in order to compare the impact of level of AMD on postural stability in order to develop training techniques for these subjects, even if these conditions are not physiological. Subjects were instructed to stay as still as possible with their arms along their body, to fix the target and stand quietly on the platform. Three randomized trials were performed for each visual condition successively. A short break was done between each condition. The total duration of the trial was 10 min.

Data Processing

To quantify the effect of AMD and visual conditions on postural control we analyzed the surface area (mm^2), the length (mm), the mean speed (mm/s), and the anteroposterior (AP) and mediolateral (ML) displacements (mm) of the CoP that are the standard deviation of the displacement. Surface area is an

TABLE 2 | Clinical characteristics of bilateral AMD subjects.

Patient (Age, years)	ETDRS		Glasses correction		AMD level		Type of AMD		Scotoma		Stereoacuity (TNO)	Dominant eye
S11 (57.1)	RE:	20/40	RE:	+5 (−0.5) 80°	RE:	4	CNV	RE:	Perimacular	/	LE
	LE:	20/20	LE:	+3.5 (−0.5) 105°	LE:	3	CNV	LE:	Paramacular		
S12 (65.9)	RE:	20/800	RE:	+1.75 (−0.5) 110°	RE:	4	CNV	RE:	Perimacular	/	LE
	LE:	20/100	LE:	+1 (−0.75) 150°	LE:	4	CNV	LE:	Perimacular		
S13 (69.6)	RE:	20/20	RE:	+2 (−0.5) 130°	RE:	3	GA	RE:	Perimacular	480″	RE
	LE:	20/25	LE:	+2 (−0.5) 50°	LE:	3	GA	LE:	Perimacular		
S14 (69.8)	RE:	20/800	RE:	/	RE:	4	CNV	RE:	Paramacular	/	LE
	LE:	20/50	LE:	/	LE:	3	CNV	LE:	Perimacular		
S15 (69.9)	RE:	20/25	RE:	+0.5 (−0.75) 95°	RE:	3	CNV	RE:	/	480″	RE
	LE:	20/63	LE:	+0.75 (−0.5) 90°	LE:	4	CNV	LE:	/		
S16 (71.7)	RE:	20/800	RE:	/	RE:	4	GA	RE:	Para- and perimacular	/	RE
	LE:	20/320	LE:	/	LE:	4	GA	LE:	Paramacular		
S17 (74.1)	RE:	20/125	RE:	/	RE:	3	GA	RE:	Perimacular	/	RE
	LE:	20/20	LE:	+0.5 (−0.25) 145°	LE:	3	CNV	LE:	Paramacular		
S18 (74.8)	RE:	20/25	RE:	+1.25 (−0.75) 100°	RE:	3	GA	RE:	/	480″	RE
	LE:	20/32	LE:	+1.25 (-0.75) 70°	LE:	3	GA	LE:	Paramacular		
S19 (76.4)	RE:	20/800	RE:	/	RE:	4	CNV	RE:	Perimacular	/	LE
	LE:	20/32	LE:	/	LE:	3	GA	LE:	Paramacular		
S20 (78.5)	RE:	20/63	RE:	/	RE:	3	CNV	RE:	Perimacular	/	RE
	LE:	20/63	LE:	/	LE:	4	CNV	LE:	/		

Data are reported for each participant with bilateral AMD. Their corrected visual acuity (ETDRS), glasses correction, AMD level, type of AMD (GA, geographic atrophy; CNV, choroidal neovascularization), stereoscopic acuity (seconds of arc, TNO test) and dominant eye are reported (LE, left eye; RE, right eye).

effective measurement of CoP variability and corresponds to an ellipse with 90% of CoP (Chiari et al., 2002; Gagey and Weber, 2004; Vuillerme et al., 2008). Length is a path of CoP. Mean speed is an efficient indicator to quantity the neuro-muscular activity required to regulate postural control (Geurts et al., 1993).

Statistical Analysis

Data were analyzed with ANOVA/MANOVA using the three groups of subjects (unilateral, bilateral AMD subjects, and control subjects) as inter- subject factor, and the four visual conditions (both eyes opens, dominant and non-dominant eye open, and both eyes closed) as within-subject factor.

In the case of significant effects *post-hoc* Bonferroni test was performed. The effect of a factor was considered as significant when the *p*-value was below 0.05.

RESULTS

ANOVA test failed to show significant age differences between the three groups [$F_{(2,27)} = 0.66$, $p = 0.54$].

Figure 1 shows the surface area of the CoP (mm^2) for each visual condition tested (BEV, DEV, NDEV, EC) for the three

groups of subjects (control, unilateral AMD, bilateral AMD). The analysis of variance (ANOVA) indicated a group effect [$F_{(2, 27)} = 3.28$, $p < 0.05$]. *Post-hoc* comparison showed a significant difference between "Control" and "Bilateral AMD" ($p < 0.05$): bilateral AMD subjects had a larger surface area than control subjects. There was a significant effect of visual condition [$F_{(3,81)} = 3.04$, $p < 0.03$]. *Post-hoc* comparison showed that surface area of CoP was significantly smaller under DEV with respect to EC ($p < 0.02$). ANOVA did not show any significant interaction between group and visual condition [$F_{(6,81)} = 0.69$, $p = 0.65$].

Figure 2 shows the length of the CoP (mm) for each visual condition tested (BEV, DEV, NDEV, EC) for the three groups of subjects (control, unilateral AMD, bilateral AMD). ANOVA did not show a significant group effect [$F_{(3,81)} = 2.29$, $p = 0.1$] but indicated a significant effect of visual condition [$F_{(3,81)} = 18.69$, $p < 10^{-6}$]. *Post-hoc* comparison showed that the length of the CoP was significantly smaller under BEV than under NDEV ($p < 0.03$) and under EC ($p < 10^{-6}$). The length of the CoP was also significantly larger under EC than under DEV ($p < 10^{-6}$) and NDEV ($p < 10^{-4}$). ANOVA did not show a significant interaction between group and visual condition [$F_{(6,81)} = 0.64$, $p = 0.67$].

TABLE 3 | Clinical characteristics of age-matched healthy subjects.

Patient (Age, years)	ETDRS			Glasses correction		AMD level		Scotoma		Stereoacuity (TNO)	Dominant eye
S21 (60.1)	RE:	20/20	RE:	(−0.75) 88°	RE:	1	RE:	/	480″	LE
	LE:	20/20	LE:	(−0.75) 100°	LE:	1	LE:	/		
S22 (63.2)	RE:	20/20	RE:	+1.50 (−0.25) 65°	RE:	1	RE:	/	480″	LE
	LE:	20/20	LE:	+2.50 (−1.5) 160°	LE:	1	LE:	/		
S23 (64.9)	RE:	20/20	RE:	+3.25 (−0.5) 105°	RE:	1	RE:	/	480″	RE
	LE:	20/20	LE:	+3.25 (−0.5) 80°	LE:	1	LE:	/		
S24 (66.5)	RE:	20/20	RE:	+0.50 (−0.5) 80°	RE:	1	RE:	/	480″	LE
	LE:	20/20	LE:	+0.25	LE:	1	LE:	/		
S25 (67.8)	RE:	20/20	RE:	+2.50 (−0.5) 60°	RE:	1	RE:	/	480″	RE
	LE:	20/20	LE:	+3 (−0.75) 105°	LE:	1	LE:	/		
S26 (69.8)	RE:	20/20	RE:	+0.25 (−0.5) 10°	RE:	1	RE:	/	480″	LE
	LE:	20/20	LE:	(−0.25) 150°	LE:	1	LE:	/		
S27 (69.9)	RE:	20/20	RE:	+1.25	RE:	1	RE:	/	480″	LE
	LE:	20/20	LE:	+1.25	LE:	1	LE:	/		
S28 (77.2)	RE:	20/20	RE:	+3	RE:	1	RE:	/	480″	RE
	LE:	20/20	LE:	+3	LE:	1	LE:	/		
S29 (79.2)	RE:	20/20	RE:	−1.5	RE:	1	RE:	/	480″	LE
	LE:	20/20	LE:	−1.75	LE:	1	LE:	/		
S30 (79.5)	RE:	20/20	RE:	+2.75 (−2) 5°	RE:	1	RE:	/	480″	RE
	LE:	20/20	LE:	+0.5 (−1.5) 20°	LE:	1	LE:	/		

Data are reported for each healthy age-matched participant. Their corrected visual acuity (ETDRS), glasses correction, AMD level, stereoscopic acuity (seconds of arc, TNO test) and dominant eye are reported (LE, left eye; RE, right eye).

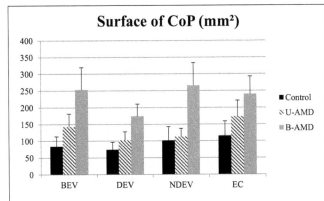

FIGURE 1 | Surface of CoP. Mean value of the surface of CoP (mm²) for each group of subject tested (control age-matched elderly, unilateral AMD and bilateral AMD), for each visual conditions, binocular eye viewing (BEV), dominant eye viewing (DEV), non-dominant eye viewing (NDEV), eyes closed (EC). Vertical bars indicate the standard error.

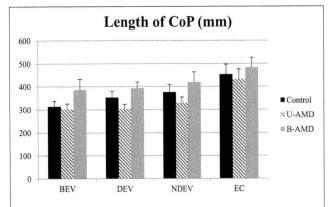

FIGURE 2 | Length of CoP. Mean of the Length of CoP (mm²) for each group of subject tested (control age-matched elderly, unilateral AMD and bilateral AMD), for each visual conditions, binocular eye viewing (BEV), dominant eye viewing (DEV), non-dominant eye viewing (NDEV), eyes closed (EC). Vertical bars indicate the standard error.

Figure 3 shows the mean speed of the CoP (mm/s) for each visual condition tested (BEV, DEV, NDEV, EC) in the three groups of subjects (control, unilateral AMD, bilateral AMD). The analysis of variance (ANOVA) did not show a significant group effect $[F_{(2, 27)} = 2.88, p = 0.07]$ but indicated an effect of visual condition $[F_{(3, 81)} = 9.68, p < 10^{-4}]$. *Post-hoc* comparison showed that the mean speed of the CoP was higher under EC than

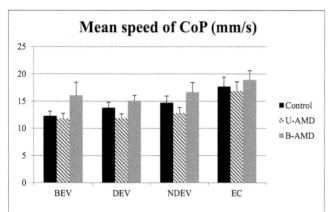

FIGURE 3 | Mean speed of CoP. Mean of the mean speed of CoP (mm²) for each group of subject tested (control age-matched elderly, unilateral AMD and bilateral AMD), for each visual conditions, binocular eye viewing (BEV), dominant eye viewing (DEV), non-dominant eye viewing (NDEV), eyes closed (EC). Vertical bars indicate the standard error.

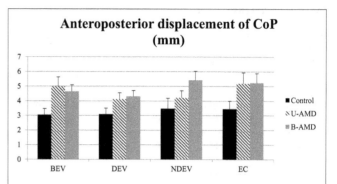

FIGURE 4 | AP displacements of CoP. AP displacements of CoP (mm) for each group of subject tested (control age-matched elderly, unilateral AMD and bilateral AMD), for each visual conditions, binocular eye viewing (BEV), dominant eye viewing (DEV), non-dominant eye viewing (NDEV), eyes closed (EC). Vertical bars indicate the standard error.

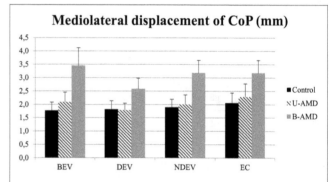

FIGURE 5 | ML displacements of CoP. ML displacements of CoP (mm) for each group of subject tested (control age-matched elderly, unilateral AMD and bilateral AMD), for each visual conditions, binocular eye viewing (BEV), dominant eye viewing (DEV), non-dominant eye viewing (NDEV), eyes closed (EC). Vertical bars indicate the standard error.

under BEV ($p < 10^{-4}$), under DEV ($p < 10^{-4}$), and under NDEV ($p < 10^{-2}$). There was no significant interaction between group and visual condition [$F_{(6, 81)} = 0.42, p = 0.85$].

Figure 4 shows the AP displacements of the CoP (mm) for each visual condition tested (BEV, DEV, NDEV, EC) in the three groups of subjects (control, unilateral AMD, bilateral AMD). The analysis of variance (ANOVA) indicated a significant group effect [$F_{(2, 27)} = 3.43, p < 0.04$]. The AP displacement was larger in AMD subjects than in healthy control age-matched subjects: *post-hoc* comparison showed that AP displacement of the CoP was shorter in control subjects than in bilateral AMD subjects ($p < 0.01$) and unilateral AMD subjects ($p < 0.05$). There was no significant effect of visual condition [$F_{(2, 27)} = 2.51, p = 0.06$] or interaction between group and visual condition [$F_{(6, 81)} = 1.4, p = 0.22$].

Figure 5 shows the ML displacements of the CoP (mm) for each visual condition tested (BEV, DEV, NDEV, EC) in the three groups of subjects (control, unilateral AMD, bilateral AMD). The analysis of variance (ANOVA) did not show any significant group effect [$F_{(2, 27)} = 2.64, p = 0.08$], or any effect of visual condition [$F_{(3, 81)} = 1.94, p = 0.1$], or any interaction between group and visual condition [$F_{(6, 81)} = 0.50, p = 0.8$].

DISCUSSION

The main findings of this study are as follows: (i) the surface area and the AP displacement of the CoP are larger in bilateral AMD subjects than in unilateral AMD subjects; (ii) postural stability in elderly subjects depends on visual conditions. These findings are discussed individually below.

Bilateral AMD Subjects Are More Unstable than Unilateral AMD Subjects

In this study we found that AMD subjects had poor postural stability with respect to controls. This finding is in agreement with others studies (Elliott et al., 1995; Kotecha et al., 2013). Moreover, two postural parameters (surface area and AP

displacement of CoP) were significantly different in bilateral AMD subjects compared with healthy elderly, and the AP displacement of CoP was significantly affected in unilateral AMD only.

Based on this finding we could assume that a postural evaluation, particularly of the surface area of the CoP, at the beginning of the AMD diagnosis may be predictive of future postural difficulties in these patients. An early postural rehabilitation care would prevent the risk of falling and in the future, studies leading with postural, and/or visual training will be necessary to improve the everyday life.

Postural balance changes throughout life. Qiu et al. (2012) studied the somatosensory system during aging and the impact of age on postural stability. Elderly patients (mean age: 72 years) have an augmentation of surface area and length of the CoP, and an augmentation of AP and ML sways, in comparison with young adults (mean age: 27 years). These authors suggested that mechanoreceptors sensibility decreases with aging as well as the capacity of treatment of sensorial information by the central nervous system. According to Faraldo-García et al. (2016), older subjects could have poor ability of adapt their body to disturbed sensory situations. Note that in younger subjects with loss of central vision (Stargardt disease) Agostini et al. (2016) found that compensatory strategies are used to control their postural stability. Such adaptive mechanisms are working well also in children with strabismus (see works of our groups, i.e., Lions et al., 2014; Bucci et al., 2016); we could make the hypothesis that in older subjects with AMD pathologies such compensations are not well developed, most likely because at this age plasticity occurs less frequently.

Postural Stability in Elderly Subjects Depends on Visual Conditions

Our results proved that AP displacements of CoP was higher in AMD subjects than controls in closed eyes condition, most likely because AMD subjects have low mobility and degraded physical performance. Such hypothesis is confirmed by previous studies (Rovner et al., 2009; Chomistek et al., 2013; Loprinzi et al., 2015). These authors suggested that physical inactivity facilitated the progression of vision loss (Chomistek et al., 2013) and cognitive loss like depressive disorders (Rovner et al., 2009). Moreover, (Loprinzi et al., 2015) showed that AMD subjects, and more generally subjects with low visual acuity increased sedentary behavior, leading to increase of risk of developing metabolic, cardiovascular, and cerebrovascular diseases.

Few studies examined postural stability under monocular viewing. (Moraes et al., 2009), studied the impact of binocular vs. monocular viewing in controlling posture in quiet stance in young adults without visual abnormalities (mean age: 22.7 years). They suggested that binocular viewing allowed a greater postural control.

Note that even if our results failed to show any interaction effect between subjects and visual condition data on monocular viewing, they suggested that AMD subjects are more stable under dominant eye viewing than under both eyes viewing condition. Studies with more patients are needed to confirm this result. We made the hypothesis that monocular visual field of the dominant eye is less disturbed than binocular visual field in AMD subjects. The confirmation of this result would open perspectives of developing of training techniques without replacing the standard follow-up of the AMD subjects by clinical ophthalmological examination. In fact, in theory, neutralization process is expected to erase some of the scotoma (no view area) in the binocular visual field. But this process is difficult for elderly people due to the age-related decrease of brain plasticity.

The role of central vs. peripheral vision information in control balance was examined in several studies. Marigold and Patla (2007) examined the role of central or peripheral vision to avoid an obstacle. These authors reported that peripheral vision was sufficient for successful obstacle avoidance during locomotion. Moreover, more recently, Timmis et al. (2016) proved, in young adults, the impact of visual field loss (to 10° compared 20°) on risk of falls. They showed that only visual field loss to 20° increased risk of falls. We could hypothesize that the size of scotoma in AMD subjects may be predictive of postural instability. According to Berencsi et al. (2005), in young adults,

central, and peripheral vision contributes to maintaining a stable standing posture. They suggested that peripheral vision control more the AP than ML displacements of CoP. Actually our result contrast this one, AP displacement of CoP is larger in AMD subjects with central field loss could be due to the different age of subjects tested in the two studies. Indeed, it is well-known that older subjects used more hip strategies to maintain postural control whereas young adults used ankle strategies (Daubney and Culham, 1999). Further studies comparing young and old subjects with poor vision are needed to explore postural strategies.

LIMITATIONS

It is important to note that in this study we used a platform with a frequency of 40 Hz and this could explain the small displacement and mean speed values reported here comparing to others studies. Secondly, a larger number of subjects with AMD will be necessary to explore further their postural instability in relationship with their scotoma measures.

CONCLUSION

The present study showed that AMD subjects, suffering from visual impairment in the central but not in the peripheral field, had worse postural performance than healthy age-matched control subjects, especially in the surface area (unilateral and bilateral AMD subjects) and AP displacements of the CoP (bilateral AMD subjects only). Because of aging, AMD subjects could have poor postural adaptive mechanisms which increase instability and risk of falls. Further studies will aim to improve knowledge and to develop reeducation techniques in these patients.

AUTHOR CONTRIBUTIONS

HC, LT, OL, AnA, AlA, TB, SS, MB: substantial contributions to the conception of the word, logistic support for the recruitment of participants, acquisition, analysis and interpretation of data for the work, drafting the work and revising critically for important intellectual content, final approval of the version to be published, Agreement to be accountable for all aspects of the work in ensuring that questions related to the accuracy or integrity of any part of the work are appropriately investigated and resolved.

ACKNOWLEDGMENTS

This study was conducted as part of Master's 2 "Recherche et Organisation en Santé spécialité Recherche en Réadaptation" (UPMC) of HC. The authors gratefully acknowledge the orthoptists, nurses, and secretaries of Centre Ophtalmologique du Val-d'Oise (OPH95) and Department of Ophthalmology, Hôtel-Dieu Hospital in Paris for their participation and their logistics support. The authors also wish to thank all participants for their kind participation.

REFERENCES

Age-Related Eye Disease Study Research Group (AREDS) (2001). The Age-Related Eye Disease Study system for classifying age-related macular degeneration from stereoscopic color fundus photographs: the Age-Related Eye Disease Study Report Number 6. *Am. J. Ophthalmol.* 132, 668–681. doi: 10.1016/S0002-9394(01)01218-1

Agostini, V., Sbrollini, A., Cavallini, C., Busso, A., Pignata, G., and Knaflitz, M. (2016). The role of central vision in posture: postural sway in Stargardt patients. *Gait Posture* 43, 233–238. doi: 10.1016/j.gaitpost.2015.10.003

Augood, C. A., Vingerling, J. R., de Jong, P. T., Chakravarthy, U., Seland, J., Soubrane, G., et al. (2006). Prevalence of age-related maculopathy in older Europeans: the European Eye Study (EUREYE). *Arch. Ophthalmol.* 124, 529–535. doi: 10.1001/archopht.124.4.529

Augustin, A., Sahel, J. A., Bandello, F., Dardennes, R., Maurel, F., Negrini, C., et al. (2007). Anxiety and depression prevalence rates in age-related macular degeneration. *Invest. Opthalmol. Vis. Sci.* 48, 1498. doi: 10.1167/iovs.06-0761

Bandello, F., Augustin, A., Sahel, J. A., Benhaddi, H., Negrini, C., Hieke, K., et al. (2008). Association between visual acuity and medical and non-medical costs in patients with wet age-related macular degeneration in France, Germany and Italy. *Drugs Aging* 25, 255–268. doi: 10.2165/00002512-200825030-00007

Berencsi, A., Ishihara, M., and Imanaka, K. (2005). The functional role of central and peripheral vision in the control of posture. *Hum. Mov. Sci.* 24, 689–709. doi: 10.1016/j.humov.2005.10.014

Brandt, T. (2003). *Vertigo: Its Multisensory Syndromes.* London; New York, NY: Springer.

Bucci, M. P., Soufi, H., Villeneuve, P., Colleville, L., Bui-Quoc, E., and Lions, C. (2016). Importance of proprioceptive information for postural control in children with strabismus before and after strabismus surgery. *Front. Syst. Neurosci.* 10:67. doi: 10.3389/fnsys.2016.00067

Campbell, A. J., Borrie, M. J., and Spears, G. F. (1989). Risk factors for falls in a community-based prospective study of people 70 years and older. *J. Gerontol.* 44, 112–117. doi: 10.1093/geronj/44.5.M112

Carroll, N. V., Slattum, P. W., and Cow, F. M. (2005). The cost of falls among the community-dwelling elderly. *J. Manag. Care Pharm.* 11, 307–316. doi: 10.18553/jmcp.2005.11.4.307

Chakravarthy, U., Augood, C., Bentham, G. C., de Jong, P. T., Rahu, M., Seland, J., et al. (2007). Cigarette smoking and age-related macular degeneration in the EUREYE Study. *Ophthalmology* 114, 1157–1163. doi: 10.1016/j.ophtha.2006.09.022

Chiari, L., Rocchi, L., and Cappello, A. (2002). Stabilometric parameters are affected by anthropometry and foot placement. *Clin. Biomech.* 17, 666–677. doi: 10.1016/S0268-0033(02)00107-9

Chomistek, A. K., Manson, J. E., Stefanick, M. L., Lu, B., Sands-Lincoln, M., and Going, S. B. (2013). Relationship of sedentary behavior and physical activity to incident cardiovascular disease: results from the Women's Health Initiative. *J. Am. Coll. Cardiol.* 61, 2346–2354. doi: 10.1016/j.jacc.2013.03.031

Christoforidis, J. B., Tecce, N., Dell'Omo, R., Mastropasqua, R., Verolino, M., and Costagliola, C. (2011). Age related macular degeneration and visual disability. *Curr. Drug Targets* 12, 221–323. doi: 10.2174/138945011794182755

Daubney, M. E., and Culham, E. G. (1999). Lower-extremity muscle force and balance performance in adults aged 65 years and older. *Phys. Ther.* 79, 1177–1185.

Elliott, D. B., Patla, A. E., Flanagan, J. G., Spaulding, S., Rietdyk, S., Strong, G., et al. (1995). The Waterloo Vision and Mobility Study: postural control strategies in subjects with ARM. *Ophthalmic. Physiol. Opt.* 15, 556–559. doi: 10.1016/0275-5408(95)00025-9

Faraldo-García, A., Santos-Pérez, S., Cruieiras, R., and Soto-Varela, A. (2016). Postural changes associated with ageing on the sensory organization test and the limits of stability in healthy subjects. *Auris Nasus Larynx* 43, 149–154. doi: 10.1016/j.anl.2015.07.001

Ferris, F. L. (1983). Senile macular degeneration: review of epidemiologic features. *Am. J. Epidemiol.* 118, 132–151. doi: 10.1093/oxfordjournals.aje.a113624

Fetter, M., and Dichgans, J. (1996). Vestibular neuritis spares the inferior division of the vestibular nerve. *Brain J. Neurol.* 119, 755–763. doi: 10.1093/brain/119.3.755

Fitzpatrick, R., and McCloskey, D. I. (1994). Proprioceptive, visual and vestibular thresholds for the perception of sway during standing in humans. *J. Physiol.* 478 (Pt 1), 173–186. doi: 10.1113/jphysiol.1994.sp020240

Friedman, D. S., O'Colmain, B. J., Muñoz, B., Tomany, S. C., McCarty, C., de Jong, P. T., et al. (2004). Prevalence of age-related macular degeneration in the United States. *JAMA Ophthalmol.* 122, 564–572. doi: 10.1001/archopht.122.4.564

Gagey, P. M., Bizzo, G., Bonnier, L., Gentaz, R., Guillaume, P., Marucchi, C., et al. (1993). *Eight Lessons Posturology, 3rd Edn.* Paris: Masson.

Gagey, P. M., and Weber, B. (1999). *Posturologie Régulation et Dérèglement de la Station Debout.* Paris: Masson.

Gagey, P. M., and Weber, B. (2004). *Posturologie: Régulation et Dérèglements de la Station Debout.* Paris: Masson.

Geurts, A. C., Nienhuis, B., and Mulder, T. W. (1993). Intrasubject variability of selected force-platform parameters in the quantification of postural control. *Arch. Phys. Med. Rehabil.* 74, 1144–1150.

Gurfinkel, V. S., and Shik, M. L. (1973). *Motor Control.* Boston, MA: Springer.

Hochberg, C., Maul, E., Chan, E. S., Van Landingham, S., Ferrucci, L., Friedman, D. S., et al. (2012). Association of vision loss in glaucoma and age-related macular degeneration with IADL disability. *Invest. Ophthalmol. Vis. Sci.* 53, 3201. doi: 10.1167/iovs.12-9469

Horak, F. B., and Shupert, C. L. (1994). Role of the vestibular system in postural control. *Vestib. Rehabil.* 13, 69–81.

Hyman, L., and Neborsky, R. (2002). Risk factors for age-related macular degeneration: an update. *Curr. Opin. Ophthalmol.* 13, 171–175. doi: 10.1097/00055735-200206000-00007

Kocur, I., and Resnikoff, S. (2002). Visual impairment and blindness in Europe and their prevention. *Br. J. Ophthalmol.* 86, 716–722. doi: 10.1136/bjo.86.7.716

Kotecha, A., Chopra, R., Fahy, R. T., and Rubin, G. S. (2013). Dual tasking and balance in those with central and peripheral vision loss. *Invest. Ophthalmol. Vis. Sci.* 54, 5408–5415. doi: 10.1167/iovs.12-12026

Leveziel, N., Delcourt, C., Zerbib, J., Dollfus, H., Kaplan, J., Benlian, P., et al. (2009). Épidémiologie de la dégénérescence maculaire liée à l'âge. *J. Fr. Ophtalmol.* 32, 440–451. doi: 10.1016/j.jfo.2009.04.009

Lions, C., Bui Quoc, E., Wiener-Vacher, S., and Bucci, M. P. (2014). Postural control in strabismic children: importance of proprioceptive information. *Front. Physiol.* 5:156. doi: 10.3389/fphys.2014.00156

Loprinzi, P. D., Swenor, B. K., and Ramulu, P. Y. (2015). Age-Related macular degeneration is associated with less physical activity among US adults: cross-sectional study. *PLoS ONE* 10:e0125394. doi: 10.1371/journal.pone.0125394

Marigold, D. S., and Patla, A. E. (2007). Visual information from the lower visual field is important for walking across multi-surface terrain. *Exp. Brain Res.* 188, 23–31. doi: 10.1007/s00221-008-1335-7

McCloud, C., and Lake, S. (2015). Understanding the patient's lived experience of neovascular age-related macular degeneration: a qualitative study. *Eye* 29, 1561–1569. doi: 10.1038/eye.2015.167

Moraes, R., Lopes, A. G., and Barela, J. A. (2009). Monocular vision and increased distance reducing the effects of visual manipulation on body sway. *Neurosci. Lett.* 460, 209–213. doi: 10.1016/j.neulet.2009.05.078

Nashner, L. M. (1979). Organization and programming of motor activity during posture control. *Prog. Brain Res.* 50, 177–184. doi: 10.1016/S0079-6123(08)60818-3

Paillard, J. (1971). Les déterminants moteurs de l'organisation de l'espace. *Cah. Psychol.* 14, 261–316.

Qiu, F., Cole, M. H., Davids, K. W., Hennig, E. M., Silburn, P. A., Netscher, H., et al. (2012). Enhanced somatosensory information decreases postural sway in older people. *Gait Posture* 35, 630–635. doi: 10.1016/j.gaitpost.2011.12.013

Rovner, B. W., Casten, R. J., Leiby, B. E., and Tasman, W. S. (2009). Activity loss is associated with cognitive decline in age-related macular degeneration. *Alzheimers Dement.* 5, 12–17. doi: 10.1016/j.jalz.2008.06.001

Sengupta, S., van Landingham, S., Solomon, S. D., Do, D. V., Friedman, D. S., and Ramulu, P. Y. (2014). Driving habits in older patients with central vision loss. *Ophthalmology* 12, 727–732. doi: 10.1016/j.ophtha.2013.09.042

Timmis, M. A., Scarfe, A. C., and Pardhan, S. (2016). How does the extent of central visual field loss affect adaptive gait? *Gait Posture* 44, 55–60. doi: 10.1016/j.gaitpost.2015.11.008

Tinetti, M. E., Speechley, M., and Ginter, S. F. (1988). Risk factors for falls among elderly persons living in the community. *N. Engl. J. Med.* 319, 1701–1707. doi: 10.1056/nejm198812293192604

Vuillerme, N., Chenu, O., Pinsault, N., Fleury, A., Demongeot, J., and Payan, Y. (2008). Can a plantar pressure-based tongue-placed electrotactile biofeedback improve postural control under altered vestibular and neck proprioceptive conditions? *Neuroscience* 155, 291–296. doi: 10.1016/j.neuroscience.2008.05.018

Walraven, J. (1975). Amblyopia screening with random-dot stereograms. *Am. J. Ophthalmol.* 80, 893–900. doi: 10.1016/0002-9394(75)90286-x

Wang, J. J., Rochtchina, E., Smith, W., Klein, R., Klein, B. E. K., Joshi, T., et al. (2009). Combined effects of complement factor H genotypes, fish consumption, and inflammatory markers on long-term risk for age-related macular degeneration in a cohort. *Am. J. Epidemiol.* 169, 633–641. doi: 10.1093/aje/kwn358

Wang, J. J., Ross, R. J., Tuo, T., Burlutsky, G., Tan, A. G., Chan, C. C., et al. (2008). The LOC387715 polymorphism, inflammatory markers, smoking, and age-related macular degeneration. A population-based case-control study. *Ophthalmology* 115, 693–699. doi: 10.1016/j.ophtha.2007.05.038

Wood, J. M., Lacherez, P., Black, A. A., Cole, M. H., Boon, M. Y., and Kerr, G. K. (2011). Risk of falls, injurious falls, and other injuries resulting from visual impairment among older adults with age-related macular degeneration. *Invest. Ophthalmol. Vis. Sci.* 52, 5088–5092. doi: 10.1167/iovs.10-6644

Wood, J. M., Lacherez, P. F., Black, A. A., Cole, M. H., Boon, M. Y., and Kerr, G. K. (2009). Postural stability and gait among older adults with age-related maculopathy. *Invest. Ophthalmol. Vis. Sci.* 50, 482–487. doi: 10.1167/iovs.08-1942

3

Imaging Posture Veils Neural Signals

Robert T. Thibault[1]* and Amir Raz[1, 2, 3]*

[1] Integrated Program in Neuroscience, Department of Neurology and Neurosurgery, McGill University, Montreal, QC, Canada,
[2] The Lady Davis Institute for Medical Research at the Jewish General Hospital, Montreal, QC, Canada, [3] Department of
Psychiatry, Institute for Community and Family Psychiatry, McGill University, Montreal, QC, Canada

Correspondence:
Robert T. Thibault
robert.thibault@mail.mcgill.ca
Amir Raz
amir.raz@mcgill.ca

Whereas modern brain imaging often demands holding body positions incongruent with everyday life, posture governs both neural activity and cognitive performance. Humans commonly perform while upright; yet, many neuroimaging methodologies require participants to remain motionless and adhere to non-ecological comportments within a confined space. This inconsistency between ecological postures and imaging constraints undermines the transferability and generalizability of many a neuroimaging assay. Here we highlight the influence of posture on brain function and behavior. Specifically, we challenge the tacit assumption that brain processes and cognitive performance are comparable across a spectrum of positions. We provide an integrative synthesis regarding the increasingly prominent influence of imaging postures on autonomic function, mental capacity, sensory thresholds, and neural activity. Arguing that neuroimagers and cognitive scientists could benefit from considering the influence posture wields on both general functioning and brain activity, we examine existing imaging technologies and the potential of portable and versatile imaging devices (e.g., functional near infrared spectroscopy). Finally, we discuss ways that accounting for posture may help unveil the complex brain processes of everyday cognition.

Keywords: posture, neuroimaging, EEG, fMRI, upright, supine, cognition, perception

INTRODUCTION

From psychiatry and cognitive science to education and marketing, many experts draw on discoveries from human brain imaging to inform their practice. However, few consumers of neuroimaging findings fully appreciate the methodological and environmental variables that these techniques often impose. For example, in a typical functional magnetic resonance imaging (fMRI) experiment, participants lie motionless in a body-sized bore while piercing screeches, thumps, and hums thunder around their head for up to an hour. In a customary electroencephalography (EEG) experiment, participants sit upright, alone, in a small, silent, and often dimly lit room, while staring at and responding to a computer screen for extended periods of time. Of the many glaring discrepancies between such imaging environments and everyday life, this review focuses on the role of body posture. We summarize important findings from research examining the relationship between posture and brain data, highlight the mechanisms underlying these postural influences, and discuss experimental techniques that can help overcome postural caveats in human brain research.

Neuroimagers seldom draw on research suggesting that environmental variables impact human cognition. Meanwhile, an entire field of research, entitled "embodied cognition," highlights the intricate relationship among our cognitive capacities, ongoing sensorimotor state, and surrounding environment (Thompson and Varela, 2001; Wilson, 2002; Thompson, 2005; Di Paolo and Thompson, 2014). Relevant postural findings highlight that slouching increases measures of helplessness and stress (Riskind and Gotay, 1982) and expansive postures increase testosterone, decrease cortisol, and amplify feelings of power and risk-tolerance (Carney et al., 2010). Static imaging environments further diminish cognitive loads related to balance, moving visual fields, and social interaction (Hari and Kujala, 2009). Considering these factors, some scientists demand a new neuroscientific model—the "embodied brain"—to better account for the ongoing interactions between brain, body, and environment (Kiverstein and Miller, 2015).

IMAGING METHODS AND IMAGING POSTURES

Popular functional neuroimaging modalities collect electromagnetic or hemodynamic brain data (**Table 1**). EEG and magnetoencephalography (MEG) record electric and magnetic signals from pyramidal neurons; fMRI measures deoxygenated blood concentrations that correlate with neural activity; and functional near infrared spectroscopy (fNIRS) measures oxygenated and deoxygenated blood flow. EEG and MEG come with spatial precision of about 1 cm, yet millisecond temporal resolution; fMRI provides millimetric spatial resolution but temporal precision of ∼1 s; fNIRS excels in neither temporal nor spatial resolution and comes with a high signal-to-noise ratio compared to fMRI (Cui et al., 2011). MEG outperforms EEG in terms of signal-to-noise ratio when accessing deeper brain regions (Goldenholz et al., 2009). Each imaging modality, moreover, permits a subset of body positions. Participants can wear EEG and fNIRS caps throughout a wide range of postures (see **Table 1**) and, with proper equipment, can move and interact with their environment; MEG restricts participants to an adjustable seat that can adopt any position between an upright chair and a horizontal bench; and most fMRI options constrain participants to horizontal positions. Compared to portable technologies (i.e., EEG and fNIRS), the large and static imaging devices (i.e., fMRI and MEG) permit fewer posture, yet provide higher-quality data. These intrinsic differences lend certain imaging modalities more advantageous for specific applications and research questions but less so for others (e.g., the postural constraints of most MRI scanners would make fMRI a good way to explore the sleeping brain, but less ideal to study the driving brain).

Two canonical imaging postures dominate brain research even though more ecological alternatives exist (see **Table 1**). These established positions include sitting upright—common in EEG, MEG, fNIRS, and most of cognitive and psychological research; and lying supine—the standard for fMRI. Whereas, a limited number of imaging experiments stray from these standardized postures, humans perform many cognitive tasks while standing and moving, yet few while lying down. Experiments leveraging non-standard body positions often ask particular questions which demand these postures. For example, researchers have participants stand or walk to better understand balance, gait, and motor disorders such as Parkinson's disease (Bakker et al., 2007; Koenraadt et al., 2014; Mahoney et al., 2016), lie supine titled 6–12° head-down past horizontal to simulate a

microgravity environment (e.g., Spironelli and Angrilli, 2011), or lie prone to investigate gravitational forces on cranial fluids (Rice et al., 2013). Whereas, the execution of these experiments fully depends on the use of non-standard imaging postures, the supine and sitting positions hardly impede researchers from conducting most neuroimaging experiments. This situation may encourage neuroimagers to continue employing standardized imaging postures even when ecological comportments could better unveil the neural mechanisms of everyday cognition.

POSTURE INFLUENCES COGNITION

Posture alters sensory perception and behavior (**Figure 1**). For example, when upright compared to supine: Olfactory thresholds increase for select odorants (e.g., Lundström et al., 2008), pain ratings amplify (e.g., Spironelli and Angrilli, 2011; Fardo et al., 2013), visual awareness improves (e.g., Goodenough et al., 1981; Marendaz et al., 1993), anticipatory anxiety heightens (e.g., Lipnicki and Byrne, 2008), approach motivation increases (Price et al., 2012), and conflicting thoughts decrease (e.g., Harmon-Jones et al., 2015). Posture further influences cognitive performance. Compared to lying supine, sitting upright improves non-verbal intelligence (e.g., Raven's Progressive Matrices; Lundström et al., 2008) and aids in composing mental images, but impairs the ability to inspect them (Mast et al., 2003). Standing compromises performance on problems requiring a burst of insight (e.g., anagrams: Lipnicki and Byrne, 2005) and improves psychomotor performance (Caldwell et al., 2000, 2003). Memories, moreover, are easier to retrieve when assuming the posture associated with the remembered event (Dijkstra et al., 2007).

The fMRI environment may alter the very phenomena researchers aim to study. This concern has motivated diverse research groups to test how posture and cognition interact (e.g., Lundström et al., 2008; Harmon-Jones and Peterson, 2009). Replication experiments, however, remain sparse, likely because posture receives more attention as a procedural caveat than a research field in its own right. Beyond posture, neuroimagers must also address several other procedural and statistical concerns before obtaining meaningful results (e.g., Eklund et al., 2016). All in all, these studies highlight the importance of considering posture across all cognitive and imaging research.

POSTURE INFLUENCES PHYSIOLOGY

Heart rate, respiratory volume, oxygen consumption, core body temperature, cortisol secretion, and other indicators of physiological arousal stabilize at higher levels when upright compared to supine (**Figure 1**; Cole, 1989; Kräuchi et al., 1997; Hennig et al., 2000; Badr et al., 2002; Jones and Dean, 2004). These physiological differences may influence the fMRI derived blood-oxygen-level dependent (BOLD) signal, regardless of whether or not brain processes actually change (Kastrup et al., 1999; Di et al., 2013). fMRI measures neuronal activity indirectly (see Shmuel, 2015); the BOLD signal stems from the hemodynamic properties of neural populations and remains

TABLE 1 | Each body posture raises particular considerations in terms of brain imaging modalities and cognitive experiments.

	Canonical imaging postures		Other everyday postures	
	Lying supine	Sitting upright	Standing erect	Sitting reclined
EEG	✓	✓	✓	✓
MEG	✓	✓	✗	✓
fMRI	✓	✗	✗	✗
fNIRS	✓	✓	✓	✓
Vigilance	Low	Medium	High	Medium/low
Assumed in waking life	Rare	Common	Common	Occasional
Associated cognitive tasks	Few	Many	Many	Few
Actions possible	Few	Many	Most	Few

To conduct fMRI beyond a horizontal body posture requires specialized scanners, which are extremely uncommon. Researchers can conduct EEG and fNIRS in any posture, but must care for occipital sensors in the supine position. Humans execute most physical and cognitive actions when sitting or standing. To better depict the posture assumed in fMRI, this photo shows a participant before entering the bore. During scanning, the head and upper body remain inside the bore, which measures about 60 cm in diameter for standard scanners.

highly sensitive to cardiopulmonary variables (Chang and Glover, 2009; Chang et al., 2009; Di et al., 2013; Weinberger and Radulescu, 2016). Thus, demonstrating that posture affects the BOLD signal falls short of confirming a change in neural activity; cardiopulmonary variables remain yoked to body position and also weigh heavily on BOLD activity.

Beyond BOLD, posture governs blood flow around the brain (Gisolf et al., 2004). A few experiments employ a stance-adjustable positron emission tomography (PET) gantry and report greater blood flow to both visual and cerebellar cortices when standing erect compared to lying supine (Ouchi et al., 1999, 2001). Using fNIRS, researchers document decreases in both oxygenated and deoxygenated cortical hemoglobin volume when participants move from lying supine to sitting upright (Edlow et al., 2010; Ozgoren et al., 2012). Due to a paucity of upright MRI scanners capable of functional sequences, researchers have yet to replicate postural fNIRS experiments with fMRI. Because fNIRS and fMRI measure similar signals (Cui et al., 2011), we can only presume that postural discrepancies would also influence fMRI data.

Beyond cardiovascular measures, posture exerts a quantifiable and direct impact on neural activity. A few EEG experiments demonstrate that, compared to lying horizontally, lying head-up on an incline between 30–45° (Cole, 1989; Vaitl and Gruppe, 1992) and sitting upright (Chang et al., 2011; Spironelli et al., 2016) increase high-frequency neural activity, associated with alertness and sensory processing, and dampen down low-frequency oscillations associated with relaxed or drowsy states. More recent studies leverage high-density EEG systems and reveal greater high-frequency power across the cortex in more upright postures (Thibault et al., 2014) as well as an 80% increase in occipital gamma power when supine compared to prone (Rice et al., 2013). Posture further alters event related potentials (ERPs) in response to standard visual paradigms (Rice et al., 2013), painful stimuli (Spironelli and Angrilli, 2011; Fardo et al., 2013), and emotional processing (Price et al., 2012; Messerotti Benvenuti et al., 2013). In contrast to these findings, a recent sensor-level MEG study revealed greater high-frequency power over common language areas only, rather than the entire cortex, when sitting upright compared to when supine or reclined (Thibault et al., 2015). Sensor-level MEG results, however, may represent only the strongest postural effects and source-level analyses of such data may reveal more widespread changes reminiscent of previous EEG findings (Lifshitz et al., under review). Whereas, the majority of these studies employ healthy young adults, posture may exert a particularly strong influence on brain function in the elderly and specific patient groups (e.g., cardiovascular disease or tramautic brain injury: Ouchi et al., 2005; Thompson et al., 2005). In this regard, converging evidence from cognitive, medical, and neuroscientific research supports the "embodied brain" hypothesis and underscores the importance of postural variables in modern imaging experiments.

UNDERLYING MECHANISMS BY WHICH POSTURE OPERATES

At least two physiological and one cognitive mechanism contribute to the influence of posture on brain data: (1) changes in noradrenalin output, (2) altered CSF thickness, and (3) a preparatory cognitive state based on the subset of interactions possible with the environment.

(1) The supine position hampers cortical excitability (Lipnicki, 2009; Spironelli et al., 2016). When lying horizontally, compared to upright, gravitational loads redistribute and stimulate arterial and cardiopulmonary baroreceptors, and in turn, lead to a reduction in sympathetic nervous system activity (Mohrman and Heller, 2003). This process appears to impede noradrenergic release from neurons in the locus coeruleus (Murase et al., 1994; Berridge and Waterhouse, 2003) and drives downstream cortical inhibition (Rau and Elbert, 2001). A cleverly designed experiment supports this theory (Cole, 1989). The researcher applied leg pressure via anti-shock trousers (normally used to treat severe blood loss) to maintain levels of baroreceptor activity between lying horizontally and lying head-up on a 40° incline. They found less high-frequency EEG activity only in the condition with reduced baroreceptor firing (i.e., 40° incline without leg pressure). Further theoretical (Lipnicki, 2009) and experimental reports (Vaitl and Gruppe, 1992; Schneider et al., 2008) support the idea that gravity initiates a physiological cascade that leads to cortical inhibition.

(2) Slight shifts in CSF thickness can drastically alter EEG data (Ramon et al., 2004, 2006; Wendel et al., 2008) and, to a lesser extent, MEG data (Vorwerk et al., 2014). Strong evidence for this interaction comes from a unique two-part multiposture MRI and EEG study (Rice et al., 2013). The researchers found that when supine compared to prone, gravity draws the brain downwards, thins out the highly conductive CSF in occipital regions by 30%, brings the brain slightly closer to posterior scalp electrodes, and in turn, amplifies high-frequency occipital EEG power by an average of 80% (Rice et al., 2013). While this study provides a wealth of information, the scarcity of erect MRI scanners likely precluded an upright condition. And yet, a complementary low-field (0.5 T) MRI study scanned participants in the seated and supine positions and found that gravity draws fluids downward into the spinal canal when upright, decreases intracranial CSF and cerebral blood flow, and amplifies intracranial compliance (Alperin et al., 2005). Measures of CSF thickness in circumscribed cortical regions, however, were not reported. Thus, the quantitative differences in CSF thickness between supine and upright postures remains largely elusive. The finding that CSF not only distorts electromagnetic brain signals, but also varies in thickness among postures, raises particular concern regarding the standard practice of using anatomical MRI data acquired in the supine posture to construct head models for EEG and MEG analyses. Whereas, postural CSF discrepancies may correlate well with brain imaging data, a clear story hardly emerges relating CSF thickness to behavioral observations. This insight suggests that factors beyond CSF likely contribute to the influence of posture on human functioning.

(3) A preparatory cognitive state, set to act on the subset of possible interactions between the current position of a participant and their surrounding environment, may partially account for the influence of posture on brain activity. For example, when lying down, the brain may be poorly prepared for locomotion (de Lange et al., 2006), to observe a moving

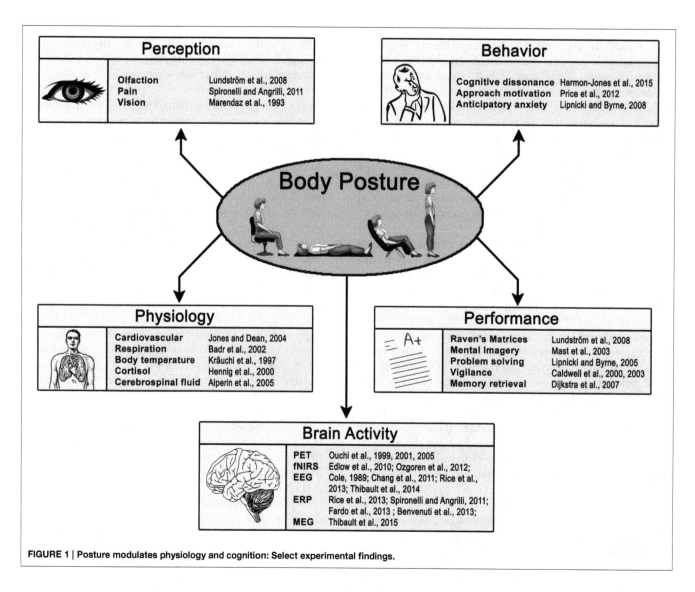

FIGURE 1 | Posture modulates physiology and cognition: Select experimental findings.

visual field (Kano, 1991), or to socially and physically interact with our environment (Hari and Kujala, 2009). Motor plans depend on ongoing limb configuration (de Lange et al., 2006), the excitability of motor cortex increases in free-standing compared to supported postures (Tokuno et al., 2009), and when sitting, compared to supine, people react more quickly to moving visual fields (Kano, 1991) and are more likely to perceive themselves as moving when exposed to a moving visual field (Guterman et al., 2012). Moreover, the supine posture decreases social behaviors (Harmon-Jones and Peterson, 2009; Price et al., 2012) and hardly invites typical social interactions known to modulate brain activity, such as eye contact (Ferri et al., 2014). These posture-dependent cognitive states may manifest in both resting-state brain oscillations (Chang et al., 2011; Thibault et al., 2014; Spironelli et al., 2016) and neural responses to stimuli (i.e., ERPs: Spironelli and Angrilli, 2011; Price et al., 2012; Fardo et al., 2013). The causality of interactions between cognition and brain activity may always remain elusive; cognitive states

propel physiological change (i.e., top-down processes) and physiological parameters also weigh on cognitive states (i.e., bottom-up effects).

Taken together, physiological cascades, cranial fluids, and cognitive set all exert varying influences on brain imaging data across postures. Whereas, noradrenergic output and cognitive processing may directly influence cortical activity measured at the neuronal level, CSF shunts the transmission of electromagnetic activity from neurons to sensors and exerts little influence on neuronal activity itself. Adopting experimental designs that evaluate and integrate these three mechanisms can only help to better understand ecological human functioning.

CORRECTING AND ACCOUNTING FOR THE EFFECTS OF POSTURE

Two paths emerge to overcome postural caveats in neuroimaging. First, we can rework standard experimental designs to minimize the influence of posture on brain activity; and second, we can embrace new imaging technologies conducive to everyday human behavior.

Accounting for the three aforementioned postural mechanisms would require a combination of innovative experimental designs, computational expertise, and a new body of research to draw upon. For example, to maintain cortical excitability in the supine posture, researchers could entertain the possibility of applying pressure to the body via anti-shock trousers to maintain baroreceptor firing (Cole, 1989), pharmacologically sustaining noradrenalin levels, or providing periodic stimulation via conversation or sensory input to sustain participant alertness. Overcoming variation in CSF thickness may require anatomical brain scans from each participant plus compensatory algorithms to calculate the standard redistribution of CSF as a function of posture. Such algorithms do not yet exist and would demand further head modeling research that taps into a database of posture-induced CSF perturbations across individuals (e.g., see Rice et al., 2013). Novel research on posture and cognition, moreover, could help future experimental designs minimize variations in cognitive state among postures. For example, research already demonstrates that poor sleep impedes working memory when supine compared to sitting (Muehlhan et al., 2014) and hampers psychomotor performance when sitting compared to standing (Caldwell et al., 2003). These findings suggest that weeding out sleep-deprived participants from supine imaging experiments could help researchers collect brain data that better reflect upright human functioning. Neuroimagers could further benefit from extending similar screening procedures to participants with mood and hormonal disturbances in response to MRI environments (Muehlhan et al., 2011) and mental performance problems in response to scanner noise (Pripfl et al., 2006). With diligence, neuroimagers can improve current research paradigms to account for a number of these postural discrepancies.

Imaging the human brain increasingly relies on smaller, lighter, and more mobile hardware. These devices hold the potential to thrust brain imaging toward investigating everyday interactive and social cognition. With the use of overhead gantries, participants undergoing EEG and fNIRS can now move and interact in a laboratory environment (Gramann et al., 2011; Mahoney et al., 2016). Recent developments, moreover, permit individuals to connect EEG electrodes to their smartphone and record brain activity in everyday contexts (Stopczynski et al., 2014). Moving while recording EEG, however, comes with caveats. Muscle activity, eye movement, and head motion all contaminate the EEG signal, especially in high-frequency bandwidths (Muthukumaraswamy, 2013). One potential concern is that researchers who are not careful may mistake these artifacts for brain oscillations themselves. The fNIRS signal also remains sensitive to motion artifacts, but responds less to muscle contamination. These portable devices sacrifice signal quality for ecological human functioning. The use of these technologies, however, is not an "either-or" dilemma. In a single experiment, we can combine data from the more precise and static imaging modalities with data from ecological yet coarser devices. Similar to how portable devices revolutionized the field of eye-tracking (Hayhoe and Ballard, 2005), wearable neuroimaging technologies hold promise to revolutionize how we study the living human brain.

CONCLUSION

Across numerous experiments, posture reliably influences brain data, core physiology, and cognitive performance. This reality rings alarm bells in a field that rarely considers postural constraints. Whereas, ecological comportments such as standing and moving recruit a host of additional brain processes and represent the base from which we perform our largest diversity of interactions, few brain imaging studies ask participants to stand or move. A pillar of neuroimaging, MRI, confines participants to a supine position seldom assumed during common wakefulness. This state of affairs brings into question the practice of using neuroimaging findings to inform our ecological behavior of everyday life. Bridging the lacuna between imaging context and ecological posture would further unveil the neural processes giving rise to the living human brain.

AUTHOR CONTRIBUTIONS

RT reviewed the literature, consulted with experts, and prepared the initial draft. RT and AR prepared the final draft together. AR provided comments throughout manuscript preparation.

FUNDING

AR acknowledges funding from the Canada Research Chair program, Discovery and Discovery Acceleration Supplement grants from the Natural Sciences and Engineering Research Council of Canada (NSERC), Canadian Institutes of Health Research, and the Bial Foundation. RT, also a Bial recipient, acknowledges an Alexander Graham Bell Canada Graduate Scholarship from NSERC. The funding sources had no involvement in reviewing the literature, writing the manuscript, or deciding to submit the paper for publication.

ACKNOWLEDGMENTS

We thank Lu Zhou for help with graphics and Drs. Xu Cui and Joseph Baker for providing the photo of fNIRS.

REFERENCES

Alperin, N., Hushek, S. G., Lee, S. H., Sivaramakrishnan, A., and Lichtor, T. (2005). MRI study of cerebral blood flow and CSF flow dynamics in an upright posture: the effect of posture on the intracranial compliance and pressure. *Acta Neurochir. Suppl.* 95, 177–181. doi: 10.1007/3-211-32318-X_38

Badr, C., Elkins, M. R., and Ellis, E. R. (2002). The effect of body position on maximal expiratory pressure and flow. *Aust. J. Physiother.* 48, 95–102. doi: 10.1016/S0004-9514(14)60203-8

Bakker, M., Verstappen, C. C. P., Bloem, B. R., and Toni, I. (2007). Recent advances in functional neuroimaging of gait. *J. Neural Transm.* 114, 1323–1331. doi: 10.1007/s00702-007-0783-8

Berridge, C. W., and Waterhouse, B. D. (2003). The locus coeruleus-noradrenergic system: modulation of behavioral state and state-dependent cognitive processes. *Brain Res. Brain Res. Rev.* 42, 33–84. doi: 10.1016/S0165-0173(03)00143-7

Caldwell, J. A., Prazinko, B., and Caldwell, J. L. (2003). Body posture affects electroencephalographic activity and psychomotor vigilance task performance in sleep-deprived subjects. *Clin. Neurophysiol.* 114, 23–31. doi: 10.1016/S1388-2457(02)00283-3

Caldwell, J. A., Prazinko, B. F., and Hall, K. K. (2000). The effects of body posture on resting electroencephalographic activity in sleep-deprived subjects. *Clin. Neurophysiol.* 111, 464–470. doi: 10.1016/S1388-2457(99)00289-8

Carney, D. R., Cuddy, A. J. C., and Yap, A. J. (2010). Power posing: brief nonverbal displays affect neuroendocrine levels and risk tolerance. *Psychol. Sci.* 21, 1363–1368. doi: 10.1177/0956797610383437

Chang, C., Cunningham, J. P., and Glover, G. H. (2009). Influence of heart rate on the BOLD signal: the cardiac response function. *Neuroimage* 44, 857–869. doi: 10.1016/j.neuroimage.2008.09.029

Chang, C., and Glover, G. H. (2009). NeuroImage relationship between respiration, end-tidal CO 2, and BOLD signals in resting-state fMRI. *Neuroimage* 47, 1381–1393. doi: 10.1016/j.neuroimage.2009.04.048

Chang, L.-J., Lin, J.-F., Lin, C.-F., Wu, K.-T., Wang, Y.-M., and Kuo, C.-D. (2011). Effect of body position on bilateral EEG alterations and their relationship with autonomic nervous modulation in normal subjects. *Neurosci. Lett.* 490, 96–100. doi: 10.1016/j.neulet.2010.12.034

Cole, R. J. (1989). Postural baroreflex stimuli may affect EEG arousal and sleep in humans. *J. Appl. Physiol.* 67, 2369–2375.

Cui, X., Bray, S., Bryant, D. M., Glover, G. H., and Reiss, A. L. (2011). A quantitative comparison of NIRS and fMRI across multiple cognitive tasks. *Neuroimage* 54, 2808–2821. doi: 10.1016/j.neuroimage.2010.10.069

de Lange, F. P., Helmich, R. C., and Toni, I. (2006). Posture influences motor imagery: an fMRI study. *Neuroimage* 33, 609–617. doi: 10.1016/j.neuroimage.2006.07.017

Di, X., Kannurpatti, S. S., Rypma, B., and Biswal, B. B. (2013). Calibrating BOLD fMRI activations with neurovascular and anatomical constraints. *Cereb. Cortex* 23, 255–263. doi: 10.1093/cercor/bhs001

Dijkstra, K., Kaschak, M. P., and Zwaan, R. A. (2007). Body posture facilitates retrieval of autobiographical memories. *Cognition* 102, 139–149. doi: 10.1016/j.cognition.2005.12.009

Di Paolo, E. A., and Thompson, E. (2014). "The enactive approach ezequiel di paolo and evan thompson forthcoming in lawrence shapiro, Edn," in *The Routledge Handbook of Embodied Cognition*, ed L. Shapiro (New York, NY: Routledge Press), 68–78.

Edlow, B. L., Kim, M. N., Durduran, T., Zhou, C., Putt, M. E., Yodh, A. G., et al. (2010). The effects of healthy aging on cerebral hemodynamic responses to posture change. *Physiol. Meas.* 31, 477–495. doi: 10.1088/0967-3334/31/4/002

Eklund, A., Nichols, T. E., and Knutsson, H. (2016). Cluster failure: why fMRI inferences for spatial extent have inflated false-positive rates. *Proc. Natl. Acad. Sci. U.S.A.* 113, 7900–7905. doi: 10.1073/pnas.1602413113

Fardo, F., Spironelli, C., and Angrilli, A. (2013). Horizontal body position reduces cortical pain-related processing: evidence from late ERPs. *PLoS ONE* 8:e81964. doi: 10.1371/journal.pone.0081964

Ferri, F., Busiello, M., Campione, G. C., De Stefani, E., Innocenti, A., Romani, G. L., et al. (2014). The eye contact effect in request and emblematic hand gestures. *Eur. J. Neurosci.* 39, 841–851. doi: 10.1111/ejn.12428

Gisolf, J., van Lieshout, J. J., van Heusden, K., Pott, F., Stok, W. J., and Karemaker, J. M. (2004). Human cerebral venous outflow pathway depends on posture and central venous pressure. *J. Physiol.* 560, 317–327. doi: 10.1113/jphysiol.2004.070409

Goldenholz, D. M., Ahlfors, S. P., Ha, M. S., Sharon, D., Ishitobi, M., Vaina, L. M., et al. (2009). Mapping the signal-to-noise-ratios of cortical sources in magnetoencephalography and electroencephalography. *Hum. Brain Mapp.* 30, 1077–1086. doi: 10.1002/hbm.20571

Goodenough, D. R., Oltman, P. K., Sigman, E., and Cox, P. W. (1981). The rod-and-frame illusion in erect and supine observers. *Percept. Psychophys.* 29, 365–370.

Gramann, K., Gwin, J. T., Ferris, D. P., Oie, K., Jung, T. P., Lin, C. T., et al. (2011). Cognition in action: imaging brain/body dynamics in mobile humans. *Rev. Neurosci.* 22, 593–608. doi: 10.1515/RNS.2011.047

Guterman, P. S., Allison, R. S., Palmisano, S., and Zacher, J. E. (2012). Influence of head orientation and viewpoint oscillation on linear vection. *J. Vestib. Res.* 22, 105–116. doi: 10.3233/VES-2012-0448

Hari, R., and Kujala, M. V., (2009). Brain basis of human social interaction: from concepts to brain imaging. *Physiol. Rev.* 89, 453–479. doi: 10.1152/physrev.00041.2007

Harmon-Jones, E., and Peterson, C. K. (2009). Supine body position reduces neural response to anger evocation. *Psychol. Sci.* 20, 1209–1210. doi: 10.1111/j.1467-9280.2009.02416.x

Harmon-Jones, E., Price, T. F., and Harmon-Jones, C. (2015). Supine body posture decreases rationalizations: testing the action-based model of dissonance. *J. Exp. Soc. Psychol.* 56, 228–234. doi: 10.1016/j.jesp.2014.10.007

Hayhoe, M., and Ballard, D. (2005). Eye movements in natural behavior. *Trends Cogn. Sci.* 9, 188–194. doi: 10.1016/j.tics.2005.02.009

Hennig, J., Friebe, J., Ryl, I., Krämer, B., Böttcher, J., and Netter, P. (2000). Upright posture influences salivary cortisol. *Psychoneuroendocrinology* 25, 69–83. doi: 10.1016/S0306-4530(99)00037-2

Jones, A., and Dean, E. (2004). Body position change and its effect on hemodynamic and metabolic status. *Heart Lung* 33, 281–290. doi: 10.1016/j.hrtlng.2004.04.004

Kano, C. (1991). An ecological theory of motion sickness and postural instability an ecological theory of motion sickness and postural instability. *Ecol. Psychol.* 3, 241–252. doi: 10.1207/s15326969eco0303

Kastrup, A., Krüger, G., Glover, G. H., and Moseley, M. E. (1999). Assessment of cerebral oxidative metabolism with breath holding and fMRI. *Magn. Reson. Med.* 42, 608–611. doi: 10.1002/(SICI)1522-2594(199909)42:3<608::AID-MRM26>3.0.CO;2-I

Kiverstein, J., and Miller, M. (2015). The embodied brain: towards a radical embodied cognitive neuroscience. *Front. Hum. Neurosci.* 9:237. doi: 10.3389/fnhum.2015.00237

Koenraadt, K. L. M., Roelofsen, E. G. J., Duysens, J., and Keijsers, N. L. W. (2014). Cortical control of normal gait and precision stepping: an fNIRS study. *Neuroimage* 85, 415–422. doi: 10.1016/j.neuroimage.2013.04.070

Kräuchi, K., Cajochen, C., and Wirz-Justice, A. (1997). A relationship between heat loss and sleepiness: effects of postural change and melatonin administration. *J. Appl. Physiol.* 83, 134–139.

Lipnicki, D. M. (2009). Baroreceptor activity potentially facilitates cortical inhibition in zero gravity. *Neuroimage* 46, 10–11. doi: 10.1016/j.neuroimage.2009.01.039

Lipnicki, D. M., and Byrne, D. G. (2005). Thinking on your back: solving anagrams faster when supine than when standing. *Brain Res. Cogn. Brain Res.* 24, 719–722. doi: 10.1016/j.cogbrainres.2005.03.003

Lipnicki, D. M., and Byrne, D. G. (2008). An effect of posture on anticipatory anxiety. *Int. J. Neurosci.* 118, 227–237. doi: 10.1080/00207450701750463

Lundström, J. N., Boyle, J. A., and Jones-Gotman, M. (2008). Body position-dependent shift in odor percept present only for perithreshold odors. *Chem. Senses* 33, 23–33. doi: 10.1093/chemse/bjm059

Mahoney, J. R., Holtzer, R., Izzetoglu, M., Zemon, V., Verghese, J., and Allali, G. (2016). The role of prefrontal cortex during postural control in Parkinsonian syndromes a functional near-infrared spectroscopy study. *Brain Res.* 1633, 126–138. doi: 10.1016/j.brainres.2015.10.053

Marendaz, C., Stivalet, P., Barraclough, L., and Walkowiac, P. (1993). Effect of gravitational cues on visual search for orientation. *J. Exp. Psychol. Hum. Percept. Perform.* 19, 1266–1277. doi: 10.1037/0096-1523.19.6.1266

Mast, F. W., Ganis, G., Christie, S., and Kosslyn, S. M. (2003). Four types of visual mental imagery processing in upright and tilted observers. *Cogn. Brain Res.* 17, 238–247. doi: 10.1016/S0926-6410(03)00111-3

Messerotti Benvenuti, S., Bianchin, M., and Angrilli, A. (2013). Posture affects emotional responses: a head down bed rest and ERP study. *Brain Cogn.* 82, 313–318. doi: 10.1016/j.bandc.2013.05.006

Mohrman, D. E., and Heller, L. J. (2003). *Cardiovascular Physiology.* New York, NY: Lange Medical Books/McGraw-Hill.

Muehlhan, M., Lueken, U., Wittchen, H. U., and Kirschbaum, C. (2011). The scanner as a stressor: evidence from subjective and neuroendocrine stress parameters in the time course of a functional magnetic resonance imaging session. *Int. J. Psychophysiol.* 79, 118–126. doi: 10.1016/j.ijpsycho.2010.09.009

Muehlhan, M., Marxen, M., Landsiedel, J., Malberg, H., and Zaunseder, S. (2014). The effect of body posture on cognitive performance: a question of sleep quality. *Front. Hum. Neurosci.* 8:171. doi: 10.3389/fnhum.2014.00171

Murase, S., Inui, K., and Nosaka, S. (1994). Baroreceptor inhibition of the locus coeruleus noradrenergic neurons. *Neuroscience* 61, 635–643. doi: 10.1016/0306-4522(94)90440-5

Muthukumaraswamy, S. D. (2013). High-frequency brain activity and muscle artifacts in MEG/EEG: a review and recommendations. *Front. Hum. Neurosci.* 7:138. doi: 10.3389/fnhum.2013.00138

Ouchi, Y., Okada, H., Yoshikawa, E., Futatsubashi, M., and Nobezawa, S. (2001). Absolute changes in regional cerebral blood flow in association with upright posture in humans: an orthostatic PET study. *J. Nucl. Med.* 42, 707–712.

Ouchi, Y., Okada, H., Yoshikawa, E., Nobezawa, S., and Futatsubashi, M. (1999). Brain activation during maintenance of standing postures in humans. *Brain* 122, 329–338.

Ouchi, Y., Yoshikawa, E., Kanno, T., Futatsubashi, M., Sekine, Y., Okada, H., et al. (2005). Orthostatic posture affects brain hemodynamics and metabolism in cerebrovascular disease patients with and without coronary artery disease: a positron emission tomography study. *Neuroimage* 24, 70–81. doi: 10.1016/j.neuroimage.2004.07.044

Ozgoren, M., Tetik, M., Izzetoglu, K., Oniz, A., and Onaral, B. (2012). "Effect of body position on NIRS based hemodynamic measures from prefrontal cortex," in *Lecture Notes in Computer Science*, eds D. Liu, C. Alippi, D. Zhao, and A. Hussain (Berlin; Heidelberg: Springer), 138–146.

Price, T. F., Dieckman, L. W., and Harmon-Jones, E. (2012). Embodying approach motivation: body posture influences startle eyeblink and event-related potential responses to appetitive stimuli. *Biol. Psychol.* 90, 211–217. doi: 10.1016/j.biopsycho.2012.04.001

Pripfl, J., Robinson, S., Leodolter, U., Moser, E., and Bauer, H. (2006). EEG reveals the effect of fMRI scanner noise on noise-sensitive subjects. *Neuroimage* 31, 332–341. doi: 10.1016/j.neuroimage.2005.11.031

Ramon, C., Schimpf, P., Haueisen, J., Holmes, M., and Ishimaru, A. (2004). Role of soft bone, CSF and gray matter in EEG simulations. *Brain Topogr.* 16, 245–248. doi: 10.1023/B:BRAT.0000032859.68959.76

Ramon, C., Schimpf, P. H., and Haueisen, J. (2006). Influence of head models on EEG simulations and inverse source localizations. *Biomed. Eng. Online* 5:10. doi: 10.1186/1475-925X-5-10

Rau, H., and Elbert, T. (2001). Psychophysiology of arterial baroreceptors and the etiology of hypertension. *Biol. Psychol.* 57, 179–201. doi: 10.1016/S0301-0511(01)00094-1

Rice, J. K., Rorden, C., Little, J. S., and Parra, L. C. (2013). Subject position affects EEG magnitudes. *Neuroimage* 64, 476–484. doi: 10.1016/j.neuroimage.2012.09.041

Riskind, J. H., and Gotay, C. C. (1982). Physical posture: could it have regulatory or feedback effects on motivation and emotion? *Motiv. Emot.* 6, 273–298. doi: 10.1007/BF00992249

Schneider, S., Brümmer, V., Carnahan, H., Dubrowski, A., Askew, C. D., and Strüder, H. K. (2008). What happens to the brain in weightlessness? A first approach by EEG tomography. *Neuroimage* 42, 1316–1323. doi: 10.1016/j.neuroimage.2008.06.010

Shmuel, A. (2015). "Locally measured neuronal correlates of functional MRI signals," in *fMRI: From Nuclear Spins to Brain Functions*, eds K. Uludağ, K. Uğurbil, and L. Berliner (New York, NY: Springer), 63–82.

Spironelli, C., and Angrilli, A. (2011). Influence of body position on cortical pain-related somatosensory processing: an ERP study. *PLoS ONE* 6:e24932. doi: 10.1371/journal.pone.0024932

Spironelli, C., Busenello, J., and Angrilli, A. (2016). Supine posture inhibits cortical activity: evidence from Delta and Alpha EEG bands. *Neuropsychologia* 89, 125–131. doi: 10.1016/j.neuropsychologia.2016.06.015

Stopczynski, A., Stahlhut, C., Larsen, J. E., Petersen, M. K., and Hansen, L. K. (2014). The smartphone brain scanner: a portable real-time neuroimaging system. *PLoS ONE* 9:e86733. doi: 10.1371/journal.pone.0086733

Thibault, R. T., Lifshitz, M., Jones, J. M., and Raz, A. (2014). Posture alters human resting-state. *Cortex* 58, 199–205. doi: 10.1016/j.cortex.2014.06.014

Thibault, R. T., Lifshitz, M., and Raz, A. (2015). Body position alters human resting-state: insights from multi-postural magnetoencephalography. *Brain Imaging Behav.* 10, 772–780. doi: 10.1007/s11682-015-9447-8

Thompson, E. (2005). Sensorimotor subjectivity and the enactive approach to experience. *Phenomenol. Cogn. Sci.* 4, 407–427. doi: 10.1007/s11097-005-9003-x

Thompson, E., and Varela, F. (2001). Radical embodiment: Neural dynamics and conscious experience. *Trends Cogn. Sci.* 5, 418–425. doi: 10.1016/S1364-6613(00)01750-2

Thompson, J., Sebastianelli, W., and Slobounov, S. (2005). EEG and postural correlates of mild traumatic brain injury in athletes. *Neurosci. Lett.* 377, 158–163. doi: 10.1016/j.neulet.2004.11.090

Tokuno, C. D., Taube, W., and Cresswell, A. G. (2009). An enhanced level of motor cortical excitability during the control of human standing. *Acta Physiol.* 195, 385–395. doi: 10.1111/j.1748-1716.2008.01898.x

Vaitl, D., and Gruppe, H. (1992). Body position and changes in EEG. *J. Psychophysiol.* 6, 111–118.

Vorwerk, J., Cho, J.-H., Rampp, S., Hamer, H., Knösche, T. R., and Wolters, C. H. (2014). A guideline for head volume conductor modeling in EEG and MEG. *Neuroimage* 100, 590–607. doi: 10.1016/j.neuroimage.2014.06.040

Weinberger, D. R., and Radulescu, E. (2016). Finding the elusive psychiatric "lesion" with 21st-Century neuroanatomy: a note of caution. *Am. J. Psychiatry.* 173, 27–33. doi: 10.1176/appi.ajp.2015.15060753

Wendel, K., Narra, N. G., Hannula, M., Kauppinen, P., and Malmivuo, J. (2008). The influence of CSF on EEG sensitivity distributions of multilayered head models. *IEEE Trans. Biomed. Eng.* 55, 1454–1456. doi: 10.1109/TBME.2007.912427

Wilson, M. (2002). Six views of embodied cognition. *Psychon. Bull. Rev.* 9, 625–636. doi: 10.3758/BF03196322

4

Regularity of Center of Pressure Trajectories in Expert Gymnasts during Bipedal Closed-Eyes Quiet Standing

Brice Isableu[1]*, Petra Hlavackova[2,3], Bruno Diot[2,4] and Nicolas Vuillerme[2,5]

[1]Aix Marseille Univ, PSYCLE, Aix-en-Provence, France, [2]Équipe d'Accueil Autonomy, Gerontology, E-health, Imaging & Society, Université Grenoble-Alpes, Grenoble, France, [3]Grenoble Alpes University Hospital, Grenoble, France, [4]Informatique de Sécurité, Montceau-les-Mines, France, [5]Institut Universitaire de France, Paris, France

*Correspondence:
Brice Isableu
brice.isableu@univ-amu.fr

We compared postural control of expert gymnasts (G) to that of non-gymnasts (NG) during bipedal closed-eyes quiet standing using conventional and nonlinear dynamical measures of center of foot pressure (COP) trajectories. Earlier findings based on COP classical variables showed that gymnasts exhibited a better control of postural balance but only in demanding stances. We examined whether the effect of expertise in Gymnastic can be uncovered in less demanding stances, from the analysis of the dynamic patterns of COP trajectories. Three dependent variables were computed to describe the subject's postural behavior: the variability of COP displacements (A_{CoP}), the variability of the COP velocities (V_{CoP}) and the sample entropy of COP (SEn_{CoP}) to quantify COP regularity (i.e., predictability). Conventional analysis of COP trajectories showed that NG and G exhibited similar amount and control of postural sway, as indicated by similar A_{CoP} and V_{CoP} values observed in NG and G, respectively. These results suggest that the specialized balance training received by G may not transfer to less challenging balance conditions such as the bipedal eyes-closed stance condition used in the present experiment. Interestingly, nonlinear dynamical analysis of COP trajectories regarding COP regularity showed that G exhibited more irregular COP fluctuations relative to NG, as indicated by the higher SEn_{CoP} values observed for the G than for the NG. The present results showed that a finer-grained analysis of the dynamic patterns of the COP displacements is required to uncover an effect of gymnastic expertise on postural control in nondemanding postural stance. The present findings shed light on the surplus value in the nonlinear dynamical analysis of COP trajectories to gain further insight into the mechanisms involved in the control of bipedal posture.

Keywords: balance, entropy

INTRODUCTION

Posture can be defined as the spatial organization of the body segments (e.g., Winter, 1995). Postural regulation is a complex skill that requires coordinating and controlling subtle rotational movements of hundreds of joints by means of several hundreds of muscles to maintain the center of mass within the base of support. The multisensory consequences of the kinematics and kinetic variations patterns of postural movements, i.e., the dynamics of postural balance, would be informative of the direction of balance (DOB, Riccio et al., 1992) and preferred modes of spatial referencing (Streepey et al., 2007a,b; Isableu et al., 2010; Slaboda and Keshner, 2012). To maintain a bipedal posture stable, central processing factors are known to play a major role insofar as the central nervous system has to process information from various sensory cues (visual, somesthetic and vestibular), and weight them in proportion to their reliabilities (Oie et al., 2002). Analysis of the center of pressure (COP) in various upright stance tasks is widely used to characterize postural control and to understand the underlying motor control mechanisms during challenging experimental conditions. Force platform is typically used to assess the location and the dynamics of the COP. COP dynamics are likely due to complex control process associated with the maintenance of postural control, as well as the inherent noise within the human neuromotor system. COP is widely used to assess the health of the postural control system, but also to learn about the effect of athletic expertise (Lion et al., 2009; Herpin et al., 2010; Paillard et al., 2011; Zemková, 2014a,b). Previous studies investigated postural control during quiet standing in expert gymnasts (G), a sport requiring high balance abilities (Vuillerme et al., 2001a,b; Asseman et al., 2004, 2008; Vuillerme and Nougier, 2004; Gautier et al., 2008). Interestingly, these studies reported no significant difference between gymnasts and non-gymnasts (NG) under relatively non-challenging conditions (bipedal eyes-open posture). Authors suggested that expertise in gymnastics only has an effect on the control of specific postures for which the practice is specifically related to (see also, Henry, 1968; Schmidt and Young, 1987). However, standing posture during an eyes-closed bipedal standing task is known, as a test condition that increases reliance on vestibular (and proprioceptive) input (Rougier, 2003; Isableu and Vuillerme, 2006; Isableu et al., 2010), but also to require attention demands in gymnast and NG (Vuillerme and Nougier, 2004). At this point, however, the common observation from these studies is that the use of conventional measures of the center of foot pressure (COP; e.g., COP surface area, COP velocity) to quantify postural control in expert gymnasts may have yielded an incomplete picture of postural control in expert gymnasts (Asseman et al., 2004; Vuillerme and Nougier, 2004). Analyses carried out on nonlinear dynamic features of the COP revealed that variability in the motor output is not randomness but structured. Further insight into the underlying dynamics of bipedal eyes-closed postural control in expert gymnasts could be obtained through the recourse to nonlinear dynamical analysis of the COP regarding its regularity (i.e., predictability) using sample entropy measures (SEn_{CoP}; Borg and Laxåback, 2010). Interestingly, a more irregular COP trajectory, as assessed by higher SEn_{CoP}, has been suggested to be associated with more automaticity and has been proposed to be viewed as a reduction of the amount of attention invested in the control of posture (e.g., Roerdink et al., 2006, 2009, 2011; Donker et al., 2007; Stins et al., 2009a,b; Manor et al., 2013; Biec et al., 2014; Wayne et al., 2014).

The present experiment was designed to address the relationship between attention invested in posture and COP regularity by comparing postural control of expert gymnasts

to that of NG during bipedal eyes-closed standing using both conventional and nonlinear dynamical measures of the COP trajectories. The two underlying hypotheses are: (A) The extensive postural control training that gymnasts receive over the years changes the requirements on their postural control system in such a way that for the same balance task they require less attentional resources than NG; and (B) If more attentional resources are invested in a postural control task, then the COP movement becomes more regular, if, on the other hand, the postural task is controlled more by automated processes, then the COP movement characteristics become more irregular or complex (e.g., Roerdink et al., 2006, 2009, 2011; Donker et al., 2007; Stins et al., 2009a,b; Manor et al., 2013; Wayne et al., 2014).

From these two hypotheses, the following prediction can be derived: if both hypotheses are correct, then the sample entropy, a measure of irregularity of a time series, calculated for the COP of gymnasts should be higher than the SEn_{CoP} of NG. Hence, the purpose of the current study was to test the two hypotheses by confirming or refuting this prediction.

As a result, taking into account the above-mentioned results (Vuillerme et al., 2001a,b; Asseman et al., 2004, 2008; Vuillerme and Nougier, 2004), no significant difference between conventional measures of the COP measured in gymnasts and those measured in NG were expected. On the other hand, and more *originally*, considering: (1) the decreased attentional demand required for regulating postural sway during quiet standing previously reported in gymnasts relative to NG using a dual-task paradigm (Vuillerme and Nougier, 2004); and (2) the proposed relationship between the amount of attention invested in posture and COP regularity (e.g., Roerdink et al., 2006, 2009, 2011; Donker et al., 2007; Stins et al., 2009a,b; Manor et al., 2013; Wayne et al., 2014), gymnasts were expected to exhibit more irregular COP trajectories, operationalized with higher SEn_{CoP}, values, than NG.

MATERIALS AND METHODS

Subjects

Two groups of athletes voluntarily participated in the experiment. They were naïve as to the purpose of the study. This study was carried out in accordance with the recommendations of the local Ethics Committee with written informed consent from all subjects. All subjects gave written informed consent to the experimental procedure in accordance with the Declaration of Helsinki. The protocol was approved by the local Ethics Committee.

The group of expert gymnasts (G) consisted of 10 males having more than 10 years of experience (8 h/week) in gymnastics competition at the regional level or higher. Females were not considered in this study to remove potential bias due to: (i) known influence of anthropometric factors and gender on postural balance in adults (Chiari et al., 2002; Farenc et al., 2003; Alonso et al., 2012); but also because (ii) mechanical, and skeletal differences known to produce different neuromuscular control of the knee joint (Shultz and Perrin, 1999) on body sway resulting in a different postural response

(Schmitz et al., 2007; Ku et al., 2012) to sensory alteration (Raffi et al., 2014); and (iii) sensory integration difference with men favoring visual dependency (Raffi et al., 2014; Persiani et al., 2015). Since our findings may originate simply from the practice of sports in general, gymnasts' performance was compared to the performance of a control group composed of 10 NG males who were also experts in sport (soccer, handball, or tennis). We also adjusted the composition of the two groups such that there was no significant difference either in age, weight and height (**Table 1**) because body properties have been demonstrated to be determinant for postural task (Chiari et al., 2002; Ruhe et al., 2010).

Experimental Procedure

Subjects stood barefoot on the force platform (Dynatronic, France) in a standardized position (feet abducted at 30°, heels separated by 3 cm), their arms hanging loosely by their sides with eyes closed. This closed eyes condition has been chosen to avoid visual information interfering with the control of bipedal posture. Indeed, given the crucial role of visual information (for a review, see Redfern et al., 2001), earlier studies provided evidence that the eyes-closed condition in evaluating postural control helps to improve the discrimination between healthy people (see Isableu and Vuillerme, 2006; Isableu et al., 2010), and patients with sensory (e.g., vestibular; Horak et al., 1990; Allum et al., 2001), somesthetic (Oppenheim et al., 1999; Nardone et al., 2001) or sensory-motor (Marigold and Eng, 2006; Blaszczyk et al., 2007) impairments. In fact, the availability of visual information allows individuals to compensate for their postural deficits (for a review, see Redfern et al., 2001) limiting the use of the eyes-open condition as a normative based clinical protocol for objective evaluation of postural control, particularly if vestibular or somesthetic functions have to be assessed (Hlavačka, 2003). As a consequence, the eyes-open condition was not measured in this study. Subject's task was to stand as still as possible during the trial.

Three 30 s trials were performed. Rest periods of 60 s were provided between successive trials during which subjects were allowed to sit down.

Data were recorded at a sampling frequency of 40 Hz which is large enough for capturing the physiological content of the postural signal localized below 5 Hz and which is equal or larger than the sampling frequency used in others studies (Cavanaugh et al., 2007; Ramdani et al., 2009, 2011; Borg and Laxåback, 2010; Rhea et al., 2011).

Collected data were protected by the MedSafe technology by the IDS Company (Montceau-les-Mines, France). IDS Company is an approved hosting provider in personal health data by the French Ministry for Social Affairs and Health.

Data Analysis

The anteroposterior and mediolateral COP time series were centered on zero mean before constructing the resultant distance COP time series. Specifically, the resultant distance is the vector distance from the center of the posturogram to each point in the posturogram and hence it is not sensitive to the orientation of the base of support on force platform (Prieto et al., 1996).

Three dependent variables computed from the resultant distance COP were used to describe the subject's postural behavior using a similar methodology as recently proposed by Roerdink et al. (2009, 2011). The "amount of sway" and the "sway control" were quantified using two conventional, scale-dependent measures (see Prieto et al., 1996; Donker et al., 2007):

(1) the variability of COP displacements (A_{CoP} in mm, expressed as the root mean square of the COP time series),
(2) the variability of the COP velocities (V_{CoP} in mm/s, expressed as the root mean square of the COP velocities time series);

To examine the dynamical structure of COP trajectories and index its regularity independent of the size or scale. To this end, the RD time series was normalized to zero mean and unit variance resultant distance by subtracting its mean from this time series and dividing it by its standard deviation. Subsequently,

(3) the sample entropy of COP (SEn_{CoP}, dimensionless) was quantified for RD distance time series (Roerdink et al., 2009, 2011). Note that sample entropy was not calculated for the resultant distance differenced time series as suggested by Ramdani et al. (2009) to eliminate the inherent non-stationary nature of COP trajectories. Indeed, Roerdink et al. (2011) showed that it yields similar results. Algorithms of Lake and colleagues (Lake et al., 2002; Richman et al., 2004) were used to estimate corresponding sample entropy values. The sample entropy in a set of data points is the negative natural logarithm of the conditional probability (CP = A/B) that a sequence of data points with length N, having repeated itself within a tolerance r for m points, will also repeat itself for $m + 1$ points, without allowing self-matches (Richman and Moorman, 2000; Lake et al., 2002). Accordingly, B represents the total number of matches of length m while A represents the subset of B that also matches for $m + 1$. Sample entropy thus follows from $-\log$ (A/B), with a low sample entropy value arising from a high probability of repeated template sequence in the data. In this context, entropy is the rate of generation of new information and the lower the entropy, the greater the regularity (predictability) of the time series in question.

The reliability of the sample entropy estimation depends on the parameter choice of m and r. Sample entropy is best estimated with m as large and r as small as possible (Roerdink et al., 2009, 2011). Lake et al. (2002) introduced a statistical criterion to optimize the parameter choice, which is based on the maximum of the relative error of sample entropy and the conditional probability estimates. This metric simultaneously penalizes the conditional probability near 0 and

TABLE 1 | Age, weight, height of Non-gymnasts (NG) and Gymnasts (G) groups.

	Non gymnasts (n = 10)	Gymnasts (n = 10)	T-test (P < 0.05)
Age (years)	22.0 ± 1.3	21.9 ± 1.0	Ns
Weight (kg)	68.3 ± 2.9	67.5 ± 2.0	Ns
Height (cm)	173.9 ± 3.3	170.9 ± 3.1	Ns

Values are means and standard deviation (±); Ns = non-significant difference between the two groups.

near 1 (Lake et al., 2002) and represents the tradeoff between accuracy and discriminative capability. The criterion was set to be no higher than 0.05, implying that the 95% confidence interval of the sample entropy estimate is maximally 10% of its value (Lake et al., 2002). Ramdani et al. (2009, 2011) recently proposed a practical graphical method based on a convergence criterion to optimize the choice of the parameter values. This optimization procedure was notably used by Roerdink et al. (2011) who found ($m = 3$, $r = 0.05$) to be the optimal couple (see Rhea et al., 2011; Hansen et al., 2017). This result is comparable to other couple of parameters previously obtained from the original optimization procedure proposed by Lake et al. (2002) for the resultant distance times series too (Donker et al., 2007; Roerdink et al., 2009). Therefore, this couple was also used in this study to perform the calculation of sample entropy (Hansen et al., 2017).

Statistical Analysis

The mean of ACoP, VCoP and SEnCoP values obtained for each of three trials were averaged for statistical analysis. COP data being normally distributed, A_{CoP}, V_{CoP} and SEn_{CoP} obtained in the NG group were compared with those obtained in the G group using t-tests for independent measures. Statistical analyses were performed using Statistica 10. Level of significance was set at 0.05.

RESULTS

Statistical difference between the NG and the G was observed neither for the A_{CoP} ($t = -1.20$, $P = 0.25$, **Figure 1A**) nor for the V_{CoP} ($t = -0.83$, $P = 0.42$, **Figure 1B**). Conversely, SEn_{CoP} was significantly higher in G than in NG ($t = -2.48$, $P = 0.023$, **Figure 1C**).

DISCUSSION

Regarding the conventional posturographic analysis of COP trajectories, our results showed that NG and G exhibited similar amount and control of postural sway, as indicated by similar A_{CoP} (**Figure 1A**) and V_{CoP} values (**Figure 1B**) observed in NG and G, respectively. These results confirmed previous observations (Vuillerme et al., 2001a,b; Asseman et al., 2004, 2008) supporting the general idea according to which, the postural control capacities are specific to the training program and the requirements of each discipline. The specialized balance training received by gymnasts may not transfer to less challenging balance conditions such as the bipedal eyes-closed stance condition used in the present experiment (see also, Henry, 1968; Schmidt and Young, 1987). However, Vuillerme and Nougier (2004), using a stimulus-responses reaction time paradigm to assess attentional investment, reported a smaller attentional involvement in balance control for expert gymnasts than for NG. Interestingly, in this study, the main effect of expertise assessed via classical COP variables was not significant. These results suggested that some variables used in conventional posturographic analysis of COP trajectories did not capture the amount of attention invested to control postural balance. One

reason is that most variables used in conventional posturographic analysis of COP trajectories are *a priori* more suited to capture linear stationary processes (i.e., additive phenomenon) hidden in signal fluctuations (Wayne et al., 2014; Gow et al., 2015), and as a consequence fail to capture complex central interaction that result from the combination of both additive and multiplicative processes (Huang et al., 2016). The results mentioned above suggest that attentional mechanisms likely involve complex neural interaction and nonlinear processes (i.e., a mixture of additive and multiplicative phenomenon). Hence, attentional-based interactions and the amount of attentional investment in postural control seem better captured in the COP fluctuations by using nonlinear (multiplicative) variables.

Regarding the nonlinear dynamical posturographic analysis of COP trajectories regarding COP regularity, our results showed indeed that G exhibited more irregular COP fluctuations relative to NG, as indicated by the higher SEn_{CoP} values observed for the G than for the NG (**Figure 1C**). This result shows that nonlinear variables (SEn_{CoP}) are more appropriate to capture nonlinear multiplicative processes in the COP signal. Following the proposed relation between COP regularity and the amount of attention invested in the control of posture (e.g., Stins et al., 2009a), these results and ours suggest less attentional investment, i.e., a more fully automatized form of balance, in experts in sports requiring fine postural control (i.e., dancers and gymnasts) than controls. Our results are in accordance with those of Vuillerme and Nougier (2004) who, using a stimulus-responses reaction time paradigm to operationalize attentional investment, reported a smaller attentional involvement in balance control for expert gymnasts than for NG. Although to the best of our knowledge, no previous study has assessed regularity of COP trajectories in expert gymnasts during bipedal eyes-closed quiet standing, our observation is in line with a recent result obtained in experts in dance (Stins et al., 2009b), a sport that also require high balance abilities. Stins et al. (2009b) reported higher SEn_{CoP} in preadolescent pre-professional dancers than age-matched non-dancers. An alternative explanation of our findings could be drawn from the Borg and Laxåback's (2010) study. The higher COP entropy observed in gymnasts relative to nongymnasts suggests they exhibited a more automatic balance control. Within this view, higher COP entropy could indicate that they deployed a more efficient balancing. The efficiency with which postural balance (low COP variability and low attentional investment) is controlled is closely tied to the selection of an appropriate mode of spatial referencing (generally proprioceptive-based; Berthoz, 1991; Paillard, 1991; Kluzik et al., 2005; Streepey et al., 2007b; Isableu et al., 2010, 2011; Mergner, 2010; Slaboda et al., 2011a,b; Brady et al., 2012; Scotto Di Cesare et al., 2015). Several authors showed that these modes of spatial referencing are known to impact the attentional investment (Goodenough et al., 1987; Marendaz et al., 1988; Marendaz, 1989; Bailleux et al., 1990; Yan, 2010; Agathos et al., 2015). Following this rationale, it is likely that with the selection of the adequate frame of reference, attentional investment should decrease, and accounts for the emergence of more irregular (more complex) COP time series (Vuillerme and Nougier, 2004), even in nondemanding stance.

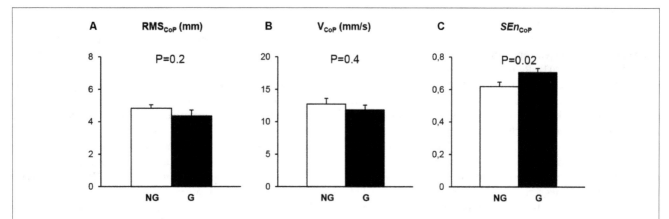

FIGURE 1 | Mean and standard error of mean of the variability of the displacements (A$_{CoP}$; **A**), the velocity (V$_{CoP}$; **B**) and the regularity (SEn$_{CoP}$; **C**) of the center of foot pressure (COP) trajectories obtained in the two groups of Non gymnasts (NG; *white bars*) and Gymnasts (G; *black bars*). The *P* values for comparisons between postural parameters computed from the NG and those computed from the G are reported.

Finally, two main conclusions can be drawn from the differential effect of expertise in gymnastics observed on the conventional (**Figures 1A,B**) and the nonlinear dynamical measure of the COP trajectory (**Figure 1C**) during bipedal eyes-closed quiet standing. First, these results suggest that, under mild challenging postural condition such as bipedal eyes-closed stance, postural control in expert gymnasts is *qualitatively*, but not *quantitatively*, different than that of controls. Although the expert population is different, the present findings are in line with those of Manor et al. (2013) and Wayne et al. (2014) on the impact of short- and long-term Tai Chi exercise training. These authors also reported that the effect of Tai Chi on postural control may be better characterized by quantifying its effects on the degree of complexity associated with the system output (i.e., COP dynamics) than by the traditional sway parameters (Manor et al., 2013; Wayne et al., 2014). Indeed, using both standard measures of postural sway and recurrence quantification analysis, these authors (Manor et al., 2013; Wayne et al., 2014) observed that trained ballet dancers exhibited similar variability and amount of postural sway, but more irregular sway and thus complex patterns than physically fit control group. Second, the observation that the balance skills of gymnasts were observed in the dynamic patterns of COP displacements (**Figure 1C**), but not in the control (**Figure 1A**) and the amount of postural sway velocity (**Figure 1B**) shed light on the surplus value in nonlinear dynamical analysis of COP trajectories to gain further insight into the mechanisms involved in the control of bipedal eyes-closed posture. Along these lines, some limitations of our study can be pointed. Nonlinear dynamics features of the COP displacements could have been explored in more depth using Multi-Scale Entropy (MSE), and Multivariate Multi-Scale Entropy (MMSE). These methods are particularly suitable to quantify the degree of regularity or predictability over multiple scales of time (see Costa et al., 2005; Gow et al., 2015). Our analyses were mainly carried out on the original time series. Additional information can be obtained from the analysis of the decremented time series (which removes the long-term correlated components from the original time series

and represent short-term complexity). Hansen et al. (2017), showed that MMSE analysis performed on the decremented time series is particularly suitable to detect signal divergence faster and can, therefore, be considered more suitable for complexity detection. Further experiments are currently performed to assess the relationship between variation of attentional ressources allocated to control potural balance and complexity of the COP at different scales, but also whether and how characteristics other than sportive expertise, such as anthropometry, neuromuscular state or preferred modes of spatial frames of reference (Streepey et al., 2007b; Isableu et al., 2010, 2011; Slaboda and Keshner, 2012; Agathos et al., 2015), that have been shown to affect balance control, could also modify the dynamical structure of the COP trajectories in terms of their regularity and complexity at different scales and frequency bands (by decomposing the original time series into intrinsic mode functions via empirical mode decomposition techniques (Costa et al., 2005; see Wei et al., 2012; Shih et al., 2015; Hansen et al., 2017).

AUTHOR CONTRIBUTIONS

BI, PH, BD and NV conceived and designed the experiment, performed the experiment, analyzed the data, contributed reagents/materials/analysis tools, wrote the article, prepared figures and/or tables, reviewed drafts of the article.

ACKNOWLEDGMENTS

Thanks to Dr. C. Franco for help analyzing data. The authors would also like to thank T. Omatomik and L. Enicka for their valuable comments and suggestions on the final manuscript. This work was supported in part by funding by IDS company, the French National Research Agency in the framework of the "Investissements d'avenir" program ANR-15-IDEX-02' and Institut Universitaire de France. The funders had no role in study design, data collection and analysis, decision to publish, or preparation of the manuscript.

REFERENCES

Agathos, C. P., Bernardin, D., Huchet, D., Scherlen, A. C., Assaiante, C., and Isableu, B. (2015). Sensorimotor and cognitive factors associated with the age-related increase of visual field dependence: a cross-sectional study. *Age (Dordr)* 37:9805. doi: 10.1007/s11357-015-9805-x

Allum, J. H., Adkin, A. L., Carpenter, M. G., Held-Ziolkowska, M., Honegger, F., and Pierchala, K. (2001). Trunk sway measures of postural stability during clinical balance tests: effects of a unilateral vestibular deficit. *Gait Posture* 14, 227–237. doi: 10.1016/s0966-6362(01)00132-1

Alonso, A. C., Luna, N. M., Mochizuki, L., Barbieri, F., Santos, S., and Greve, J. M. (2012). The influence of anthropometric factors on postural balance: the relationship between body composition and posturographic measurements in young adults. *Clinics (Sao Paulo)* 67, 1433–1441. doi: 10.6061/clinics/2012(12)14

Asseman, F., Caron, O., and Crémieux, J. (2004). Is there a transfer of postural ability from specific to unspecific postures in elite gymnasts? *Neurosci. Lett.* 358, 83–86. doi: 10.1016/j.neulet.2003.12.102

Asseman, F. B., Caron, O., and Crémieux, J. (2008). Are there specific conditions for which expertise in gymnastics could have an effect on postural control and performance? *Gait Posture* 27, 76–81. doi: 10.1016/j.gaitpost.2007.01.004

Bailleux, C., Marendaz, C., and Ohlmann, T. (1990). Selection of reference frames in form orientation task in relation to postural-gravitational constraints. *Perception* 19:381A.

Berthoz, A. (1991). "Reference frames for the perception and control of movement," in *Brain and Space*, ed. J. Paillard (Oxford: Oxford University Press), 81–110.

Bieć, E., Zima, J., Wójtowicz, D., Wojciechowska-Maszkowska, B., Kręcisz, K., and Kuczyński, M. (2014). Postural stability in young adults with down syndrome in challenging conditions. *PLoS One* 9:e94247. doi: 10.1371/journal.pone.0094247

Blaszczyk, J. W., Orawiec, R., Duda-Kodowska, D., and Opala, G. (2007). Assessment of postural instability in patients with Parkinson's disease. *Exp. Brain Res.* 183, 107–114. doi: 10.1007/s00221-007-1024-y

Borg, F. G., and Laxåback, G. (2010). Entropy of balance-some recent results. *J. Neuroeng. Rehabil.* 7:38. doi: 10.1186/1743-0003-7-38

Brady, R. A., Peters, B. T., Batson, C. D., Ploutz-Snyder, R., Mulavara, A. P., and Bloomberg, J. J. (2012). Gait adaptability training is affected by visual dependency. *Exp. Brain Res.* 220, 1–9. doi: 10.1007/s00221-012-3109-5

Cavanaugh, J. T., Mercer, V. S., and Stergiou, N. (2007). Approximate entropy detects the effect of a secondary cognitive task on postural control in healthy young adults: a methodological report. *J. Neuroeng. Rehabil.* 4:42. doi: 10.1186/1743-0003-4-42

Chiari, L., Rocchi, L., and Cappello, A. (2002). Stabilometric parameters are affected by anthropometry and foot placement. *Clin. Biomech. (Bristol, Avon)* 17, 666–677. doi: 10.1016/s0268-0033(02)00107-9

Costa, M., Goldberger, A. L., and Peng, C. K. (2005). Multiscale entropy analysis of biological signals. *Phys. Rev. E Stat. Nonlin. Soft Matter Phys.* 71:021906. doi: 10.1103/physreve.71.021906

Donker, S. F., Roerdink, M., Greven, A. J., and Beek, P. J. (2007). Regularity of center-of-pressure trajectories depends on the amount of attention invested in postural control. *Exp. Brain Res.* 181, 1–11. doi: 10.1007/s00221-007-0905-4

Farenc, I., Rougier, P., and Berger, L. (2003). The influence of gender and body characteristics on upright stance. *Ann. Hum. Biol.* 30, 279–294. doi: 10.1080/0301446031000068842

Gautier, G., Thouvarecq, R., and Vuillerme, N. (2008). Postural control and perceptive configuration: influence of expertise in gymnastics. *Gait Posture* 28, 46–51. doi: 10.1016/j.gaitpost.2007.09.007

Goodenough, D. R., Oltman, P. K., and Cox, P. W. (1987). The nature of individual differences in field dependence. *J. Res. Pers.* 21, 81–99. doi: 10.1016/0092-6566(87)90028-6

Gow, B. J., Peng, C. K., Wayne, P. M., and Ahn, C. A. (2015). Multiscale entropy analysis of center-of-pressure dynamics in human postural control: methodological considerations. *Entropy* 17, 7926–7947. doi: 10.3390/e17127849

Hansen, C., Wei, Q., Shieh, J. S., Fourcade, P., Isableu, B., and Majed, L. (2017). Sample entropy, univariate, and multivariate multi-scale entropy in comparison with classical postural sway parameters in young healthy adults. *Front. Hum. Neurosci.* 11:206. doi: 10.3389/fnhum.2017.00206

Henry, F. M. (1968). "Specificity versus generality in learning motor skill," in *Classical Studies on Physical Activities*, eds R. C. Brown and G. S. Kenyon (Englewood Cliffs, NJ: Prentice Hall), 340–350.

Herpin, G., Gauchard, G. C., Lion, A., Collet, P., Keller, D., and Perrin, P. P. (2010). Sensorimotor specificities in balance control of expert fencers and pistol shooters. *J. Electromyogr. Kinesiol.* 20, 162–169. doi: 10.1016/j.jelekin.2009.01.003

Hlavačka, F. (2003). Human postural responses to sensory stimulations: measurements and model. *Meas. Sci. Rev.* 3, Section 2.

Horak, F. B., Nashner, L. M., and Diener, H. C. (1990). Postural strategies associated with somatosensory and vestibular loss. *Exp. Brain Res.* 82, 167–177. doi: 10.1007/bf00230848

Huang, N. E., Hu, K., Yang, C. C. A., Chang, H.-C., Jia, D., Liang, K.-W., et al. (2016). On Holo-Hilbert spectral analysis: a full informational spectral representation for nonlinear and non-stationary data. *Philos. Trans. A Math. Phys. Eng. Sci.* 374:20150206. doi: 10.1098/rsta.2015.0206

Isableu, B., Fourre, B., Vuillerme, N., Giraudet, G., and Amorim, M. A. (2011). Differential integration of visual and kinaesthetic signals to upright stance. *Exp. Brain Res.* 212, 33–46. doi: 10.1007/s00221-011-2693-0

Isableu, B., Ohlmann, T., Cremieux, J., Vuillerme, N., Amblard, B., and Gresty, M. A. (2010). Individual differences in the ability to identify, select and use appropriate frames of reference for perceptuo-motor control. *Neuroscience* 169, 1199–1215. doi: 10.1016/j.neuroscience.2010.05.072

Isableu, B., and Vuillerme, N. (2006). Differential integration of kinaesthetic signals to postural control. *Exp. Brain Res.* 174, 763–768. doi: 10.1007/s00221-006-0630-4

Kluzik, J., Horak, F. B., and Peterka, R. J. (2005). Differences in preferred reference frames for postural orientation shown by after-effects of stance on an inclined surface. *Exp. Brain Res.* 162, 474–489. doi: 10.1007/s00221-004-2124-6

Ku, P. X., Abu Osman, N. A., Yusof, A., and Wan Abas, W. A. (2012). The effect on human balance of standing with toe-extension. *PLoS One* 7:e41539. doi: 10.1371/journal.pone.0041539

Lake, D. E., Richman, J. S., Griffin, M. P., and Moorman, J. R. (2002). Sample entropy analysis of neonatal heart rate variability. *Am. J. Physiol. Regul. Integr. Comp. Physiol.* 283, R789–R797. doi: 10.1152/ajpregu.00069.2002

Lion, A., Gauchard, G. C., Deviterne, D., and Perrin, P. P. (2009). Differentiated influence of off-road and on-road cycling practice on balance control and the related-neurosensory organization. *J. Electromyogr. Kinesiol.* 19, 623–630. doi: 10.1016/j.jelekin.2008.03.008

Manor, B., Lipsitz, L. A., Wayne, P. M., Peng, C. K., and Li, L. (2013). Complexity-based measures inform Tai Chi's impact on standing postural control in older adults with peripheral neuropathy. *BMC Complement. Altern. Med.* 13:87. doi: 10.1186/1472-6882-13-87

Marendaz, C. (1989). Selection of reference frames and the 'vicariance' of perceptual systems. *Perception* 18, 739–751. doi: 10.1068/p180739

Marendaz, C., Bailleux, C., and Chassouant, N. (1988). Dynamics of management of spatial reference frames: perceptual mode substitutions and functional habits. *Bull. Psychol.* 42, 31–39.

Marigold, D. S., and Eng, J. J. (2006). The relationship of asymmetric weight-bearing with postural sway and visual reliance in stroke. *Gait Posture* 23, 249–255. doi: 10.1016/j.gaitpost.2005.03.001

Mergner, T. (2010). A neurological view on reactive human stance control. *Annu. Rev. Control* 34, 177–198. doi: 10.1016/j.arcontrol.2010.08.001

Nardone, A., Galante, M., Lucas, B., and Schieppati, M. (2001). Stance control is not affected by paresis and reflex hyperexcitability: the case of spastic patients. *J. Neurol. Neurosurg. Psychiatry* 70, 635–643. doi: 10.1136/jnnp.70.5.635

Oie, K. S., Kiemel, T., and Jeka, J. J. (2002). Multisensory fusion: simultaneous re-weighting of vision and touch for the control of human posture. *Cogn. Brain Res.* 14, 164–176. doi: 10.1016/s0926-6410(02)00071-x

Oppenheim, U., Kohen-Raz, R., Alex, D., Kohen-Raz, A., and Azarya, M. (1999). Postural characteristics of diabetic neuropathy. *Diabetes Care* 22, 328–332. doi: 10.2337/diacare.22.2.328

Paillard, J. (Ed.). (1991). "Motor and representational framing in space," in *Brain and Space*, (Oxford: Oxford University Press), 163–182.

Paillard, T., Margnes, E., Portet, M., and Breucq, A. (2011). Postural ability reflects the athletic skill level of surfers. *Eur. J. Appl. Physiol.* 111, 1619–1623. doi: 10.1007/s00421-010-1782-2

Persiani, M., Piras, A., Squatrito, S., and Raffi, M. (2015). Laterality of stance during optic flow stimulation in male and female young adults. *Biomed Res. Int.* 2015:542645. doi: 10.1155/2015/542645

Prieto, T. E., Myklebust, J. B., Hoffmann, R. G., Lovett, E. G., and Myklebust, B. M. (1996). Measures of postural steadiness: differences between healthy young and elderly adults. *IEEE Trans. Biomed. Eng.* 43, 956–966. doi: 10.1109/10.532130

Raffi, M., Piras, A., Persiani, M., and Squatrito, S. (2014). Importance of optic flow for postural stability of male and female young adults. *Eur. J. Appl. Physiol.* 114, 71–83. doi: 10.1007/s00421-013-2750-4

Ramdani, S., Seigle, B., Lagarde, J., Bouchara, F., and Bernard, P. L. (2009). On the use of sample entropy to analyze human postural sway data. *Med. Eng. Phys.* 31, 1023–1031. doi: 10.1016/j.medengphy.2009.06.004

Ramdani, S., Seigle, B., Varoqui, D., Bouchara, F., Blain, H., and Bernard, P. L. (2011). Characterizing the dynamics of postural sway in humans using smoothness and regularity measures. *Ann. Biomed. Eng.* 39, 161–171. doi: 10.1007/s10439-010-0137-9

Redfern, M. S., Yardley, L., and Bronstein, A. M. (2001). Visual influences on balance. *J. Anxiety Disord.* 15, 81–94. doi: 10.1016/s0887-6185(00)00043-8

Rhea, C. K., Silver, T. A., Hong, S. L., Ryu, J. H., Studenka, B. E., Hughes, C. M., et al. (2011). Noise and complexity in human postural control: interpreting the different estimations of entropy. *PLoS One* 6:e17696. doi: 10.1371/journal.pone.0017696

Riccio, G. E., Martin, E. J., and Stoffregen, T. A. (1992). The role of balance dynamics in the active perception of orientation. *J. Exp. Psychol. Hum. Percept. Perform.* 18, 624–644. doi: 10.1037//0096-1523.18.3.624

Richman, J. S., Lake, D. E., and Moorman, J. R. (2004). Sample entropy. *Methods Enzymol.* 384, 172–184. doi: 10.1016/S0076-6879(04)84011-4

Richman, J. S., and Moorman, J. R. (2000). Physiological time-series analysis using approximate entropy and sample entropy. *Am. J. Physiol. Heart Circ. Physiol.* 278, H2039–H2049.

Roerdink, M., De Haart, M., Daffertshofer, A., Donker, S. F., Geurts, A. C., and Beek, P. J. (2006). Dynamical structure of center-of-pressure trajectories in patients recovering from stroke. *Exp. Brain Res.* 174, 256–269. doi: 10.1007/s00221-006-0441-7

Roerdink, M., Geurts, A. C., de Haart, M., and Beek, P. J. (2009). On the relative contribution of the paretic leg to the control of posture after stroke. *Neurorehabil. Neural Repair* 23, 267–274. doi: 10.1177/1545968308323928

Roerdink, M., Hlavackova, P., and Vuillerme, N. (2011). Center-of-pressure regularity as a marker for attentional investment in postural control: a comparison between sitting and standing postures. *Hum. Mov. Sci.* 30, 203–212. doi: 10.1016/j.humov.2010.04.005

Rougier, P. (2003). The influence of having the eyelids open or closed on undisturbed postural control. *Exp. Brain Res.* 47, 73–83. doi: 10.1016/s0168-0102(03)00187-1

Ruhe, A., Fejer, R., and Walker, B. (2010). The test-retest reliability of centre of pressure measures in bipedal static task conditions—a systematic review of the literature. *Gait Posture* 32, 436–445. doi: 10.1016/j.gaitpost.2010.09.012

Schmitz, R. J., Kulas, A. S., Perrin, D. H., Riemann, B. L., and Shultz, S. J. (2007). Sex differences in lower extremity biomechanics during single leg landings. *Clin. Biomech. (Bristol, Avon)* 22, 681–688. doi: 10.1016/j.clinbiomech.2007.03.001

Schmidt, R. A., and Young, D. E. (1987). "Transfer of movement control in motor learning," in *Transfer of Learning*, eds S. M. Cormier and J. D. Hagman (Orlando, FL: Academic Press), 47–79.

Scotto Di Cesare, C., Macaluso, T., Mestre, D. R., and Bringoux, L. (2015). Slow changing postural cues cancel visual field dependence on self-tilt detection. *Gait Posture* 41, 198–202. doi: 10.1016/j.gaitpost.2014.09.027

Shih, M.-T., Doctor, F., Fan, S.-Z., Jen, K.-K., and Shieh, J.-S. (2015). Instantaneous 3D EEG signal analysis based on empirical mode decomposition and the hilbert-huang transform applied to depth of anaesthesia. *Entropy* 17, 928–949. doi: 10.3390/e17030928

Shultz, S. J., and Perrin, D. H. (1999). Using surface electromyography to assess sex differences in neuromuscular response characteristics. *J. Athl. Train.* 34, 165–176.

Slaboda, J. C., and Keshner, E. A. (2012). Reorientation to vertical modulated by combined support surface tilt and virtual visual flow in healthy elders and adults with stroke. *J. Neurol.* 259, 2664–2672. doi: 10.1007/s00415-012-6566-7

Slaboda, J. C., Lauer, R., and Keshner, E. A. (2011a). Time series analysis of postural responses to combined visual pitch and support surface tilt. *Neurosci. Lett.* 491, 138–142. doi: 10.1016/j.neulet.2011.01.024

Slaboda, J. C., Lauer, R. T., and Keshner, E. A. (2011b). Continuous visual field motion impacts the postural responses of older and younger women during and after support surface tilt. *Exp. Brain Res.* 211, 87–96. doi: 10.1007/s00221-011-2655-6

Stins, J. F., Ledebt, A., Emck, C., van Dokkum, E. H., and Beek, P. J. (2009a). Patterns of postural sway in high anxious children. *Behav. Brain Funct.* 5:42. doi: 10.1186/1744-9081-5-42

Stins, J. F., Michielsen, M. E., Roerdink, M., and Beek, P. J. (2009b). Sway regularity reflects attentional involvement in postural control: effects of expertise, vision and cognition. *Gait Posture* 30, 106–109. doi: 10.1016/j.gaitpost.2009.04.001

Streepey, J. W., Kenyon, R. V., and Keshner, E. A. (2007a). Field of view and base of support width influence postural responses to visual stimuli during quiet stance. *Gait Posture* 25, 49–55. doi: 10.1016/j.gaitpost.2005.12.013

Streepey, J. W., Kenyon, R. V., and Keshner, E. A. (2007b). Visual motion combined with base of support width reveals variable field dependency in healthy young adults. *Exp. Brain Res.* 176, 182–187. doi: 10.1007/s00221-006-0677-2

Vuillerme, N., Danion, F., Marin, L., Boyadjian, A., Prieur, J. M., Weise, I., et al. (2001a). The effect of expertise in gymnastics on postural control. *Neurosci. Lett.* 303, 83–86. doi: 10.1016/s0304-3940(01)01722-0

Vuillerme, N., Teasdale, N., and Nougier, V. (2001b). The effect of expertise in gymnastics on proprioceptive sensory integration in human subjects. *Neurosci. Lett.* 311, 73–76. doi: 10.1016/s0304-3940(01)02147-4

Vuillerme, N., and Nougier, V. (2004). Attentional demand for regulating postural sway: the effect of expertise in gymnastics. *Brain Res. Bull.* 63, 161–165. doi: 10.1016/j.brainresbull.2004.02.006

Wayne, P. M., Gow, B. J., Costa, M. D., Peng, C. K., Lipsitz, L. A., Hausdorff, J. M., et al. (2014). Complexity-based measures inform effects of tai chi training on standing postural control: cross-sectional and randomized trial studies. *PLoS One* 9:e114731. doi: 10.1371/journal.pone.0114731

Wei, Q., Liu, D.-H., Wang, K.-H., Liu, Q., Abbod, M. F., Jiang, B. C., et al. (2012). Multivariate multiscale entropy applied to center of pressure signals analysis: an effect of vibration stimulation of shoes. *Entropy* 14, 2157–2172. doi: 10.3390/e14112157

Winter, D. A. (1995). Human balance and posture control during standing and walking. *Gait Posture* 3, 193–214. doi: 10.1016/0966-6362(96)82849-9

Yan, J. H. (2010). Cognitive styles affect choice response time and accuracy. *Pers. Individ. Dif.* 48, 747–751. doi: 10.1016/j.paid.2010.01.021

Zemková, E. (2014a). Author's reply to Paillard T: "sport-specific balance develops specific postural skills". *Sports Med.* 44, 1021–1023. doi: 10.1007/s40279-014-0175-9

Zemková, E. (2014b). Sport-specific balance. *Sports Med.* 44, 579–590. doi: 10.1007/s40279-013-0130-1

5

Anticipatory Postural Control of Stability during Gait Initiation Over Obstacles of Different Height and Distance Made Under Reaction-Time and Self-Initiated Instructions

Eric Yiou[1,2]*, Romain Artico[1,2], Claudine A. Teyssedre[1,2], Ombeline Labaune[1,2] and Paul Fourcade[1,2]

[1] CIAMS, Université Paris Sud, Université Paris-Saclay, Orsay, France, [2] CIAMS, Université d'Orléans, Orléans, France

*Correspondence:
Eric Yiou
eric.yiou@u-psud.fr

Despite the abundant literature on obstacle crossing in humans, the question of how the central nervous system (CNS) controls postural stability during gait initiation with the goal to clear an obstacle remains unclear. Stabilizing features of gait initiation include anticipatory postural adjustments (APAs) and lateral swing foot placement. To answer the above question, 14 participants initiated gait as fast as possible in three conditions of obstacle height, three conditions of obstacle distance and one obstacle-free (control) condition. Each of these conditions was performed with two levels of temporal pressure: reaction-time (high-pressure) and self-initiated (low-pressure) movements. A mechanical model of the body falling laterally under the influence of gravity and submitted to an elastic restoring force is proposed to assess the effect of initial (foot-off) center-of-mass position and velocity (or "initial center-of-mass set") on the stability at foot-contact. Results showed that the anticipatory peak of mediolateral (ML) center-of-pressure shift, the initial ML center-of-mass velocity and the duration of the swing phase, of gait initiation increased with obstacle height, but not with obstacle distance. These results suggest that ML APAs are scaled with swing duration in order to maintain an equivalent stability across experimental conditions. This statement is strengthened by the results obtained with the mechanical model, which showed how stability would be degraded if there was no adaptation of the initial center-of-mass set to swing duration. The anteroposterior (AP) component of APAs varied also according to obstacle height and distance, but in an opposite way to the ML component. Indeed, results showed that the anticipatory peak of backward center-of-pressure shift and the initial forward center-of-mass set decreased with obstacle height, probably in order to limit the risk to trip over the obstacle, while the forward center-of-mass velocity at foot-off increased with obstacle distance, allowing a further step to be taken. These effects of obstacle height and distance were globally similar under low and high-temporal pressure. Collectively, these findings imply that the CNS is able to predict the potential instability elicited by the obstacle clearance and that it scales the spatiotemporal parameters of APAs accordingly.

Keywords: stability, anticipatory postural adjustments, obstacle clearance, mechanical modeling, temporal pressure, gait initiation, motor coordination, human

INTRODUCTION

The control of postural stability is crucial for the efficient performance of day-to-day motor tasks. Like all terrestrial species, humans move around in a gravity field that permanently induces postural destabilization through its attracting effect towards the center of the earth. Major questions in motor control relate to the way in which humans are able to maintain stability during motor tasks that involve whole body progression, such as locomotor tasks, and how they adapt to environmental constraints, e.g., when clearing an obstacle. Gait initiation, which corresponds to the transient period between quiet standing and swing foot contact with the ground, is a classical paradigm for studying balance control mechanisms during complex whole body movement (e.g., Brenière et al., 1987; Lyon and Day, 1997, 2005; McIlroy and Maki, 1999; Yiou et al., 2012a for a recent review; Caderby et al., 2014). The act of lifting the swing foot from the ground to step in the desired direction does indeed induce a reduction in the size of the mediolateral (ML) base of support, moving from a bipedal to a unipedal stance. If the center of mass is not repositioned above (or closer to) the limits of the new base of support -i.e., the stance foot-, the body will topple towards the swing leg side during the single stance phase (or "swing phase") of gait initiation under the effect of gravity, which may cause lateral instability at foot contact. This instability is invariably attenuated during volitional stepping by the development of dynamic postural phenomena that occur before the swing phase. These dynamic phenomena correspond to "anticipatory postural adjustments" (APAs). They include a center of pressure shift towards the swing leg side which serves to accelerate the center of mass in the opposite direction, i.e., towards the stance leg side (Do et al., 1991; Jian et al., 1993; McIlroy and Maki, 1999; Nouillot et al., 2000; Caderby et al., 2014; Yiou et al., 2016). If not enough APAs are generated in the ML direction, a strategy of base of support enlarging, associated with a more lateral swing foot placement, has been shown to be triggered to maintain stability (Zettel et al., 2002; Caderby et al., 2014). In addition to this putative stabilizing function, APAs have been shown to provide the dynamic conditions for whole body progression in the desired direction. For example, during gait initiation, APAs in the anteroposterior (AP) direction include a backwards center of pressure shift that promotes the forward propulsive forces necessary to reach the intended center of mass velocity and step length (Brenière et al., 1987; Lepers and Brenière, 1995; Michel and Chong, 2004).

Postural stability during gait initiation might be further challenged by the presence of an obstacle that needs to be cleared. There has been extensive literature on the control of obstacle crossing during ongoing locomotion, especially in regards to the role of vision (e.g., Mohagheghi et al., 2004; Patla and Greig, 2006; Marigold et al., 2007). In comparison, the question how the postural and the focal components of gait initiation over an obstacle are coordinated to ensure safe body progression has received much less attention (e.g., Brunt et al., 1999; Yiou et al., 2016). Yet, it is known that gait initiation is among the motor activities associated with the highest proportion of

falls in the elderly (Robinovitch et al., 2013). In addition, the most frequent cause of falling in this population is an incorrect weight transfer, which, as stated above, is one of the major functions of APAs. In addition to the risk of tripping over the obstacle, the presence of an obstacle gives rise to an increase in the duration of the swing phase and therefore an increase in the potential for lateral instability (Zettel et al., 2002; Yiou et al., 2016). Hence, it is surprising that previous studies on the influence of an obstacle on the lateral motion of the center of mass during ongoing walking have reported that lateral stability remained unchanged when the height of the obstacle was varied (Chou et al., 2001; Hahn and Chou, 2004). This result led the authors to suggest the existence of some forms of adaptive postural mechanisms aimed at compensating for the increased potential instability related to obstacle height. However, these mechanisms remain to be clarified. To date, the question of whether or not the stabilizing mechanisms of gait initiation can accommodate obstacle constraints has been investigated in only one study (Yiou et al., 2016). This study showed that the amplitude of ML APAs was larger in the obstacle condition than in the obstacle free (control) condition. It was suggested that this increase was responsible for the maintenance of postural stability at swing foot contact. Similar results were obtained by Zettel et al. (2002) during their comparison of reactive stepping over an obstacle in response to a brisk plate-form shift with the same reactive stepping in an obstacle-free condition. However, these studies are all limited by the fact that only one obstacle height and distance were tested. Thus, one can question the generalizability of these results and more specifically, the extent to which the central nervous system (CNS) is able to adjust the stabilizing features of gait initiation (including ML APAs and base of support enlargement) to match changes in obstacle height and distance and the related potential for instability. Moreover, subjects of these studies invariably increased ML APAs when stepping (voluntarily or reactively) over the obstacle; thus, it could not be established that the absence of such an increase would have necessarily led to instability at foot contact. Lyon and Day (1997, 2005) used a single-segment mechanical model in which the body falls freely under the influence of gravity to predict the magnitude of the lateral center of mass fall during the swing phase of step initiation. In the present study, we elaborated on a mechanical model that was based on these last two studies in order to investigate how changes in the parameters of ML APAs can impact on postural stability at foot contact. Such modeling may thus provide further insight into the adaptability of the postural system to environmental constraints.

This study aims to investigate how the CNS controls postural stability during gait initiation when clearing obstacles of different heights and distances. Changes in obstacle height and distance were expected to bring about modulation of the swing phase and give rise to instability. In addition, as daily motor tasks may be performed under various temporal pressure constraints, gait initiation trials were performed in reaction-time (high pressure) and self-initiated (low pressure) conditions. Our previous study (Yiou et al., 2016) showed that the duration of APAs associated with gait initiation when faced with an obstacle was shorter under high pressure than under low pressure. This difference in duration was compensated by an increase in the amplitude of ML APAs. As only one obstacle height and distance were used (one 20 cm high obstacle, placed at a 20% body height distance from the participant), it can be questioned whether the CNS uses a similar anticipatory postural adaptation to temporal pressure when the obstacle constraints are manipulated. This is particularly the case when height and distance are increased, thereby placing a higher level of stress on the postural system.

This question might be addressed in regards to current theory on motor control, according to which our nervous system would possess neural structures (or internal models) that predict the future state of a system given the current state and the sensorimotor control signals (Wolpert and Flanagan, 2001). Such prediction would allow us to achieve rapid and accurate voluntary behavior despite the difficulties presented by motor noise, delayed sensory feedback, and a complex musculoskeletal apparatus. As stressed in Mille et al. (2012), it is clear that "the anticipatory nature of the APAs involves a role for motor prediction". Specifically, APAs structure would reflect the existence of internal models that predicts the destabilizing effect associated with the stepping (Lyon and Day, 1997, 2005). When stepping over an obstacle, it can therefore be expected that APAs will be scaled according to the potential destabilization associated with obstacle constraints. We thus hypothesize that the stabilizing features of gait initiation are scaled according to the changes in the swing phase duration that is associated with obstacle height and/or distance. More specifically, it is expected that a greater swing phase duration will be associated with larger ML APAs and eventually, a larger base of support in order to maintain unchanged postural stability at swing foot contact. Similar effects of obstacle constraints are expected under low and high temporal pressure conditions. However, APAs of larger amplitude and lower duration are expected in the high pressure condition compared with the low pressure condition. Mechanical modeling of the whole body during gait initiation is expected to reveal the extent to which postural stability at foot contact may be degraded in case ML APAs are not adequately scaled to modifications in swing duration induced by obstacle constraints.

MATERIALS AND METHODS

Participants

Fourteen subjects (eight males and six females, aged 23.2 ± 4 years [mean $\pm$ SD], height 173.4 ± 7.3 cm and weight 65.8 ± 8.7 kg) participated in the experiment. All were free of any known neuromuscular disorders. They gave written informed consent after being instructed as to the nature and purpose of the experiment, which was approved by the local ethics committee. The study conformed to the standards set by the Declaration of Helsinki.

Experimental Protocol

Participants were requested to initiate gait as fast as possible with their preferred limb while clearing an obstacle placed in front of them (**Figure 1**). Three conditions of obstacle

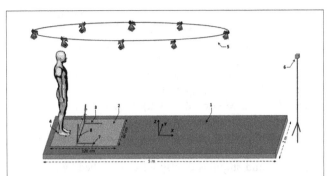

FIGURE 1 | Schematic illustration of the experimental set-up. Key: (1) walkway; (2) force-plate; (3) obstacle; (4) reflective marker; (5) Vicon camera; (6) visual target; (7) obstacle distance marker; and (8) obstacle height marker.

height (2.5%, 5% and 10% of each subject's height), three conditions of obstacle distance (10%, 20% and 30% of each subject's height) and an obstacle-free control condition were used. The three obstacle distances corresponded to 21%, 42% and 63% of the step length obtained in the control condition, respectively. Each condition of obstacle height and distance was realized in two blocks, which differed in terms of their level of temporal pressure constraint: a reaction-time and a self-initiated block. In the reaction-time block (high temporal pressure), participants were instructed to initiate gait "as soon as possible" after an acoustic signal was given. In the self-initiated block (low temporal pressure), they were instructed to initiate gait when they felt ready, after receiving an "all set" signal; it was made clear that the "all set" signal was not a "go" signal and that they could take as much time as they needed to prepare their movements. The order of conditions within one given block and the order of the blocks were randomized between participants. In each condition, subjects were allowed two familiarization trials. Five trials were then recorded. A 3-min rest was imposed between two successive conditions to avoid fatigue. In each condition, the participants initially stood upright with their feet hip-width apart, their arms hanging loosely either side of their body and their body weight evenly distributed between their legs. The boundaries of their feet in the initial posture were outlined on the force plate, and participants were instructed to systematically reposition their feet within these marks under supervision. They were repeatedly reminded of the task instructions.

Materials

Gait was initiated on a force plate (600 × 1200 mm, AMTI, Watertown, MA, USA) located at the beginning of a five-meter track (**Figure 1**). The force plate was embedded in the track and was large enough to allow the participant's swing foot to systematically land on it at the end of gait initiation. After crossing the obstacle, participants walked to the end of the track, then stood still for a few seconds before returning to their starting position. The obstacle consisted of a lightweight wooden rod (length: 65 cm; diameter: 1 cm) that rested on two adjustable upright standards. The participant's toes served as the reference point for positioning the obstacle at the various distances. Reflective skin markers (9 mm in diameter) were placed bilaterally at the hallux (toe marker), head of the fifth metatarsal (metatarsal marker), posterior calcaneus (heel marker) and at the middle of the top of the obstacle (obstacle marker). A V8i VICON eight-camera (Mcam2) motion capture system (Oxford Metrics Ltd., UK) with 64 analog channels was used to record the movement of the foot markers and to detect the position of the obstacle. Kinematic and kinetic data were collected simultaneously at a rate of 500 Hz. Data acquisition and stimulus display were controlled by a custom-made program written in Matlab^{TM} (R2009b, The MathWorks Inc., Natick, MA, USA).

Data Analysis

Kinematic and force plate data were low-pass filtered using a Butterworth filter with a 15 Hz (Mickelborough et al., 2000) and a 10 Hz (Caderby et al., 2014) cut-off frequency, respectively. The ML (yP) and AP (xP) coordinates of the center of pressure were computed from force plate data as follows:

$$yP = \frac{Mx + Fy \times dz}{Fz} \tag{1}$$

$$xP = \frac{-My + Fx \times dz}{Fz} \tag{2}$$

where Mx and My are the moments around the AP and ML axes, respectively; Fy, Fx and Fz are the ML, AP and vertical ground reaction forces, respectively; and dz is the distance between the surface of the force plate and its origin.

Instantaneous acceleration of the center of mass along the AP and ML axes was determined from the ground reaction force according to Newton's second law. Center of mass velocity and displacement were computed by successive numerical integrations of center of mass acceleration using integration constants equal to zero, i.e., initial velocity and displacement null (Brenière et al., 1987). The following instants were determined from biomechanical traces: gait initiation onset (t_0), swing heel off, swing toe off and swing foot contact. T_0 and foot contact were determined from force plate data, whereas heel off and toe off were determined from VICON data. Two t_0 times were estimated, one for the ML axis and one for the AP axis. The t_0 times corresponded to the instants when the ML or AP center of pressure trace deviated 2.5 standard deviations from its baseline value. Heel off and toe off corresponded to the instants when the vertical position of the swing heel marker and the anterior position of the swing toe marker increased by 3 mm from their position in the initial static posture. Foot contact corresponded to the instant when the ML and AP center of pressure traces shifted abruptly laterally towards the swing leg side, and forwardly, respectively (this abrupt shift occurred at the same instant in the two traces).

Mechanical Model

In the present study, the human body was modeled during the swing phase of gait initiation (from toe off to foot contact) as

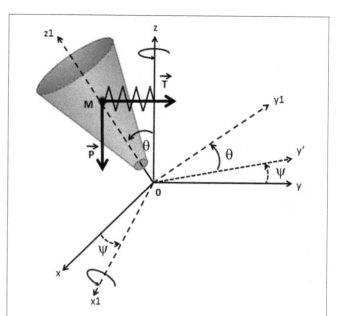

FIGURE 2 | Mechanical model. The mechanical model is represented as a conic inverted pendulum which pivots about a fixed point 0. Body displacement during the swing phase (from toe off to foot contact) presents five degrees of freedom on the absolute referential (0; x; y; z). (0; x_1; y_1; z_1) are the main axes of the inertia momentum of the solid body after precession ψ around z and nutation θ around x_1. The center of mass m falls under the influence of the gravity force P and the elastic restoring force T. The initial position and velocity of the cone correspond to the position and velocity of the subject's center of mass at toe off.

a single conic inverted pendulum which rotates about a fixed point 0 (**Figure 2**). This model was based on work carried out in earlier studies (Jian et al., 1993; MacKinnon and Winter, 1993; Lyon and Day, 1997, 2005). The displacement of this cone had five degrees of freedom on the absolute referential (0, x, y, z), i.e., three translations and two rotations. A new referential (0, x_1, y_1, z_1) was considered after precession ψ around z and nutation θ around x_1, in which the inertia momentum of the body was expressed with its eigenvalues (Winter et al., 1990). The proper rotation ψ around z_1 with respect to ψ and θ was neglected. During the swing phase, we considered that the center of mass was falling laterally under the influence of two forces: the gravity force $P = mg$ (where m is the mass of the solid, and g is the gravitational acceleration) and an elastic restoring force T that reflects active muscular control of the movement (Farley and Morgenroth, 1999; Morasso and Schieppati, 1999), with $T = k|yM|$ (where k is the stiffness of the hip abductor muscles acting on the stance leg side during the swing phase (Winter, 1995) and $|yM|$ is the absolute value of the ML center of mass shift, which was systematically oriented towards the swing leg side (positive values) during the swing phase). The initial position and velocity of the cone corresponded to the position and velocity of the subject's center of mass at toe off. The addition of a restoring force on the conic model was necessary in order to control the initial velocity at toe off. Without this supplementary force, the conic pendulum would fall towards the stance leg side in most trials.

The equation of motion in $(0, x_1, y_1, z_1)$ was:

$$OM \times \left(mg + k\,|yM|\right) = \frac{d\sigma_{/0}}{dt} \tag{3}$$

Where $OM = l_M\, z_1$, with l_M: distance of the center of mass along z_1, and $\sigma_{/0}$: angular momentum computed as $\sigma_{/0} = I_{/0}\,\Omega$, where $I_{/0}$ is the diagonal matrix of inertia along the main axes (x_1, y_1, z_1) and Ω is the total angular velocity:

$$\Omega = \dot{\theta}x_1 + \dot{\psi}\sin\theta\, y_1 + \dot{\psi}\cos\theta\, z_1 \tag{4}$$

Finally, the differential equations of angular movement were:

$$\ddot{\theta} = \frac{mgl_M\sin\theta + k\,|yM|\,l_M\sin\psi\cos\theta - \dot{\psi}^2\cos\theta\sin\theta\left(I_{oz_1} - I_{ox_1}\right)}{I_{ox_1}} \tag{5}$$

$$\ddot{\psi} = \frac{k\,|yM|\,l_M\cos\psi\sin\theta - 2\dot{\theta}\dot{\psi}\cos\theta\sin\theta\left(I_{ox_1} - I_{oz_1}\right)}{I_{ox_1}\sin^2\theta + I_{oz_1}\cos^2\theta} \tag{6}$$

The subsequent motion of the model's center of mass was predicted by solving numerically the differential equations of motion using a fourth order Runge-Kutta algorithm. The spherical coordinates numerically computed (l_M, θ, ψ) were then transformed into Cartesian coordinates (x, y, z) in order to compare experimental data with the model's theoretical data.

Dependant Variables

Experimental Variables

Gait initiation was divided into three phases: APAs (from t_0 to heel off), swing foot lift (from heel off to toe off) and swing phase (from toe off to foot contact, **Figure 3**). The duration of APAs along the ML and AP axes were computed separately, because the t_0 times for these two axes did not necessarily occur simultaneously (Caderby et al., 2014). The amplitude of APAs was characterized by the peaks of the backward and lateral center of pressure shift obtained during the APAs time window. Center of mass velocity and displacement along the ML and AP axes were quantified at toe off and foot contact. The ML and AP center of mass position in the initial upright static posture was estimated by averaging the center of pressure position during the 250 ms period preceding the "all set" or the "go" signal, depending on the temporal pressure condition (Yiou et al., 2016). Spatiotemporal features of the swing phase of gait initiation that were investigated included: swing phase duration, AP center of mass velocity at foot contact, step length, step width, and dynamic stability at foot contact. Step length corresponded to the distance covered by the heel marker of the swing leg from the initial posture to foot contact. In addition, the vertical distance between the obstacle and the swing heel and swing toe markers was measured at the time when these markers passed over the obstacle. For each trial in the obstacle condition, the shorter of these two vertical distances was reported; this corresponded to the "foot clearance". An adaptation of the "margin of stability" (MOS) introduced by

Hof et al. (2005) was used to quantify ML dynamic stability at foot contact (thereafter referred to as "stability"). The MOS corresponded to the difference between the ML boundary of the base of support (BOS$_{ymax}$) and the ML position of the "extrapolated center of mass" at swing foot contact (YcoM$_{FC}$). Thus:

$$MOS = BOS_{ymax} - YcoM_{FC} \tag{7}$$

Because kinematic data showed that participants first landed on the force plate with the swing heel or the swing toe, BOS$_{ymax}$ was estimated using the ML position of the swing heel or metatarsal marker at foot contact. The ML distance between the position of the swing foot marker at foot contact (heel or toe) and the position of the stance metatarsal marker at t_0 represented step width, and was representative of the size of the ML base of support. Based on the study by Hof et al. (2005) and the results from our previous studies (Caderby et al., 2014; Yiou et al., 2016), the ML position of the extrapolated center of mass at foot contact (YcoM$_{FC}$) was calculated as follows:

$$YcoM_{FC} = yM_{FC} + \frac{y'M_{FC}}{\omega_0} \tag{8}$$

where yM_{FC} and $y'M_{FC}$ are respectively the ML center of mass position and velocity at foot contact, and ω_0 is the eigen frequency of the body, modeled as an inverted pendulum and calculated as follows:

$$\omega_0 = \sqrt{\frac{g}{l}} \tag{9}$$

where $g = 9.81$ m/s^2 is the gravitational acceleration and l is the length of the inverted pendulum, which in this study correspond to 57.5% of body height (Winter et al., 1990).

ML dynamic stability at foot contact is preserved on the condition that YcoM$_{FC}$ is within BOS$_{ymax}$, which corresponds to a positive MOS. A negative MOS indicates a ML instability and implies that a corrective action (e.g., in the form of an additional lateral step) is required to maintain balance.

Theoretical Variables

In order to test the validity of the model, the theoretical ML position and velocity of the center of mass at foot contact were computed by implementing the model with the initial center of mass set (ML center of mass position and velocity at foot off) and the swing phase duration obtained in each of the experimental trials. This gave theoretical values which were then compared with the experimental ones. The ML APAs were found to be scaled with swing duration in the experimental conditions (see "Results" Section); thus, these theoretical values are referred to the "theoretical conditions with APAs scaling". The model was then used to assess whether postural stability at foot contact would be degraded if the ML APAs were not scaled to swing duration, i.e., if there was no adaptation of the initial center of mass set to the obstacle height and distance. For this purpose, the theoretical ML position and velocity of

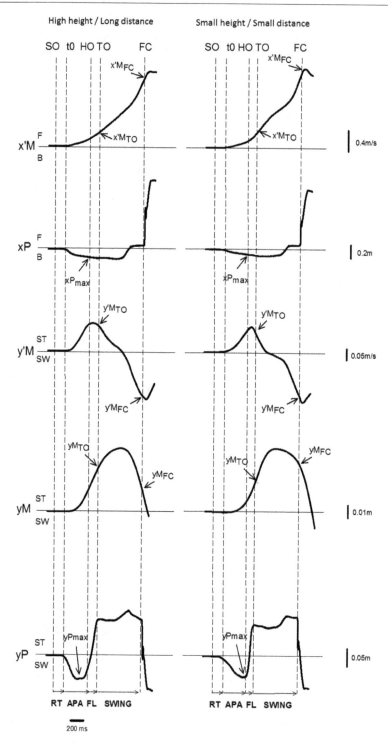

FIGURE 3 | Example of biomechanical traces and representation of the main experimental variables obtained for one representative subject initiating gait (one trial) in the reaction-time condition with the high height/long distance condition (left) and the small height/small distance condition (right). *Anteroposterior (AP) direction* x'M: center of mass (COM) velocity; x'M$_{TO}$, x'M$_{FC}$: COM velocity at foot off and at foot contact. xP: center of pressure (COP) displacement; xPmax: peak of COP displacement during APAs; F: forward; B: backward. *Mediolateral (ML) direction* y'M: ML COM velocity; y'M$_{TO}$, y'M$_{FC}$: COM velocity at foot off and foot contact; yM: ML COM displacement; yM$_{FC}$: COM displacement at foot contact; yP: ML COP displacement; yPmax: peak of COP displacement during APAs; and ST: stance limb; SW: swing limb. *Vertical dashed lines* SO: Go signal onset (in the reaction-time condition only); t$_0$ onset variation of biomechanical traces; HO: swing heel off; FO: swing foot off; FC: swing foot contact. *Horizontal arrows*: RT: time-windows for reaction-time; APA: anticipatory postural adjustments FL: foot lift; SWING: swing phase.

the center of mass at foot contact were again computed, but this time by implementing the model with: (i) the mean ML position and velocity of the center of mass at foot off obtained for each subject in the reaction-time and self-initiated obstacle-free (control) conditions; and (ii) the swing phase duration obtained in each experimental trial. The theoretical extrapolated center of mass position and the theoretical MOS at foot contact were then calculated by following the same procedure used for the experimental data. The theoretical values obtained with this procedure are referred to as the "theoretical conditions without APA scaling".

Statistics

Mean values and standard deviations were calculated for each variable in the experimental and theoretical conditions. The normality of data was checked using the Kolmogorov-Smirnov test and the homogeneity of variances was checked using the Bartlett test. To test the influence of obstacle height, obstacle distance and temporal pressure, a [3 ("obstacle height": 2.5%, 5% and 10% of the subject's height) × 3 ("obstacle distance": 10%, 20% and 30% of the subject's height) × 2 ("temporal pressure": reaction-time and self-initiated)] ANOVA with repeated measures was used on each experimental variable.

To test the validity of the model, a [3 ("obstacle height") × 3 ("obstacle distance") × 2 ("temporal pressure") × 2 ("modeling with APAs scaling": experimental conditions vs. theoretical conditions with APA scaling)] was used on the following variables: ML center of mass position and velocity, ML extrapolated center of mass, and MOS at foot contact. Linear correlations between these experimental and theoretical variables were calculated using Pearson's correlation coefficient. Finally, to test the effect of APA scaling on postural stability, a [3 ("obstacle height") × 3 ("obstacle distance") × 2 ("Modeling without APA scaling": experimental conditions vs. theoretical conditions with no APA scaling)] RM ANOVA was used on the following variables: ML center of mass position and velocity, ML extrapolated center of mass, and MOS at foot contact. The alpha level was set at 0.05. A Tukey *post hoc* test was used when necessary.

RESULTS

Description of the Biomechanical Traces in the Experimental Conditions

The time course of the biomechanical traces was globally similar in the different temporal and obstacle conditions. The traces obtained in two representative conditions are reported in **Figure 3**. Swing heel off was systematically preceded by postural dynamics that corresponded to APAs. During these APAs, the center of pressure displacement reached a peak value in a backward direction (see the negative variation of the xP trace in **Figure 3**) and towards the swing leg side (negative variation of the yP trace), while the center of mass velocity was directed forwards (positive variation of the x'M trace) and towards the stance leg side (positive variation of the y'M trace). The ML center of mass velocity trace reached a first peak value

towards the stance leg side at around heel off. This trace, then fell towards the swing leg side and a second peak value towards this side was reached a few milliseconds after foot contact. The ML center of mass shift trace was bell-shaped and reached a peak value toward the stance leg side at the beginning of the swing phase. The AP center of mass velocity increased progressively until it reached a peak value a few milliseconds after swing foot contact, while the center of mass was continuously shifted forward. Differences across the conditions are reported in the paragraphs below.

Stability
Height Effect
Stability can be evaluated from foot clearance and the MOS. The risk of the swing foot striking the obstacle, which might then endanger balance, increased as foot clearance decreased. The MOS is used to quantify ML dynamic stability at foot contact. The results showed that the foot clearance significantly decreased with obstacle height ($F_{(2,26)} = 9.25$, $p < 0.001$; **Figure 4**). In contrast, there was no significant effect of the obstacle height on the MOS value ($F_{(2,26)} = 2.57$, $p > 0.05$) and related center of mass components, i.e., the ML center of mass shift ($F_{(2,26)} = 0.31$, $p > 0.05$) and velocity ($F_{(2,26)} = 0.46$, $p > 0.05$), and extrapolated center of mass position at foot contact ($F_{(2,26)} = 1.95$, $p > 0.05$).

Distance Effect
The results showed that foot clearance also significantly decreased with obstacle distance ($F_{(2,26)} = 30.07$, $p < 0.001$; **Figure 4**). There was no effect of the obstacle distance on the MOS ($F_{(2,26)} = 0.01$, $p > 0.05$), the ML center of mass shift ($F_{(2,26)} = 0.99$, $p > 0.05$) and velocity ($F_{(2,26)} = 0.64$, $p > 0.05$), and the extrapolated center of mass position at foot contact ($F_{(2,26)} = 0.11, p > 0.05$).

Temporal Pressure Effect
There was no significant effect of the temporal pressure on the following variables: foot clearance ($F_{(1,13)} = 3.77$, $p > 0.05$), MOS value ($F_{(1,13)} = 0.96$, $p > 0.05$), ML center of mass shift ($F_{(1,13)} = 0.95$, $p > 0.05$) and velocity ($F_{(1,13)} = 0.55$, $p > 0.05$) and extrapolated center of mass position at foot contact ($F_{(1,13)} = 0.35, p > 0.05$).

Postural and Foot Lift Phase
Height Effect
The results showed that there was a significant effect of the obstacle height on the duration of APAs along the ML axis ($F_{(2,26)} = 5.63$, $p < 0.01$, **Figure 5**) and the AP axis ($F_{(2,26)} = 9.38$, $p < 0.001$), and on the duration of the foot-lift phase ($F_{(2,26)} = 6.18$, $p < 0.01$). Each of these temporal variables decreased when the obstacle height increased. With regard to the spatial variables, results showed that both the peak of anticipatory ML center of pressure shift ($F_{(2,26)} = 21.44$, $p < 0.001$) and the ML center of mass velocity at toe off ($F_{(2,26)} = 4.36$, $p < 0.05$) significantly increased with obstacle height. In contrast, the peak of anticipatory backward center

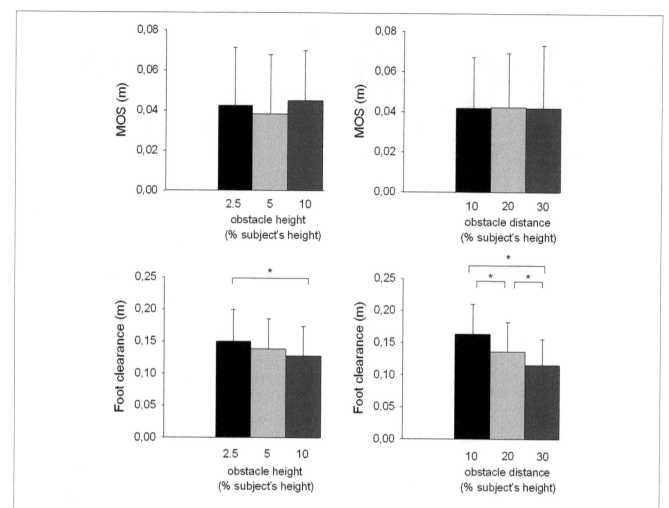

FIGURE 4 | Effects of obstacle height and distance on stability parameters. Reported are mean values (all participants together) ± 1 SD. MOS, margin of stability. *Indicates a significant difference between bars.

of pressure shift ($F_{(2,26)} = 11.43$, $p < 0.001$), the differential between the center of pressure and the center of mass position $F_{(2,26)} = 8.15$, $p < 0.01$) and the forward center of mass velocity at toe off ($F_{(2,26)} = 13.86$, $p < 0.001$) significantly decreased with obstacle height. The obstacle height constraint therefore had a similar effect on the temporal component of APAs along the AP and ML axes, but had an opposite effect on the spatial component of APAs along these two axes.

Distance Effect

Increasing the obstacle distance had a very different effect on the postural and foot lift phases compared with increasing the obstacle height. Indeed, the results showed that obstacle distance had no significant effect on the duration of APAs along the ML axis ($F_{(2,26)} = 1.44$, $p > 0.05$). However, it did have a significant effect on the APA duration along the AP axis ($F_{(2,26)} = 3.77$, $p < 0.05$) and on the duration of the foot lift ($F_{(2,26)} = 21.53$, $p < 0.001$). Specifically, these two variables increased with obstacle distance. The results further showed that there was no

significant effect of the obstacle distance on the following spatial variables: peak of anticipatory ML ($F_{(2,26)} = 0.62$, $p > 0.05$) and AP center of pressure shift ($F_{(2,26)} = 1.00$, $p > 0.05$), ML ($F_{(2,26)} = 1.78$, $p > 0.05$) and AP ($F_{(2,26)} = 2.18$, $p > 0.05$) center of mass shift at toe off, and ML center of mass velocity at toe off ($F_{(2,26)} = 1.30$, $p > 0.05$). In contrast, the forward center of mass velocity at toe off increased significantly with obstacle distance ($F_{(2,26)} = 30.51$, $p < 0.001$).

Temporal Pressure Effect

The results showed that the following temporal variables were significantly shorter in the reaction-time block than in the self-initiated block: duration of APAs along the AP axis ($F_{(1,13)} = 61.63$, $p < 0.001$) and ML axis ($F_{(1,13)} = 31.6$, $p < 0.001$), and duration of foot lift ($F_{(1,13)} = 16.99$, $p < 0.01$). The following spatial variables reached a significantly larger value in the reaction-time block than in the self-initiated block: peak of anticipatory ML ($F_{(1,13)} = 20.04$, $p < 0.001$) and AP ($F_{(1,13)} = 41.82$, $p < 0.001$) center of pressure shift, and ML center of mass velocity at foot off ($F_{(1,13)} = 11.60$,

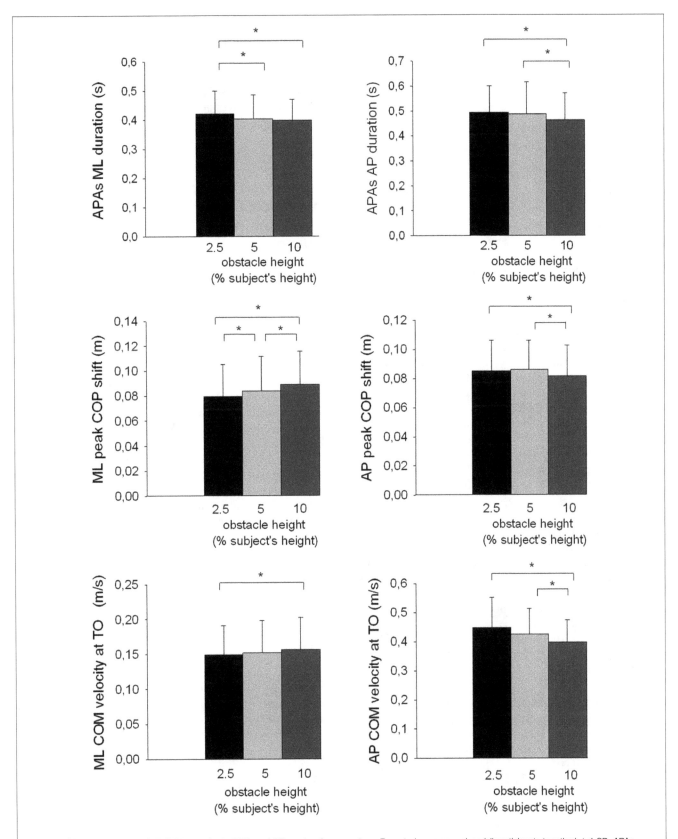

FIGURE 5 | Effects of obstacle height on selected ML and AP postural parameters. Reported are mean values (all participants together) ± 1 SD. APAs, anticipatory postural adjustments; TO, toe off; COP, center of pressure; COM, center of mass. *Indicates a significant difference between bars.

$p < 0.01$). In contrast, the ML ($F_{(1,13)} = 1.98$, $p > 0.05$) and AP ($F_{(1,13)} = 2.45$, $p > 0.05$) shift of the center of mass at foot off were not significantly different for the two temporal pressure blocks.

Swing Phase

Height Effect

The results showed that the duration of the swing phase significantly increased with obstacle height ($F_{(2,26)} = 58.07$, $p < 0.001$). In contrast, there was no significant effect of the obstacle height on the step length ($F_{(2,26)} = 2.77$, $p > 0.05$), step width ($F_{(2,26)} = 0.59$, $p > 0.05$) and motor performance (in terms of forward center of mass velocity at swing foot contact; $F_{(2,26)} = 0.74$, $p > 0.05$). Finally, the results showed that there was no change in swing foot strike patterns with changes to obstacle height; here, subjects landed on the force plate with the heel first in 85% of the trials.

Distance Effect

The results showed that there was no effect of the obstacle distance on the duration of the swing phase ($F_{(2,26)} = 2.57$, $p > 0.05$) and step width $F_{(2,26)} = 0.05$, $p > 0.05$). In contrast, there was a significant effect of the obstacle distance on the step length ($F_{(2,26)} = 23.05$, $p < 0.001$) and motor performance ($F_{(2,26)} = 6.72$, $p < 0.01$). Both variables increased with distance. Finally, the results showed that there was a significant effect of obstacle distance on the foot strike pattern, with the ratio of forefoot strike increasing with obstacle distance ($F_{(2,26)} = 7.37$, $p < 0.01$). This ratio increased from 6.7% for the small distance obstacle condition to 20.7% for the long distance obstacle condition.

Temporal Pressure Effect

The results showed that there was a significant effect of the temporal pressure on the duration of the swing phase ($F_{(1,13)} = 10.81$, $p < 0.01$). This duration was longer in the reaction-time block than in the self-initiated block. In contrast, there was no effect of the temporal pressure on the following variables: step length ($F_{(1,13)} = 0.58$, $p > 0.05$), step width ($F_{(1,13)} = 0.20$, $p > 0.05$), motor performance ($F_{(1,13)} = 0.04$, $p > 0.05$) and foot strike pattern (the mean percentage of the heel-strike pattern was 86%).

Validation of the Mechanical Model

A visual analysis of **Figure 6** illustrates the excellent fit between the experimental traces and those obtained with the mechanical model. The best fit between experimental (dashed line) and theoretical (full line) data was obtained for a stiffness of the hip abductor muscles of about 1000 N/m. This value corroborates with previous data in the literature (Morasso and Schieppati, 1999). This corresponds to a restoring force of approximately $T = 50$ N, applied at the center of mass. This close fit was further strengthened by the finding that there was no significant effect of the factor "modeling with APA scaling" on the MOS and on the related center of mass

components. In addition, there was no interaction between this factor and obstacle height, obstacle distance and temporal pressure for any of these variables. In contrast, there was a significant positive correlation between the theoretical data (obtained in the conditions with ML APA scaling) and the experimental data for the MOS ($r = 0.42$, $p < 0.05$), the ML center of mass position ($r = 0.94$, $p < 0.001$) and the ML center of mass velocity ($r = 0.72$, $p < 0.001$) at foot contact. Collectively, these results validate the mechanical model.

Comparison of Experimental Data and Theoretical Data Obtained in the Conditions Without Mediolateral APA Scaling

In the theoretical conditions without ML APA scaling, the same initial ML center of mass set used in the control condition (obstacle-free condition) was introduced into the conditions where an obstacle had to be cleared (see "Materials and Methods" Section). The results showed there was a significant effect of the factor "modeling without APA scaling" on the MOS ($F_{(2,26)} = 4.77$, $p < 0.05$) and with the exception of the ML center of mass position at foot contact ($F_{(2,26)} = 1.63$, $p > 0.05$), on each of the MOS-related center of mass components, i.e., peak of ML velocity ($F_{(2,26)} = 8.73$, $p < 0.001$) and extrapolated center of mass ($F_{(2,26)} = 4.84$, $p < 0.05$) at foot contact. Specifically, the mean MOS value was significantly lower in the theoretical conditions compared with the experimental conditions, and the extrapolated center of mass reached positions closer to the lateral boundary of the base of support. In addition, the peak of ML center of mass velocity at foot contact—which was directed towards the swing leg side—reached a greater value in the theoretical conditions than in the experimental conditions. Also, there was a "modeling without APA scaling" × "obstacle height" interaction on the MOS ($F_{(2,26)} = 4.77$, $p < 0.05$) and on each related variable. Most interestingly, the difference in the MOS value between the experimental and theoretical conditions without APA scaling increased progressively when the obstacle height increased (**Figure 7**). A negative MOS value was even reached for the middle height obstacle. Finally, the results showed that there was no significant "modeling without APA scaling" × "obstacle distance" interaction ($F_{(2,26)} = 0.22$, $p > 0.05$) or "modeling without APA scaling" × "temporal pressure" interaction ($F_{(2,26)} = 0.16$, $p > 0.05$). These results thus illustrate how postural stability can be expected to degrade in cases where ML APAs are not scaled according to swing duration.

DISCUSSION

The goal of the present study was to investigate how the CNS controls postural stability during gait initiation when negotiating obstacles of different heights and distances under low and high temporal pressure constraints. Based on a mechanical model of the body falling laterally under the

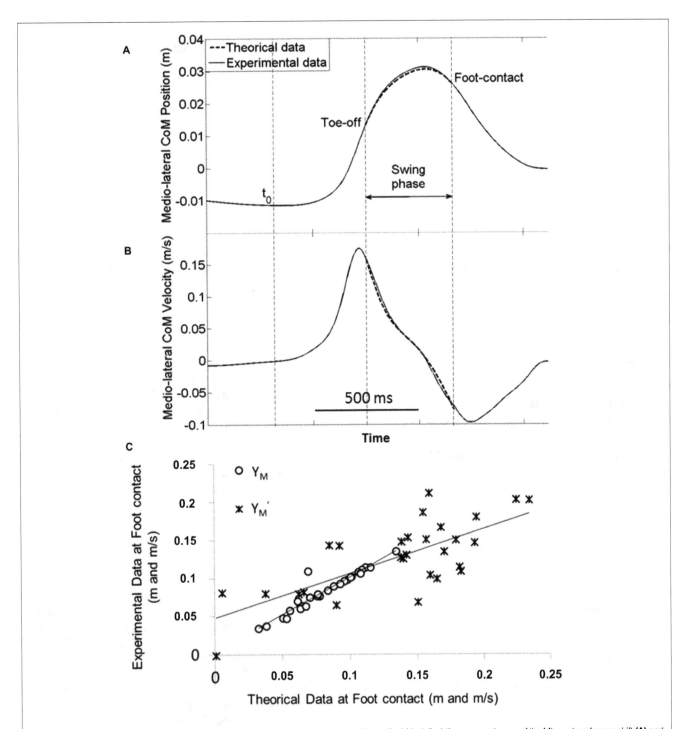

FIGURE 6 | Validation of the mechanical model. Typical experimental (full line) and theoretical (dash line) time-course traces of the ML center of mass shift **(A)** and velocity **(B)** are superimposed during the swing phase (from swing foot off to foot contact). Traces are obtained from one representative subject in the reaction-time condition with the medium height and short distance obstacle. **(C)** Example of linear regression between experimental vs. theoretical data obtained in the obstacle free (control) condition. Each point represents the average value of the ML center of mass position (Y_M) and velocity (Y'_M) at foot contact in the control conditions (self-initiated and reaction-time conditions pooled together) for each of the 14 subjects. Note the excellent fit between the experimental and theoretical data.

influence of gravity and submitted to an elastic restoring force, the functional link between the observed ML APA scaling and the maintenance of postural stability across the experimental conditions was first discussed. This was followed by a discussion of the way in which the AP and ML components of APAs need to be coordinated to ensure safe body progression. Globally, the results illustrate the capacity of the CNS to adapt coordination between the postural and focal

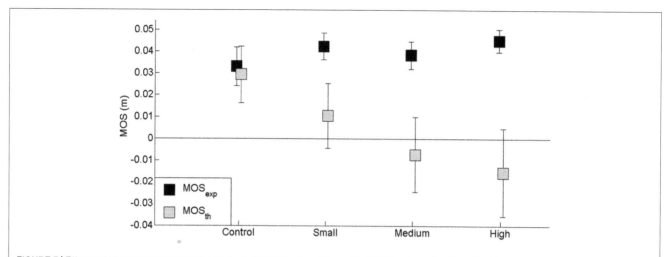

FIGURE 7 | Effects of obstacle height on the experimental (MOS_{exp}) and theoretical (MOS_{th}) "margin of stability" (MOS) values computed in the conditions with no APA scaling. The height of the obstacle is indicated in the abscissa (small, medium and high). In the control condition, there was no obstacle. Reported are mean values (all participants together) ± 1 SD. Note that the experimental MOS values remained unchanged, while theoretical MOS values decreased with obstacle height.

components of a motor task to meet various spatial and temporal constraints.

Scaling Mediolateral APAs to Swing Duration Allows the Maintenance of Postural Stability

As expected, increasing the obstacle height resulted in a significant increase in swing duration (Chou et al., 2001; Hahn and Chou, 2004), thereby mechanically increasing the potential for lateral imbalance during the swing phase of gait initiation. Indeed, previous studies have reported that the swing phase of gait initiation could be assimilated to a ML (Lyon and Day, 1997, 2005) and forward (Lepers and Brenière, 1995) ballistic center of mass fall around the stance ankle, with gravity being the main motor of action. Increasing the duration of this phase may therefore theoretically lead to a larger center of mass motion and velocity at the end of this ballistic phase, i.e., at foot contact. The original model of the whole body falling towards the swing leg side after swing foot off, which was developed in the present study, is in accordance with this statement. Indeed, when the initial center of mass set (i.e., center of mass shift and velocity at foot off) remained the same as in the obstacle-free condition, it was found that artificially increasing the swing phase duration directly impacted on the center of mass set at foot contact. As a consequence, postural stability at this instant was degraded, as revealed by a decrease in the theoretical MOS values. In contrast to this effect of obstacle height, increasing the obstacle distance did not result in any significant change in the swing phase duration. This is coherent with the finding that both step length and step velocity increased with obstacle distance. Thus, as expected, the theoretical center of mass set at foot contact and the related degree of postural stability remained unchanged when this distance increased.

Although the theoretical model revealed the potential for increased instability with obstacle height, the results obtained in the experimental conditions showed that there was no main effect of obstacle height on the center of mass set at foot contact and on the related level of stability. Similar findings were observed in recent studies (Chou et al., 2001; Hahn and Chou, 2004) that examined the clearance of obstacles of varying height during steady walking. This led the authors to suggest the existence of some forms of adaptive postural mechanisms, although these mechanisms were not described. The present results show that the anticipatory peak of ML center of pressure shift increased along with obstacle height. This increase is responsible for a subsequent increase in the ML center of mass velocity at toe off. As stated above, it is clear from the theoretical model that if such an increase in the initial center of mass set had not occurred when the obstacle height increased, a lower state of postural stability would have been reached at foot contact, as shown by the lower theoretical MOS values. Thus, in order to maintain an equivalent stability in the experimental conditions, the additive strategy would be needed to compensate for insufficient APAs, e.g., in the form of lateral stepping so as to increase the base of support width (Zettel et al., 2002; Caderby et al., 2014). If this is still insufficient, because not enough time is available to position the swing foot laterally, a strategy of lateral leg crossover stepping, linked with a high risk of lateral falling (Patton et al., 2006), may be necessary to recover balance. Our results thus show that the CNS precisely scales the ML APAs to the duration of the swing phase, so as to maintain an equivalent postural stability at foot contact across the experimental conditions. The finding that obstacle distance had no influence on ML APAs parameters and the related initial center of mass set (in contrast with obstacle height) is in line with this statement, because swing duration did not vary with this obstacle feature.

The present findings are in accordance with the notion that postural stability at the end of a voluntary leg movement is a major parameter taken into account during the programming of APAs (Do et al., 1991; Nouillot et al., 2000). Do et al. (1991) used a lower limb flexion-extension executed as fast as possible to test the influence of final stability on APAs. The initial body posture was bipedal, while the final one was either bipedal (stable posture) or unipedal (unstable posture). The biomechanical and electromyographic data showed that ML APAs were larger when the final posture was unstable, because of the need to propel the center of mass further (i.e., above the stance foot) to maintain stability in the final posture. Similarly, the amplitude of the ML APAs in the present study increased along with the potential for instability at foot contact, which corresponded to the end of the gait initiation process. In contrast to the study by Do et al. (1991), the potential for increased instability at the end of gait initiation was masked in our study, because the MOS remained the same across the experimental conditions. A similar remark can be made with regard to previous studies which focused on the effect of various environmental (Chou et al., 2001; Hahn and Chou, 2004; Yiou et al., 2011, 2016) or temporal constraints (Yiou et al., 2012b; Hussein et al., 2013; Caderby et al., 2014) on the control of ML stability during dynamic tasks (e.g., leg flexion, gait initiation and steady walking). In the present study, this potential for instability was revealed in the theoretical trials, where it was found that without APA scaling the MOS values decreased when obstacle height was increased. The present results thus demonstrate the imperative need to adequately scale the ML APAs features to the swing phase duration in order to maintain an optimal stability. Moreover, the invariance of the MOS value across the experimental conditions, despite the presence of potential instability, adds to the growing evidence that this parameter may function as a balance control parameter, as previously suggested in the literature (e.g., Yiou et al., 2011, 2012b; Caderby et al., 2014; Nakano et al., 2016).

This invariance implies that the CNS is able to precisely predict the potential instability elicited by obstacle clearance and that it scales the spatiotemporal parameters of the ML APAs accordingly. The results of this study are thus in accordance with the view that in programming APAs, the CNS uses internal models that takes into account the dynamic consequences of an expected perturbation and generates responses to counter their effect (e.g., Flanagan and Wing, 1997; Wing et al., 1997). More specifically, internal models would be used to predict the effect of the gravitational forces acting on the whole-body during obstacle clearance. This prediction would serve to program, adaptive APAs so as to maintain unchanged stability despite the variations in obstacle constraints. The notion that internal models integrate external forces (such as gravity or Coriolis forces) acting on body segments to plan and execute movements, has been classically proposed for various voluntary upper limb movements, such as grip force with load during object manipulation (e.g., Johansson and Cole, 1992; Flanagan and Wing, 1997; Kawato, 1999; Wolpert and Flanagan, 2001), arm movement in the vertical plane (e.g., Papaxanthis et al., 2005; Gaveau and Papaxanthis, 2011), arm reaching (Cohn et al., 2000) etc. The results of the current study further suggest that such internal models of gravity may also be used to plan and execute the postural component of a whole body motor task.

Coordination Between Mediolateral and Anteroposterior Components of APAs Allows Safe Body Progression

Surprisingly, the results also showed that the duration of both the ML APAs and the foot lift phase decreased with obstacle height. Less time was therefore allocated by participants to propelling the center of mass laterally before triggering the ballistic phase of gait initiation. This reduction in time may seem at odds with the need to increase the ML center of mass set at foot off, as argued above. We propose that it is linked to the spatial constraints exerted on the progression velocity in the AP direction. It can indeed reasonably be speculated that delaying the time of swing foot off in the presence of a high obstacle would increase the forward fall of the center of mass (allowing participants to get closer to the obstacle), as well as the amplitude of the forward center of mass velocity at foot off (Lepers and Brenière, 1995). By so doing, less time would then be allocated for clearing the obstacle with the trailing leg during the following swing phase, with a consequent increased risk of tripping over the obstacle. Instead, the results showed that the forward center of mass shift and velocity at foot off both decreased with obstacle height, which might be a combined effect of this shortened delay for swing foot off with the reduced amplitude of the anticipatory backward center of pressure shift. The amplitude of AP and ML APAs were thus both scaled according to swing duration but in an opposite way. Note that a similar strategy for AP APAs attenuation has already been reported in a study that compared stepping over an obstacle in reaction to rapid surface translation with stepping when there is no obstacle to be cleared (Zettel et al., 2002). The reduction in time taken to lift the swing foot might reflect a protective strategy directed to clear the obstacle safely by reducing the chances of contact between the trailing leg and the obstacle. It is however noteworthy that the vertical distance between the swing foot and the top of the obstacle at the time of obstacle clearance (i.e., the "foot clearance") decreased with obstacle height. In our trials, we did not observe any obstacle contact; thus, we believe that the obstacle (height and distance) and the velocity constraints of the present study were not putting young, healthy participants at risk of forward tripping.

Given the precise scaling of the initial ML center of mass set required to maintain stability across the obstacle conditions (see **Figure 7**), the present findings suggest that the CNS must necessarily have taken into account the reduction in time allocated to lift the swing foot to program the ML APAs' amplitude. Part of the observed increase in the peak of anticipatory ML center of pressure shift may therefore serve to compensate for this shortened duration so that an adequate initial ML center of mass set can be reached to maintain stability. In other words, it is likely that constraints imposed on the progression direction (which are likely responsible for the reduction in time allocated for swing toe off, as argued above) were integrated into the programming of APAs in the ML direction. This statement adds to the growing evidence that the CNS exerts a global control over the anticipatory postural dynamics in the horizontal plane (Caderby et al., 2014) rather than an independent control of APAs along the AP and ML axes and on the associated postural function (forward body progression and ML stability, respectively). This coordination between the ML and AP components of APAs thus seems to be an imperative condition for both safely clearing the obstacle and reaching a stable state at foot contact. Thus, in addition to the need to coordinate each postural component of the task (the AP and the ML postural components) with the focal one, the CNS also needs to coordinate the postural components between them so that participants can safely clear the obstacle.

Temporal Pressure-Induced Adaptive Changes of Mediolateral and Anteroposterior APAs

Compensation for a reduced ML APAs duration by an increase in the ML APAs amplitude was found in the present study when comparing the high and low temporal pressure conditions. Specifically, the duration of APAs in the high pressure condition was shorter and the peaks of anticipatory ML and AP center of pressure shift were larger than in the low pressure condition. A similar effect of temporal pressure was previously reported in the literature for various stepping tasks such as gait initiation with or without an obstacle to clear (Yiou et al., 2016), or rapid leg flexion (Yiou et al., 2012b; Hussein et al., 2013). It is presumed that these changes in the spatiotemporal APAs parameters under high temporal pressure reflect a strategy to hasten the onset of the voluntary movement (swing foot off) so as to meet the instruction to initiate the step as soon as possible after the GO signal, while maintaining the same stability and progression velocity. Obstacle height and temporal pressure, thus induced similar adaptive changes in the ML APAs parameters. This similitude could be explained by the fact that increasing the obstacle height and the temporal pressure level both required an earlier swing foot off and induced a longer swing phase duration. For this reason, combining these two constraints in one single condition (i.e., clearing a high obstacle within a high temporal pressure) may have been particularly challenging for the postural control system. The fact that postural stability was maintained in such a challenging condition further reveals the adaptability of this system.

The present results may be discussed in regards to recent studies which focused on the effect of temporal pressure on ML stability during ongoing walking with the goal to cross an obstacle (e.g., Moraes et al., 2007; Nakano et al., 2015, 2016). In these studies, participants avoided a virtual planar obstacle that could suddenly appear one step before the obstacle crossing, thus inducing a temporal pressure. In the condition without temporal pressure (control condition), the obstacle could be seen by participants when they stood in their initial posture. Under temporal pressure, the authors found that the extrapolated center of mass position at the swing foot contact was located further toward the swing leg side as compared to the control condition. The MOS however, remained unchanged because of a greater lateral step placement. In the present study, no such effect of temporal pressure on the actual and extrapolated center of mass position or on foot placement was observed. The MOS and the related center of mass components remained, however the

same as in the low temporal pressure condition. This invariance was due to the above reported changes in APAs parameters with temporal pressure. These discrepancies between the present study and the literature might possibly be ascribed to the time allocated to plan an efficient anticipatory strategy to maintain postural stability. In the present study, participants could indeed visually catch the features of the obstacle largely before the imperative "go" signal in the high pressure condition. In other words, they had plenty of time to predict the postural disturbance associated with the forthcoming task, and they could thus plan the APAs parameters accordingly. In line, MacKinnon et al. (2007) reported that the spatiotemporal features of APAs for gait initiation were progressively assembled before the deliverance of the "go" signal. In contrast, in the above reported studies, the obstacle appeared just one step before it had to be cleared. Participants had therefore much less time than in the present study to plan in advance the level of anticipatory postural dynamics required to maintain stability at foot-contact. Such a situation may potentially be detrimental to stability since it is known that vision is used in a feedforward rather than in on-line mode to regulate obstacle clearance during ongoing locomotion (Patla and Vickers, 1997). To maintain stability, participants in these studies thus needed to use an additive strategy of lateral foot placement to maintain stability. Future studies will investigate this hypothesis by enabling participants to catch the obstacle features with various delays before and after the deliverance of the "go" signal.

CONCLUSION

The results of this study show that the CNS is able to scale and coordinate the ML and AP components of APAs according to obstacle constraints and related variations in swing duration. This capacity allows participants to safely clear the obstacle and maintain optimal postural stability. These results were strengthened by the findings obtained with the mechanical model, which revealed how stability would be degraded if the ML APAs were not scaled to swing duration. These findings imply that the CNS is able to precisely predict the potential instability elicited by obstacle clearance and that it scales the spatiotemporal parameters of APAs according to this prediction. The results offer a better understanding of how the body adapts to environmental constraints in order to ensure safe and efficient whole-body progression. In a future study, we will investigate the strategies of young, healthy adults and compare them with those adopted by older adults (fallers and non-fallers) in the maintenance of stability in a similarly complex environment.

AUTHOR CONTRIBUTIONS

EY, RA, CT, OL, PF: designed the study; collected, analyzed and interpreted the data; drafted and revised the manuscript; gave final approval.

FUNDING

This research was funded by the French Government.

REFERENCES

Brenière, Y., Do, M. C., and Bouisset, S. (1987). Are dynamic phenomena prior to stepping essential to walking? *J. Mot. Behav.* 19, 62–76. doi: 10.1080/00222895.1987.10735400

Brunt, D., Liu, S. M., Trimble, M., Bauer, J., and Short, M. (1999). Principles underlying the organization of movement initiation from quiet stance. *Gait Posture* 10, 121–128. doi: 10.1016/s0966-6362(99)00020-x

Caderby, T., Yiou, E., Peyrot, N., Begon, M., and Dalleau, G. (2014). Influence of gait speed on the control of mediolateral dynamic stability during gait initiation. *J. Biomech.* 47, 417–423. doi: 10.1016/j.jbiomech.2013.11.011

Chou, L., Kaufman, K. R., Brey, R. H., and Draganich, L. F. (2001). Motion of the whole body's center of mass when stepping over obstacles of different heights. *Gait Posture* 13, 17–26. doi: 10.1016/s0966-6362(00)00087-4

Cohn, J. V., DiZio, P., and Lackner, J. R. (2000). Reaching during virtual rotation: context specific compensations for expected coriolis forces. *J. Neurophysiol.* 83, 3230–3240.

Do, M. C., Nouillot, P., and Bouisset, S. (1991). Is balance or posture at the end of a voluntary movement programmed? *Neurosci. Lett.* 130, 9–11. doi: 10.1016/0304-3940(91)90215-f

Farley, C. T., and Morgenroth, D. C. (1999). Leg stiffness primarily depends on ankle stiffness during human hopping. *J. Biomech.* 32, 267–273. doi: 10.1016/s0021-9290(98)00170-5

Flanagan, J. R., and Wing, A. M. (1997). The role of internal models in motion planning and control: evidence from grip force adjustments during movements of hand-held loads. *J. Neurosci.* 17, 1519–1528.

Gaveau, J., and Papaxanthis, C. (2011). The temporal structure of vertical arm movements. *PLoS One* 6:e22045. doi: 10.1371/journal.pone.0022045

Hahn, M. E., and Chou, L. (2004). Age-related reduction in sagittal plane center of mass motion during obstacle crossing. *J. Biomech.* 37, 837–844. doi: 10.1016/j.jbiomech.2003.11.010

Hof, A., Gazendam, M., and Sinke, W. (2005). The condition for dynamic stability. *J. Biomech.* 38, 1–8. doi: 10.1016/j.jbiomech.2004.03.025

Hussein, T., Yiou, E., and Larue, J. (2013). Age-related differences in motor coordination during simultaneous leg flexion and finger extension: influence of temporal pressure. *PLoS One* 8:e83064. doi: 10.1371/journal.pone.0083064

Jian, Y., Winter, D., Ishac, M., and Gilchrist, L. (1993). Trajectory of the body COG and COP during initiation and termination of gait. *Gait Posture* 1, 9–22. doi: 10.1016/0966-6362(93)90038-3

Johansson, R. S., and Cole, K. J. (1992). Sensory-motor coordination during grasping and manipulative actions. *Curr. Opin. Neurobiol.* 2, 815–823. doi: 10.1016/0959-4388(92)90139-c

Kawato, M. (1999). Internal models for motor control and trajectory planning. *Curr. Opin. Neurobiol.* 9, 718–727. doi: 10.1016/s0959-4388(99)00028-8

Lepers, R., and Brenière, Y. (1995). The role of anticipatory postural adjustments and gravity in gait initiation. *Exp. Brain Res.* 107, 118–124. doi: 10.1007/bf00228023

Lyon, I. N., and Day, B. L. (1997). Control of frontal plane body motion in human stepping. *Exp. Brain Res.* 115, 345–356. doi: 10.1007/pl00005703

Lyon, I. N., and Day, B. L. (2005). Predictive control of body mass trajectory in a two-step sequence. *Exp. Brain Res.* 161, 193–200. doi: 10.1007/s00221-004-2058-z

MacKinnon, C. D., Bissig, D., Chiusano, J., Miller, E., Rudnick, L., Jager, C., et al. (2007). Preparation of anticipatory postural adjustments prior to stepping. *J. Neurophysiol.* 97, 4368–4379. doi: 10.1152/jn.01136.2006

MacKinnon, C. D., and Winter, D. A. (1993). Control of whole body balance in the frontal plane during human walking. *J. Biomech.* 26, 633–644. doi: 10.1016/0021-9290(93)90027-c

Marigold, D. S., Weerdesteyn, V., Patla, A. E., and Duysens, J. (2007). Keep looking ahead? Re-direction of visual fixation does not always occur during an unpredictable obstacle avoidance task. *Exp. Brain Res.* 176, 32–42. doi: 10.1007/s00221-006-0598-0

McIlroy, W. E., and Maki, B. E. (1999). The control of lateral stability during rapid stepping reactions evoked by antero-posterior perturbation: does anticipatory control play a role? *Gait Posture* 9, 190–198. doi: 10.1016/s0966-6362(99)00013-2

Michel, V., and Chong, R. (2004). The strategies to regulate and to modulate the propulsive forces during gait initiation in lower limb amputees. *Exp. Brain Res.* 158, 356–365. doi: 10.1007/s00221-004-1908-z

Mickelborough, J., Linden, M. V., Richards, J., and Ennos, A. (2000). Validity and reliability of a kinematic protocol for determining foot contact events. *Gait Posture* 11, 32–37. doi: 10.1016/s0966-6362(99)00050-8

Mille, M. L., Creath, R. A., Prettyman, M. G., Johnson Hilliard, M., Martinez, K. M., Mackinnon, C. D., et al. (2012). Posture and locomotion coupling: a target for rehabilitation interventions in persons with Parkinson's disease. *Parkinsons Dis.* 2012:754186. doi: 10.1155/2012/754186

Mohagheghi, A. A., Moraes, R., and Patla, A. E. (2004). The effects of distant and on-line visual information on the control of approach phase and step over an obstacle during locomotion. *Exp. Brain Res.* 155, 459–468. doi: 10.1007/s00221-003-1751-7

Moraes, R., Allard, F., and Patla, A. E. (2007). Validating determinants for an alternate foot placement selection algorithm during human locomotion in cluttered terrain. *J. Neurophysiol.* 98, 1928–1940. doi: 10.1152/jn.00044.2006

Morasso, P. G., and Schieppati, M. (1999). Can muscle stiffness alone stabilize upright standing? *J. Neurophysiol.* 82, 1622–1626.

Nakano, W., Fukaya, T., Kanai, Y., Akizuki, K., and Ohashi, Y. (2015). Effects of temporal constraints on medio-lateral stability when negotiating obstacles. *Gait Posture* 42, 158–164. doi: 10.1016/j.gaitpost.2015.05.004

Nakano, W., Fukaya, T., Kobayashi, S., and Ohashi, Y. (2016). Age effects on the control of dynamic balance during step adjustments under temporal constraints. *Hum. Mov. Sci.* 47, 29–37. doi: 10.1016/j.humov.2016.01.015

Nouillot, P., Do, M. C., and Bouisset, S. (2000). Are there anticipatory segmental adjustments associated with lower limb flexions when balance is poor in humans? *Neurosci. Lett.* 279, 77–80. doi: 10.1016/s0304-3940(99)00947-7

Papaxanthis, C., Pozzo, T., and McIntyre, J. (2005). Kinematic and dynamic processes for the control of pointing movements in humans revealed by short-term exposure to microgravity. *Neuroscience* 135, 371–383. doi: 10.1016/j.neuroscience.2005.06.063

Patla, A. E., and Greig, M. (2006). Any way you look at it, successful obstacle negotiation needs visually guided on-line foot placement regulation during the approach phase. *Neurosci. Lett.* 397, 110–114. doi: 10.1016/j.neulet.2005.12.016

Patla, A. E., and Vickers, J. N. (1997). Where and when do we look as we approach and step over an obstacle in the travel path? *Neuroreport* 8, 3661–3665. doi: 10.1097/00001756-199712010-00002

Patton, J. L., Hilliard, M. J., Martinez, K., Mille, M., and Rogers, M. W. (2006). A simple model of stability limits applied to sidestepping in young, elderly and elderly fallers. *Conf. Proc. IEEE Eng. Med. Biol. Soc.* 1, 3305–3308. doi: 10.1109/iembs.2006.260199

Robinovitch, S. N., Feldman, F., Yang, Y., Schonnop, R., Leung, P. M., Sarraf, T., et al. (2013). Video capture of the circumstances of falls in elderly people residing in long-term care: an observational study. *Lancet* 381, 47–54. doi: 10.1016/j.jemermed.2013.03.011

Wing, A. M., Flanagan, J. R., and Richardson, J. (1997). Anticipatory postural adjustments in stance and grip. *Exp. Brain Res.* 116, 122–130. doi: 10.1007/pl00005732

Winter, D. (1995). Human balance and posture control during standing and walking. *Gait Posture* 3, 193–214. doi: 10.1016/0966-6362(96)82849-9

Winter, D. A., Patla, A. E., and Frank, J. S. (1990). Assessment of balance control in humans. *Med. Prog. Technol.* 16, 31–51.

Wolpert, D. M., and Flanagan, J. R. (2001). Motor prediction. *Curr. Biol.* 11, R729–R732. doi: 10.1016/S0960-9822(01)00432-8

Yiou, E., Caderby, T., and Hussein, T. (2012a). Adaptability of anticipatory postural adjustments associated with voluntary movement. *World J. Orthop.* 3, 75–86. doi: 10.5312/wjo.v3.i6.75

Yiou, E., Hussein, T., and Larue, J. (2012b). Influence of temporal pressure on anticipatory postural control of medio-lateral stability during rapid leg flexion. *Gait Posture* 35, 494–499. doi: 10.1016/j.gaitpost.2011.11.015

Yiou, E., Deroche, T., Do, M. C., and Woodman, T. (2011). Influence of fear of falling on anticipatory postural control of medio-lateral stability during rapid leg flexion. *Eur. J. Appl. Physiol.* 111, 611–620. doi: 10.1007/s00421-010-1680-7

Yiou, E., Fourcade, P., Artico, R., and Caderby, T. (2016). Influence of temporal pressure constraint on the biomechanical organization of gait initiation made with or without an obstacle to clear. *Exp. Brain Res.* 234, 1363–1375. doi: 10.1007/s00221-015-4319-4

Zettel, J. L., Mcilroy, W. E., and Maki, B. E. (2002). Environmental constraints on foot trajectory reveal the capacity for modulation of anticipatory postural adjustments during rapid triggered stepping reactions. *Exp. Brain Res.* 146, 38–47. doi: 10.1007/s00221-002-1150-5

6

Higher Precision in Pointing Movements of the Preferred vs. Non-Preferred Hand is Associated with an Earlier Occurrence of Anticipatory Postural Adjustments

Carlo Bruttini, Roberto Esposti, Francesco Bolzoni and Paolo Cavallari*

Human Motor Control and Posture Laboratory, Human Physiology Section of the DePT, Università degli Studi di Milano, Milan, Italy

Correspondence:
Paolo Cavallari
paolo.cavallari@unimi.it

It is a common experience to exhibit a greater dexterity when performing a pointing movement with the preferred limb (PREF) vs. the non-preferred (NON-PREF) one. Here we provide evidence that the higher precision in pointing movements of the PREF vs. NON-PREF hand is associated with an earlier occurrence of the anticipatory postural adjustments (APAs). In this aim, we compared the APAs which stabilize the left or the right arm when performing a pen-pointing movement (prime mover flexor carpi radialis (FCR)). Moreover, we analyzed the elbow and wrist kinematics as well as the precision of the pointing movement. The mean kinematics of wrist movement and its latency, with respect to prime mover recruitment, were similar in the two sides, while APAs in triceps brachii (TB), biceps brachii (BB) and anterior deltoid (AD) were more anticipated when movements were performed with the PREF than with the NON-PREF hand (60–70 vs. 20–30 ms). APAs amplitudes were comparable in the muscles of the two sides. Earlier APAs in the preferred limb were associated with a better fixation of the elbow, which showed a lower excursion, and with a less scattered pointing error (PREF: 10.1 ± 0.8 mm; NON-PREF: 16.3 ± 1.7). Present results suggest that, by securing the more proximal joints dynamics, an appropriate timing of the intra-limb APAs is necessary for refining the voluntary movement precision, which is known to be scarce on the NON-PREF side.

Keywords: motor control, posture, APAs, handedness, precision, human

INTRODUCTION

Anticipatory postural adjustments (APAs) are commonly defined as unconscious muscular activities aimed to counterbalance the perturbation caused by the primary movement. In this respect, they have been shown to ensure whole-body balance (Massion, 1992; Bouisset and Do, 2008) and to stabilize body segments (Patla et al., 2002). They are also involved in initiating the displacement of the body center of mass when starting gait (Brenière et al., 1987) and forward reaching (Stapley et al., 1998, 1999). The APAs originate from a feed-forward command (Belen'kiĭ et al., 1967; Aruin and Latash, 1995), tailored on several kinematical aspects of the primary movement. Within a few trials, the central nervous system (CNS) is able to adapt APAs to changes in the desired movement speed (Shiratori and Aruin, 2007; Esposti et al., 2015), amplitude of motor action (Aruin and Shiratori, 2004) and the expected mass of the moving segment (Friedli et al., 1984; Toussaint et al., 1998). APAs have been first illustrated in movements that involve a relatively large mass, such as a shoulder flexion, that would produce a backward displacement of the center of mass projection on the ground (Bouisset and Zattara, 1987). Such perturbation may lead to the loss of the whole body equilibrium (Hess, 1943; Bouisset and Zattara, 1987); therefore, in order to counteract it, the recruitment of the prime mover muscles is normally preceded by *inter-limb APAs* in lower limbs, hips and trunk, which in turn induce a forward displacement of the center of mass, preventing falling.

More recently, Aoki (1991) reported that a pattern of postural activity in arm muscles also precedes voluntary wrist movements (*intra-limb APAs*), and that this pattern is related to the movement direction in space, just as similar to the inter-limb APAs described above. In this path, Caronni and Cavallari (2009) reported that also when voluntarily flexing a single segment of tiny mass, such as the index-finger, an intra-limb APA chain develops in several upper-limb muscles, to stabilize the *segmental* equilibrium of the whole arm. Similarly to the APAs preceding wrist flexion, the APA pattern associated to a finger flexion changes according to the direction of the focal movement. Indeed, with the prone hand, both wrist and index-finger flexions are preceded by an excitatory burst in triceps brachii (TB), while biceps brachii (BB) and anterior deltoid (AD) show a concomitant inhibition. Instead, with the hand supine, the opposite occurs: BB and AD show excitatory APAs, while TB undergoes a concomitant inhibition. From these last data, an additional role of APAs may be envisaged: besides maintaining the whole-body equilibrium, it seems that APAs may be important in refining voluntary movement precision. In fact, according to the results obtained in a four-joint software mechanical model and confirmed by an electrical stimulation of the median nerve, Caronni and Cavallari (2009) suggested that intra-limb APAs not only guarantee the maintenance of the arm posture, but may be also very important in controlling the trajectory and the final position of the moving segment. However, up to now, no direct evidence of such a conclusion has been reached when dispatching a voluntary motor command.

To shed further light on the relationship between APAs and movement precision, we studied pointing movements performed by flexing the wrist while holding a digitizer pen, so as to ascertain whether the well known imprecision of the non-preferred (NON-PREF) vs. preferred (PREF) arm (Woodworth, 1899) leading to smaller pointing errors with the PREF limb (Roy et al., 1994; Ypsilanti et al., 2009), may be correlated to a worse control of APAs. Considering that APAs are scaled according to the mass of the moving segment and given that the two hands have a similar mass, it would be surprising to observe differently structured APAs accompanying similar movements of the two sides. On the other hand, a different APAs programming between the two sides, e.g., in timing and/or amplitude, would demonstrate that APAs are essential in refining movement precision.

MATERIALS AND METHODS

Experiments were carried out in 13 adult healthy volunteers (4 females); mean age 31.7 ± 9.4 years. All subjects were right-handed, as confirmed by their scores on the 10-item version of the Edinburgh Handedness Inventory (Oldfield, 1971). The procedure was conducted in accordance to the Declaration of Helsinki. All subjects provided written informed consent; none of them had any history of orthopedic or neurological diseases. No ethical approval was required because the experimental procedure was non-invasive, did not require any drug administration and was carried out on healthy volunteers.

Experimental Procedure

Subjects sat on a chair with both arms along the body, elbows flexed at 90°, the wrists prone and in axis with the forearm. The moving wrist was kept unsupported and slightly extended, with the dorsum of the first metacarpo-phalangeal joint in contact with a proximity switch (CJ10–30GK-E2, Pepperl+Fuchs®, Mannheim, Germany). Subjects were explicitly asked to keep their back supported, the arm/forearm still and to look at the target during the experiment, to be aware of their movement performance. Subjects were asked to hold a digitizer pen with the most natural pinch grip and to briskly flex their wrist so as to point to the target with the pen tip as quick and precise as possible (pen-pointing). The target consisted in two orthogonal lines drawn on a white paper, taped on the pen tablet (Intuos Pen and Touch small, Wacom®, Saitama, Japan; active tablet area 152 × 95 mm; pen weight 12.5 g). The lines were 1 mm thick × 2 cm long, so that the target center was clearly visible. The chair was height adjustable, while the proximity switch and the pen tablet were screwed on articulated arms (Manfrotto 143 MAGIC ARM® + 035 Superclamp Kit, Manfrotto®, Cassola, Italy), so as to adapt to the different body dimensions of the subjects. In the initial position, the pen tip was held approximately 6–7 cm above the cross.

Each pen-pointing movement was self-paced and performed after an acoustic signal. The time between the beep and the movement onset varied according to the subject will; this procedure was adopted to exclude any reaction time.

In each experiment, two sessions of 60 pen-pointing movements were performed, one with each hand (PREF vs. NON-PREF); each session was divided into four sequences of 15 movement trials. The 15 trials were accomplished in a temporal window of about 2 min, and then the subject had time to rest (about 3 min) before undergoing a new sequence. Subjects never complained about fatigue.

At the end of each session, the EMGs of the BB, TB and AD muscles of each side were separately evaluated during a maximal press against a fixed support, which changed according to the tested muscle. The upper limb was kept in the same posture adopted during the pen-pointing experiments, so as not to alter the positioning of the recording electrodes with respect to the muscles. Subjects were thus asked to push as hard as possible upon a fixation point and maintain the push for 5 s. When testing the AD, the fixation point was positioned in front of the arm, at the level of the cubital fossa, and subjects had to push forward against it by trying to flex the arm at the shoulder. When testing the TB, the fixation point was positioned under the wrist and subjects had to push downward against it by trying to extend the forearm at the elbow. When testing the BB, the fixation point was positioned over the wrist and subjects had to push upward against it by trying to flex the forearm at the elbow.

Movement and EMG Recordings

The onset of the wrist flexion was monitored by the proximity switch. Flexion-extension of wrist and elbow joints was recorded by strain-gauge goniometers (mod. SG65 and SG110 respectively, Biometrics Ltd®, Newport, UK) taped to the skin over the respective joint. Angular displacements were DC amplified (P122, Grass Technologies®, West Warwick, RI, USA), A/D converted at 2 KHz with 12 bit resolution (PCI-6024E, National Instruments®, Austin, TX, USA) and stored. Goniometer calibration was undertaken before each experimental session.

Pairs of pre-gelled surface electrodes, 24 mm apart, (H124SG, Kendall ARBO, Tyco Healthcare, Neustadt/Donau, Germany) were used to record the EMG signal from the prime mover flexor carpi radialis (FCR) and from some of the ipsilateral postural muscles: BB, TB and AD. A good selectivity of the EMG recordings was achieved both by a careful positioning of the electrodes over the skin covering the muscle belly and by checking that the activity from the recorded muscle, during its phasic contraction, was not contaminated by signals from other sources. EMG was AC amplified (IP511, Grass Technologies®, West Warwick, RI, USA; gain 2–10 k) and band-pass filtered (30–1000 Hz, to minimize both movement artifacts and high frequency noise). Goniometric and EMG signals were A/D converted at 2 kHz with 12-bit resolution (PCI-6024E, National Instruments®, Austin, TX, USA), visualized online and stored for further analysis.

The position of the subject was always visually controlled by the experimenter, who also evaluated the amplitude and duration of each pointing movement by looking at the wrist angle trace on the computer screen, so as to remind the subject to speed-up the movement, if necessary.

Data Analysis

For each tested hand, the 60 EMG traces of the prime mover and those simultaneously recorded from the postural muscles were digitally rectified and integrated (time constant: 25 ms). All the EMG and goniometric traces were then averaged in a fixed temporal window: from −1000 to +300 ms with respect to the onset of the FCR EMG, identified by a software threshold set at +2 SD of the initial excitation level (from 1000 to 500 ms prior to movement onset).

On each experiment, latency and amplitude of the postural activity was measured off-line on the averaged traces, after subtracting from them the initial excitation level. Since the initial EMG level represented the tonic activity required to keep the upper limb in the experimental position, the APAs

superimposed on it and should therefore be measured as changes (either positive or negative) in postural muscles activity. Also the peak-to-peak amplitude of wrist and elbow movements were measured off-line on the averaged traces, after subtracting their initial level for illustration purposes. The EMG onset in each postural muscle was identified by a software threshold set at ±2 SD of the initial excitation level, and visually validated. Latency of the APA was referred to the FCR EMG onset, with negative values indicating a time-advance. In order to measure the amplitude of each APA, the rectified EMG was first integrated from the APA onset to the movement onset. The resulting value was then normalized to the corresponding reference value, which was calculated as the mean value of the rectified EMG during the 5 s maximal press multiplied by the APA duration. APA amplitudes (normalized EMGi) were thus expressed in % of the reference value.

The peak-to-peak angular displacement of the elbow joint was measured from the onset of wrist flexion, signaled by the proximity switch, to the moment when flexion started to be braked, i.e., when wrist acceleration zeroed. The time of first contact between the pen tip and the tablet signaled the movement end; the distance between the pen-tip position and the target center at that moment being the pointing error. APA latencies and APA amplitudes (absolute values) were compared by a repeated measures analysis of variance (ANOVA) with factors *muscle* (BB vs. TB vs. AD) and *side* (PREF vs. NON-PREF). All other PREF vs. NON-PREF comparisons were performed by using paired t-tests. Statistical significance was set at $p < 0.05$.

RESULTS

When pointing while holding a pen with the PREF hand the FCR muscle activation was preceded by clear inhibitory postural adjustments in BB and AD muscles, and by an excitatory postural adjustment in TB (**Figure 1**, representative subject). This APA pattern preceded wrist flexion of about 60 ms. Instead, when the same subject pointed with the NON-PREF hand, APAs showed a similar pattern (excitation in TB and inhibition in BB and AD), but were clearly less anticipated. This change in the APA timing was associated to an increased elbow angular displacement during the movement, with respect to the PREF side. Thus, thanks to a better stabilization of the proximal joint, the representative subject was more precise in PREF than in NON-PREF. Indeed, this is apparent when comparing the final position of the pen-tip in the two sides.

Figure 2 illustrates the mean latency and amplitudes of APAs, the average latency, duration and amplitude of the wrist movement, as well as the average elbow displacement and pointing error in the whole sample. Note that the latency, amplitude and duration of wrist movement were at all similar in the PREF vs. NON-PREF hand (latency: $t_{(12)} = 0.19$, $p = 0.84$; duration: $t_{(12)} = 0.32$, $p = 0.75$; amplitude: $t_{(12)} = 0.17$, $p = 0.86$). Despite the invariance of average kinematics of the focal movement, the excitatory APA in TB and inhibitory APAs in BB and AD were delayed of about 20–30 ms in NON-PREF

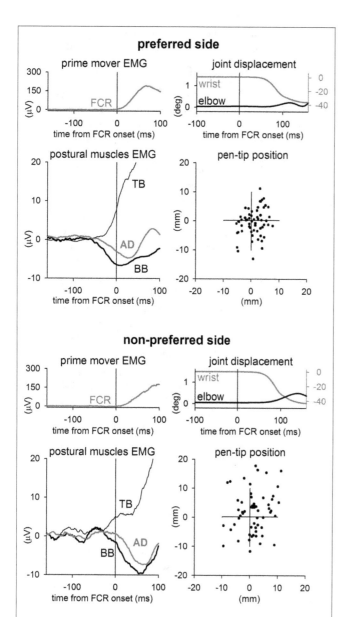

FIGURE 1 | Sample recordings from a representative subject. Rectified and integrated average recordings of EMG in Flexor Carpi Radialis (FCR, prime mover), Biceps Brachii (BB), Triceps Brachii (TB), Anterior Deltoid (AD), together with wrist flexion, elbow excursion and ensuing final position of pen-tip. Time 0 = FCR onset. When pointing with the preferred wrist (upper panels), the right elbow equilibrium was preserved thanks to excitatory APAs in TB and inhibitory APAs in BB and AD, which precede the FCR activation by about 65 ms. In the non-preferred side (lower panels) APAs were delayed, indeed they advanced the prime mover onset by just 20–30 ms. This was associated with an increase of the elbow excursion during the wrist movement. The effect that the different APA timing and the associated elbow stabilization had on the pen-tip final position is shown on the right-lowermost panels.

with respect to PREF, the time shift being similar in all muscles. Indeed, two-way ANOVA only found a main effect of *side* ($F_{(1,12)} = 18.43$, $p = 0.001$), with no effect of *muscles* ($F_{(2,24)} = 2.90$, $p = 0.075$), nor *interaction* ($F_{(2,24)} = 0.71$, $p = 0.50$). The absolute values of APA amplitude were different

in the three muscles but did not show any significant PREF vs. NON-PREF difference. Indeed, two-way ANOVA only found a main effect of *muscle* ($F_{(2,24)} = 16.65$, $p < 0.0001$; Tukey *post hoc* revealed that APA was lower in BB than in TB and AD, with no difference among the latter two), with no effect of *side* ($F_{(1,12)} = 1.23$, $p = 0.29$) nor *interaction* ($F_{(2,24)} = 2.05$, $p = 0.15$).

When pointing with the NON-PREF hand, the delay of the APA chain was associated to a greater displacement of the elbow joint with respect to the PREF side ($t_{(12)} = 3.68$, $p = 0.0035$) and to a larger and more scattered pointing error ($t_{(12)} = 5.18$, $p < 0.0002$).

DISCUSSION

This article illustrates an asymmetry in the temporal organization of the intra-limb APAs that stabilize the arm when producing a pen-pointing movement, performed by flexing one or the other wrist. Indeed, when pointing with the NON-PREF side, the APA chain in BB, TB and AD was less anticipated with respect to FCR recruitment. Considering that the mechanical perturbations induced by the focal movements were similar in the two sides, as witnessed by the similarities of wrist kinematics, the change in the APA timing was associated to the less efficient fixation of the elbow joint, which led to the reduced precision of the pointing movement. Therefore, we propose that the increased precision of the PREF hand stems from a more precise tailoring of APAs timing in that side.

Considerations About APA Amplitude Measurements

Given the difference in APA latency, statistics about APA amplitude should be interpreted carefully. In fact, they are based on data which do not represent comparable portions of the feedforward postural commands in the two sides. The onset of this command clearly produces the APA onset, but its end may occur either before or after the movement onset. As an example, the AD inhibitory APA, illustrated in **Figure 1**, seems to decay before wrist flexion in the PREF side while it decays after such movement in the NON-PREF side. Therefore, the APA amplitude in the PREF side fully quantifies the expression of the feedforward command, but it represents only a fraction of it in the NON-PREF side. In other words, the feedforward postural command does not necessarily end within the APA but may as well continue during the movement, when the simultaneous postural adjustments (SPAs) occur. In this case, SPAs become expression of a compound feedforward-feedback signal, in which it is impossible to identify the end of the feedforward component.

To overcome this problem, it could have been possible to choose a fixed time-window, ending before the movement onset. However, amplitude measurements would have been again inconclusive. Indeed, if the time window had ended before the APA peak, the measurement would have approximated the slope (rate of change) of the feedforward command, not its real

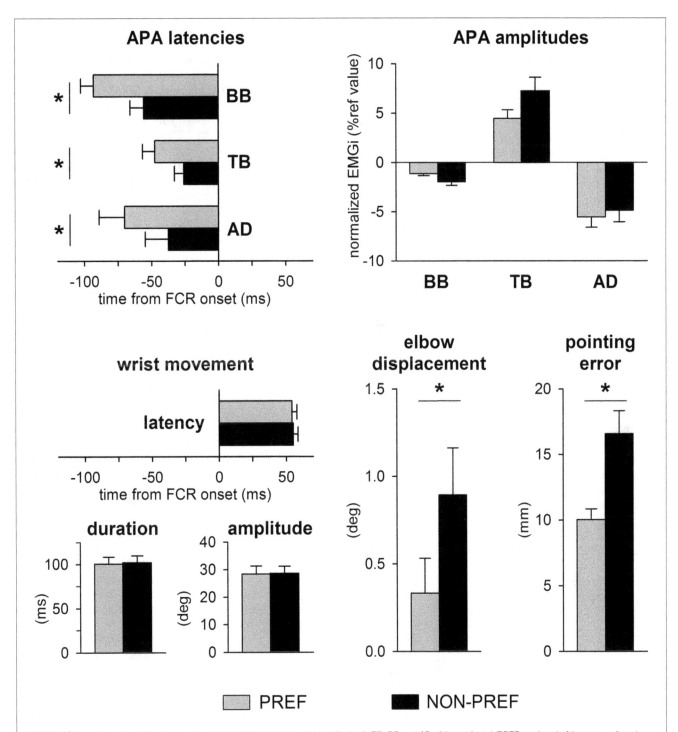

FIGURE 2 | Data from all subjects. Top panels show APAs latencies and amplitudes in TB, BB and AD of the preferred (PREF, gray) and of the non-preferred (NON-PREF, black) sides. Bottom panels report the latency, duration and amplitude of the wrist movement, as well as the elbow displacement and the pointing error on each side. Changes in APA latency were associated to a significant increase of the elbow displacement and pointing error. Time 0 = EMG onset in the prime mover Flexor Carpi Radialis (FCR). Mean values ± SEM. *$p < 0.05$.

amplitude. If instead the time-window had included the APA peak but not its decay, the measurement would have mixed-up amplitude and slope, in variable proportions.

In conclusion, the absence of statistical differences between the APAs amplitudes in the two sides does not grant that

the respective feedforward commands were also comparable. Instead, since the APAs onset is the direct expression of the onset of the feedforward command, the observed change in latency grants for a different the temporal organization of the APAs.

APAs Accompanying Preferred and Non-Preferred Limb Movements

Literature about *lateralization* of motor control shows a greater skill in the PREF vs. NON-PREF side for arm, wrist and finger movements (Todor et al., 1982). Substantial differences were illustrated in the coordination of muscular recruitment and intersegmental torques in the two sides, which in turn implied a more efficient strategy for the dominant (PREF) arm (Sainburg and Kalakanis, 2000; Sainburg, 2014) as well as a right-hand superiority in task such as throwing (Watson and Kimura, 1989), and a superiority in control of body stabilization during rapid step initiation with the PREF-leg (Yiou and Do, 2010). In particular, Bagesteiro and Sainburg (2002) illustrated that the more efficient strategy for the dominant arm was associated to different EMG profiles and therefore, they suggested that manual asymmetries result from differences between the two sides in controlling the effects of limb dynamics (see also Oliveira and Sanders, 2015).

Little is known instead about APAs and lateralization, since the large majority of studies on APAs have been conducted on voluntary movements performed with the PREF hand/side. Only a few studies have addressed the lateralization question (e.g., Teyssèdre et al., 2000; Mezaour et al., 2009; Yiou and Do, 2010). Teyssèdre et al. (2000), as an example, investigated whether lateral preference for one upper limb could involve side differences in APAs of postural muscles, showing an earlier occurrence of APAs for pointing movements performed with the PREF upper limb, and concluding that lateral preference is associated with postural laterality.

On the other hand, with regard to the central organization of the postural control, it has been recently shown that the left hemisphere in right-handers was more involved in the predictive control of the body and the consequent environmental dynamics. Instead, the right hemisphere of the same subjects was more involved during the deceleration phase of motion, as an impedance control mechanism to terminate the movement (Yadav and Sainburg, 2014). Consequently, it could be argued that the enhanced predictive control of body and environmental dynamics, driven by the left hemisphere, led to the more efficient anticipatory postural strategy, as we observed in the PREF side of our right-handed subjects. Recently, by studying long-latency stretch reflexes as a mechanism that permits the postural control, it has been suggested that handedness affects more the feedforward strategies than those based on sensory feed-back (Walker and Perreault, 2015).

In summary, the *lateralization* of APAs observed in the present study is in accordance with all the above described articles and provides novel evidence in favor of a functional linkage between the timing of intra-limb APAs, the resulting stability of elbow joint and the ensuing precision of pen-pointing movements.

APAs and Precision

According to shooting coaches and athletes, good postural balance is a vital component of a successful shooting performance. During bipedal standing, top-level rifle shooters stabilized their whole body balance better than naive shooters (Aalto et al., 1990); the capability to reduce the oscillation, especially in the last few seconds before pulling the trigger, expresses the better control of posture in athletes and was associated with a better shooting performance (Era et al., 1996; Mononen et al., 2007). Ypsilanti et al. (2009) illustrated a better stabilization of the center of pressure (CoP) and an improvement in the movement precision for pointing movements performed with the PREF than NON-PREF upper-limb, but did not provide results regarding the APAs chain. More recently, Furuya et al. (2011) demonstrated that professional pianists tended to play using less muscular activity and to take greater advantage of shoulder joint rotation during a keystroke than did novice.

The idea that the precision of a voluntary movement relies on proper APAs was first proposed for what concerns the *inter-limb* APAs. To the best of our knowledge, this idea was forwarded by studies that analyzed the linkage between APAs and movement precision in pointing to targets of different sizes (Nana-Ibrahim et al., 2008; Bertucco and Cesari, 2010). However, these results might be an outcome of the relationship between APAs and intended movement speed (Shiratori and Aruin, 2007; Esposti et al., 2015), since the speed of voluntary movements varies as a function of the target width, according to the Fitts (1954) law. In order to get rid of the possible bias due to changes in movement speed, Caronni et al. (2013) studied inter-limb APAs during an upper limb pointing movement before and after donning prismatic lenses, which are known to shift the binocular eye field and cause the subject to miss the target (Redding et al., 2005). By using this experimental paradigm, these authors showed that, despite similar kinematics of the focal movement, pointing errors occurred when lower limb APAs were out of proportion with respect to the recruitment of prime mover muscles in the shoulder. It has been also recently demonstrated that training induce improvement in the correct tailoring of the APA chain with respect to the prime mover recruitment, both in young adults (Kanekar and Aruin, 2015) and elderly (Kubicki et al., 2012; Aruin et al., 2015). Thus, the increased precision of voluntary movement observed after training (Hamman et al., 1995; Yang et al., 2013) might be partly due to a more appropriate tuning of APAs on the prime mover recruitment. The linkage between APAs and movement precision was also suggested for *intra-limb* APAs by Caronni and Cavallari (2009). Indeed, these authors showed that when simulating an index-finger flexion using a software mechanical model of the arm, a clear disturbance of both focal movement and upper-limb posture was observed, with relevant changes at wrist and elbow level. In the model, the only way to prevent these effects was to block all segments but the finger, preventing the proximal joints from rotating (*fictive* APAs). Since this observation derived from a very simplified system, Caronni and Cavallari (2009) also looked for a more realistic model: a finger tap was thus evoked in a real arm by electrical stimulation of the median nerve. This experiment showed similar recordings to those predicted by the software mechanical model. However, both the software stimulation and the electrically evoked tap did not faithfully represent the physiological pointing movement, since in the two cases no voluntary command was generated. Thus, considering that the experimental paradigm used in the present article involved subjects who voluntarily performed a pointing movement, present results are helpful for completing the framework originally proposed by Caronni and Cavallari (2009).

Further Considerations on the Motor Program for APAs and Prime Mover Recruitment

Present data should be discussed in the framework of the suggestion of a *shared motor command* for both APAs and prime mover recruitment (Aruin and Latash, 1995; Stapley et al., 1999; Leonard et al., 2011; Caronni et al., 2013). In particular, it was recently demonstrated that the intra-limb APAs stabilizing the arm when producing a brisk index-finger flexion were still present under an ischemic block of the forearm that suppressed the prime mover EMG, the finger movement and the related mechanical perturbation. Indeed, APAs remained tailored to the intended movement, i.e., to the expected perturbation, even after 60 movement trials in which that perturbation did not occur (Bruttini et al., 2014). Furthermore, in the same article, it was illustrated that intra-limb APAs were strongly attenuated when adding a fixation point to the wrist, i.e., closer to the voluntary moving segment (index-finger), a result that agrees with arm-pull experiments in standing subjects (Cordo and Nashner, 1982; Dietz and Colombo, 1996). Altogether, those results support the idea that the recruitment of postural and prime mover muscles should be driven by a *shared motor command*, according to a well-acquired pattern, which drives the muscular chain starting from the fixation point(s) and including the moving segment. Indeed, the shared motor command theory states that the central command to postural muscles and prime movers is "unique", so that the postural and voluntary components cannot be decoupled. However, this does not imply that a given voluntary command is always coupled to the same postural command. Thus, the observed time difference in postural commands between the PREF and NON-PREF limb can simply be the expression of a *badly* matched timing within the shared motor command (postural vs. focal components) in the NON-PREF side, which in turn may simply result from the reduced motor experience in that side. This latter interpretation seems the one to be PREF, also considering that a similar

timing disruption was observed in some pathological studies, in particular for what concerns cerebellar dysfunction. Indeed ataxic patients, who typically display dysmetria (i.e., the inability to precisely reach a given target), showed a temporal disruption of intra-limb APAs both during finger flexions (Bruttini et al., 2015) and in the bimanual unloading task (Diedrichsen et al., 2005). Data from these pathological studies further strengthen the linkage between APA timing and movement precision we observed in the present study. Considering that physical exercise enhances APAs (Kubicki et al., 2012; Aruin et al., 2015; Kanekar and Aruin, 2015) and movement precision (Aalto et al., 1990; Era et al., 1996; Mononen et al., 2007), while a short-term immobilization alters the APAs control (Bolzoni et al., 2012), it is more than probable that training the NON-PREF side would effectively improve APAs timing and movement precision.

Taking into account all these considerations, the classical definition of APA (Massion, 1992) might be extended, for instance, to: motor activities *starting from a fixation point*, aiming to *produce the necessary dynamics* so as to *refine the precision and accuracy of a voluntary movement*, thus implicitly taking into account the perturbation induced by the primary movement.

CONCLUSION

Present results showed a lateralization of the intra-limb APAs stabilizing the arm when producing a pen-pointing movement. The APAs delay in movements performed with the NON-PREF hand, in comparison to the recordings of the preferred side, were associated to an impaired stability of the elbow joint, with similar kinematics of the focal movement in the two sides. As a result, the focal movement perturbation caused an increased elbow excursion in the NON-PREF upper-limb, eventually leading to the diminished movement precision on that side. These data strengthen the idea that the APA chain is essential for an appropriate stabilization of the joints involved in the posture-focal chain and therefore, allows refining the precision of the focal movement.

AUTHOR CONTRIBUTIONS

All authors contributed in conceptualizing and designing the experiment, acquiring and analyzing the data, interpreting the results and writing the article. All authors approved the final version and agree to be accountable for all aspects of this work.

REFERENCES

Aalto, H., Pyykkö, I., Ilmarinen, R., Kähkönen, E., and Starck, J. (1990). Postural stability in shooters. *ORL J. Otorhinolaryngol. Relat. Spec.* 52, 232–238. doi: 10.1159/000276141

Aoki, F. (1991). Activity patterns of upper arm muscles in relation to direction of rapid wrist movement in man. *Exp. Brain Res.* 83, 679–682. doi: 10.1007/bf00229847

Aruin, A. S., Kanekar, N., Lee, Y. J., and Ganesan, M. (2015). Enhancement of anticipatory postural adjustments in older adults as a result of a single session of ball throwing exercise. *Exp. Brain Res.* 233, 649–655. doi: 10.1007/s00221-014-4144-1

Aruin, A. S., and Latash, M. L. (1995). The role of motor action in anticipatory postural adjustments studied with self-induced and externally triggered perturbations. *Exp. Brain Res.* 106, 291–300. doi: 10.1007/bf00241125

Aruin, A. S., and Shiratori, T. (2004). The effect of the amplitude of motor action on anticipatory postural adjustments. *J. Electromyogr. Kinesiol.* 14, 455–462. doi: 10.1016/j.jelekin.2003.12.002

Bagesteiro, L. B., and Sainburg, R. L. (2002). Handedness: dominant arm advantages in control of limb dynamics. *J. Neurophysiol.* 88, 2408–2421. doi: 10.1152/jn.00901.2001

Belen'kiĭ, V. E., Gurfinkel', V. S., and Pal'tsev, E. I. (1967). Control elements of voluntary movements. *Biofzika* 12, 135–141.

Bertucco, M., and Cesari, P. (2010). Does movement planning follow Fitts' law? Scaling anticipatory postural adjustments with movement speed and accuracy. *Neuroscience* 171, 205–213. doi: 10.1016/j.neuroscience.2010.08.023

Bolzoni, F., Bruttini, C., Esposti, R., and Cavallari, P. (2012). Hand immobilization affects arm and shoulder postural control. *Exp. Brain Res.* 220, 63–70. doi: 10.1007/s00221-012-3115-7

Bouisset, S., and Do, M. C. (2008). Posture, dynamic stability and voluntary movement. *Neurophysiol. Clin.* 38, 345–362. doi: 10.1016/j.neucli.2008.10.001

Bouisset, S., and Zattara, M. (1987). Biomechanical study of the programming of anticipatory postural adjustments associated with voluntary movement. *J. Biomech.* 20, 735–742. doi: 10.1016/0021-9290(87)90052-2

Brenière, Y., Cuong Do, M., and Bouisset, S. (1987). Are dynamic phenomena prior to stepping essential to walking? *J. Mot. Behav.* 19, 62–76. doi: 10.1080/00222895.1987.10735400

Bruttini, C., Esposti, R., Bolzoni, F., and Cavallari, P. (2014). Ischemic block of the forearm abolishes finger movements but not their associated anticipatory postural adjustments. *Exp. Brain Res.* 232, 1739–1750. doi: 10.1007/s00221-014-3866-4

Bruttini, C., Esposti, R., Bolzoni, F., Vanotti, A., Mariotti, C., and Cavallari, P. (2015). Temporal disruption of upper-limb anticipatory postural adjustments in cerebellar ataxic patients. *Exp. Brain Res.* 233, 197–203. doi: 10.1007/s00221-014-4103-x

Caronni, A., Bolzoni, F., Esposti, R., Bruttini, C., and Cavallari, P. (2013). Accuracy of pointing movements relies upon a specific tuning between APAs and prime mover activation. *Acta Physiol.* 208, 111–124. doi: 10.1111/apha.12081

Caronni, A., and Cavallari, P. (2009). Anticipatory postural adjustments stabilise the whole upper-limb prior to a gentle index-finger tap. *Exp. Brain Res.* 194, 59–66. doi: 10.1007/s00221-008-1668-2

Cordo, P. J., and Nashner, L. M. (1982). Properties of postural adjustments associated with rapid arm movements. *J. Neurophysiol.* 47, 287–302.

Diedrichsen, J., Verstynen, T., Lehman, S., and Ivry, R. (2005). Cerebellar involvement in anticipating the consequences of self-produced actions during bimanual movements. *J. Neurophysiol.* 93, 801–812. doi: 10.1152/jn.00662.2004

Dietz, V., and Colombo, G. (1996). Effects of body immersion on postural adjustments to voluntary arm movements in humans: role of load receptor input. *J. Physiol. Lond.* 497, 849–856. doi: 10.1113/jphysiol.1996.sp021815

Era, P., Konttinen, N., Mehto, P., Saarela, P., and Lyytinen, H. (1996). Postural stability and skilled performance—a study on top-level and naive rifle shooters. *J. Biomech.* 29, 301–306. doi: 10.1016/0021-9290(95)00066-6

Esposti, R., Bruttini, C., Bolzoni, F., and Cavallari, P. (2015). Intended rather than actual movement velocity determines the latency of anticipatory postural adjustments. *Exp. Brain Res.* 233, 397–403. doi: 10.1007/s00221-014-4122-7

Fitts, P. M. (1954). The information capacity of the human motor system in controlling the amplitude of movement. *J. Exp. Psychol.* 47, 381–391. doi: 10.1037/h0055392

Friedli, W. G., Hallett, M., and Simon, S. R. (1984). Postural adjustments associated with rapid voluntary arm movements 1. Electromyographic data. *J. Neurol. Neurosurg. Psychiatry* 47, 611–622. doi: 10.1136/jnnp.47.6.611

Furuya, S., Goda, T., Katayose, H., Miwa, H., and Nagata, N. (2011). Distinct inter-joint coordination during fast alternate keystrokes in pianists with superior skill. *Front. Hum. Neurosci.* 5:50. doi: 10.3389/fnhum.2011.00050

Hamman, R., Longridge, N. S., Mekjavic, I., and Dickinson, J. (1995). Effect of age and training schedules on balance improvement exercises using visual biofeedback. *J. Otolaryngol.* 24, 221–229.

Hess, W. R. (1943). Teleokinetisches und ereismatisches Kraftsystem in Biomotorik. *Helv. Physiol. Pharmacol. Acta* 1, C62–C63.

Kanekar, N., and Aruin, A. S. (2015). Improvement of anticipatory postural adjustments for balance control: effect of a single training session. *J. Electromyogr. Kinesiol.* 25, 400–405. doi: 10.1016/j.jelekin.2014.11.002

Kubicki, A., Petrement, G., Bonnetblanc, F., Ballay, Y., and Mourey, F. (2012). Practice-related improvements in postural control during rapid arm movement in older adults: a preliminary study. *J. Gerontol. A Biol. Sci. Med. Sci.* 67, 196–203. doi: 10.1093/gerona/glr148

Leonard, J. A., Gritsenko, V., Ouckama, R., and Stapley, P. J. (2011). Postural adjustments for online corrections of arm movements in standing humans. *J. Neurophysiol.* 105, 2375–2388. doi: 10.1152/jn.00944.2010

Massion, J. (1992). Movement, posture and equilibrium: interaction and coordination. *Prog. Neurobiol.* 38, 35–56. doi: 10.1016/0301-0082(92)90034-c

Mezaour, M., Yiou, E., and Le Bozec, S. (2009). Does symmetrical upper limb task involve symmetrical postural adjustments? *Gait Posture* 30, 239–244. doi: 10.1016/j.gaitpost.2009.05.007

Mononen, K., Konttinen, N., Viitasalo, J., and Era, P. (2007). Relationships between postural balance, rifle stability and shooting accuracy among novice rifle shooters. *Scand. J. Med. Sci. Sports* 17, 180–185. doi: 10.1111/j.1600-0838.2006.00549.x

Nana-Ibrahim, S., Vieilledent, S., Leroyer, P., Viale, F., and Zattara, M. (2008). Target size modifies anticipatory postural adjustments and subsequent elementary arm pointing. *Exp. Brain Res.* 184, 255–260. doi: 10.1007/s00221-007-1178-7

Oldfield, R. C. (1971). The assessment and analysis of handedness: the Edinburgh inventory. *Neuropsychologia* 9, 97–113. doi: 10.1016/0028-3932(71)90067-4

Oliveira, N., and Sanders, R. H. (2015). Kinematic and kinetic evidence for functional lateralization in a symmetrical motor task: the water polo eggbeater kick. *Exp. Brain Res.* 233, 947–957. doi: 10.1007/s00221-014-4166-8

Patla, A. E., Ishac, M. G., and Winter, D. A. (2002). Anticipatory control of center of mass and joint stability during voluntary arm movement from a standing posture: interplay between active and passive control. *Exp. Brain Res.* 143, 318–327. doi: 10.1007/s00221-001-0968-6

Redding, G. M., Rossetti, Y., and Wallace, B. (2005). Applications of prism adaptation: a tutorial in theory and method. *Neurosci. Biobehav. Rev.* 29, 431–444. doi: 10.1016/j.neubiorev.2004.12.004

Roy, E. A., Kalbfleisch, L., and Elliott, D. (1994). Kinematic analyses of manual asymmetries in visual aiming movements. *Brain Cogn.* 24, 289–295. doi: 10.1006/brcg.1994.1017

Sainburg, R. L. (2014). Convergent models of handedness and brain lateralization. *Front. Psychol.* 5:1092. doi: 10.3389/fpsyg.2014.01092

Sainburg, R. L., and Kalakanis, D. (2000). Differences in control of limb dynamics during dominant and non dominant arm reaching. *J. Neurophysiol.* 83, 2661–2675.

Shiratori, T., and Aruin, A. (2007). Modulation of anticipatory postural adjustments associated with unloading perturbation: effect of characteristics of a motor action. *Exp. Brain Res.* 178, 206–215. doi: 10.1007/s00221-006-0725-y

Stapley, P. J., Pozzo, T., Cheron, G., and Grishin, A. (1999). Does the coordination between posture and movement during human whole-body reaching ensure center of mass stabilization? *Exp. Brain Res.* 129, 134–146. doi: 10.1007/s002210050944

Stapley, P., Pozzo, T., and Grishin, A. (1998). The role of anticipatory postural adjustments during whole body forward reaching movements. *Neuroreport* 9, 395–401. doi: 10.1097/00001756-199802160-00007

Teyssèdre, C., Lino, F., Zattara, M., and Bouisset, S. (2000). Anticipatory EMG patterns associated with preferred and non-preferred arm pointing movements. *Exp. Brain Res.* 134, 435–440. doi: 10.1007/s002210000490

Todor, J. I., Kyprie, P. M., and Price, H. L. (1982). Lateral asymmetries in arm, wrist and finger movements. *Cortex* 18, 515–523. doi: 10.1016/s0010-9452(82)80050-6

Toussaint, H. M., Michies, Y. M., Faber, M. N., Commissaris, D. A., and van Dieën, J. H. (1998). Scaling anticipatory postural adjustments dependent on confidence of load estimation in a bi-manual whole-body lifting task. *Exp. Brain Res.* 120, 85–94. doi: 10.1007/s002210050380

Walker, E. H., and Perreault, E. J. (2015). Arm dominance affects feedforward strategy more than feedback sensitivity during a postural task. *Exp. Brain Res.* 233, 2001–2011. doi: 10.1007/s00221-015-4271-3

Watson, N. V., and Kimura, D. (1989). Right-hand superiority for throwing but not for intercepting. *Neuropsychologia* 27, 1399–1414. doi: 10.1016/0028-3932(89)90133-4

Woodworth, R. S. (1899). Accuracy of voluntary movement. *Psychol. Rev. Monogr. Suppl.* 3, i-114. doi: 10.1037/h0092992

Yadav, V., and Sainburg, R. L. (2014). Limb dominance results from asymmetries in predictive and impedance control mechanisms. *PLoS One* 9:e93892. doi: 10.1371/journal.pone.0093892

Yang, W. W., Liu, Y. C., Lu, L. C., Chang, H. Y., Chou, P. P., and Liu, C. (2013). Performance enhancement among adolescent players after 10 weeks of pitching training with appropriate baseball weights. *J. Strength Cond. Res.* 27, 3245-3251. doi: 10.1519/JSC.0b013e31828ddfeb

Yiou, E., and Do, M. C. (2010). Control of mediolateral stability during rapid step initiation with preferred and non-preferred leg: is it symmetrical? *Gait Posture* 32, 145-147. doi: 10.1016/j.gaitpost.2010.03.018

Ypsilanti, A., Hatzitaki, V., and Grouios, G. (2009). Lateralized effects of hand and eye on anticipatory postural adjustments in visually guided aiming movements. *Neurosci. Lett.* 462, 121-124. doi: 10.1016/j.neulet.2009.06.044

7

Rigid Ankle Foot Orthosis Deteriorates Mediolateral Balance Control and Vertical Braking during Gait Initiation

Arnaud Delafontaine[1]*, Olivier Gagey[1,2], Silvia Colnaghi[3], Manh-Cuong Do[1] and Jean-Louis Honeine[3]

[1]CIAMS, Université Paris-Sud Université Paris-Saclay, Orsay, France; CIAMS, Université d'Orléans, Orléans, France, [2]Service de Chirurgie Orthopédique, C.H.U Kremlin Bicêtre, Kremlin Bicêtre, France, [3]CSAM Laboratory, Department of Public Health, University of Pavia, Pavia, Italy

*Correspondence:
Arnaud Delafontaine
arnaud.delafontaine@u-psud.fr

Rigid ankle-foot orthoses (AFO) are commonly used for impeding foot drop during the swing phase of gait. They also reduce pain and improve gait kinematics in patients with weakness or loss of integrity of ankle-foot complex structures due to various pathological conditions. However, this comes at the price of constraining ankle joint mobility, which might affect propulsive force generation and balance control. The present study examined the effects of wearing an AFO on biomechanical variables and electromyographic activity of tibialis anterior (TA) and soleus muscles during gait initiation (GI). Nineteen healthy adults participated in the study. They initiated gait at a self-paced speed with no ankle constraint as well as wearing an AFO on the stance leg, or bilaterally. Constraining the stance leg ankle decreased TA activity ipsilaterally during the anticipatory postural adjustment (APA) of GI, and ipsilateral soleus activity during step execution. In the sagittal plane, the decrease in the stance leg TA activity reduced the backward displacement of the center of pressure (CoP) resulting in a reduction of the forward velocity of the center of mass (CoM) measured at foot contact (FC). In the frontal plane, wearing the AFO reduced the displacement of the CoP in the direction of the swing leg during the APA phase. The mediolateral velocity of the CoM increased during single-stance prompting a larger step width to recover balance. During step execution, the CoM vertical downward velocity is normally reduced in order to lessen the impact of the swing leg with the floor and facilitates the rise of the CoM that occurs during the subsequent double-support phase. The reduction in stance leg soleus activity caused by constraining the ankle weakened the vertical braking of the CoM during step execution. This caused the absolute instantaneous vertical velocity of the CoM at FC to be greater in the constrained conditions with respect to the control condition. From a rehabilitation perspective, passively- or actively-powered assistive AFOs could correct for the reduction in muscle activity and enhance balance control during GI of patients.

Keywords: ankle-foot orthosis, ankle rigidity, gait initiation, balance control, vertical braking

INTRODUCTION

Ankle joint plays a critical role during locomotion and is frequently prone to injury (Fuchs et al., 2003). The "traditional" ankle-foot orthoses (AFO) are rigid and designed to immobilize the ankle joint at a right angle. Such an approach is effective for preventing foot drop during swing phase ensuring toe clearance and proper contact with the heel (Yamamoto et al., 1997; Shorter et al., 2013; Alam et al., 2014). Immobilization of the ankle joint, henceforth referred to as ankle rigidity, has also been documented to reduce pain (Leung and Moseley, 2003; Thoumie et al., 2004; Richie, 2007), stimulate proprioception (Feuerbach et al., 1994; Nigg, 2001; Richie, 2007) and enhance gait for a wide range of patients suffering from severe locomotive disorders (Danielsson and Sunnerhagen, 2004; Lucareli et al., 2007; Wang et al., 2007; Brehm et al., 2008; Abe et al., 2009; Fatone et al., 2009). The current modern design of AFOs include articulated devices capable of assisting plantarflexion during stance. Whereas some studies confirmed the benefits of assistive AFOs (Guillebastre et al., 2009; Bregman et al., 2011; Eddison and Chockalingam, 2013; Petrucci et al., 2013; Kerkum et al., 2014; Kim et al., 2015), other studies have asserted a minimal effect of traditional AFOs on global gait kinematics in hemiplegic patients (Yamamoto et al., 1997; Mulroy et al., 2010). Therefore, taken into consideration the economic cost and the bulkiness of some articulated AFOs, the standard rigid model is still commonly used in rehabilitation practices.

While the effects of wearing AFOs on the general kinematic of gait during steady-state walking have been studied to a certain extent, little is known about their effects on the kinematics and EMG parameters of gait initiation (GI). GI is now a well-established experimental paradigm which has led to numerous fundamental findings. It comprises of an anticipatory postural adjustment (APA) phase and step execution phase (Carlsöö, 1966; Brenière and Do, 1986, 1991; Brenière et al., 1987). In GI, an APA has two objectives. The first is to create a disequilibrium torque in the sagittal plane which allows to initiate forward movement of the center of mass (CoM) from immobile posture. The motor strategy involves inhibition of antigravity background muscle activity of soleus (Sol) and bilateral activation of tibialis anterior (TA) which induce backward displacement of the center of pressure (CoP) relative to CoM, creating the disequilibrium torque (Crenna and Frigo, 1991; Lepers and Brenière, 1995). The magnitude of the disequilibrium torque plays a crucial role in determining global kinematic of GI (Honeine et al., 2014). The second objective of APA is to displace the CoM in the direction of the stance leg prior to step execution (Mille et al., 2014). The CoM lateral displacement towards the swing leg allows modulating the disequilibrium torque in the frontal plane to prevent a rapid medial fall and control mediolateral kinematic variables (Lyon and Day, 1997; Honeine et al., 2016; Yiou et al., 2016a,b). The CoM displacement during APA has been shown to result from loading the swing leg whilst unloading the other (Carlsöö, 1966; Winter, 1995). Loading the swing leg causes the ipsilateral movement of the CoP and contralateral movement of CoM.

Honeine et al. (2016) showed that during APA, stance leg TA activity ipsilaterally flexes the knee, contributing to hip abductor activity in loading the swing leg which produces the typical displacement of CoP in the frontal plane. During step execution, stance leg Sol is activated in order to resist the action of gravity and brake the fall of the CoM (Honeine et al., 2013, 2014). Braking the fall of CoM could ease the impact of the swing limb at foot contact (FC), reducing the stress on the leg joints and providing postural stability during the subsequent double-stance phase (Kuo, 2007; Welter et al., 2007; Chong et al., 2009).

Lower leg proprioceptive afferent inputs play a major role in modulating lower leg activity during the APA phase of GI (Ruget et al., 2008, 2010; Mouchnino and Blouin, 2013). By constraining the ankle joint, an AFO would necessarily alter this somatosensory information and could thus have a deteriorating effect on motor performance during APA. Delafontaine et al. (2015) showed that ankle hypomobility induced by means of strapping the joint deteriorated both the APA and step execution phases. In addition, strapping the ankle had a tendency to impair mediolateral balance control and braking of CoM fall during single-stance.

In the present study, we investigated the effect of firm ankle rigidity caused by wearing a solid "standard" AFO on GI. We hypothesized that immobilizing the ankle should cause an ipsilateral reduction in TA dorsiflexor muscle activity during APA and Sol plantarflexor muscle activity during step execution. The reduction in TA activity during APA is expected to produce a reduction in forward and lateral CoM velocity throughout GI (Honeine et al., 2013, 2014, 2016). We also postulate that the reduction in stance leg Sol activity during step execution should impede the braking of the CoM downward fall (Honeine et al., 2013, 2014). If our hypothesis is confirmed, then this study would favor the use of articulated plantar-flexion-assisting AFOs in order to enhance dynamic balance during locomotive tasks of patients.

MATERIALS AND METHODS

Subjects

Nineteen healthy adults (10 men and 9 women, mean age 30.3 $\pm$ 4.4 years, height 1.7 $\pm$ 0.07 m and body-mass 69.8 $\pm$ 6.2 kg) participated in this study. All subjects gave informed written consent as required by the Declaration of Helsinki. The experiment was approved by the local ethic committee of the University Paris-Saclay (EA 4532).

Experimental Protocol

Subjects stood on a force platform (0.9 × 1.80 m, AMTI, Watertown, MA, USA). They were asked to initiate gait at a self-paced speed following an acoustic signal. Subjects were specifically instructed not to start walking in a reaction-time mode, but to start when they felt ready (this usually occurred following an interval of 0.5–1 s). They performed GI under three experimental conditions: GI without wearing an orthosis

(Ctrl), GI while wearing the orthosis on the stance leg ankle (O-St), and GI while wearing the orthoses on both ankles (O-Bi). The order of the conditions was randomly assigned. Before recording, preferential starting leg of the subjects was established. Subjects were asked to stand still eyes closed, and a small thrust was applied to their back forcing them to make a step forward. This was repeated three times. Subjects were instructed to initiate gait with the stepping leg that was used during this test. Each experimental condition comprised 10 trials. Biomechanical variables, obtained from each trial, were calculated (see below). The mean of the 10 trials for each variable was then computed. Subjects were asked to wear everyday sneaker shoes. In the O-St conditions, subjects kept wearing the shoe on the swing side in order to match the elevation of the orthosis and mimic real life situation. A rigid "standard" short ankle foot orthosis ("botte de marche courte MaxTrax® Ankle", Donjoy®) was used in this study (**Figure 1**). The orthosis was designed to prevent plantar/dorsi flexion and eversion/inversion movements of the ankle (Thoumie et al., 2004).

Acquisition and Measurements

Ground reaction forces and CoP data were obtained from the force platform. Surface EMG activity of TA and Sol was recorded using bipolar Ag-AgCl electrodes via wireless preamplifiers (Zero-wire, Aurion, Milan, Italy). Electrode sites and preparation was performed according to the SENIAM protocol (Merletti and Hermens, 2000). EMG raw traces were bandpass filtered (10–500 Hz) with a second order Butterworth no-lag filter. Force platform and EMG data were digitized with an analog to digital converter at a sampling frequency of 1000 Hz and saved on a PC for off-line analysis.

The mediolateral (ML) CoP instantaneous position curve was used to determine the onset of GI ($t0$), first foot off (FO1) and FC, in addition to the second foot off (FO2; **Figure 2**). The instant of $t0$ was determined as the instant when the ML CoP trace deviated 2 standard deviations

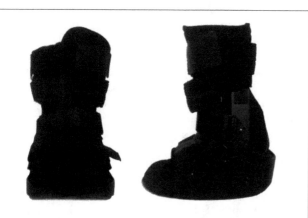

FIGURE 1 | "Standard" short ankle foot orthosis. The figure portrays a frontal and side view of the rigid orthosis that was used in this study. The orthosis can block dorsi- and plantarflexion of the ankle in addition to reducing the eversion and inversion of the foot.

from its baseline value. The moments of foot offs and that of FC were determined as the local minimums of the second derivative of the ML CoP trace. Visual inspection was conducted on all trials to verify the correctness of the algorithm.

The APA phase was considered to be the time-window spanning from $t0$ until FO1. The step execution phase was considered as the period between foot off and FC. Step length was approximated as the distance between the anteroposterior (AP) position of CoP at the instants of $t0$ and the FO2 (**Figure 2**). Step width was considered to be the distance between the ML position of the CoP at the instants of the FO1 and FO2 (**Figure 2**). The CoM acceleration in the ML and AP directions were calculated by dividing the respective ground reaction forces by the subjects' mass. The CoM vertical acceleration was obtained by subtracting the subjects' bodyweight from the vertical ground reaction force and dividing by the subjects mass. The CoM velocity in all three directions was then obtained by integrating the respective acceleration with respect to time. The magnitude of the vertical braking during step execution was measured as the difference between the minimum vertical velocity of CoM during single support and its vertical velocity at FC (**Figure 3**).

EMG raw traces were rectified and then low-pass filtered at a cut-off frequency of 25 Hz with a no-lag second order Butterworth filter. Amplitudes of EMG activity of each muscle were calculated by integrating the respective EMG filtered trace. Amplitudes of TA activity of both legs were calculated from the moment of onset until the instant of foot off. Amplitudes of stance leg Sol activity were calculated from the moment of onset until the instant of FC. The moment of muscle onset was calculated using a custom-made algorithm based on continuous (Morlet) wavelets transform (see Honeine et al., 2016).

Statistical Analyses

The Shapiro-Wilk test was used to determine if the studied variables were normally distributed. If Shapiro-Wilk test was significant (i.e., SW-p < 0.05), then the hypothesis that the data is normally distributed should be excluded. In the result section, the normality distribution tests are presented in the following condition order: Ctrl, O-St and O-Bi. Repeated-measures analysis of variances (ANOVAs) were used to test the effect of the three experimental conditions on the kinematics and EMG parameters. A significant outcome was followed up with the Bonferroni correction *post hoc* test. The threshold of significance was set at p < 0.05.

RESULTS

We first analyzed general kinematic variables of GI. **Table 1** contains the grand mean and standard deviation of the duration of APA and step execution. Wearing the AFO, i.e., in the O-St and O-Bi conditions, had a significant effect on the durations of both the APA and step execution phases (SW-p: 0.16, 0.44, 0.22—$F_{(2,36)}$ = 38, p < 0.001; SW-p: 0.24, 0.11, 0.82—$F_{(2,36)}$ = 55, p < 0.001, respectively). *Post hoc* analyses showed that wearing

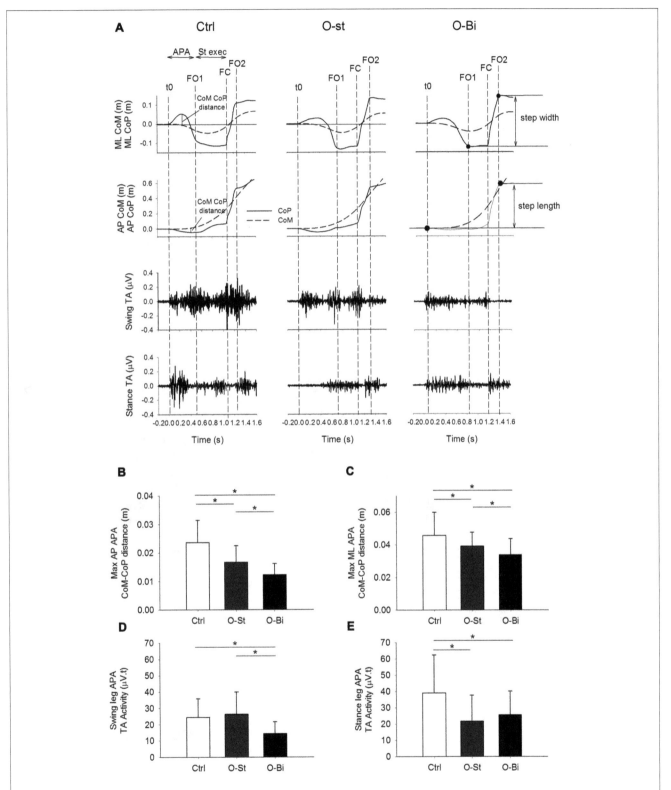

FIGURE 2 | Anteroposterior (AP) and mediolateral (ML) center of mass (CoM)-center of pressure (CoP) distance and the bilateral tibialis anterior (TA) activity. Panel **(A)** shows, from top to bottom the timelines of the ML and AP CoP (solid lines) and CoM (dashed lines) trajectories in addition of the raw traces of swing and stance TA activity during gait initiation (GI). The traces were obtained from a single trial of a representative subject in the Ctrl (left), O-St (middle) and O-Bi (right) conditions. The vertical dash lines represent the instant of t0, first foot off (FO1), foot contact (FC) second foot off (FO2). Panels **(B–E)** show the grand means (N = 19) and standard deviations of the maximum AP and ML distance between the CoM and CoP, the swing and stance TA activity. The histograms show that wearing the ankle-foot orthoses (AFO) decreases the activity of TA and ML and AP CoP and CoM excursions. *Indicates significant difference ($p < 0.05$).

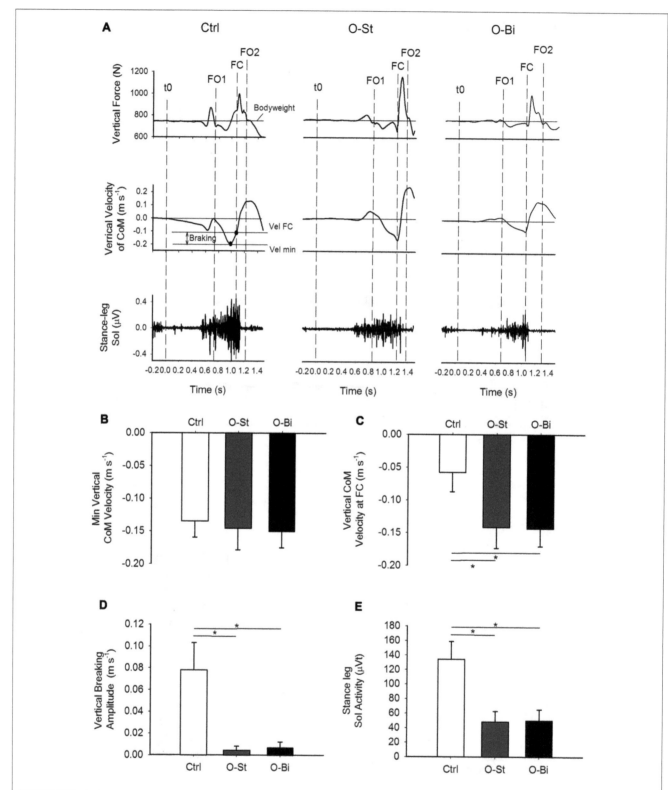

FIGURE 3 | Vertical ground reaction force and CoM velocity and the stance leg Sol activity. Panel **(A)** shows, from top to bottom) the timelines of the vertical ground reaction forces and vertical CoM velocity in addition of the raw traces of stance Sol activity during GI. The traces were obtained from a single trial of a representative subject in the Ctrl (left), O-St (middle) and O-Bi (right) conditions. The vertical dash lines represent the instant of t0, first foot off (FO1), FC second foot off (FO2). Panels **(B–E)** show the grand means (N = 19) and standard deviations of the minimum vertical velocity of CoM, the vertical velocity of CoM at FC, the vertical braking of CoM vertical fall and the stance Sol activity during step execution. It can be noted that wearing the AFO decreases the activity of Sol, which affects the braking action on the CoM vertical fall. *Indicates significant difference (p < 0.05).

TABLE 1 | Grand means (N = 19) and standard deviations of the durations of gait initiation (GI) phases.

	Duration of APA (s)	Duration of step execution (s)
Ctrl	0.62 ± 0.04	0.37 ± 0.02
O-St	0.74 ± 0.05*	0.31 ± 0.03*
O-Bi	0.67 ± 0.05*◇	0.38 ± 0.03◇

*Significantly different than Ctrl, ◇ significantly different than O-St.

the orthosis increased the duration of APA, more so when the AFO was worn on the stance leg than bilaterally ($p < 0.001$ for both comparisons). The duration of step execution decreased only in the O-St condition ($p < 0.001$).

APA in the Anteroposterior Direction

The time-profiles of the CoM (dashed line) and CoP (solid line) during the first step in the sagittal plane in addition to the TA activity of both legs are presented in **Figure 2A** top panels. The traces were obtained from one subject during all three conditions: Ctrl (left), O-St (middle) and O-Bi (left). As seen in the figure, CoP is displaced backwards during APA. The displacement is accompanied by bilateral activation of the TA muscles. Grand mean and standard deviation of the maximal distance between CoM and CoP during APA in AP direction in addition to the amplitude of EMG activity of both TA muscles are shown in the **Figures 2B,D,E.**

ANOVA showed a significant effect of wearing the orthosis on the maximum CoM-CoP distance in the AP direction during the APA phase (SW-p for the Ctrl, O-St and O-Bi respectively: 0.95, 0.18, 0.24—$F_{(2,36)} = 30.3$, $p < 0.001$). Post hoc analyses showed that the maximum AP CoM-CoP distances observed during APA were greatest in the Ctrl condition and smallest in the O-Bi condition ($p < 0.05$ for all comparisons). ANOVA also showed an effect of wearing the orthosis on the activity of TA (swing leg: SW-p: 0.67, 0.72, 0.15—$F_{(2,36)} = 18.7$, $p < 0.001$; stance leg: SW-p: 0.14, 0.31, 0.38—$F_{(2,36)} = 24.4$, $p < 0.001$). Post hoc analyses showed that the activity of TA was always smaller when the ankles were constrained by the orthosis with respect to not wearing it ($p < 0.001$ for all comparisons).

APA in the Mediolateral Direction

Figure 2A also portrays the displacement time profiles of the CoM (dashed line) and CoP (solid line) in the frontal plane in all three conditions. During APA, CoP is displaced laterally in the direction of the swing foot. The displacement of CoP causes a movement of the CoM

in the opposite direction. ANOVA showed a significant effect of wearing the orthosis on the maximum ML CoM-CoP distance during the APA phase (SW-p: 0.16, 0.4, 0.73—$F_{(2,36)} = 21.6$, $p < 0.001$, respectively). Post hoc analyses showed that the maximum ML CoM-CoP distances measured during APA were greatest in the Ctrl condition and smallest in the O-Bi condition ($p < 0.05$ for all comparisons). Grand means and standard deviations are shown in **Figure 2C**.

Kinematic Variables of Step Execution

Grand means and standard deviations of the AP and ML velocity of CoM measured at FC, as well as step length, and step width are shown in **Table 2**. Wearing the orthosis significantly changed the instantaneous AP velocity measured at the instant of FC (SW-p: 0.19, 0.75, 0.28—$F_{(2,36)} = 37.9$, $p < 0.001$). Post hoc tests revealed that the AP velocity of the CoM decreased in both the O-St and O-Bi conditions ($p < 0.001$ in both comparisons). However, the AP CoM velocity was higher in the O-Bi condition with respect to O-St ($p < 0.05$). The orthosis did not modify step length (SW-p: 0.46, 0.21, 0.11—$F_{(2,36)} = 0.32$, $p = 0.74$). Wearing the rigid AFO also changed the ML velocity of CoM measured at FC (SW-p: 0.07, 0.12, 0.39—$F_{(2,36)} = 60.3$, $p < 0.001$). Post hoc analyses showed an increase in ML velocity of the CoM, more so when it was applied bilaterally than to the stance leg alone ($p < 0.05$ for all comparisons). Step width was also significantly affected as a result of wearing the AFO (SW-p: 0.47, 0.69, 0.67—$F_{(2,36)} = 55$, $p < 0.001$). Post hoc analyses showed that step width increased in O-St with respect to Ctrl and was largest in the O-Bi condition ($p < 0.01$ for both comparisons).

Active Vertical Braking during Step Execution

The time-profiles of the vertical ground reaction force, the CoM vertical velocity curves (upper panels) and of the EMG activity of the stance leg soleus (lower panels) obtained from one trial of a single subject in the Ctrl (left), O-St (middle) and O-Bi (left) conditions are shown in panel A of **Figure 3**. As can be seen in the figure, following foot off, the CoM accelerated downward (negative velocity indicates downward movement of CoM) and then reversed. In fact, during single support, the CoM velocity shows a "V" shape indicating that the CoM fall was braked. In Ctrl condition, the braking action, which is accompanied by a surge in stance soleus activity, caused a reduction in the absolute of vertical velocity of the CoM measured at FC. In the O-St and O-Bi conditions,

TABLE 2 | Grand means (N = 19) and standard deviations of general kinematics variables of GI.

	AP velocity at foot contact (m/s)	ML velocity at foot contact (m/s)	Step length (m)	Step width (m)
Ctrl	1.05 ± 0.10	0.16 ± 0.05	0.55 ± 0.04	0.17 ± 0.04
O-St	0.87 ± 0.11*	0.19 ± 0.06*	0.53 ± 0.05	0.21 ± 0.05*
O-Bi	0.912 ± 0.12*◇	0.23 ± 0.06*◇	0.55 ± 0.07	0.24 ± 0.05*◇

*Significantly different than Ctrl, ◇ significantly different than O-St.

the soleus activity of stance leg was reduced and minimum absolute velocity at FC, in most cases, was recorded at FC. This reveals that constraining the stance leg with a rigid AFO has a deteriorating effect on the active vertical braking that occurs during unconstrained GI.

Grand means and standard deviations of the minimum vertical velocity of CoM during single-support, the vertical velocity of CoM measured at the instant of FC, the active vertical braking of CoM and the amplitude of the stance leg Sol activity during single-support are shown in **Figure 3** (lower panels). ANOVA showed no effect of the orthosis on the absolute minimum vertical velocity of CoM during single-support across the conditions (SW-p: 0.34, 0.52, 0.14—$F_{(2,36)}$ = 0.28, p = 0.54). However, wearing the orthosis had an effect on the vertical velocity of CoM measured at the instant of FC (SW-p: 0.12, 0.6, 0.19—$F_{(2,36)}$ = 106.7, p < 0.001) and the magnitude of vertical braking of CoM during single-stance (SW-p: 0.52, 0.57, 0.07—$F_{(2,36)}$ = 266.1, p < 0.001). *Post hoc* analyses revealed that both the absolute vertical velocity of CoM at FC and the amplitude of vertical braking of CoM were significantly smaller in the O-St and O-Bi condition with respect to the Ctrl conditions (p < 0.001). *Post hoc* analyses showed that the absolute vertical minimum velocity of CoM and the absolute velocity at FC measured in O-St and O-Bi conditions were comparable (p > 0.05). Wearing the orthosis also had an effect on the amplitude of the stance leg Sol activity during single-support (SW-p: 0.18, 0.31, 0.26—$F_{(2,36)}$ = 101.4, p < 0.001). *Post hoc* analyses showed that the amplitude of the stance leg Sol activity was lowest in the O-St and O-Bi (p < 0.001).

DISCUSSION

The results of the present study show that AFOs cause an ipsilateral reduction in TA activity during APA, and ipsilateral decrease of Sol activity during step execution. The decrease in muscle activity is accompanied by a decrease in AP CoM velocity and an increase in ML CoM velocity. In addition, constraining the stance leg ankle joint reduced the vertical braking of the CoM fall that is observed in the single-stance phase of normal GI.

Foot and ankle proprioceptive inputs are known to play a role in modulating lower leg activity during the APA phase of GI (Ruget et al., 2008, 2010; Mouchnino and Blouin, 2013). The modification of lower limb muscle activity in this study may be linked to alteration in the proprioceptive foot and ankle inputs that are caused by constraining the ankle with a rigid AFO. In line with Delafontaine et al. (2015), the reduction in AP velocity measured at FC, with respect to control, is greater in the O-St than in the O-Bi condition. Delafontaine et al. (2015) suggested that the higher AP CoM velocity in the double-constrained condition is probably due to the better capacity of the brain to deal with a symmetrical change of proprioceptive inputs, as opposed to the asymmetrical somatosensory modification that occurs when only one ankle is constrained. The increase in AP velocity in the O-Bi condition could also be caused by adjusting

trunk position in order to advance the position of the CoM relative to the base of support and increase forward momentum, which is thought to occur in lower limb amputees (Michel and Do, 2002).

Our evidence that induced stance leg ankle rigidity reduces the activity of the TA is consistent with the results of Geboers et al. (2002). During the APA phase of GI, the bilateral increase in TA activity accompanied by the silencing of both Sol muscles is responsible for generating a forward momentum (Crenna and Frigo, 1991; Honeine et al., 2013, 2014). It may be noted that the decrease in TA activity was compensated by an increase in the duration of APA in order to allow the gravitational torque to accumulate more pace and reach higher forward velocity. Nonetheless, the forward velocity reached at FC when the stance leg was constrained is lower than in the control condition. In addition, Honeine et al. (2016) have shown that TA activity during APA is greater in the stance leg than the contralateral limb. This causes a slight stance leg knee flexion which assists the hip abductor activity in loading the future swing leg and displacing the CoP in the direction of the swinging leg (Carlsöö, 1966; Winter, 1995). In the present study, reduction of the activity of stance TA activity also results in a decrease in ML CoP displacement during APA, corroborating the results of Honeine et al. (2016). In line with Caderby et al. (2014) and Honeine et al. (2016), for the same initial stance width, a smaller CoP displacement during APA causes the ML distance between the CoM and CoP to be larger during the subsequent step execution. This produces a larger gravitational torque during the single-support phase. As a result, the velocity of the medial fall during single-stance increases, prompting a rise in step width to restore stability in the frontal plane.

The results of this study also show that wearing the AFO on the stance leg (i.e., in the O-St and O-Bi condition) reduces the activity of the stance leg soleus EMG during single-support, as shown in studies investigating steady-state walking (Yamamoto et al., 1993; Boninger and Leonard, 1996; Miyazaki et al., 1997; Akizuki et al., 2001). In normal gait, during the single-stance phase, the body rotates around the ankle-forefoot articulation system causing the CoM to accelerate downwards. In healthy individuals, the CoM downward velocity is reduced prior to FC (Chong and Do, 2003). This active braking of CoM during single-stance is the result of triceps-surae activity (Honeine et al., 2013, 2014). In our study, the decrease of the stance leg soleus activity reduces the effectiveness of vertical braking of the CoM fall during the step-execution phase and substantially increases the shock between the swing leg and the ground at FC. In other words, the downward fall of the CoM is halted mechanically by the impact of the swing foot with the ground. On the one hand, Chong and Do (2003) and Welter et al. (2007) state that the main aim of the active braking is to reduce the shock between the heel of the swing leg and the ground. On the other hand, the dynamic inverted pendulum model provided by Kuo (2007) suggest that the vertical braking action observed in late single-stance is required to minimize the work that is necessary to lift the CoM during the subsequent double-support phase. Hence, the triceps surae braking action is necessary for the proper execution of the step-to-step transition.

Furthermore, it should be kept in mind that AFOs are traditionally designed with the main objective of preventing foot-drop in order to allow for toe clearance and promote contacting the floor with the heel instead of the metatarsals (Yamamoto et al., 1997; Shorter et al., 2013; Alam et al., 2014). Nonetheless, many "modern" AFOs have been designed in order to assist plantarflexion. Such devices can be broadly classified into two categories: passive and active devices. Passive AFOs generally employ spring mechanisms in order to store energy during single-stance, later releasing it in order to assist plantarflexion. The types of springs in passive AFO vary from mechanical (Guillebastre et al., 2009), pneumatic (Ferris et al., 2005), carbon composites material (Zou et al., 2014), oil damper (Ohata et al., 2011), and magneto reological damper (Svensson and Holmberg, 2008). Active AFOs operate an actuator in order to perform a torque across the ankle joint. Most common actuators are small electric motors (Bai et al., 2015) or pneumatic pumps (Chin et al., 2009). Furthermore, some actively-powered AFOs are designed to be controlled through EMG activity (Ferris et al., 2005; Cain et al., 2007; Wentink et al., 2013). Such a control system is thought to increase the efficiency of the AFO by enhancing the timing during which the assistive torque is generated (Alam et al., 2014).

Assistive AFOs have been shown to enhance push-off which restores active braking during late single-stance. The effect of those assistive AFOs have been shown to be beneficial for cerebral palsy patients (Eddison and Chockalingam, 2013; Kerkum et al., 2014) and hemiplegic patients following a stroke (Kim et al., 2015). In addition, Bregman et al. (2011) have shown that wearing a spring-assisted AFO decreases the energy cost of gait in stroke patients by about 10%. Their result corroborates with the hypothesis of Kuo (2007) who states that vertical force applied during late single-stance helps to reduce the energetic cost required to raise the CoM during double stance. In addition, Petrucci et al. (2013) showed that mechanically-generating plantarflexion across the swing leg ankle during APA increases the mediolateral displacement of the CoP. It is important to note that the negative effects that were induced by the rigid AFO are comparable to those described in impaired gait consecutive to different diseases. For instance, in hemiparetic stroke subjects, the preparatory ML displacement of CoP is reduced when gait is initiated with the affected limb (Hesse et al., 1997). In addition, progressive supranuclear palsy patients (Welter et al., 2007), parkinsonians (Chastan et al., 2009a,b) and elderly subjects (Chong et al., 2009) have been already documented to have deficits in braking the downward acceleration of the CoM during single-stance. It is thought that such locomotive symptoms are due to supraspinal complications affecting the central command responsible for the proper generation of APA (Rocchi et al., 2012) and step execution (Demain et al., 2014). In this study, a population of healthy young subjects was tested and the effects were obtained by mechanically constraining the ankle joint. Based on our data alone it is not possible to state whether constraining the stance leg further deteriorates the central command of patients which could worsen balance control and the active

braking of gait. For instance, Chen et al. (2015) have shown that wearing an anterior (flexible) AFO improves lateral CoM displacement in stroke patients during upright stance. Further research should be performed in order to investigate whether rigid AFO could have an increased negative effect on patients and whether assistive AFO could restore balance control and active braking.

Limitations

Wearing AFO enlarges the area of the base of support of the subjects. In addition, the same AFO was used regardless of the subjects' shoe size. Our present data do not allow to differentiate between the influence of the enlargement of the base of support and that of constraining the ankle. In addition, wearing the AFO also increases the volume of the whole shank. Therefore, it could be possible that the increase in step-width in the O-St and O-Bi conditions is a precautious strategy aimed at preventing the ankle to bump into the AFO or a collision between the two AFOs during the execution of the second step. Future experiments including a variation of initial feet-width and/or wearing slimmer AFOs should untangle this problem. In impaired locomotive neurological patients such as Parkinsonians, this technical problem could have two ambivalent effects. Indeed, it could further deteriorate balance control or improve it, as subjects should walk with enlarged step-width. Future experiments should shed light on this question.

CONCLUSIONS

Blocking ankle movement or limiting it disturbs kinematics gait parameters, balance control in the frontal plane and deteriorates the vertical braking action during single-stance. It would be interesting to test whether utilization of assistive AFO devices could permit to regain normal or nearly normal gait, i.e., walking with normal equilibrium and without ankle pain.

AUTHOR CONTRIBUTIONS

AD contributed with project creation, data collection, data analysis and drafted the manuscript. OG contributed with project creation, data analysis. SC contributed with project creation, data analysis. M-CD and J-LH contributed with project creation, data collection, data analysis. All authors discussed the results and participated in the revision of the manuscript.

FUNDING

This study was supported in part by the grant "Projet Attractivité" from the Paris-Sud University.

ACKNOWLEDGMENTS

The authors would like to thank Dr. David Gibas for editing and proofreading the final version of the manuscript.

REFERENCES

Abe, H., Michimata, A., Sugawara, K., Sugaya, N., and Izumi, S. (2009). Improving gait stability in stroke hemiplegic patients with a plastic ankle-foot orthosis. *Tohoku J. Exp. Med.* 218, 193–199. doi: 10.1620/tjem.218.193

Akizuki, K. H., Gartman, E. J., Nisonson, B., Ben-Avi, S., and McHugh, M. P. (2001). The relative stress on the Achilles tendon during ambulation in an ankle immobiliser: implications for rehabilitation after Achilles tendon repair. *Br. J. Sports Med.* 35, 329–333; discussion 333–334. doi: 10.1136/bjsm. 35.5.329

Alam, M., Choudhury, I. A., and Bin Mamat, A. (2014). Mechanism and design analysis of articulated ankle foot orthoses for drop-foot. *ScientificWorldJournal* 2014:867869. doi: 10.1155/2014/867869

Bai, Y., Gao, X., Zhao, J., Jin, F., Dai, F., and Lv, Y. (2015). A portable ankle-foot orthosis powered by electric motor. *Open Mech. Eng. J.* 9, 982–991. doi: 10.2174/1874155x01509010982

Boninger, M. L., and Leonard, J. A. Jr. (1996). Use of bivalved ankle-foot orthosis in neuropathic foot and ankle lesions. *J. Rehabil. Res. Dev.* 33, 16–22.

Bregman, D. J. J., van der Krogt, M. M., de Groot, V., Harlaar, J., Wisse, M., and Collins, S. H. (2011). The effect of ankle foot orthosis stiffness on the energy cost of walking: a simulation study. *Clin. Biomech. (Bristol Avon)* 26, 955–961. doi: 10.1016/j.clinbiomech.2011.05.007

Brehm, M. A., Harlaar, J., and Schwartz, M. (2008). Effect of ankle-foot orthoses on walking efficiency and gait in children with cerebral palsy. *J. Rehabil. Med.* 40, 529–534. doi: 10.2340/16501977-0209

Brenière, Y., Cuong Do, M., and Bouisset, S. (1987). Are dynamic phenomena prior to stepping essential to walking? *J. Mot. Behav.* 19, 62–76. doi: 10.1080/00222895.1987.10735400

Brenière, Y., and Do, M. C. (1986). When and how does steady state gait movement induced from upright posture begin? *J. Biomech.* 19, 1035–1040. doi: 10.1016/0021-9290(86)90120-x

Brenière, Y., and Do, M. C. (1991). Control of gait initiation. *J. Mot. Behav.* 23, 235–240. doi: 10.1080/00222895.1991.9942034

Caderby, T., Yiou, E., Peyrot, N., Begon, M., and Dalleau, G. (2014). Influence of gait speed on the control of mediolateral dynamic stability during gait initiation. *J. Biomech.* 47, 417–423. doi: 10.1016/j.jbiomech.2013. 11.011

Cain, S. M., Gordon, K. E., and Ferris, D. P. (2007). Locomotor adaptation to a powered ankle-foot orthosis depends on control method. *J. Neuroeng. Rehabil.* 4:48. doi: 10.1186/1743-0003-4-48

Carlsöö, S. (1966). The initiation of walking. *Acta Anat. (Basel)* 65, 1–9. doi: 10.1159/000142864

Chastan, N., Do, M. C., Bonneville, F., Torny, F., Bloch, F., Westby, G. W., et al. (2009a). Gait and balance disorders in Parkinson's disease: impaired active braking of the fall of centre of gravity. *Mov. Disord.* 24, 188–195. doi: 10.1002/mds.22269

Chastan, N., Westby, G. W., Yelnik, J., Bardinet, E., Do, M. C., Agid, Y., et al. (2009b). Effects of nigral stimulation on locomotion and postural stability in patients with Parkinson's disease. *Brain* 132, 172–184. doi: 10.1093/brain/awn294

Chen, C. L., Chen, F. F., Lin, C. H., Lou, S. Z., Chang, H. Y., and Yeung, K. T. (2015). Effect of anterior ankle-foot orthoses on weight shift in persons with stroke. *Arch. Phys. Med. Rehabil.* 96, 1795–1801. doi: 10.1016/j.apmr.2015. 05.003

Chin, R., Hsiao-Wecksler, E. T., Loth, E., Kogler, G., Manwaring, S. C., Tyson, S. N., et al. (2009). A pneumatic power haversting ankle-foot orthosis to prevent foot-drop. *J. Neuroeng. Rehabil.* 6:19. doi: 10.1186/1743-0003-6-19

Chong, R. K. Y., Chastan, N., Welter, M. L., and Do, M. C. (2009). Age-related changes in the center of mass velocity control during walking. *Neurosci. Lett.* 458, 23–27. doi: 10.1016/j.neulet.2009.04.022

Chong, R. K., and Do, M. C. (2003). "Control of center of mass velocity during walking," in *Recent Research Developments in Biomechanics*, ed. S. G. Pandalai (India: Transworld Research Network), 65–72.

Crenna, P., and Frigo, C. (1991). A motor program for the initiation of forward oriented movements in man. *J. Physiol.* 437, 635–653. doi: 10.1113/jphysiol. 1991.sp018616

Danielsson, A., and Sunnerhagen, K. S. (2004). Energy expenditure in stroke subjects walking with a carbon composite ankle foot orthosis. *J. Rehabil. Med.* 36, 165–168. doi: 10.1080/16501970410025126

Delafontaine, A., Honeine, J. L., Do, M. C., Gagey, O., and Chong, R. K. Y. (2015). Comparative gait initiation kinematics between simulated unilateral and bilateral ankle hypomobility: does bilateral constraint improve speed performance? *Neurosci. Lett.* 603, 55–59. doi: 10.1016/j.neulet.2015. 07.016

Demain, A., Westby, G. W., Fernandez-Vidal, S., Karachi, C., Bonneville, F., Do, M. C., et al. (2014). High-level gait and balance disorders in the elderly: a midbrain disease? *J. Neurol.* 261, 196–206. doi: 10.1007/s00415-013-7174-x

Eddison, N., and Chockalingam, N. (2013). The effect of tuning ankle foot orthoses-footwear combination on the gait parameters of children with cerebral palsy. *Prosthet. Orthot. Int.* 37, 95–107. doi: 10.1177/0309364612450706

Fatone, S., Gard, S. A., and Malas, B. S. (2009). Effect of ankle-foot orthosis alignment and foot-plate length on the gait of adults with poststroke hemiplegia. *Arch. Phys. Med. Rehabil.* 90, 810–818. doi: 10.1016/j.apmr.2008. 11.012

Ferris, D. P., Czerniecki, J. M., and Hannaford, B. (2005). An ankle-foot orthosis powered by artificial pneumatic muscles. *J. Appl. Biomech.* 21, 189–197. doi: 10.1123/jab.21.2.189

Feuerbach, J. W., Grabiner, M. D., Koh, T. J., and Weiker, G. G. (1994). Effect of an ankle orthosis and ankle ligament anesthesia on ankle joint proprioception. *Am. J. Sports Med.* 22, 223–229. doi: 10.1177/036354659402200212

Fuchs, S., Sandmann, C., Skwara, A., and Chylarecki, C. (2003). Quality of life 20 years after arthrodesis of the ankle. *J. Bone Joint Surg. Br.* 85, 994–998. doi: 10.1302/0301-620x.85b7.13984

Geboers, J. F., Drost, M. R., Spaans, F., Kuipers, H., and Seelen, H. A. (2002). Immediate and long-term effects of ankle-foot orthosis on muscle activity during walking: a randomized study of patients with unilateral foot drop. *Arch. Phys. Med. Rehabil.* 83, 240–245. doi: 10.1053/apmr.2002. 27462

Guillebastre, B., Calmels, P., and Rougier, P. (2009). Effects of rigid and dynamic ankle-foot orthoses on normal gait. *Foot Ankle Int.* 30, 51–56. doi: 10.3113/FAI. 2009.0051

Hesse, S., Reiter, F., Jahnke, M., Dawson, M., Sarkodie-Gyan, T., and Mauritz, K. H. (1997). Asymmetry of gait initiation in hemiparetic stroke subjects. *Arch. Phys. Med. Rehabil.* 78, 719–724. doi: 10.1016/s0003-9993(97)90079-4

Honeine, J. L., Schieppati, M., Crisafulli, O., and Do, M. C. (2016). The neuro-mechanical processes that underlie goal-directed medio-lateral APA during gait initiation. *Front. Hum. Neurosci.* 10:445. doi: 10.3389/fnhum.2016. 00445

Honeine, J. L., Schieppati, M., Gagey, O., and Do, M. C. (2013). The functional role of triceps surae muscle during human locomotion. *PLoS One* 8:e52943. doi: 10.1371/journal.pone.0052943

Honeine, J. L., Schieppati, M., Gagey, O., and Do, M. C. (2014). By counteracting gravity, triceps surae sets both kinematics and kinetics of gait. *Physiol. Rep.* 2:e00229. doi: 10.1002/phy2.229

Kerkum, Y. L., Brehm, M. A., Buizer, A. I., van den Noort, J. C., Becher, J. G., and Harlaar, J. (2014). Defining the mechanical properties of a spring-hinged ankle foot orthosis to assess its potential use in children with spastic cerebral palsy. *J. Appl. Biomech.* 30, 728–731. doi: 10.1123/jab.2014-0046

Kim, E. S., Yoon, Y.-S., Sohn, M. K., Kwak, S.-H., Choi, J. H., and Oh, J. S. (2015). Effect of pneumatic compressing powered orthosis in stroke patients: preliminary study. *Ann. Rehabil. Med.* 39, 226–233. doi: 10.5535/arm.2015.39. 2.226

Kuo, A. D. (2007). The six determinants of gait and the inverted pendulum analogy: a dynamic walking perspective. *Hum. Mov. Sci.* 26, 617–656. doi: 10.1016/j.humov.2007.04.003

Lepers, R., and Brenière, Y. (1995). The role of anticipatory postural adjustments and gravity in gait initiation. *Exp. Brain Res.* 107, 118–124. doi: 10.1007/bf00228023

Leung, J., and Moseley, A. (2003). Impact of ankle-foot orthoses on gait and leg muscle activity in adults with hemiplegia. *Physiotherapy* 89, 39–55. doi: 10.1016/s0031-9406(05)60668-2

Lucareli, P., Lima, M., Lucarelli, J., and Lima, F. (2007). Changes in joint kinematics in children with cerebral palsy while walking with and without a floor reaction ankle-foot orthosis. *Clinics (Sao Paulo)* 62, 63–68. doi: 10.1590/s1807-59322007000100010

Lyon, I. N., and Day, B. L. (1997). Control of frontal plane body motion in human stepping. *Exp. Brain Res.* 115, 345–356. doi: 10.1007/pl00005703

Merletti, R., and Hermens, J. (2000). Introduction to the special issue on the SENIAM european concerted action. *J. Electromyogr. Kinesiol.* 10, 283–286. doi: 10.1016/s1050-6411(00)00019-5

Michel, V., and Do, M. C. (2002). Are stance ankle plantar flexor muscles necessary to generate propulsive force during human gait initiation? *Neurosci. Lett.* 325, 139–143. doi: 10.1016/s0304-3940(02)00255-0

Mille, M. L., Simoneau, M., and Rogers, M. W. (2014). Postural dependence of human locomotion during gait initiation. *J. Neurophysiol.* 112, 3095–3103. doi: 10.1152/jn.00436.2014

Miyazaki, S., Yamamoto, S., and Kubota, T. (1997). Effect of ankle-foot orthoses on active ankle moment in patients with hemiparesis. *Med. Biol. Eng. Comput.* 35, 381–385. doi: 10.1007/bf02534094

Mouchnino, L., and Blouin, J. (2013). When standing on a moving support, cutaneous inputs provide sufficient information to plan the anticipatory postural adjustments for gait initiation. *PLoS One* 8:e55081. doi: 10.1371/journal.pone.0055081

Mulroy, S. J., Eberly, V. J., Gronely, J. K., Weiss, W., and Newsam, C. J. (2010). Effect of AFO design on walking after stroke: impact of ankle plantar flexion contracture. *Prosthet. Orthot. Int.* 34, 277–292. doi: 10.3109/03093646.2010. 501512

Nigg, B. M. (2001). The role of impact forces and foot pronation: a new paradigm. *Clin. J. Sport Med.* 11, 2–9. doi: 10.1097/00042752-200101000-00002

Ohata, K., Yasui, T., Tsuboyama, T., and Ichihashi, N. (2011). Effects of an ankle-foot orthosis with oil damper on muscle activity in adults after stroke. *Gait Posture* 33, 102–107. doi: 10.1016/j.gaitpost.2010.10.083

Petrucci, M. N., MacKinnon, C. D., and Hsiao-Wecksler, E. T. (2013). Modulation of anticipatory postural adjustments of gait using a portable powered ankle-foot orthosis. *IEEE Int. Conf. Rehabil. Robot.* 2013:6650450. doi: 10.1109/ICORR. 2013.6650450

Richie, D. H. Jr. (2007). Effects of foot orthoses on patients with chronic ankle instability. *J. Am. Podiatr. Med. Assoc.* 97, 19–30. doi: 10.7547/0970019

Rocchi, L., Carlson-Kuhta, P., Chiari, L., Burchiel, K. J., Hogarth, P., and Horak, F. B. (2012). Effects of deep brain stimulation in the subthalamic nucleus or globus pallidus internus on step initiation in Parkinson disease: laboratory investigation. *J. Neurosurg.* 117, 1141–1149. doi: 10.3171/2012.8. JNS112006

Ruget, H., Blouin, J., Coyle, T., and Mouchnino, L. (2010). Modulation of proprioceptive inflow when initiating a step influences postural adjustments. *Exp. Brain Res.* 201, 297–305. doi: 10.1007/s00221-009-2035-7

Ruget, H., Blouin, J., Teasdale, N., and Mouchnino, L. (2008). Can prepared anticipatory postural adjustments be updated by proprioception? *Neuroscience* 155, 640–648. doi: 10.1016/j.neuroscience.2008.06.021

Shorter, K. A., Xia, J., Hsiao-Wecksler, E. T., Durfee, W. K., and Kogler, G. F. (2013). Technologies for powered ankle-foot orthotic systems: possibilities and challenges. *IEEE/ASME Trans. Mechatronics.* 18, 337–347. doi: 10.1109/tmech. 2011.2174799

Svensson, W., and Holmberg, U. (2008). Ankle-foot-orthosis control in inclinations and stairs. *IEEE Int. Conf. Rehabil. Robot.* 2008, 301–306. doi: 10.1109/ramech.2008.4681479

Thoumie, P., Sautreuil, P., and Faucher, M. (2004). Evaluation des propriétés physiologiques des orthèses de cheville. Revue de littérature. *Ann. Readapt. Med. Phys.* 47, 225–232. doi: 10.1016/j.annrmp.2004.02.010

Wang, R. Y., Lin, P. Y., Lee, C. C., and Yang, Y. R. (2007). Gait and balance performance improvements attributable to ankle-foot orthosis in subjects with hemiparesis. *Am. J. Phys. Med. Rehabil.* 86, 556–562. doi: 10.1097/phm. 0b013e31806dd0d3

Welter, M. L., Do, M. C., Chastan, N., Torny, F., Bloch, F., du Montcel, S. T., et al. (2007). Control of vertical components of gait during initiation of walking in normal adults and patients with progressive supranuclear palsy. *Gait Posture* 26, 393–399. doi: 10.1016/j.gaitpost.2006.10.005

Wentink, E. C., Beijen, S. I., Hermens, H. J., Rietman, J. S., and Veltink, P. H. (2013). Intention detection of gait initiation using EMG and kinematic data. *Gait Posture* 37, 223–228. doi: 10.1016/j.gaitpost.2012.07.013

Winter, D. (1995). Human balance and posture control during standing and walking. *Gait Posture* 3, 193–214. doi: 10.1016/0966-6362(96) 82849-9

Yamamoto, S., Ebina, M., Kubo, S., Kawai, H., Hayashi, T., Iwasaki, M., et al. (1993). Quantification of the effect of dorsi-/ plantar flexibility of ankle-foot orthoses on hemiplegic gait: a preliminary report. *J. Prosthet. Orthot.* 5, 88–94. doi: 10.1097/00008526-199307000-00006

Yamamoto, S., Ebina, M., Miyazaki, S., Kawai, H., and Kubota, T. (1997). Development of a new ankle-foot orthosis with dorsiflexion assist, part 1: desirable characteristics of ankle-foot orthoses for hemiplegic patients. *J. Prosthet. Orthot.* 9, 174–179. doi: 10.1097/00008526-199700940-00009

Yiou, E., Artico, R., Teyssedre, C. A., Labaune, O., and Fourcade, P. (2016a). Anticipatory postural control of stability during gait initiation over obstacles of different height and distance made under reaction-time and self-initiated instructions. *Front. Hum. Neurosci.* 10:449. doi: 10.3389/fnhum.2016. 00449

Yiou, E., Teyssèdre, C., Artico, R., and Fourcade, P. (2016b). Comparison of base of support size during gait initiation using force-plate and motion-capture system: a Bland Altman analysis. *J. Biomech.* 49, 4168–4172. doi: 10.1016/j.jbiomech. 2016.11.008

Zou, D., He, T., Dailey, M., Smith, K. E., Silva, M. J., Sinacore, D. R., et al. (2014). Experimental and computational analysis of composite ankle-foot orthosis. *J. Rehabil. Res. Dev.* 51, 1525–1536. doi: 10.1682/JRRD.2014-02-0046

8

Short-Term Effects of Thoracic Spine Manipulation on the Biomechanical Organisation of Gait Initiation

Sébastien Ditcharles[1,2,3], Eric Yiou[1,2]*, Arnaud Delafontaine[1,2,3] and Alain Hamaoui[4,5]

[1]CIAMS, Université Paris-Sud, Université Paris-Saclay, Orsay, France, [2]CIAMS, Université d'Orléans, Orléans, France, [3]Ecole Nationale de Kinésithérapie et Rééducation (ENKRE), Saint-Maurice, France, [4]Laboratoire de Physiologie de la Posture et du Mouvement (PoM Lab), Université JF Champollion, Albi, France, [5]Laboratoire Activité Physique, Performance et Santé (MEPS), Université de Pau et des Pays de l'Adour (UPPA), Tarbes, France

Correspondence:
Eric Yiou
eric.yiou@u-psud.fr

Speed performance during gait initiation is known to be dependent on the capacity of the central nervous system to generate efficient anticipatory postural adjustments (APA). According to the posturo-kinetic capacity (PKC) concept, any factor enhancing postural chain mobility and especially spine mobility, may facilitate the development of APA and thus speed performance. "Spinal Manipulative Therapy High-Velocity, Low-Amplitude" (SMT-HVLA) is a healing technique applied to the spine which is routinely used by healthcare practitioners to improve spine mobility. As such, it may have a positive effect on the PKC and therefore facilitate gait initiation. The present study aimed to investigate the short-term effect of thoracic SMT-HVLA on spine mobility, APA and speed performance during gait initiation. Healthy young adults ($n = 22$) performed a series of gait initiation trials on a force plate *before* ("pre-manipulation" condition) and *after* ("post-manipulation" condition) a sham manipulation or an HVLA manipulation applied to the ninth thoracic vertebrae (T9). Participants were randomly assigned to the sham ($n = 11$) or the HVLA group ($n = 11$).The spine range of motion (ROM) was assessed in each participant immediately after the sham or HVLA manipulations using inclinometers. The results showed that the maximal thoracic flexion increased in the HVLA group after the manipulation, which was not the case in the sham group. In the HVLA group, results further showed that each of the following gait initiation variables reached a significantly lower mean value in the post-manipulation condition as compared to the pre-manipulation condition: APA duration, peak of anticipatory backward center of pressure displacement, center of gravity velocity at foot-off, mechanical efficiency of APA, peak of center of gravity velocity and step length. In contrast, for the sham group, results showed that none of the gait initiation variables significantly differed between the pre- and post-manipulation conditions. It is concluded that HVLA manipulation applied to T9 has an immediate beneficial effect on spine mobility but a detrimental effect on APA development and speed performance during gait initiation. We suggest that a neural effect induced by SMT-HVLA, possibly mediated by a transient alteration in the early sensory-motor integration, might have masked the potential mechanical benefits associated with increased spine mobility.

Keywords: anticipatory postural adjustments, gait initiation, spinal manipulation HVLA, T9 vertebrae, range of motion, posturo-kinetic capacity

INTRODUCTION

The coordination between posture and movement is known to be a key factor in motor performance. Gait initiation, which is the transient phase between quiet standing posture and ongoing walking, is a classical model used in the literature to investigate this coordination (e.g., Mann et al., 1979; Brenière et al., 1987; Yiou et al., 2007; Honeine et al., 2016). It is composed of a postural phase preceding the swing foot-off, which corresponds to the "anticipatory postural adjustments (APA)". The postural phase is followed by an execution phase ending when the peak of forward center of gravity (COG) velocity (or speed performance) is reached (Brenière et al., 1987; Lepers and Brenière, 1995). During these APA, the forward propulsive forces required to reach the peak COG velocity are generated by an anticipatory backward center of pressure (COP) shift. The larger this shift, the greater the speed performance (Brenière et al., 1987; Lepers and Brenière, 1995). The relationship between APA and speed performance during gait initiation illustrates the biomechanical concept of "Posturo-kinetic capacity (PKC)" (Bouisset and Zattara, 1987; Bouisset and Do, 2008), according to which the motor performance of any motor task (in terms of speed, force or precision) depends on the capacity of the central nervous system to generate appropriate APA. According to this concept, any factors that would impair (or conversely enhance) APA development may impair (or enhance) the motor performance. This PKC concept was substantiated by experimental studies which investigated the relationship between postural chain mobility, APA and motor performance during various motor tasks such as isometric ramp push (Le Bozec and Bouisset, 2004), pointing (Lino et al., 1992; Teyssèdre et al., 2000), and more recently, trunk flexion (Diakhaté et al., 2013) or sit-to-stand (Diakhaté et al., 2013; Alamini-Rodrigues and Hamaoui, 2016; Hamaoui and Alamini-Rodrigues, 2017a,b). In these studies, postural chain mobility was varied by changing the seat-thigh contact (Teyssèdre et al., 2000; Le Bozec and Bouisset, 2004; Diakhaté et al., 2013), by increasing the muscular tension along the torso (Hamaoui et al., 2004, 2011; Hamaoui and Le Bozec, 2014) or by restraining the spine mobility at different levels by means of splints (Alamini-Rodrigues and Hamaoui, 2016; Hamaoui and Alamini-Rodrigues, 2017a,b). These studies showed that the restriction of the postural chain mobility, and especially the spine mobility, has a negative influence on APA and motor performance. Conversely, according to the PKC concept, enhancing the postural chain mobility should have a positive influence on these parameters. Besides this purely mechanical influence, APA associated with stepping initiation are also known to be finely tuned to the continuous proprioceptive (Ruget et al., 2010) and cutaneous inflow (Do and Gilles, 1992; Ruget et al., 2008) arising from the postural body segments. Perturbations of this sensory inflow, e.g., by reducing the plantar support or by vibrating the ankle muscles, have been shown to alter APA and motor performance.

"Spinal Manipulative Therapy High-Velocity, Low-Amplitude" (SMT-HVLA) is a healing technique applied to the spine that has been used for centuries by healthcare practitioners including Osteopaths, Chiropractors and Physiotherapists to relieve symptomatic patients from acute and chronic low back/neck pain and/or to improve spine mobility (Wiese and Callender, 2005). As such, SMT-HVLA may have the potential to improve the PKC and thus motor performance. As stressed in the literature (e.g., the review of Pickar and Bolton, 2012), a number of sustained changes in the spinal biomechanics have been thought to occur as a result of SMT-HVLA. For example, the impulsive thrust delivered during the manipulation may alter the segmental biomechanics by releasing trapped meniscoïds, releasing adhesions, or by diminishing distortion in the intervertebral disc. In addition, recent studies reported relaxation of paraspinal muscles following SMT-HVLA as revealed with decreased electromyographic (EMG) activity (DeVocht et al., 2005; Lehman, 2012). Increased spine mobility might result from such changes in the spinal biomechanics and/or EMG activity. Interestingly, this technique is nowadays widely used by healthy athletes (runners, footballers, sprinters etc.) just before a competition in order to reach their "peak performance" (Leonardi, 1994). However, it must be noted that the effect of SMT-HVLA on the articular free play is still controversial (for review see Millan et al., 2012a), with mitigated results on sports performance (Miners, 2010). Shrier et al. (2006) compared jump height and running velocity with and without pre-event SMT-HVLA in elite healthy athletes. These authors found that there was no significant effect of SMT-HVLA on the countermovement jump height and sprint times. However, they also stressed that the direction and magnitude of the observed changes were consistent with a clinically relevant performance enhancement. A similar conclusion was stated by Humphries et al. (2013) with regard to the immediate effect of lower cervical spine manipulation on handgrip strength and free-throw accuracy of asymptomatic basketball players. These authors reported a slight increase in free-throw percentage, which according to them, deserved further investigation.

Besides the potential increase in spine mobility, movement kinematics may also be potentially influenced by neurophysiological changes induced by SMT-HVLA. For example, studies on the anesthetized cat have shown that spinal manipulation induced changes in the discharge of somatosensory afferents from the paraspinal region (Pickar, 2002; Pickar and Bolton, 2012; Reed et al., 2015), including those afferents innervating muscle spindles, Golgi Tendon Organs and high threshold mechanoreceptors. There are currently no unequivocal data regarding whether SMT-HVLA activates nociceptors. In humans, changes in the sensori-motor pathways following SMT-HVLA have been reported in the literature, but with sometimes contradictory results. For example, studies using the Hoffman reflex (H-reflex) technique indicated that spinal manipulation induced a decreased motoneuronal excitability in asymptomatic subjects (Murphy et al., 1995; Dishman and Burke, 2003) and in low back pain patients (Suter et al., 2005), while Niazi et al. (2015) indicated, on the contrary, an increased excitability. Data collection and data analysis methodology of the H-reflex have been evoked by these latter authors to explain this discrepancy with the literature. At the cortical level, it seems that there exists a consensus concerning the alteration of the sensorimotor processing and sensorimotor integration following spinal manipulation, as evidenced with the somatosensory-evoked potential technique (e.g., Haavik-Taylor and Murphy, 2007; Taylor and Murphy, 2008; Haavik Taylor and Murphy, 2010; see "Discussion" Section on this aspect).

As stressed in the literature (e.g., Pickar and Bolton, 2012), the extent to which these mechanical and neurophysiological responses to spinal manipulation reflect beneficial outcomes (e.g., pain relief or enhanced spine mobility) remains unclear. However, each of these responses has the potential to induce changes in the coordination between posture and movement, which strongly relies on both sensory inputs from the postural limbs and postural joint mobility as stressed above. The present study, therefore, aimed to investigate the short-term effect of SMT-HVLA on spine mobility, APA and speed performance during gait initiation in young healthy adults. We first hypothesized that a SMT-HVLA applied to the ninth thoracic vertebra (T9) will increase the spine range of motion and facilitate APA development in the gait initiation paradigm, which is known to involve spine mobility (e.g., Ceccato et al., 2009). Second, we also assumed that the various short-term neurological effects of this manipulation may either improve or reduce the PKC and task performance.

MATERIALS AND METHODS

Subjects

The study was a randomized investigation that included 22 right-handed young healthy adults. The non-probability convenience method was used, i.e., participants were randomly assigned to one of the two following groups using the envelope method (**Figure 1**): 11 participants (six female, five male; 28 ± 4 years [mean ± SD]; 64 ± 8 kg; 169 ± 8 cm) were assigned to the HVLA group and eleven participants (five female, six male; 29 ± 4 years; 63 ± 8 kg; 170 ± 8 cm) to the sham group. Participants were blinded to their group allocation. They had no known contraindications to spinal manipulation such as recent history of trauma, known metabolic disorders, inflammatory infectious arthropathies, or bone malignancies. None of them suffered from back pain during the experiment or have suffered in the past months. In addition, participants were all naïve about SMT-HVLA manipulation. They all gave written consent after having been informed of the nature and purpose of the experiment which was approved by local ethics committees from the CIAMS Research Unit, Equipe d'Accueil (EA) 4532. The study complied with the standards established by the Declaration of Helsinki. Our study was assigned the following trial registration number: 2017-002389-34.

Experimental Task and Conditions

All experiments took place in the Biomechanics laboratory of the Paris Saclay University which is located within the Kremlin Bicêtre Hospital (Paris, France). Physical conditions (room temperature and time of the day) were common to all

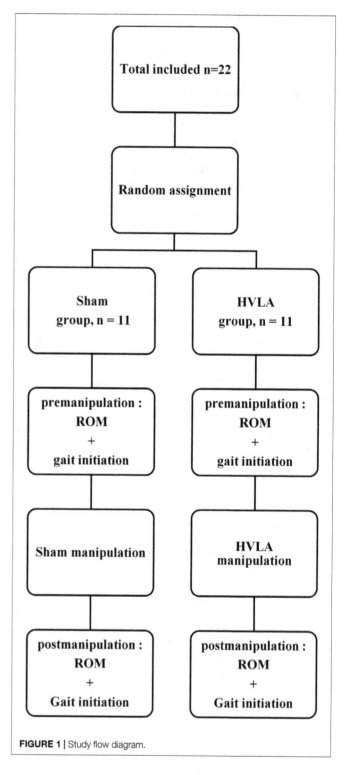

FIGURE 1 | Study flow diagram.

treatment groups (see below), and also constant before/after the manipulation.

Participants initially stood barefoot in a natural upright posture on a force plate embedded at the beginning of a 6 m walkway track. The feet were shoulder-width apart, with the arms alongside the trunk and the gaze directed forward to a small target at eye level and out of reach (2 cm diameter, 5 m distant). The locations of the heel and big toe of each foot in the initial posture were marked with sections of adhesive tape placed on the force plate and were used as a visual reference on which participants positioned themselves under the supervision of the experimenters. From the initial posture, participants performed two series of ten gait initiation trials: one just before, and a second one immediately after a specific manipulation (pre- and post-manipulation conditions, respectively) depending on their group (HVLA or sham). All ten trials within each condition were averaged. In these two conditions, participants initiated gait at a spontaneous velocity and at their own initiative following an auditory signal delivered by the experimenter, and then continued walking straight until the end of the track. Participants initiated gait with their preferred leg in all trials. One blank trial was provided in the pre-manipulation condition (not recorded) to ensure that the instructions were well understood by the participant and that the material was operational. The rest time was approximately 10 s between trials. The Range of Motion (ROM) of the thoracic spine was assessed (see description below) for each participant in the HVLA and sham groups immediately before and after the HVLA or sham manipulations (see description below), respectively.

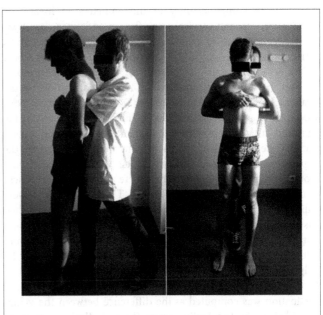

FIGURE 2 | Profile (left) and front (right) views of the participant's and the practitioner's initial postures in the sham and HVLA manipulations. The written informed consent was obtained from the participants depicted in the images.

HVLA and Sham Manipulations

The HVLA and sham manipulations complied with the 2016 Consensus on Interventions Reporting Criteria List for Spinal Manipulative Therapy (CIRCLE SMT; Groeneweg et al., 2017). Both manipulation procedures were performed by one of the authors of the present study, an experienced professional physiotherapist and osteopath practitioner with 10 years of clinical experience in his own practice. The practitioner is also a teacher at the Ecole Nationale de Kinésithérapie et Rééducation (France). He has received extensive training in the study protocols and was certified for both thoracic lift manipulation and sham procedure by simulating multiple study visit scenarios overseen by research team members.

SMT-HVLA was applied to the ninth thoracic vertebra (T9) since this vertebra is described as the "walking vertebra", a concept arising from the classical article of Wernham (1985). This concept is based on the fact that the T9 vertebra is the inflexion point of the curvature change of thoracic cyphosis in lumbar lordosis. This vertebra ensures the junction between the thoracic and lumbar segments, mainly in their counter-rotation movement, especially during walking. In this plane, the center of rotation between the thoracic and the pelvic belts is presumably positioned between L3 and T7 (Konz et al., 2006).

In the HVLA group, the spinous process of the ninth thoracic vertebrae (T9) of the participant was identified by the practitioner and was marked with a pen. The participant stood upright with the hands positioned on the transverse processes of the selected vertebra with palms facing the back. The practitioner stood behind him/her with the front foot positioned between the participant's feet. The practitioner circled the participant's trunk by passing his arms under his/her armpits, and his chest was in contact with the palms of the participant's hands. From this posture, he applied a single manual rapid horizontal pressure to the T9 vertebrae, followed by a single rapid vertical traction of the vertebral column. This technique corresponds to the standing thoracic "lift-off" technique. Before the manipulation, the practitioner systematically informed the participant that the sound of a cavitation was not a sign of success, and after the manipulation, that the manipulation was successful.

In the sham group, the experimental protocol was exactly the same as in the HVLA group with regard to the T9 marking, the initial/final postures, and the information given to the participant on the efficacy of the manipulation (positive verbal reinforcement). This guaranteed the blindness of participants with respect to their group allocation. Only the manipulation differed between the two groups. The manipulation used in the sham group corresponded to the "light touch methodology" validated by the North Texas Chronic Low Pain Trial (Licciardone et al., 2013). In this manipulation, the practitioner did not apply any compression or traction of the vertebral column but solely maintained the above-described posture with the participant for 10 s.

The HVLA and sham manipulations took place beside the force plate to ensure minimal time between the end of the manipulation procedure and the beginning of the first gait initiation trial of the post-manipulation condition. A brief overview of the practitioner's and the participant's postures adopted for the manipulations is provided in **Figure 2**.

Evaluation of Spine ROM

Spine ROM was evaluated before the series of gait initiation trials in the pre- and post-manipulation conditions (**Figure 1**). Two inclinometers (Bubble® Inclinometer, Fabrication Enterprises, White Plains, NY, USA) were used to evaluate spine ROM.

The reliability and accuracy of inclinometers in measuring lumbar lordosis and cervical spine flexion and extension ROM have been assessed in previous studies (Lewis and Valentine, 2010; Garmabi et al., 2012). The measurement of the spine ROM was conducted according to the standard protocol set out in the American Medical Association guide to the evaluation of permanent impairment (Doege and Houston, 1993; Cocchiarela and Andersson, 2001). The spinous process of the first and last thoracic vertebrae (T1 and T12) and the second sacral vertebrae (S2) of the participant were identified by the experimenter and marked with a pen while the participant stood upright. The inclinometers were then placed on these marks two by two (T1 and T12 or T12 and S2) and were calibrated to zero in this position. The participant was then instructed to perform maximum trunk flexion and extension with legs stretched. Each movement was repeated two times with the inclinometer positioned at T1/T12 then at T12/S2 (**Figure 3**). The mean ROM value obtained in these two trials was computed. For each movement direction, trunk inclination was computed as the difference between the values provided by the two inclinometers (thoracic flexion/extension: T1/T12; lumbar flexion/extension: T12/S2). The thoraco-lumbar flexion and extension were calculated from the sum of the thoracic and lumbar values in flexion and extension, respectively.

Materials

External forces and moments applied to the participants were recorded from a force plate (600 × 1200 mm, AMTI, Watertown, MA, USA). Before analysis, the force-plate signals were filtered using a low-pass Butterworth filter with a 10 Hz cutoff frequency (Caderby et al., 2017). Biomechanical data were sampled at 500 Hz and stored on a hard disk for off-line analysis. Data acquisition and stimulus display were controlled by a custom-made program written in Matlab^{TM} (R2009b, The MathWorks Inc., Natick, MA, USA). Only the postural dynamics along the anteroposterior axis were considered in the present study as we were mainly interested in the speed performance of gait initiation. Instantaneous COG acceleration was obtained with the ratio [ground reaction forces/subject's mass] following Newton's second law ($\Sigma F = m\gamma$, where ΣF, the sum of external forces applied to the whole body; m, body mass; γ, COG acceleration). The COG velocity was obtained through simple integration of the COG acceleration trace. The instantaneous COP displacement (xP) was computed using the formula:

$$xP = \frac{-My + Fx \times dz}{Fz}$$

where My, Fx, Fz are the moment around the mediolateral axis, the anteroposterior and vertical ground reaction forces, respectively; dz is the distance between the surface of the force plate and its origin, located at the center of the force plate.

Swing toe-off (TO) and foot-contact (FC) instants were detected with force plate data (Caderby et al., 2013) and with foot switches (Force Sensing Resistor, 1 cm^2 surface, Biometrics, France) affixed under the heel and big toe of the swing foot.

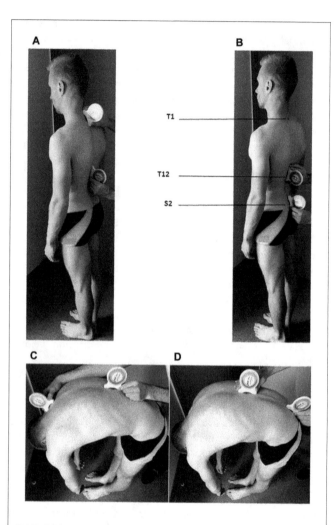

FIGURE 3 | Positioning of the two inclinometers for the evaluation of the spine range of motion. **(A)** Inclinometers are positioned over the spinous process of the first and last thoracic vertebrae (T1 and T12, respectively) and are calibrated in this position for the evaluation of the maximal thoracic flexion **(C)**. **(B)** Inclinometers are positioned over T12 and the spinous process of the second sacral vertebrae (S2) and are calibrated in this position for the evaluation of the maximal lumbar flexion **(D)**. The written informed consent was obtained from the participants depicted in the images.

The "biomechanical traces" (see **Figure 4**) will refer to the COP displacement and COG velocity traces obtained from the force plate recordings.

Gait Initiation Variables

Data acquisition was triggered 200 ms prior to the auditory signal, which allowed *post hoc* calculation of the COP position in the initial posture. The anteroposterior component of the COP initial position was computed as the mean COP value obtained during these 200 ms. APA duration corresponded to the time between the onset rise of the COP trace to the time of swing TO (e.g., Yiou et al., 2011; Delafontaine et al., 2015). The APA onset was detected when the COP trace deviated 2.5 standard deviations from its baseline value (e.g., Caderby et al., 2017). APA amplitude was estimated with

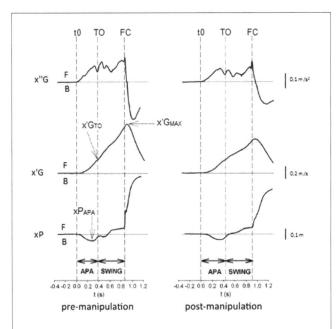

FIGURE 4 | Biomechanical profiles of gait initiation in the pre- and post-manipulation conditions in one representative participant of the HVLA group. x"G, x'G, xP: anteroposterior center of gravity (COG) acceleration, COG velocity, and center of pressure (COP) displacement, respectively. t0, TOT, foot-contact (FC): onset rise of x"G trace, swing toe-off (TO) and swing FC. Anticipatory postural adjustments (APA), SWING: APA and swing phase. x'G$_{MAX}$, x'G$_{TOT}$, xP$_{APA}$: peak of COG velocity, COG velocity at TO, peak of anticipatory backward COP displacement. F: forward displacement, velocity or acceleration, B: backward displacement, velocity or acceleration.

the forward COG velocity at the TO time and with the maximal backward COP displacement during APA (**Figure 4**). Swing phase duration corresponded to the time between swing TO and swing FC. Step motor performance (speed performance) was quantified with the maximal COG velocity. Step length corresponded to distance between the peak backward COP position obtained during the APA and the COP position at the time of the rear TO (Yiou et al., 2016). Finally, the mechanical efficiency of the APA was quantified with the ratio [COG velocity at TO/APA duration] (Yiou et al., 2011). It is assumed that the greater this ratio, the greater the mechanical efficiency.

The experimenter who analyzed the data and performed the ROM measures (pre and post treatment) was different from the practitioner and was blinded to the treatment group so as to ensure absence of expectation bias and optimize the reliability of the test procedure.

Statistics

Mean values and standard deviations of ROM and gait initiation variables were computed in each condition for all subjects. The normality of data was checked using the Kolmogorov-Smirnov test and the homogeneity of variances was checked using the Bartlett test. A 2 × 2 mixed-model analysis of variance (ANOVA) was used, with GROUP (HVLA vs. sham) as the between-subject factor and CONDITION (pre-manipulation

vs. post-manipulation) as the within-subject factor. For each ANOVA, the hypothesis of interest was the 2-way-interaction (GROUP × CONDITION). Significant outcomes were followed up with the Tukey *post hoc* test. In addition, the participants' anthropometrical characteristics were compared between groups using independent Student's *t*-tests for continuous data, and chi-square tests of independence were used for categorical data to evaluate the adequacy of the randomization. The level of statistical significance was set at alpha = 0.05. Data analysis was performed using Statistica 12, statsoft®.

RESULTS

Anthropometrical Characteristics of Participants

Participants were randomly assigned to the sham or HVLA groups. Their anthropometrical characteristics are reported in **Table 1**. Statistical analysis showed that the two groups were homogenous in terms of mean age, gender, height and weight.

Comparison of Spine ROM between Groups and Conditions

The results showed that there was no significant main effect of GROUP, CONDITION or GROUP × CONDITION interaction on any of the spine ROM values, except on the thoracic flexion. For this variable, there was a significant main effect of GROUP ($F_{(1,21)} = 4.53, p < 0.05$), CONDITION ($F_{(1,21)} = 15.73, p < 0.01$) and GROUP × CONDITION interaction ($F_{(1,21)} = 14.55, p < 0.01$). For the HVLA group, the *post hoc* analysis further indicated that this variable was significantly larger in the post-manipulation condition (mean value: 24 ± 12°) than in the pre-manipulation condition (20 ± 12°) ($p < 0.05$). In contrast, for the sham group, it was not significantly different. Finally, it is noteworthy that there was no significant difference in any of the spine ROM values (including the thoracic flexion) between the HVLA and the sham group in the pre-manipulation condition. The spine mobility was therefore equivalent between the two groups before the manipulation.

Description of Typical Biomechanical Traces Obtained during Gait Initiation

The time-course of the biomechanical traces obtained during gait initiation was globally similar in the pre- and the post-manipulation condition for both the HVLA and sham groups. As classically reported in the literature, the swing TO was

TABLE 1 | Anthropometrical characteristics of participants.

	HVLA group (*n* = 11)	Sham group (*n* = 11)	P Value
Age (years)	28 ± 4	29 ± 4	0.633[†] NS
Gender	Females 6	Females 5	0.670[‡] NS
	Males 5	Males 6	
Height (cm)	169 ± 8	170 ± 8	0.913[†] NS
Weight (kg)	64 ± 8	63 ± 8	0.815[†] NS

Values given are means ± 1 standard deviation, except for gender; [†]Independent samples t test; [‡]Chi-square test. NS: non-significant difference.

systematically preceded by dynamic phenomena corresponding to APA (**Figure 4**). These APA included the backward COP displacement along with the forward COG acceleration. The COG velocity increased progressively until it reached a maximum value a few milliseconds after the time of swing FC.

Comparison of Gait Initiation Variables between Groups and Conditions

The results showed that there was a significant main effect of GROUP on every gait initiation variables investigated in this study, i.e., APA duration ($F_{(1,21)} = 6.25$, $p < 0.01$), peak of anticipatory backward COP displacement ($F_{(1,21)} = 19.07$, $p < 0.001$), COG velocity at TO ($F_{(1,21)} = 6.92$, $p < 0.01$), mechanical efficiency of APA ($F_{(1,21)} = 10.05$, $p < 0.01$), peak COG velocity ($F_{(1,21)} = 19.75$, $p < 0.001$), step length ($F_{(1,21)} = 11.81$, $p < 0.001$) and swing phase duration ($F_{(1,21)} = 5.87, p < 0.01$). In addition, there was a significant main effect of CONDITION on each of the following variables: APA duration ($F_{(1,21)} = 3.95, p < 0.05$), peak of anticipatory backward COP displacement ($F_{(1,21)} = 19.73, p < 0.001$), COG velocity at TO ($F_{(1,21)} = 12.40, p < 0.001$), mechanical efficiency of APA ($F_{(1,21)} = 9.39, p < 0.01$), peak COG velocity ($F_{(1,21)} = 12.04$, $p < 0.001$) step length ($F_{(1,21)} = 22.22, p < 0.001$) and swing phase duration ($F_{(1,21)} = 2.39, p < 0.05$). Finally, there was a significant GROUP X CONDITION interaction on each of the following variables: APA duration ($F_{(1,21)} = 2.92, p < 0.05$),

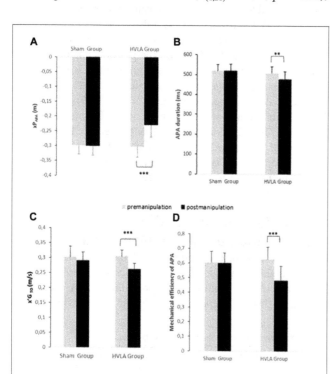

FIGURE 5 | Comparison of APAs related variables between the pre- and post-manipulation conditions in the sham and HVLA groups. **(A)** xP$_{APA}$: peak of anticipatory backward center of pressure displacement, **(B)** APA duration, **(C)** x'G$_{TOT}$: center of gravity velocity at TO and **(D)** mechanical efficiency of APAs. **, *** Statistical difference with $p < 0.01$, $p < 0.001$, respectively. Values given are means ± 1 standard error.

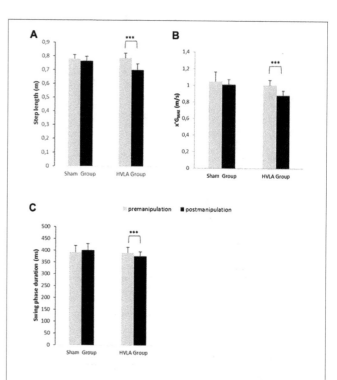

FIGURE 6 | Comparison of swing phase-related parameters of gait initiation between the pre- and post-manipulation conditions in the sham and HVLA groups. **(A)** Step length, **(B)** x'G$_{MAX}$: peak center of gravity velocity and **(C)** swing phase duration. *** Statistical difference with $p < 0.01$, $p < 0.001$, respectively. Values given are means ± 1 standard error.

peak of anticipatory backward COP displacement ($F_{(1,21)} = 11.92$, $p < 0.01$), COG velocity at TO ($F_{(1,21)} = 4.22$, $p < 0.05$), mechanical efficiency of APA ($F_{(1,21)} = 8.51, p < 0.01$), peak COG velocity ($F_{(1,21)} = = 3.27, p < 0.05$), step length ($F_{(1,21)} = 9.66$, $p < 0.01$) and swing phase duration ($F_{(1,21)} = 6.29, p < 0.05$).

The *post hoc* analysis further indicated that, for the HVLA group, each of the gait initiation variables investigated in this study was significantly lower in the post-manipulation condition than in the pre-manipulation condition (see **Figures 5, 6** for details on the *post hoc* analysis). In contrast, regarding the sham group, none of these variables significantly differed between the pre- and post-manipulation condition. Finally, it is noteworthy that none of the gait initiation variables significantly differed between the sham and the HVLA groups in the pre-manipulation condition. The two groups were therefore homogeneous with respect to these variables before the manipulation.

DISCUSSION

This study investigated the effect of SMT-HVLA manipulation applied to T9 on spine ROM and on the biomechanical organisation of gait initiation. Participants purposely performed series of gait initiation trials before and after sham or SMT-HVLA manipulations. Spine ROM and classical biomechanical gait initiation parameters were compared in the pre- and post-manipulation conditions.

The results showed that the spine ROM, and especially the maximal thoracic flexion, was larger post-manipulation than pre-manipulation in the HVLA group, which was not the case in the sham group. The mean increase was 20%. The HVLA manipulation applied to T9 had, therefore, a beneficial effect on spine mobility, even in a group composed of young adults with no known spine pathologies. A similar result was found in the sole study to date that tested the effect of thoracic HVLA manipulation on spine ROM (Schiller, 2001). However, this study only examined right and left thoracic lateral flexion using a goniometer (BROM 2), and the population tested included patients with thoracic back pain. To our knowledge, the other studies focusing on thoracic HVLA measured the cervical ROM, and reported small or no beneficial effects (González-Iglesias et al., 2009; Suvarnnato et al., 2013). These negligible variations have led us to exclude the cervical section from spine ROM measurement.

SMT-HVLA has been shown to have a beneficial effect on spine-related pain, both clinically and in experimentally-induced pain (for reviews see Millan et al., 2012a,b). However, it remains unclear from the literature if it has an immediate noticeable biomechanical effect on spinal motion that can be measured in terms of an increased ROM (Millan et al., 2012a). One of the main goals of healthcare practitioners applying SMT-HVLA manipulation is to increase spine ROM, e.g., in athletes before competition or in patients with spine stiffness. A recent review on this aspect emphasized that some studies found spinal manipulation to have limited effect on the ROM, while others found it had none (Millan et al., 2012a). These mitigated effects could probably stem from many factors such as the different tools used in research and in clinical practice to measure ROM (single/double/triple inclinometers, goniometers, a rangiometer, tape measures, visual estimation, spine motion analyzer, etc.), the direction, duration and force applied to the participant's spine, the expertise of the practitioner etc. The present study shows that analogical inclinometers may be used to detect an increased spine ROM following thoracic SMT-HVLA.

Postural mobility, and especially spine mobility, is known to be a key factor of the PKC (Bouisset and Zattara, 1987; Bouisset and Do, 2008). According to the PKC concept, any factor that may enhance (or conversely, alter) this capacity would favor (or hinder) the motor performance and postural stability. This concept has been substantiated by many recent experimental studies which manipulated spine mobility using various means, e.g., by the application of splints at different levels of the spine (Alamini-Rodrigues and Hamaoui, 2016), by experimentally-induced trunk muscular tension (Hamaoui et al., 2004, 2011; Hamaoui and Le Bozec, 2014), or by changing the contact surface between the thighs and seat in the sitting posture (Lino et al., 1992; Teyssèdre et al., 2000; Le Bozec and Bouisset, 2004; Diakhaté et al., 2013). It has been shown that constraining spine mobility may disturb postural equilibrium when maintaining erect posture as revealed by measuring the COP. In dynamical tasks, such as sit-to-stand (Diakhaté et al., 2013; Alamini-Rodrigues and Hamaoui, 2016), maximal

isometric ramp push (Le Bozec and Bouisset, 2004), arm pointing (Lino et al., 1992; Teyssèdre et al., 2000) or trunk flexion (Diakhaté et al., 2013) from the sitting posture, facilitating spine mobility has been shown to favor APA development and thus motor performance. Based on the results of these studies—and given that spine mobility is known to be highly solicited during locomotion and gait initiation (e.g., Thorstensson et al., 1984; Ceccato et al., 2009; Cusin et al., 2017), APA development and motor performance could have been expected to be facilitated following SMT-HVLA. It is also noteworthy that T9 is described as the "walking vertebra", a concept arising from the classical article of Wernham (1985). This concept is based on the fact that the T9 vertebra is the inflexion point of the curvature change of thoracic cyphosis in lumbar lordosis. This vertebra ensures the junction of the thoracic and lumbar segments, mainly in their counter-rotation movement, especially while walking. As such, the T9 HVLA manipulation is commonly used by healthcare practitioners in patients with locomotor deficiencies. However, its impact on the locomotor function has to date never been evaluated in systematic studies. In contrast to our expectations, APA amplitude and duration decreased following manipulation in the HVLA group, by 24% and 6%, respectively. This was not the case in the sham group, which shows that this result could not be ascribed to a placebo effect. Not only were the APA parameters reduced, but their efficiency (computed as the ratio [COG velocity at foot-off/APA duration]) was reduced (by 23% as compared to the pre-manipulation condition). In other words, the capacity of the postural system to generate forward propulsive forces during the limited duration of APA was less efficient post-manipulation. As a consequence of the lower initial (foot-off) COG velocity, the peak COG velocity (speed performance) and step length both reached lower values post-manipulation in the HVLA group (compared to the pre-manipulation condition, the decrease was 14%, 12% and 11%, respectively). This finding was expected since it is well-known that the two latter step parameters are positively correlated with the amplitude of APA, i.e., the higher the peak anticipatory backward COP shift is, the higher the speed performance and step lengths are (Brenière et al., 1987). Because there was no change in APA parameters post-manipulation in the sham group, step length and speed performance remained the same as in the pre-manipulation condition. Because in the present study, spine mobility was increased following the HVLA manipulation, which is known to be a factor of improved motor performance, the question arises as to why APA development and speed performance were impaired instead of being improved.

Besides its mechanical effect on spine mobility (for reviews see Pickar, 2002; Millan et al., 2012a), SMT-HVLA is known to induce transient changes in the sensorimotor pathways and structures involved in the coordination between posture and movement. As stressed in the "Introduction" Section, studies using the H-reflex technique to investigate the effect of SMT-HVLA on motoneuronal excitability reported controversial findings, i.e., both an increased (Niazi et al., 2015) and a decreased excitability (Murphy et al., 1995; Dishman and Burke, 2003; Suter et al., 2005) have been found. It seems however that there exists a consensus concerning the effects of spinal manipulation on the sensorimotor processing and integration at the cortical level, as evidenced with the somatosensory evoked potential technique (SEP). Specifically, recent studies reported an alteration of the amplitude of the cortical SEP peaks N20 and N30 following SMT-HVLA (Haavik and Murphy, 2012; Lelic et al., 2016). The N20 peak is known to represent the arrival of the afferent volley at the primary somatosensory cortex (Desmedt and Cheron, 1980; Nuwer et al., 1994; Mauguière, 1999), while later peaks such as the N30 SEP peak are thought to reflect early sensory-motor integration (Rossi et al., 2003; regarding the possible generators of this peak, see Haavik and Murphy, 2012; Lelic et al., 2016). In addition, studies in the anesthetized cat have shown that spinal manipulation induced changes in the discharge of mechanoreceptors from the paraspinal region, especially group Ia spindle afferents (Pickar, 2002; Reed et al., 2015). The extent to which the cortical and afferent responses to spinal manipulation reflect beneficial outcomes (e.g., pain relief), remains largely unclear in the literature; however, what is clear, is that these responses have the potential to induce changes in the coordination between posture and movement, which is known to strongly rely on proprioceptive inputs from the postural limbs, and even more importantly, on how the CNS processes, interprets and transforms this afferent information into motor commands (Paulus and Brumagne, 2008; Haavik and Murphy, 2012). Lelic et al. (2016) recently speculated that since spinal manipulation is known to reduce pain and improve function in clinical trials (Botelho and Andrade, 2012; Mieritz et al., 2014; Schneider et al., 2015), the observed reduction of the N30 amplitude following SMT-HVLA may reflect a beneficial change. However, it should be noted (as the authors did) that reduced N30 SEP peak amplitudes have also been found in the literature in pathological populations such as Parkinson's disease (Cheron et al., 1994; Kang and Ma, 2016), known to have deficits in APA production during both voluntary lower (e.g., Delval et al., 2014) and upper limb tasks (e.g., Bazalgette et al., 1987). Kang and Ma (2016) even reported that frontal N30 status indicated the motor severity of Parkinson's disease. During gait initiation, disturbances in Parkinson's disease include reduced APA and abnormal APA timing (Delval et al., 2014). During arm elevation, postural movements are known to be less anticipatory in Parkinson's patients than in controls (Bazalgette et al., 1987). In the present study, APA were also less anticipatory, had a smaller amplitude and were less efficient in the HVLA group following manipulation than prior to manipulation. Globally taken, the results from the literature may thus suggest that a reduction of the N30 amplitude after HVLA manipulation may reflect a transitory alteration in the cortical integration of sensory-motor information, and may thus reflect a negative change. If so, such alteration has the potential to affect motor coordination during locomotor tasks such as gait initiation. In other words, we propose that a neural effect, possibly mediated by a transient alteration in the early sensory-motor integration following SMT-HVLA could be one of the mechanisms responsible for the present results. This neural effect may have masked the potential mechanical benefits associated with increased spine mobility.

STUDY LIMITATIONS

There are some limitations to the present study that should be pointed out. First, this study only focused on a biomechanical investigation. It is clear that studies linking the changes in motor behavior observed in the present study, to the changes of activity in the neural structures and pathways reported in the literature should be carried out to further substantiate the data interpretation. This is why we used the term "pilot" in the title of this article. Second, it should be emphasized that only short-term effects were investigated. It is not excluded that thoracic HVLA manipulation may have a long-term beneficial effect on APA and speed performance. Third, the biomechanical responses described in this study were obtained from young healthy participants and may not be generalizable to other populations, including patients with spinal pain. Finally, it is known that a manipulation is rarely specific to only the adjustment site (Ross et al., 2004). This non-specificity is amplified by the technique used in this article as it is an indirect technique. There is no direct contact of the practitioner with the chosen vertebra since the compressive force is indirectly transmitted by the hand of the patient between his own vertebrae and the thorax of the practitioner. We point out that the role of T9 vertebra and the interest of its manipulation is based solely on empirical knowledge although these notions are still taught in physiotherapy and osteopathy schools. Currently, some studies suggest that the center of rotation of the thoracic zone in the horizontal plane corresponds to a very wide area (T7–L3; Konz et al., 2006).

CONCLUSION

The present results showed that thoracic HVLA manipulation in young healthy participants has an immediate beneficial effect on spine mobility but a detrimental effect on APA development and speed performance during gait initiation. It thus seems that HVLA manipulation should be considered with caution by participants who seek an immediate increase of speed performance during locomotor tasks.

AUTHOR CONTRIBUTIONS

SD and EY designed the study; collected, analyzed and interpreted the data; drafted and revised the manuscript; gave final approval. AH and AD interpreted the data; drafted and revised the manuscript.

FUNDING

This research was funded by the French Government.

ACKNOWLEDGMENTS

We greatly thank the two reviewers for scrutinizing our manuscript and for their relevant comments.

REFERENCES

Alamini-Rodrigues, C., and Hamaoui, A. (2016). Effect of three different lumbar splints on posturokinetic capacity when performing the sit-to-stand task. *Ann. Phys. Rehabil. Med.* doi: 10.1016/j.rehab.2016.09.003 [Epub ahead of print].

Bazalgette, D., Zattara, M., Bathien, N., Bouisset, S., and Rondot, P. (1987). Postural adjustments associated with rapid voluntary arm movements in patients with Parkinson's disease. *Adv. Neurol.* 45, 371–374.

Botelho, M. B., and Andrade, B. B. (2012). Effect of cervical spine manipulative therapy on judo athletes' grip strength. *J. Manipulative Physiol. Ther.* 35, 38–44. doi: 10.1016/j.jmpt.2011.09.005

Bouisset, S., and Do, M.-C. (2008). Posture, dynamic stability and voluntary movement. *Neurophysiol. Clin.* 38, 345–362. doi: 10.1016/j.neucli.2008.10.001

Bouisset, S., and Zattara, M. (1987). Biomechanical study of the programming of anticipatory postural adjustments associated with voluntary movement. *J. Biomech.* 20, 735–742.

Brenière, Y., Cuong Do, M., and Bouisset, S. (1987). Are dynamic phenomena prior to stepping essential to walking? *J. Mot. Behav.* 19, 62–76. doi: 10.1080/00222895.1987.10735400

Caderby, T., Yiou, E., Peyrot, N., de Viviés, X., Bonazzi, B., and Dalleau, G. (2017). Effects of changing body weight distribution on mediolateral stability control during gait initiation. *Front. Hum. Neurosci.* 11:127. doi: 10.3389/fnhum.2017.00127

Caderby, T., Yiou, E., Peyrot, N., Bonazzi, B., and Dalleau, G. (2013). Detection of swing heel-off event in gait initiation using force-plate data. *Gait Posture* 37, 463–466. doi: 10.1016/j.gaitpost.2012.08.011

Ceccato, J.-C., de Sèze, M., Azevedo, C., and Cazalets, J.-R. (2009). Comparison of trunk activity during gait initiation and walking in humans. *PLoS One* 4:e8193. doi: 10.1371/journal.pone.0008193

Cheron, G., Piette, T., Thiriaux, A., Jacquy, J., and Godaux, E. (1994). Somatosensory evoked potentials at rest and during movement in Parkinson's disease: evidence for a specific apomorphine effect on the frontal N30 wave. *Electroencephalogr. Clin. Neurophysiol.* 92, 491–501.

Cocchiarela, L., and Andersson, G. B. J. (2001). *Guides to the Evaluation of Permanent Impairment.* 5th Edn. Chicago, IL: American Medical Association.

Cusin, E., Do, M.-C., and Rougier, P. R. (2017). How does wearing a lumbar orthosis interfere with gait initiation? *Ergonomics* 60, 837–843. doi: 10.1080/00140139.2016.1206214

Delafontaine, A., Honeine, J. L., Do, M. C., Gagey, O., and Chong, R. K. (2015). Comparative gait initiation kinematics between simulated unilateral and bilateral ankle hypomobility: Does bilateral constraint improve speed performance? *Neurosci. Lett.* 603, 55–59. doi: 10.1016/j.neulet.2015.07.016

Delval, A., Tard, C., and Defebvre, L. (2014). Why we should study gait initiation in Parkinson's disease. *Neurophysiol. Clin.* 44, 69–76. doi: 10.1016/j.neucli.2013.10.127

Desmedt, J. E., and Cheron, G. (1980). Central somatosensory conduction in man: neural generators and interpeak latencies of the far-field components recorded from neck and right or left scalp and earlobes. *Electroencephalogr. Clin. Neurophysiol.* 50, 382–403. doi: 10.1016/0013-4694(80)90006-1

DeVocht, J. W., Pickar, J. G., and Wilder, D. G. (2005). Spinal manipulation alters electromyographic activity of paraspinal muscles: a descriptive study. *J. Manipulative Physiol. Ther.* 28, 465–471. doi: 10.1016/j.jmpt.2005.07.002

Diakhaté, D. G., Do, M. C., and Le Bozec, S. (2013). Effects of seat-thigh contact on kinematics performance in sit-to-stand and trunk flexion tasks. *J. Biomech.* 46, 879–882. doi: 10.1016/j.jbiomech.2012.12.022

Dishman, J. D., and Burke, J. (2003). Spinal reflex excitability changes after cervical and lumbar spinal manipulation: a comparative study. *Spine J.* 3, 204–212. doi: 10.1016/s1529-9430(02)00587-9

Do, M. C., and Gilles, M. (1992). Effects of reducing plantar support on anticipatory postural and intentional activities associated with flexion of the lower limb. *Neurosci. Lett.* 148, 181–184. doi: 10.1016/0304-3940(92)90834-t

Doege, Theodore C., American Medical Association, and Houston, Thomas P. (1993). *Guides to the Evaluation of Permanent Impairment.* 4th Edn. Chicago, IL: American Medical Association.

Garmabi, S., Mohseni-Bandpei, M. A., Abdollahi, I., and Tabatabaei, S. S. (2012). Reliability of measuring lumbar lordosis, flexion and extension using dual inclinometer in healthy subjects and patients with non-specific chronic low back pain. *Archiv. Rehabil.* 13, 8–17. Available online at: http://rehabilitationj.uswr.ac.ir/article-1-1001-en.html

González-Iglesias, J., Fernández-de-las-Peñas, C., Cleland, J. A., and Gutiérrez-Vega Mdel, R. (2009). Thoracic spine manipulation for the management of patients with neck pain: a randomized clinical trial. *J. Orthop. Sports Phys. Ther.* 39, 20–27. doi: 10.2519/jospt.2009.2914

Groeneweg, R., Rubinstein, S. M., Oostendorp, R. A. B., Ostelo, R. W. J. G., and van Tulder, M. W. (2017). Guideline for reporting interventions on spinal manipulative therapy: consensus on interventions reporting criteria list for spinal manipulative therapy (CIRCLe SMT). *J. Manipulative Physiol. Ther.* 40, 61–70. doi: 10.1016/j.jmpt.2016.10.013

Haavik, H., and Murphy, B. (2012). The role of spinal manipulation in addressing disordered sensorimotor integration and altered motor control. *J. Electromyogr. Kinesiol.* 22, 768–776. doi: 10.1016/j.jelekin.2012.02.012

Haavik Taylor, H., and Murphy, B. (2010). The effects of spinal manipulation on central integration of dual somatosensory input observed after motor training: a crossover study. *J. Manipulative Physiol. Ther.* 33, 261–272. doi: 10.1016/j.jmpt.2010.03.004

Haavik-Taylor, H., and Murphy, B. (2007). Cervical spine manipulation alters sensorimotor integration: a somatosensory evoked potential study. *Clin. Neurophysiol.* 118, 391–402. doi: 10.1016/j.clinph.2006.09.014

Hamaoui, A., and Alamini-Rodrigues, C. (2017a). Effect of experimentally-induced trunk muscular tensions on the sit-to-stand task performance and associated postural adjustments. *Front. Hum. Neurosci.* 11:32. doi: 10.3389/fnhum.2017.00032

Hamaoui, A., and Alamini-Rodrigues, C. (2017b). Influence of cervical spine mobility on the focal and postural components of the sit-to-stand task. *Front. Hum. Neurosci.* 11:129. doi: 10.3389/fnhum.2017.00129

Hamaoui, A., and Le Bozec, S. (2014). Does increased muscular tension along the torso disturb postural equilibrium more when it is asymmetrical? *Gait Posture* 39, 333–338. doi: 10.1016/j.gaitpost.2013.07.131

Hamaoui, A., Do, M. C., and Bouisset, S. (2004). Postural sway increase in low back pain subjects is not related to reduced spine range of motion. *Neurosci. Lett.* 357, 135–138. doi: 10.1016/j.neulet.2003.12.047

Hamaoui, A., Friant, Y., and Le Bozec, S. (2011). Does increased muscular tension along the torso impair postural equilibrium in a standing posture? *Gait Posture* 34, 457–461. doi: 10.1016/j.gaitpost.2011.06.017

Honeine, J.-L., Schieppati, M., Crisafulli, O., and Do, M.-C. (2016). The neuro-mechanical processes that underlie goal-directed medio-lateral APA during gait initiation. *Front. Hum. Neurosci.* 10:445. doi: 10.3389/fnhum.2016.00445

Humphries, K. M., Ward, J., Coats, J., Nobert, J., Amonette, W., and Dyess, S. (2013). Immediate effects of lower cervical spine manipulation on handgrip strength and free-throw accuracy of asymptomatic basketball players: a pilot study. *J. Chiropr. Med.* 12, 153–159. doi: 10.1016/j.jcm.2013.10.008

Kang, S. Y., and Ma, H.-I. (2016). N30 somatosensory evoked potential is negatively correlated with motor function in Parkinson's disease. *J. Mov. Disord.* 9, 35–39. doi: 10.14802/jmd.15038

Konz, R. J., Fatone, S., Stine, R. L., Ganju, A., Gard, S. A., and Ondra, S. L. (2006). A kinematic model to assess spinal motion during walking. *Spine* 31, E898–E906. doi: 10.1097/01.brs.0000245939.97637.ae

Le Bozec, S., and Bouisset, S. (2004). Does postural chain mobility influence muscular control in sitting ramp pushes? *Exp. Brain Res.* 158, 427–437. doi: 10.1007/s00221-004-1918-x

Lehman, G. (2012). Kinesiological research: the use of surface electromyography for assessing the effects of spinal manipulation. *J. Electromyogr. Kinesiol.* 22, 692–696. doi: 10.1016/j.jelekin.2012.02.010

Lelic, D., Niazi, I. K., Holt, K., Jochumsen, M., Dremstrup, K., Yielder, P., et al. (2016). Manipulation of dysfunctional spinal joints affects sensorimotor integration in the prefrontal cortex: a brain source localization study. *Neural Plast.* 2016:3704964. doi: 10.1155/2016/3704964

Leonardi, L. (1994). Achieving peak athletic performance. *Today's Chiropr.* 25, 94–95.

Lepers, R., and Brenière, Y. (1995). The role of anticipatory postural adjustments and gravity in gait initiation. *Exp. Brain Res.* 107, 118–124. doi: 10.1007/bf00228023

Lewis, J. S., and Valentine, R. E. (2010). Clinical measurement of the thoracic kyphosis. a study of the intra-rater reliability in subjects with and without shoulder pain. *BMC Musculoskelet. Disord.* 11:39. doi: 10.1186/1471-2474-11-39

Licciardone, J. C., Minotti, D. E., Gatchel, R. J., Kearns, C. M., and Singh, K. P. (2013). Osteopathic manual treatment and ultrasound therapy for chronic low back pain: a randomized controlled trial. *Ann. Fam. Med.* 11, 122–129. doi: 10.1370/afm.1468

Lino, F., Duchêne, J. L., and Bouisset, S. (1992). "Effect of seat contact area on the velocity of a pointing task," in *Biomechanics*, eds P. Bellotti and A. Capozzo (Rome: Università La Sapienza), 232.

Mann, R. A., Hagy, J. L., White, V., and Liddell, D. (1979). The initiation of gait. *J. Bone Joint Surg. Am.* 61, 232–239.

Mauguière, F. (1999). Utility of somatosensory evoked potentials (SEPs) in spinal cord lesions and functional surgery of pain and spasticity. *Electroencephalogr. Clin. Neurophysiol. Suppl.* 50, 31–39.

Mieritz, R. M., Hartvigsen, J., Boyle, E., Jakobsen, M. D., Aagaard, P., and Bronfort, G. (2014). Lumbar motion changes in chronic low back pain patients: a secondary analysis of data from a randomized clinical trial. *Spine J.* 14, 2618–2627. doi: 10.1016/j.spinee.2014.02.038

Millan, M., Leboeuf-Yde, C., Budgell, B., Descarreaux, M., and Amorim, M.-A. (2012a). The effect of spinal manipulative therapy on spinal range of motion: a systematic literature review. *Chiropr. Man. Ther.* 20:23. doi: 10.1186/2045-709x-20-23

Millan, M., Leboeuf-Yde, C., Budgell, B., and Amorim, M.-A. (2012b). The effect of spinal manipulative therapy on experimentally induced pain: a systematic literature review. *Chiropr. Man. Ther.* 20:26. doi: 10.1186/2045-709x-20-26

Miners, A. L. (2010). Chiropractic treatment and the enhancement of sport performance: a narrative literature review. *J. Can. Chiropr. Assoc.* 54, 210–221.

Murphy, B. A., Dawson, N. J., and Slack, J. R. (1995). Sacroiliac joint manipulation decreases the H-reflex. *Electromyogr. Clin. Neurophysiol.* 35, 87–94.

Niazi, I. K., Türker, K. S., Flavel, S., Kinget, M., Duehr, J., and Haavik, H. (2015). Changes in H-reflex and V-waves following spinal manipulation. *Exp. Brain Res.* 233, 1165–1173. doi: 10.1007/s00221-014-4193-5

Nuwer, M. R., Aminoff, M., Desmedt, J., Eisen, A. A., Goodin, D., Matsuoka, S., et al. (1994). IFCN recommended standards for short latency somatosensory evoked potentials. report of an IFCN committee. international federation of clinical neurophysiology. *Electroencephalogr. Clin. Neurophysiol.* 91, 6–11. doi: 10.1016/0013-4694(94)90012-4

Paulus, I., and Brumagne, S. (2008). Altered interpretation of neck proprioceptive signals in persons with subclinical recurrent neck pain. *J. Rehabil. Med.* 40, 426–432. doi: 10.2340/16501977-0189

Pickar, J. G. (2002). Neurophysiological effects of spinal manipulation. *Spine J.* 2, 357–371. doi: 10.1016/s1529-9430(02)00400-x

Pickar, J. G., and Bolton, P. S. (2012). Spinal manipulative therapy and somatosensory activation. *J. Electromyogr. Kinesiol.* 22, 785–794. doi: 10.1016/j.jelekin.2012.01.015

Reed, W. R., Long, C. R., Kawchuk, G. N., and Pickar, J. G. (2015). Neural responses to the mechanical characteristics of high velocity, low amplitude spinal manipulation: effect of specific contact site. *Man. Ther.* 20, 797–804. doi: 10.1016/j.math.2015.03.008

Ross, J. K., Bereznick, D. E., and McGill, S. M. (2004). Determining cavitation location during lumbar and thoracic spinal manipulation: is spinal manipulation accurate and specific? *Spine* 29, 1452–1457. doi: 10.1097/01.brs.0000129024.95630.57

Rossi, S., della Volpe, R., Ginanneschi, F., Ulivelli, M., Bartalini, S., Spidalieri, R., et al. (2003). Early somatosensory processing during tonic muscle pain in humans: relation to loss of proprioception and motor "defensive" strategies. *Clin. Neurophysiol.* 114, 1351–1358. doi: 10.1016/s1388-2457(03)00073-7

Ruget, H., Blouin, J., Teasdale, N., and Mouchnino, L. (2008). Can prepared anticipatory postural adjustments be updated by proprioception? *Neuroscience* 155, 640–648. doi: 10.1016/j.neuroscience.2008.06.021

Ruget, H., Blouin, J., Coyle, T., and Mouchnino, L. (2010). Modulation of proprioceptive inflow when initiating a step influences postural adjustments. *Exp. Brain Res.* 201, 297–305. doi: 10.1007/s00221-009-2035-7

Schiller, L. (2001). Effectiveness of spinal manipulative therapy in the treatment of mechanical thoracic spine pain: a pilot randomized clinical trial. *J. Manipulative Physiol. Ther.* 24, 394–401. doi: 10.1067/mmt.2001.116420

Schneider, M., Haas, M., Glick, R., Stevans, J., and Landsittel, D. (2015). Comparison of spinal manipulation methods and usual medical care for acute and subacute low back pain: a randomized clinical trial. *Spine* 40, 209–217. doi: 10.1097/brs.0000000000000724

Shrier, I., Macdonald, D., and Uchacz, G. (2006). A pilot study on the effects of pre-event manipulation on jump height and running velocity. *Br. J. Sports Med.* 40, 947–949. doi: 10.1136/bjsm.2006.029439

Suter, E., McMorland, G., and Herzog, W. (2005). Short-term effects of spinal manipulation on H-reflex amplitude in healthy and symptomatic subjects. *J. Manipulative Physiol. Ther.* 28, 667–672. doi: 10.1016/j.jmpt.2005.09.017

Suvarnnato, T., Puntumetakul, R., Kaber, D., Boucaut, R., Boonphakob, Y., Arayawichanon, P., et al. (2013). The effects of thoracic manipulation versus mobilization for chronic neck pain: a randomized controlled trial pilot study. *J. Phys. Ther. Sci.* 25, 865–871. doi: 10.1589/jpts.25.865

Taylor, H. H., and Murphy, B. (2008). Altered sensorimotor integration with cervical spine manipulation. *J. Manipulative Physiol. Ther.* 31, 115–126. doi: 10.1016/j.jmpt.2007.12.011

Teyssèdre, C., Lino, F., Zattara, M., and Bouisset, S. (2000). Anticipatory EMG patterns associated with preferred and non-preferred arm pointing movements. *Exp. Brain Res.* 134, 435–440. doi: 10.1007/s002210000490

Thorstensson, A., Nilsson, J., Carlson, H., and Zomlefer, M. R. (1984). Trunk movements in human locomotion. *Acta Physiol. Scand.* 121, 9–22. doi: 10.1111/j.1748-1716.1984.tb10452.x

Wernham, J. (1985). *Mechanics of the Spine*. Maidstone: Year Book.

Wiese, G., and Callender, A. (2005). "A history of spinal manipulation," in *Principles and Practice of Chiropractic*, eds S. Haldeman, S. Dagenasis, and B. Budgell (New York, NY: McGraw-Hill), 5–22.

Yiou, E., Hamaoui, A., and Le Bozec, S. (2007). Influence of base of support size on arm pointing performance and associated anticipatory postural adjustments. *Neurosci. Lett.* 423, 29–34. doi: 10.1016/j.neulet.2007.06.034

Yiou, E., Ditcharles, S., and Le Bozec, S. (2011). Biomechanical reorganisation of stepping initiation during acute dorsiflexor fatigue. *J. Electromyogr. Kinesiol.* 21, 727–733. doi: 10.1016/j.jelekin.2011.04.008

Yiou, E., Teyssèdre, C., Artico, R., and Fourcade, P. (2016). Comparison of base of support size during gait initiation using force-plate and motion-capture system: a bland and altman analysis. *J. Biomech.* 49, 4168–4172. doi: 10.1016/j.jbiomech.2016.11.008

9

Accelerometer-Based Step Regularity is Lower in Older Adults with Bilateral Knee Osteoarthritis

John M. Barden[1]*, Christian A. Clermont[2], Dylan Kobsar[2] and Olivier Beauchet[3]

[1] Faculty of Kinesiology and Health Studies, Neuromechanical Research Centre, University of Regina, Regina, SK, Canada,
[2] Faculty of Kinesiology, University of Calgary, Calgary, AB, Canada, [3] Division of Geriatric Medicine, Department of Medicine, McGill University, Montreal, QC, Canada

*Correspondence:
John M. Barden
john.barden@uregina.ca

Purpose: To compare the regularity and symmetry of gait between a cohort of older adults with bilateral knee osteoarthritis (OA) and an age and sex-matched control group of older adults with healthy knees.

Methods: Fifteen (8 females) older adults with knee OA (64.7 ± 6.7 years) and fifteen (8 females) pain-free controls (66.1 ± 10.0 years) completed a 9-min. walk at a self-selected, comfortable speed while wearing a single waist-mounted tri-axial accelerometer. The following gait parameters were compared between the two groups according to sex: mean step time, mean stride time, stride and step regularity (defined as the consistency of the stride-to-stride or step-to-step pattern) and the symmetry of gait (defined as the difference between step and stride regularity) as determined by an unbiased autocorrelation procedure that analyzed the pattern of acceleration in the vertical, mediolateral and anteroposterior directions.

Results: Older adults with knee OA displayed significantly less step regularity in the vertical ($p < 0.05$) and anteroposterior ($p < 0.05$) directions than controls. Females with knee OA were also found to have significantly less mediolateral step regularity than female controls ($p < 0.05$), whereas no difference was found between males.

Conclusion: The results showed that the regularity of the step pattern in individuals with bilateral knee OA was less consistent compared to similarly-aged older adults with healthy knees. The findings suggest that future studies should investigate the relationship between step regularity, sex and movement direction as well as the application of these methods to the clinical assessment of knee OA.

Keywords: knee osteoarthritis, accelerometry, gait regularity, gait symmetry

INTRODUCTION

The ability to locomote is a fundamental activity for all humans, and is an essential component of maintaining independence and a healthy quality of life. However, it is understood that the physiological changes that accompany aging in the last decades of life increasingly challenge the neuromuscular system to maintain consistent levels of mobility. Often these changes are exacerbated by other disease mechanisms or processes in one or more systems, to the extent that gait function can be severely compromised. Osteoarthritis (OA) is a debilitating disease that involves the progressive degradation of articular cartilage in the body's major weight bearing joints

(Baliunas et al., 2002). It affects millions of people worldwide, with knee OA being the most common in terms of prevalence (6% of adults > 30 years of age) (Zhang and Jordan, 2008). It is widely reported that knee OA is associated with compromised gait function in that it exacerbates the altered spatiotemporal gait parameters caused by aging, such as reduced stride length and speed and increased stride time, stance phase duration and double support time (Al-Zahrani and Bakheit, 2002; Astephen et al., 2008; Mills et al., 2013a). In addition to changes in mean spatiotemporal gait parameters, other studies have shown that knee OA is associated with changes in the variability of these parameters and the basic movement patterns that comprise the gait cycle (Kiss, 2011; Tochigi et al., 2012).

Research that has investigated the variability of one or more aspects of the gait cycle defines the area of study known as gait variability. Numerous studies have shown that gait variability is particularly sensitive to differences between healthy individuals and those with mild to moderate gait impairments. Evidence suggests that too much or too little variability is disadvantageous to the stability of the system, as has been shown by studies that have found both increased and decreased gait variability in different populations (Hausdorff, 2009; Tochigi et al., 2012). Studies on gait variability have largely investigated the regulation and timing of the gait pattern in various pathological conditions, including Parkinson's disease (Hausdorff, 2009), multiple sclerosis (Kalron, 2016), Alzheimer's disease (Wittwer et al., 2013), ALS (Hausdorff et al., 2000) and the changes in gait associated with healthy aging (Hausdorff et al., 1997; Kobsar et al., 2014a). A variety of different methods (cameras, pressure-sensitive mats and accelerometry) have been used to investigate a range of parameters that typically include linear measures such as the standard deviation (SD) or coefficient of variation of mean spatiotemporal gait parameters (e.g., stride time SD), or more sophisticated non-linear methods that aim to quantify the complexity of the gait cycle across different time spans (e.g., sample entropy, fractal scaling index) (Hausdorff et al., 1997; Tochigi et al., 2012; Kobsar et al., 2014a; Alkjaer et al., 2015). The application of accelerometry for gait variability analysis is advantageous because it allows for the collection of large amounts of data (i.e., potentially thousands of gait cycles) using unobtrusive sensors under natural walking conditions (Kobsar et al., 2014a). Conducting a similar analysis using a lab-based 3D camera system (for example) requires the use of a treadmill, which potentially alters the participant's internal rhythm (and consequently their gait variability) due to the external pacing imposed by the constant speed of the belt. It also provides the opportunity to take advantage of advanced analytical methods such as autocorrelation analysis (Moe-Nilssen and Helbostad, 2004), which can be used to extract discrete parameters such as the stride time and step time, in addition to using the entire acceleration waveform to determine the regularity (consistency of the stride-to-stride or step-to-step pattern) and symmetry (difference between step and stride regularity) of the gait cycle (Moe-Nilssen and Helbostad, 2004; Kobayashi et al., 2014; Kobsar et al., 2014a).

In general, studies that have investigated gait variability have produced favorable results that have advanced the understanding

of the effect of different pathologies on gait function; however, the majority of these studies have focused on the effects of neural pathology (Moon et al., 2016) as opposed to diseases that directly affect the musculoskeletal system such as hip and knee OA. Several studies have found differences in select measures of gait variability (Yakhdani et al., 2010; Kiss, 2011; Tochigi et al., 2012; Gustafson et al., 2015) and gait symmetry (Mills et al., 2013b) in patients with unilateral and bilateral knee OA, respectively, presumably because pathophysiologically-induced changes to the morphology of the joint (e.g., decreased joint space, decreased range of motion, and increased pain) produce altered gait patterns as a result of CNS-mediated compensation strategies that develop over time to avoid pain, re-distribute joint loads and/or maintain dynamic stability under adverse conditions. Other studies have shown that sex and laterality (i.e., unilateral vs. bilateral incidence) are important factors that should be considered when investigating step regularity and gait symmetry in older adults with and without knee OA. Recently, Kobayashi et al. (2014) found differences in step regularity between older adult males and females, while Kiss (2011) found differences in cadence and step length variability between males and females with knee OA. With respect to gait symmetry, Mills et al. (2013b) have shown that between-limb kinematic asymmetries are greater for individuals with bilateral knee OA as opposed to unilateral knee OA. Consequently, the purpose of this study was to use an accelerometry-based unbiased autocorrelation procedure to determine the stride regularity, step regularity and gait symmetry of individuals with bilateral knee OA, and to compare these values to a group of age and sex-matched pain-free controls. It was hypothesized that males and females with knee OA would display less step and stride regularity than control participants and that their gait would be less symmetric. Based on the results of Kobayashi et al. (2014), it was also hypothesized that male participants in both groups would have lower step regularity than females.

METHODS

Participants

Fifteen adults, 55 years of age or older (8 females, 7 males; 64.7 ± 6.8 years), with bilateral knee OA participated in the study. In addition, fifteen age and sex-matched older adults (8 females, 7 males; 66.1 ± 10.0 years) who presented with no knee pain or diagnosis of knee OA were recruited as control participants. **Table 1** provides further information concerning the participant demographics. Inclusion criteria for the knee OA group consisted of having received a medical diagnosis of knee OA in addition to being able to walk comfortably for at least 9 min without the use of an assistive device (e.g., cane or walker). The severity of knee OA (as determined by the Kellgren-Lawrence grading scale) varied across participants, in that five participants had a K-L grade of 4 (in the most severe knee), eight had a grade of 3, and two had a grade of 2. Participants in the control group were selected using the same criteria as those for the knee OA group except for the presence of knee OA. Participants in either group were excluded if they had any recent surgery that affected their legs or lumbar spine, if they possessed

TABLE 1 | Demographic and temporal gait parameter data for knee OA and control group participants.

Parameter	Control (Mean ± SD)			Knee OA (Mean ± SD)		
	Female (n = 8)	Male (n = 7)	Total (n = 15)	Female (n = 8)	Male (n = 7)	Total (n = 15)
Age (years)	66.8 ± 10.5	65.3 ± 10.2	66.1 ± 10.0	63.9 ± 8.7	65.6 ± 4.0	64.7 ± 6.8
Height (cm)	**159.3 ± 4.0**[†]	**176.8 ± 8.5**[†]	167.5 ± 11.0	**160.7 ± 7.6**[†]	**174.6 ± 5.4**[†]	167.2 ± 9.7
Mass (kg)	**61.9 ± 9.5**[†]	**84.3 ± 16.2**[†]	**72.4 ± 17.1***	**78.5 ± 10.0**[†]	**92.7 ± 6.6**[†]	**85.2 ± 11.0***
BMI (kg/m^2)	24.4 ± 3.9	26.8 ± 3.4	**25.5 ± 3.8***	30.5 ± 4.4	30.6 ± 3.8	**30.6 ± 4.0***
Stride time (ms)	979 ± 74	1029 ± 73	1002 ± 76	1055 ± 76	1046 ± 73	1051 ± 72
Step time (ms)	489 ± 37	515 ± 37	501 ± 38	527 ± 38	523 ± 37	525 ± 36

Results of the two-way ANOVA (group × sex) indicating significant differences between groups (p < 0.01) in bold. [†] Significant differences between sexes (p < 0.01) are marked in bold.

OA in any other lower extremity joint (e.g., hip), if they had any neuromuscular disorders (e.g., Parkinson's disease, multiple sclerosis, etc.), history of stroke, cardiovascular disease, or any other medical condition or physical impairment that would affect their gait, balance, and/or their ability to walk at a steady pace for 10 min. This study was carried out in accordance with the recommendations of the University of Regina Research Ethics Board (REB) with written informed consent from all subjects. All subjects gave written informed consent in accordance with the Declaration of Helsinki. The protocol was approved by the University of Regina Research Ethics Board (REB-71S112).

Apparatus and Procedure

The height and weight of each participant was recorded for the purpose of calculating the body mass index (BMI). The test procedure required the participants to walk around an oval 200-m indoor track at a consistent, self-selected speed for a period of 9 min. Self-selected speeds were chosen because they most accurately represent the natural gait pattern according to each participant's stature and other physical factors such as strength and flexibility (Clermont and Barden, 2016). A single triaxial accelerometer (GENEActiv, Cambridgeshire, UK) was attached to a belt that was located firmly at the lower back (L3) to approximate the total body center of mass (Moe-Nilssen and Helbostad, 2004; Kobsar et al., 2014b). For a depiction of the experimental setup please refer to Kobsar et al. (2014b). The accelerometer recorded continuous acceleration at a sampling rate of 100 Hz during the 9-min walking trial, which is consistent with sampling frequencies used by previous studies to determine measures of gait variability (Hartmann et al., 2009; Kobsar et al., 2014a).

Data Analysis

The data sets from the 9-min walking trials were reduced to 6 min by removing the first and last 90 s of each trial. The average number of steps for 6 min of walking was 682.1 (SD ± 45.1) for knee OA participants and 710.1 (SD ± 36.5) for control participants. This was done to ensure that the participants had sufficient time to achieve a steady-state walking speed prior to the analysis and to remove any potential gait irregularities associated with anticipating the termination of the trial (Lindemann et al., 2008). All data processing and

gait parameter calculations were done using MATLAB version R2016A (The MathWorks Inc., Natick, MA). The signals from all three accelerometer axes were initially processed using a zero-lag, 4th order Butterworth low-pass filter with a cut-off frequency of 10 Hz. Subsequently, a negative peak-detection (local minima) method on the anteroposterior axis was used to identify each individual step to determine the step times for the 6-min time series (Terrier and Dériaz, 2011). From this series of step times, the mean step time and stride time were determined. Mean step time was defined as the average of all step times (i.e., right and left combined) and stride time was obtained by combining each set of subsequent left and right steps together. As per previous studies, a median filter was used to remove any potential outliers (defined as step times greater than three SDs from the median) in each subject's step time series (Hausdorff and Edelberg, 1997; Kobsar et al., 2014a).

To determine stride and step regularity, an unbiased autocorrelation procedure (see **Figure 1**) was used to measure the correlation of the acceleration signal for each step (first dominant period) or stride (second dominant period) at different periods of time (i.e., phase shifts) across each of the three accelerometer axes (Moe-Nilssen and Helbostad, 2004; Kobsar et al., 2014a). Step regularity was defined as the correlation between the original acceleration signal and the acceleration signal phase shifted to the average step time, whereas stride regularity was shifted to the average stride time (Kobsar et al., 2014a). These phase shifts were consistent with the first and second dominant periods of the unbiased autocorrelation coefficient, respectively (Moe-Nilssen and Helbostad, 2004; Kobayashi et al., 2014; Kobsar et al., 2014a). Gait symmetry (Sym) was defined as the percent difference between the regularity of steps (StpReg) and the regularity of strides (StrReg) for each of the three axes, with zero being perfect symmetry and larger values depicting greater levels of asymmetry (the difference between the consistency of strides and the consistency of steps) in the accelerometer waveform (Kobsar et al., 2014a).

$$Symmetry = \left\{ \frac{|StpReg - StrReg|}{(StpReg + StrReg)/2} \right\} * 100$$

Consequently, the accelerometer waveforms in the vertical (V), anteroposterior (AP), and mediolateral (ML) directions were

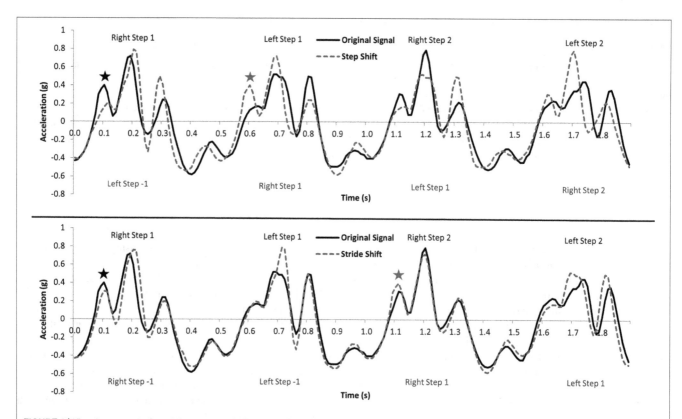

FIGURE 1 | Visual representation of the autocorrelation procedure for a series of four steps. The top panel shows the correlation between the original signal and the signal shifted equivalent to the average step time, which defines step regularity. The bottom panel shows the correlation between the original signal and the signal shifted equivalent to the average stride time, which defines stride regularity. The ★ shows the original and step/stride shifted waveforms in the top and bottom panels, respectively. Adapted from Kobsar et al. (2014a), with permission from Elsevier.

phase-shifted using the autocorrelation procedure to determine the step regularity (StpV, StpAP, StpML), stride regularity (StrV, StrAP, StrML) and symmetry (SymV, SymAP, SymML) of knee OA and control group participants.

Statistical Analysis

Separate two-way (group × sex) ANOVAs were used to compare dependent variables for participant demographics (age, height, mass, and BMI), temporal gait parameters (stride time and step time) as well as stride regularity (StrRegV, StrRegAP, StrRegML), step regularity (StpRegV, StpRegAP, StpRegML) and gait symmetry (SymV, SymAP, SymML). Post-hoc comparisons using Fisher's LSD test were used to further identify any significant interaction effects. Effect sizes (partial η^2) were determined for all comparisons according to the following categories: small (<0.06), moderate (0.06–0.14) and large (>0.14) (Cohen, 1988). All statistical analyses were performed using IBM SPSS Statistics 19.0 (SPSS Inc., Armonk, NY) with the significance level set to $p < 0.05$.

RESULTS

Mean values for age, height, mass, and BMI along with the temporal gait variables (step and stride time) for both groups are presented in **Table 1**.

Significant between group differences were found for mass $[F_{(1, 26)} = 9.65, p = 0.005, \eta_p^2 = 0.271]$, and BMI $[F_{(1, 26)} = 12.01, p = 0.002, \eta_p^2 = 0.317]$, indicating that participants with knee OA had a higher mass and a greater BMI than control group participants. Significant differences were also found between males and females of both groups for height $[F_{(1, 26)} = 43.00, p = 0.000, \eta_p^2 = 0.623]$ and mass $[F_{(1, 26)} = 20.61, p = 0.000, \eta_p^2 = 0.442]$, demonstrating that male participants were heavier and taller than their female counterparts. Mean differences between groups for stride time $[F_{(1,26)} = 2.91, p = .100, \eta_p^2 = 0.101]$ and step time $[F_{(1, 26)} = 2.91, p = 0.100, \eta_p^2 = 0.101]$ approached significance with moderate effect sizes, suggesting that the strides and steps of knee OA participants took longer, which is indicative of slower walking speeds.

The two-way ANOVA results for stride regularity, step regularity and gait symmetry are summarized in **Table 2**. The mean values for stride regularity, step regularity and gait symmetry for participants in both groups (for each axis) are presented in **Figure 2**. Significant group main effects were found for step regularity in the vertical $[F_{(1,26)} = 5.28, p = 0.030, \eta_p^2 = 0.169]$ and anteroposterior directions $[F_{(1,26)} = 5.77, p = 0.024, \eta_p^2 = 0.182]$, indicating that the steps of both males and females with knee OA were completed with less regularity (i.e., were associated with less similar waveforms) than control participants. No significant main or interaction

TABLE 2 | ANOVA results for stride regularity, step regularity and gait symmetry based on accelerometer axis (i.e., direction).

Factor	Stride regularity						Step regularity						Gait symmetry					
	V		AP		ML		V		AP		ML		V		AP		ML	
	p	η_p^2	p	η_p^2	p	η_p^2	p	η_p^2	p	η_p^2	p	η_p^2	p	η_p^2	p	η_p^2	p	η_p^2
Group	0.06	**0.13**[†]	0.79	0.00	0.93	0.00	**0.03***	0.17	**0.02***	0.18	0.17	0.07	0.22	0.06	0.07	**0.12**[†]	0.22	0.06
Sex	0.62	0.01	0.86	0.00	0.46	0.02	0.60	0.01	0.79	0.00	0.52	0.02	0.38	0.03	0.14	0.08	0.52	0.02
Group*Sex	0.99	0.00	0.57	0.01	0.24	0.05	0.83	0.00	0.60	0.01	**0.03***	0.18	0.96	0.00	0.65	0.01	0.08	**0.12**[†]

*V, vertical; AP, anteroposterior; ML, mediolateral. *Significant differences (p < 0.05) are indicated in bold. Effect sizes (partial η2) were determined for all comparisons according to the following categories: small (<0.06), moderate (0.06–0.14) and large (>0.14) (Hartmann et al., 2009). [†]Differences approaching significance with moderate effect sizes are indicated in bold.*

effects were found for stride regularity or gait symmetry in any of the three directions. A significant interaction effect [$F_{(1,26)}$ = 5.50, $p = 0.027$, $\eta_p^2 = 0.175$] was also found for step regularity in the mediolateral direction. *Post-hoc* comparisons revealed that mediolateral step regularity was significantly higher for female controls than for females with knee OA ($p < 0.05$), whereas the difference between males was non-significant. Further, mediolateral step regularity was significantly higher for female controls than for males ($p < 0.05$), whereas the difference between males and females in the knee OA group was not significant. All significant differences were associated with large effect sizes ($\eta_p^2 > 0.14$). **Table 2** also shows that several additional comparisons (specifically, group *StrRegV*, group *SymAP*, and group*sex *SymML*) were associated with moderate effect sizes ($\eta_p^2 = 0.06$–0.14) and *p*-values that approached significance ($p < 0.06$, $p < 0.07$, and $p < 0.08$, respectively).

DISCUSSION

The purpose of this study was to compare the stride regularity, step regularity and gait symmetry of individuals with knee OA to age and sex-matched control participants, using an unbiased autocorrelation procedure based on data obtained from a triaxial accelerometer. It was hypothesized that males and females with knee OA would display less step and stride regularity than control participants and that their gait would be less symmetric. It was also hypothesized that male participants in both groups would have lower step regularity than females. Participants with knee OA had a higher mass and a greater BMI than control group participants ($p < 0.01$), which is consistent with the findings of other studies on knee OA (Landry et al., 2007). More importantly, the hypothesis with respect to step regularity was supported in that significant differences were found between knee OA and control group participants in the vertical and anteroposterior directions. Significant differences were also found for mediolateral step regularity between females with and without knee OA, and between males and females in the control group. To the best of our knowledge, this is the first study to have investigated stride and step regularity in individuals with knee OA using accelerometry-based autocorrelation analysis. Two other studies have investigated step and stride regularity in

healthy older adults and the current findings are consistent with those results (Kobayashi et al., 2014; Kobsar et al., 2014a).

This study found significant differences in vertical and anteroposterior step regularity between participants with and without knee OA. This finding demonstrates that the similarity of step-to-step trunk acceleration waveforms was less regular (more variable) for individuals with knee OA compared to similarly-aged older adults with healthy knees. Only a limited number of studies have investigated gait variability in knee OA, and the findings of this study are generally consistent (in terms of increased variability) with the study by Kiss (2011) who found that knee OA participants demonstrated greater variability in step length, stance time, cadence, and double-support time than controls. However, these findings conflict with the results of Tochigi et al. (2012) and Yakhdani et al. (2010), who found that participants with knee OA possessed reduced variability of leg and knee motion compared to controls. In relation to this difference, it is important to note that Tochigi et al. (2012) and Yakhdani et al. (2010) not only used different methods (Sample Entropy and Lyapunov exponents, respectively), but more importantly quantified the variability of the affected limb as opposed to the variability of the approximate total body center of mass as was the case in this study. From a dynamical systems perspective, the variability of an injured limb may be inherently different from that of the center of mass during gait (Hamill et al., 2012). It is also important to note that significant differences in mass and BMI were found between knee OA and control group participants. To our knowledge, no studies have investigated the effect of body mass on step and stride regularity in older adults (or in younger adults), and as such it is not possible to know whether this had any effect on the results. Given that body mass and BMI are both important risk factors for knee OA (and are therefore common in this population), it is important that future studies take these factors into account. Further research is also needed to investigate the effect of knee OA on joint specific (knee) and total body variability to provide further insights into gait coordination and stability in this population. Additionally, a study by Lewek et al. (2006) found no difference in knee motion variability between unilateral knee OA participants and controls, but an increase in variability of the unaffected limb within the knee OA group. These mixed results demonstrate that additional research is needed to determine the relationship between knee OA and the various measures of gait variability.

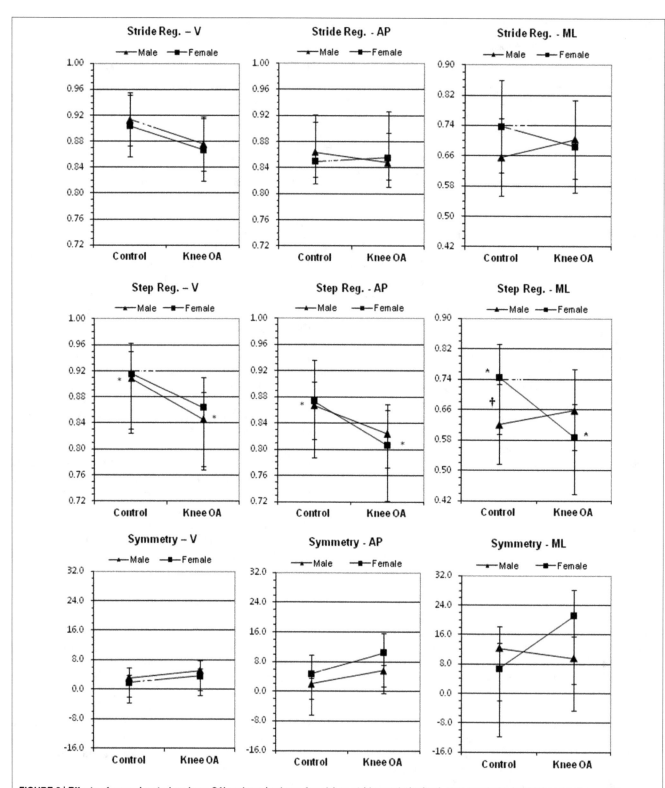

FIGURE 2 | Effects of group (control vs. knee OA) and sex (male vs. female) on stride regularity (top), step regularity (middle) and gait symmetry (bottom) in the vertical (V), anteroposterior (AP) and mediolateral (ML) directions. The * indicates a significant difference ($p < 0.05$) between groups whereas the [†]indicates a significant difference ($p < 0.05$) between male and female controls. Error bars = ± 1 standard deviation of the mean.

With respect to the current findings, it is important to interpret the differences in anteroposterior step regularity in combination with the differences in stride regularity (Moe-Nilssen and Helbostad, 2004). Specifically, anteroposterior stride regularity was essentially the same for both groups, whereas step regularity was significantly less for the knee OA group. Low values for step regularity in combination with similarly low values for stride regularity indicate low regularity for both steps and strides, whereas low step regularity with a higher stride regularity indicates better regularity for strides than steps, which suggests bilateral asymmetry between left and right steps (Moe-Nilssen and Helbostad, 2004). This difference between step and stride regularity is also reflected in the gait symmetry measure, which in the case of the anteroposterior direction was associated with a moderate effect size ($\eta_p^2 = 0.12$) that approached significance ($p < 0.07$). Together these findings suggest that individuals with knee OA possessed greater bilateral step asymmetry than individuals with healthy knees. This indicates that the variability of the anteroposterior trunk acceleration pattern on a step-to-step basis was greater than normal in individuals with knee OA. It is possible that this may have occurred because of differences in knee OA severity between the two limbs, resulting in a less consistent pattern of motion between right and left steps. In relation to this point, it should be noted that the participants in this study possessed bilateral knee OA, and while it might seem reasonable to speculate that a similar study on unilateral knee OA participants would find an even more pronounced difference in anteroposterior step regularity, a recent study by Mills et al. (2013b) demonstrated that bilateral joint kinematic asymmetries were more prevalent in individuals with bilateral knee OA than unilateral knee OA. Mills et al. suggested that this may occur because individuals with unilateral disease maintain kinematic symmetry further into the knee OA process than those with bilateral disease (Mills et al., 2013b). Concerning the importance of the anteroposterior direction, it has also been suggested that differences in anteroposterior stride and step regularity may reflect differences in the control of the propulsion and braking phases of gait (Kobsar et al., 2014a), whereas Moe-Nilssen et al. (2010) found that anteroposterior step autocorrelation (i.e., anteroposterior step regularity) was highly associated (negatively correlated) with step length variability. Consequently, in addition to bilateral asymmetry, it is possible that reduced anteroposterior step regularity indicates a diminished capacity to control step length in individuals with bilateral knee OA.

With respect to the difference in vertical step regularity, it is important to note that the vertical stride regularity of knee OA participants was also lower than that of the control group (which approached significance at $p < 0.06$ with a moderate effect size of $\eta_p^2 = 0.13$), suggesting that a more general lack of regularity for both steps and strides existed in this direction for those with knee OA. This is supported by the fact that the gait symmetry values for the knee OA group were lower for the vertical direction (indicating greater symmetry between steps and strides) than for the anteroposterior direction. Consequently, the findings for the vertical direction suggest a more general lack of consistency in the overall pattern of gait for individuals with knee OA. In terms of what these results might signify, it

is conceivable that they could reflect inconsistencies in loading and/or differences in step time variability. Evidence exists to suggest the latter as Moe-Nilssen et al. (2010) have shown that vertical step autocorrelation (i.e., step regularity) is highly related to step time variability. Therefore, in addition to greater bilateral step asymmetry, it is conceivable that the differences in anteroposterior and vertical step regularity together indicate that individuals with knee OA possess greater step length and step time variability than participants with healthy knees. If supported by future research, these findings suggest that waist-mounted accelerometry and autocorrelation analysis could be used to conduct clinical assessments of gait variability in individuals with knee OA using a simple, non-invasive, self-paced walking test. Such assessments have the potential to evaluate differences in gait between individuals with different levels of knee OA severity, to evaluate individuals before and after knee replacement surgery and to evaluate the functional outcomes of post-surgical physical therapy. Given the advantages of using accelerometers to determine measures of gait variability (i.e., small size, low cost, collection of large amounts of data and easily placed on the body in multiple locations, not to mention their ubiquity in most modern smart phones), the potential for clinical application is substantial. This potential will be realized if future studies can demonstrate that gait variability parameters, such as step and stride regularity, have practical value as clinical outcome measures that can be applied to the assessment and treatment of knee OA.

This study also found a significant interaction effect for mediolateral step regularity, such that females with knee OA had significantly lower mediolateral step regularity than female controls, while females within the control group had significantly higher mediolateral step regularity than males. These findings were surprising because it was not hypothesized that group differences in step regularity, stride regularity or gait symmetry would be dependent on sex. For control participants, the data clearly shows that an important difference exists between males and females for both mediolateral step and stride regularity, such that males had lower step and stride regularity than females. This is in contrast to the vertical and anteroposterior directions in which the mean values were quite similar. It is interesting to note that a recent study by Kobayashi et al. (2014), which investigated step and stride regularity in young and older adults, found differences in step regularity for the vertical and anteroposterior directions between males and females in the older adult group, but not for the young group. Unfortunately, Kobayashi et al. (2014) did not provide data for the mediolateral direction, but the findings for step regularity are consistent with the current study in terms of older adult males displaying lower step regularity than females, albeit for different directions. This study did not find any differences in vertical and anteroposterior step regularity between older adult male and female controls as Kobayashi et al. (2014) did; however, it is possible that this could be the result of the small number of steps that were used to determine step and stride regularity in the Kobayashi et al. (2014) study (participants walked the length of a 7 m walkway twice, which likely amounted to approximately 20–30 steps, as opposed to the approximately 700 steps used in this study).

Given that Moe-Nilssen et al. (2010) found no relationship between mediolateral step regularity and other gait variability parameters such as step time and step length variability, it is possible that mediolateral trunk variability may serve a different purpose in locomotor control compared to the other two directions. This is consistent with the observations made by Kobsar et al. (2014a), who suggested that mediolateral step regularity may be indicative of dynamic balance control. Regardless of what the difference signifies, to our knowledge this is the first study to have found a significant difference in mediolateral step regularity between older adult males and females and between females with and without knee OA. If this parameter is representative of dynamic balance control, it suggests that older adult females have better postural stability in the mediolateral direction than men. This may occur because men on average tend to be taller than women, and in theory maintaining dynamic stability with an aging neuromuscular control system should be more challenging for those individuals with a higher center of mass. However, it is also interesting that the relationship between male and female mediolateral step regularity appears to be negated in the presence of knee OA. Given that no previous research exists on step or stride regularity in knee OA it is difficult to speculate about what the cause of this might be. Nevertheless, it can be inferred that knee OA appears to affect the consistency of mediolateral trunk acceleration patterns more for women than for men, suggesting that women with knee OA may experience a greater loss of dynamic balance control than men. It is also conceivable that mediolateral step regularity might be associated with fall risk and/or the etiology of knee OA (given that knee OA is more common in women than in men), and as such this is an important finding that should be investigated further, both in healthy older adults and in adults with knee OA.

While the main strength of this study is the use of an accelerometer-based approach to investigate step/stride regularity and gait symmetry in older adults with knee OA, there were several limitations that should be considered. First, the participants were not matched according to body mass or BMI, and given that significant differences existed between the groups for these parameters, it is conceivable that these differences may have affected the results. Second, the sample size was relatively small and limited to participants with bilateral knee OA. The sample was also heterogeneous with respect to knee OA severity (i.e., K-L grade range of 2–4), both between limbs and between participants, and as such these factors may have also affected the results. Given that this study provides preliminary evidence to suggest a relationship between knee OA and step regularity,

future studies should attempt to stratify participants according to severity.

CONCLUSION

This study found that males and females with knee OA possessed significantly less vertical and anteroposterior step regularity than similarly-aged control group participants with pain-free knees. The findings suggest that the presence of knee OA affects the control of gait such that the consistency of the step pattern (more than the stride pattern) is compromised. Based on these results, it is not possible to know whether this is a direct consequence of the effects of knee OA itself (for e.g., pain and reduced range of motion), or if the increased variability is reflective of one or more compensation strategies employed by the CNS to manage the pathomechanics caused by the structural deficiencies of the joint. The study also found that mediolateral step regularity was lower for females with knee OA and lower for males than for females in the control group, suggesting that the relationship between mediolateral step regularity and knee OA is different in males and females. To our knowledge this is the first study to investigate stride regularity, step regularity and gait symmetry in individuals with knee OA, and the findings suggest that future research is needed to determine the specific aspects of gait control that are represented by these parameters (for e.g., is there a relationship between mediolateral step regularity and step width variability or dynamic balance control?). Given that this study found differences in step regularity with a relatively small number of bilateral knee OA participants, future studies (with larger sample sizes) should investigate unilateral knee OA and the effect of knee OA severity on step and stride regularity. The application of accelerometry-based gait regularity analysis for the assessment and treatment of knee OA in the clinical setting should also be investigated.

AUTHOR CONTRIBUTIONS

JB authored the manuscript and was involved with all aspects of the study, CC was involved with the data collection and analysis, DK conducted the data analysis and OB assisted with manuscript preparation and revision.

ACKNOWLEDGMENTS

The authors would like to acknowledge the University of Regina President's Publication Fund for their support of this manuscript.

REFERENCES

Alkjaer, T., Raffalt, P. C., Dalsgaard, H., Simonsen, E. B., Petersen, N. C., Bliddal, H., et al. (2015). Gait variability and motor control in people with knee osteoarthritis. *Gait Posture* 42, 479–484. doi: 10.1016/j.gaitpost.2015.07.063

Al-Zahrani, K. S., and Bakheit, A. M. (2002). A study of the gait characteristics of patients with chronic osteoarthritis of the knee. *Disabil. Rehabil.* 24, 275–280. doi: 10.1080/09638280110087098

Astephen, J. L., Deluzio, K. L., Caldwell, G. E., and Dunbar, M. J. (2008). Biomechanical changes at the hip, knee, and ankle joints during gait are associated with knee osteoarthritis severity. *J. Orthop. Res.* 26, 332–341. doi: 10.1002/jor.20496

Baliunas, A. J., Hurwitz, D. E., Ryals, A. B., Karrar, A., Case, J. P., Block, J. A., et al. (2002). Increased knee joint loads during walking are present in subjects with knee osteoarthritis. *Osteoarthr. Cartil.* 10, 573–579. doi: 10.1053/joca.2002.0797

Clermont, C. A., and Barden, J. M. (2016). Accelerometer-based determination of gait variability in older adults with knee osteoarthritis. *Gait Posture* 50, 126–130. doi: 10.1016/j.gaitpost.2016.08.024

Cohen, J. (1988). *Statistical Power Analysis for the Behavioral Sciences*. Hillsdale, NJ: Lawrence Erlbaum.

Gustafson, J. A., Robinson, M. E., Fitzgerald, G. K., Tashman, S., and Farrokhi, S. (2015). Knee motion variability in patients with knee osteoarthritis: the effect of self-reported instability. *Clin. Biomech.* 30, 475–480. doi: 10.1016/j.clinbiomech.2015.03.007

Hamill, J., Palmer, C., and Van Emmerik, R. E. (2012). Coordinative variability and overuse injury. *Sports Med. Arthrosc. Rehabil. Ther. Technol.* 4:45. doi: 10.1186/1758-2555-4-45

Hartmann, A., Luzi, S., Murer, K., de Bie, R. A., and de Bruin, E. D. (2009). Concurrent validity of a trunk tri-axial accelerometer system for gait analysis in older adults. *Gait Posture* 29, 444–448. doi: 10.1016/j.gaitpost.2008.11.003

Hausdorff, J. M. (2009). Gait dynamics in Parkinson's disease: common and distinct behavior among stride length, gait variability, and fractal-like scaling. *Chaos* 19, 026113. doi: 10.1063/1.3147408

Hausdorff, J. M., and Edelberg, H. K. (1997). Increased gait unsteadiness in community-dwelling elderly fallers. *Arch. Phys. Med. Rehabil.* 78, 278–283. doi: 10.1016/S0003-9993(97)90034-4

Hausdorff, J. M., Lertratanakul, A., Cudkowicz, M. E., Peterson, A. L., Kaliton, D., and Goldberger, A. L. (2000). Dynamic markers of altered gait rhythm in amyotrophic lateral sclerosis. *J. Appl. Physiol.* 88, 2045–2053.

Hausdorff, J. M., Mitchell, S. L., Firtion, R., Peng, C. K., Cudkowicz, M. E., Wei, J. Y., et al. (1997). Altered fractal dynamics of gait: reduced stride-interval correlations with aging and Huntington's disease. *J. Appl. Physiol.* 82, 262–269.

Kalron, A. (2016). Gait variability across the disability spectrum in people with multiple sclerosis. *J. Neurol. Sci.* 361, 1–6. doi: 10.1016/j.jns.2015.12.012

Kiss, R. M. (2011). Effect of severity of knee osteoarthritis on the variability of gait parameters. *J. Electromyogr. Kinesiol.* 21, 695–703. doi: 10.1016/j.jelekin.2011.07.011

Kobayashi, H., Kakihana, W., and Kimura, T. (2014). Combined effects of age and gender on gait symmetry and regularity assessed by autocorrelation of trunk acceleration. *J. Neuroeng. Rehabil.* 11:109. doi: 10.1186/1743-0003-11-109

Kobsar, D., Olson, C., Paranjape, R., and Barden, J. M. (2014b). The validity of gait variability and fractal dynamics obtained from a single, body-fixed triaxial accelerometer. *J. Appl. Biomech.* 30, 343–347. doi: 10.1123/jab.2013-0107

Kobsar, D., Olson, C., Paranjape, R., Hadjistavropoulos, T., and Barden, J. M. (2014a). Evaluation of age-related differences in the stride-to-stride fluctuations, regularity and symmetry of gait using a waist-mounted tri-axial accelerometer. *Gait Posture* 39, 553–557. doi: 10.1016/j.gaitpost.2013.09.008

Landry, S. C., McKean, K. A., Hubley-Kozey, C. L., Stanish, W. D., and Deluzio, K. J. (2007). Knee biomechanics of moderate OA patients measured during gait at a self-selected and fast walking speed. *J. Biomech.* 40, 1754–1761. doi: 10.1016/j.jbiomech.2006.08.010

Lewek, M. D., Scholz, J., Rudolph, K. S., and Snyder-Mackler, L. (2006). Stride-to-stride variability of knee motion in patients with knee osteoarthritis. *Gait Posture* 23, 505–511. doi: 10.1016/j.gaitpost.2005.06.003

Lindemann, U., Najafi, B., Zijlstra, W., Hauer, K., Muche, R., Becker, C., et al. (2008). Distance to achieve steady state walking speed in frail elderly persons. *Gait Posture* 27, 91–96. doi: 10.1016/j.gaitpost.2007.02.005

Mills, K., Hettinga, B. A., Pohl, M. B., and Ferber, R. (2013b). Between-limb kinematic asymmetry during gait in unilateral and bilateral mild to moderate knee osteoarthritis. *Arch. Phys. Med. Rehabil.* 94, 2241–2247. doi: 10.1016/j.apmr.2013.05.010

Mills, K., Hunt, M. A., and Ferber, R. (2013a). Biomechanical deviations during level walking associated with knee osteoarthritis: a systematic review and meta-analysis. *Arthritis Care Res.* 65, 1643–1665. doi: 10.1002/acr.22015

Moe-Nilssen, R., Aaslund, M. K., Hodt-Billington, C., and Helbostad, J. L. (2010). Gait variability measures may represent different constructs. *Gait Posture* 32, 98–101. doi: 10.1016/j.gaitpost.2010.03.019

Moe-Nilssen, R., and Helbostad, J. L. (2004). Estimation of gait cycle characteristics by truck accelerometry. *J. Biomech.* 37, 121–126. doi: 10.1016/S0021-9290(03)00233-1

Moon, Y., Sung, J., An, R., Hernandez, M. E., and Sosnoff, J. J. (2016). Gait variability in people with neurological disorders: a systematic review and meta-analysis. *Hum. Mov. Sci.* 47, 197–208. doi: 10.1016/j.humov.2016.03.010

Terrier, P., and Dériaz, O. (2011). Kinematic variability, fractal dynamics and local dynamic stability of treadmill walking. *J. Neuroeng. Rehabil.* 8:12. doi: 10.1186/1743-0003-8-12

Tochigi, Y., Segal, N. A., Vaseenon, T., and Brown, T. D. (2012). Entropy analysis of tri-axial leg acceleration signal waveforms for measurement of decrease of physiological variability in human gait. *J. Orthop. Res.* 30, 897–904. doi: 10.1002/jor.22022

Wittwer, J. E., Webster, K. E., and Hill, K. (2013). Reproducibility of gait variability measures in people with Alzheimer's disease. *Gait Posture* 38, 507–510. doi: 10.1016/j.gaitpost.2013.01.021

Yakhdani, H. R., Bafghi, H. A., Meijer, O. G., Bruijn, S. M., van den Dikkenberg, N., Stibbe, A. B., et al. (2010). Stability and variability of knee kinematics during gait in knee osteoarthritis before and after replacement surgery. *Clin. Biomech.* 25, 230–236. doi: 10.1016/j.clinbiomech.2009.12.003

Zhang, Y., and Jordan, J. M. (2008). Epidemiology of osteoarthritis. *Rheum. Dis. Clin. N. Am.* 34, 515–529. doi: 10.1016/j.rdc.2008.05.007

10

Head Stability and Head-Trunk Coordination in Horseback Riders: The Contribution of Visual Information According to Expertise

Agnès Olivier [1,2,3]*, Elise Faugloire [3], Laure Lejeune [3], Sophie Biau [4] and Brice Isableu [5]

[1] CIAMS, Univ Paris-Sud, Université Paris-Saclay, Orsay, France, [2] CIAMS, Université d'Orléans, Orléans, France,
[3] Normandie Univ, UNICAEN, CESAMS, Caen, France, [4] ENE, Institut Français du Cheval et de l'Equitation, Saumur, France,
[5] Aix Marseille Univ, PSYCLE, Aix-en-Provence, France

*Correspondence:
*Agnès Olivier
agnes.olivier@u-psud.fr;
olivieragnes1@hotmail.com*

Maintaining equilibrium while riding a horse is a challenging task that involves complex sensorimotor processes. We evaluated the relative contribution of visual information (static or dynamic) to horseback riders' postural stability (measured from the variability of segment position in space) and the coordination modes they adopted to regulate balance according to their level of expertise. Riders' perceptual typologies and their possible relation to postural stability were also assessed. Our main assumption was that the contribution of visual information to postural control would be reduced among expert riders in favor of vestibular and somesthetic reliance. Twelve Professional riders and 13 Club riders rode an equestrian simulator at a gallop under four visual conditions: (1) with the projection of a simulated scene reproducing what a rider sees in the real context of a ride in an outdoor arena, (2) under stroboscopic illumination, preventing access to dynamic visual cues, (3) in normal lighting but without the projected scene (i.e., without the visual consequences of displacement) and (4) with no visual cues. The variability of the position of the head, upper trunk and lower trunk was measured along the anteroposterior (AP), mediolateral (ML), and vertical (V) axes. We computed discrete relative phase to assess the coordination between pairs of segments in the anteroposterior axis. *Visual field dependence-independence* was evaluated using the Rod and Frame Test (RFT). The results showed that the Professional riders exhibited greater overall postural stability than the Club riders, revealed mainly in the AP axis. In particular, head variability was lower in the Professional riders than in the Club riders in visually altered conditions, suggesting a greater ability to use vestibular and somesthetic information according to task constraints with expertise. In accordance with this result, RFT perceptual scores revealed that the Professional riders were less dependent on the visual field than were the Club riders. Finally, the Professional riders exhibited specific coordination modes that, unlike the Club riders, departed from pure in-phase and anti-phase patterns and depended on visual conditions. The present findings provide evidence of major differences in the sensorimotor processes contributing to postural control with expertise in horseback riding.

Keywords: head stability, postural stability, head-trunk coordination, visual information, field dependence-independence, horseback rider, expertise, riding simulator

INTRODUCTION

Horseback riding is a challenging task that requires regulating postural balance while sitting on a moving base of support. To control their balance, riders need to adapt their movements to those of the horse while picking up information in the environment to direct the horse toward the intended goal. Stabilizing the head in this context is very challenging and yet crucial for motor performance. Because the head contains the visual and vestibular systems that play a decisive role in balance control, its stabilization in space is important for optimal processing of visual and vestibular information (e.g., Gresty and Bronstein, 1992; Amblard et al., 2001) and therefore, to provide a stable base for action (e.g., Ripoll et al., 1986; Clément et al., 1988; Pozzo et al., 1990). In the present study, we sought to assess whether (i) postural stability[1], and more specifically head stability, is a signature of expertise in horseback riders, (ii) the contribution of visual information to riders' postural stability is reduced among expert riders in favor of vestibular and somesthetic reliance, and (iii) expert riders adopt specific postural coordination modes to preserve head stability.

Balance control involves the visual, vestibular and somesthetic systems. The contribution of vision to balance has received the greatest attention in the literature and has been tested in numerous conditions including the suppression of visual afferences by eye closure (e.g., Perrin et al., 1998; Perrot et al., 1998; Callier et al., 2001; Rougier et al., 2003), the stimulation of the central or peripheral visual field (e.g., Berencsi et al., 2005), the deterioration of visual acuity or the reduction of the visual field (e.g., Laurent et al., 1989; Schmid et al., 2008), the inclination or displacement of the visual environment (Isableu et al., 1997, 2010, 2011; Gautier et al., 2008), the selective suppression of dynamic visual cues by stroboscopic illumination (e.g., Amblard et al., 1985) or their gain in a ground optical flow (e.g., Baumberger et al., 2004). The results of these studies highlighted the importance of vision in balance control, but these conclusions should be moderated in the context of sporting expertise. Indeed, sports activities involve complex sensorimotor skills and constrain the subjects to act and process multiple information sources (proprioceptive, tactile, auditory, etc.) with a particularly high level of accuracy and rapidity.

To be efficient, the expert develops, through years of training, optimal responses to both external and internal constraints (Ericsson et al., 1993; Ericsson and Lehmann, 1996). In particular, the contribution of sensory information to postural control evolves with training and differs according to the level of practice (Era et al., 1996; Perrot et al., 1998; Bringoux et al., 2000), the type of physical activity (Hosseinimehr et al., 2009), and the specificity of gesture, support, task, or position in the environment within the same sport or sport family (Robert

et al., 2004; Bizid and Paillard, 2006; Stambolieva et al., 2011). Overall, these studies showed that the contribution of vision to the regulation of postural balance tends to decrease with expertise, while somesthetic and vestibular information become more critical. For example, experts in soccer, surfing, dance, and gymnastics can use the remaining sensory modalities to compensate for a lack of vision in unstable postures (e.g., Perrin et al., 1998; Vuillerme et al., 2001a,b; Paillard et al., 2006, 2011).

Studies on horseback riding have investigated various topics such as equine gait (e.g., Galloux et al., 1994; Peham et al., 2004), horse-rider interactions (e.g., Lagarde et al., 2005; Byström et al., 2009; Wolframm et al., 2013; Münz et al., 2014), rider muscle activity (e.g., Terada, 2000; Terada et al., 2004), rider joint position (e.g., Kang et al., 2010), and rider body movements (e.g., Münz et al., 2013; Byström et al., 2015; Eckardt and Witte, 2016; Engell et al., 2016). However, very little research has been devoted to the use of sensory information in horseback riding and none has been devoted to the contribution of sensory information to rider postural stability. Some authors have suggested that expert riders use mainly proprioceptive information rather than visual information to control the horse's pace (Laurent and Pailhous, 1982; Laurent et al., 1989). Others have emphasized the importance of haptic information for coordination between the rider's movements and those of the horse (e.g., Lagarde et al., 2005). Indeed, various contacts (e.g., with the saddle, rein, stirrup) and pressures (between the rider's pelvis and the horse's saddle, primarily) are produced during the horse/rider interaction in riding. They provide rich and patterned somesthetic information (proprioceptive and tactile) that are of utmost importance to the rider in regulating and coordinating his/her movements with those of the horse. Thus, an interesting question is whether the contribution of somesthetic information to postural stability increases with expertise in horseback riding at the expense of vision, as was observed in other sports activities.

A related question concerns interindividual differences in the use of sensory information for spatial orientation, and more specifically the visual field dependence-independence (e.g., Witkin, 1950; Oltman, 1968; Paillard, 1971; Isableu et al., 1997, 2010). It has been proposed that Field Dependence (FD) or Independence (FI) reflects the weight each individual assigns to visual or non-visual information (Isableu et al., 1997, 2003, 2010, 2011; Bringoux et al., 2016). At one extreme, field-dependent subjects are affected by the surrounding visual field and are thus assumed to rely predominantly on visual information, while, at the opposite end of the continuum, field-independent subjects are less affected by the visual surroundings and so are assumed to rely more on somesthetic and vestibular cues. The influence of this perceptual typology has been observed regularly in both perceptual orientation and postural tasks (e.g., Witkin, 1950; Crémieux and Mesure, 1994; Collins and De Luca, 1995; Luyat et al., 1997; Golomer et al., 1999; Kluzik et al., 2005; Rousseu and Crémieux, 2005; Slaboda et al., 2011).

Visual field dependence-independence is of particular interest for the present study as it has been shown both to be related to expertise in sport (e.g., Liu, 2003; Guillot and Collet, 2004; Rousseu and Crémieux, 2005) and to induce interindividual differences in postural control (e.g., Golomer et al., 1999; Isableu

---

[1] In the dynamical systems perspective, stability has a precise definition related to a system's response to a change in initial conditions or to a perturbation (e.g., Strogatz, 1994). In this view, the term postural stability refers to the stability of the underlying movement dynamics (e.g., Newell et al., 1993). In the present paper, we use the term "postural stability" in its most widespread sense in the literature on postural control, which supposes a reduced amount of variability of the segments in space.

et al., 2003, 2010). Several studies have shown that experts tend to be more field-independent in a number of physical activities such as acrobatic sports (e.g., Liu, 2003; Guillot and Collet, 2004; Rousseu and Crémieux, 2005). Moreover, some studies have highlighted a relationship between perceptual typologies and postural performance (e.g., Isableu et al., 1997; Golomer et al., 1999; Isableu et al., 2003, 2010) showing that field-dependent subjects were less stable than field-independent subjects in postural tasks, in particular when visual conditions were altered (through the inclination of the visual frame, the suppression of dynamic visual information using stroboscopic illumination or the suppression of visual information).

To date, no study has investigated interindividual differences or the relationship between perceptual typologies and sensorimotor performance in horseback riders (Olivier et al., 2012). Addressing these questions could help understand the differences between expert and non-expert riders in the weight they assign to visual information and in their ability to use non-visual information to regulate balance. Based on the results of previous studies, it can be expected that expert riders would be less dependent on the visual field, leading them to better stabilize their head compared to novice riders.

Beyond perceptual aspects, addressing the question of postural stability in riders also raises the question of the coordination modes used to regulate balance. Postural coordination during upright stance has been studied intensively in various contexts and according to different theoretical approaches (e.g., Nashner and McCollum, 1985; Assaiante and Amblard, 1993, 1995; Bardy et al., 1999; Faugloire et al., 2005). Overall, these studies have shown that head stability—and more generally postural stability—can be achieved through different coordination modes which were found to evolve with development (Assaiante and Amblard, 1995), motor learning (e.g., Zanone and Kelso, 1992; Vereijken et al., 1997; Faugloire et al., 2006, 2009), and expertise in sports activities (Marin et al., 1999; Gautier et al., 2009). In particular, Marin et al. (1999) compared the postural coordination modes adopted by novices and experts in gymnastics in terms of hip-ankle relative phase. Their results showed that increasing the difficulty of the postural task produced a change from an in-phase pattern between the ankle and the hips (almost synchronized flexion-extension of the joints) to an anti-phase pattern (joints moving in opposite directions) occurring earlier in non-gymnasts than in gymnasts. The fact that expert gymnasts were able to maintain the in-phase pattern at greater task difficulties than non-gymnasts demonstrates that expertise in gymnastics leads to a functional modification of existing postural coordination modes.

In horseback riding, riders have to anticipate and compensate for the horse's movements in a sitting posture. While the maintenance of stance in an upright posture, either on a stable or an unstable base of support, involves mainly the ankle, hip and knee joints (e.g., Nashner and McCollum, 1985; Bardy et al., 1999), riders primarily regulate balance through movements of the pelvis, trunk and neck (Vitte et al., 1995; Silva e Borges et al., 2011; Janura et al., 2015). Thus, the results obtained in studies on postural coordination in an upright stance do not apply to horseback riding situations. Interesting insights

are provided by studies on postural regulation in a sitting position (e.g., Forssberg and Hirschfeld, 1994; Vibert et al., 2001; Keshner, 2003, 2004). In these studies, participants sat on a sled that was translated in anteroposterior directions (Forssberg and Hirschfeld, 1994; Vibert et al., 2001; Keshner, 2003, 2004), sideways (Vibert et al., 2001), or rotated in the sagittal plane (Forssberg and Hirschfeld, 1994). In most studies, the participants' legs and shins were resting horizontally in front of them (Forssberg and Hirschfeld, 1994; Keshner, 2003, 2004) and visual information was suppressed (Vibert et al., 2001; Keshner, 2003, 2004). Overall, the results showed that the head lagged behind the trunk in response to the perturbation (e.g., Forssberg and Hirschfeld, 1994; Vibert et al., 2001; Keshner, 2003, 2004) and that somatosensory information generated at the pelvis level, and not vestibular information from the head, appears to trigger postural responses during sitting (e.g., Forssberg and Hirschfeld, 1994; Keshner, 2003, 2004). These interesting results do not help to understand the contribution of vision because the availability of visual information was not manipulated: vision was either suppressed by eye closure (Vibert et al., 2001) or darkness (Keshner, 2003, 2004), or was available in all conditions (Forssberg and Hirschfeld, 1994). Also, the important differences between these studies and horseback riding situations in terms of the sitting position (closed vs. open coxo-femoral angle), the nature of the movements of the base of support (linear translation in the horizontal plane vs. pitch and vertical movements) and their rhythmicity (discrete vs. cyclic) do not allow to generalize these results to riders' postural coordination modes.

The purpose of the present study was to evaluate the relative contribution of visual information to head and trunk stability in Club and Professional horseback riders and the coordination modes adopted to regulate balance depending on expertise. With this aim, the participants were asked to ride a riding simulator while facing a dynamic virtual scene under four visual conditions: in normal lighting allowing the participants to access dynamic visual cues (*continuous simulated scene condition*), under stroboscopic illumination, preventing access to dynamic visual cues (*stroboscopic simulated scene condition*), in normal lighting with full visual access to the fixed surroundings but without the projected scene and thus without the visual consequences of the displacements corresponding to the context of a ride (*no simulated scene condition*) and with no visual cues (*no vision condition*).

(i)   Our first hypothesis was that expert riders produce lower postural displacements and deploy more efficient postural control from the top of the head to the lower trunk leading them to better stabilize their head.

(ii) Our second hypothesis was that the contribution of visual information to riders' postural stability is reduced among expert riders in favor of vestibular and somesthetic reliance, leading experts to maintain head stability better in visually altered conditions than less experienced riders. This differential reliance is also expected to be revealed by specific perceptual typologies according to expertise, with Professional riders being less dependent on the visual field than Club riders.

(iii) Our third hypothesis was that expert horseback riders exhibit specific coordination modes to maintain a high level of postural stability, as has been observed in studies on postural coordination and expertise in other sports (Marin et al., 1999; Gautier et al., 2009).

METHODS

Participants

Twenty-five participants were divided into two groups based on their level of horseback riding expertise. The characteristics of the two groups of participants are presented in **Table 1**. One group was composed of 12 elite Professional riders who specialized in show jumping and cross country riding. These members of the French National Horseback Riding School had a minimum of 20 years of practice and had participated in international competitions. The other group was composed of 13 Club riders who were ranked "Galop 5" by the French Riding Federation and had no particular specialty in any of the equestrian sports. Some of them had participated in competitions at a regional level. All of the participants were novices in the use of a riding simulator.

All of the participants had normal or corrected-to-normal vision, and reported no balance disorder, injury or pathology that might affect their ability to perform tests on a riding simulator. Local ethical approval from the Université Paris-Sud EA 4532 ethics committee was granted for this study. Each participant signed an informed consent statement after receiving oral and written descriptions of the procedure.

Apparatus

Figure 1 illustrates the set-up used in this experiment. The participants rode the riding simulator Persival (Persival Industrie, Saumur, France) from the French National Horseback Riding School at a simulated gallop (stride cycle frequency of 1.4 Hz, vertical displacement amplitude of 17 cm). The use of a riding simulator ensured that the same motion of the base of support was applied to every participant. Displacements of the participants' head and trunk were measured with an electromagnetic tracking system (Fastrack, Polhemus Inc., Colchester, VT, USA), sampled at 40 Hz. Three receivers were placed on the participants: on the top of the head, on the seventh cervical vertebra (C7), corresponding to the base of the neck, and on the third lumbar vertebra (L3), which corresponds to the center of the lordotic curve of the lower back. The receiver on the top of the head was attached to the rider's helmet and the other two were attached directly to the skin using double-sided adhesive and medical cloth tape. The transmitter was located 90 cm above and 35 cm behind the back of the simulator saddle, on a shelf attached to the ceiling. The receivers attached to the head, C7, and L3 were within 52, 72, and 112 cm of the transmitter, respectively, leading to a positional resolution of 0.0025, 0.0163, and 0.095 cm, respectively (the resolution of electromagnetic tracking system measurement is affected by the distance between the transmitter and the receiver).

The participants sat on the saddle of the Persival simulator at a distance of 3.20 m from the projection screen (1.92 × 1.36 m), creating a visual angle of about 33.40° horizontally and 23.99°

TABLE 1 | Mean characteristics of the Professional and Club riders (standard deviation in parentheses).

	Professional riders	Club riders
Number of participants	12 [2 women]	13 [7 women]
Age	38.33 years (7.05)	29.85 years (6.07)
Height	179.58 cm (8.47)	171.23 cm (10.43)
Weight	70.75 kg (8.62)	64.54 kg (9.65)
Years of practice	29.67 years (5.48)	10.23 years (6.02)
Years of practice in competition	16.67 years (6.14)	1.54 years (2.18)
Amount of practice per week	36.17 h/week (6.56)	1.31 h/week (1.75)

vertically. In order to minimize peripheral visual information, opaque black curtains were placed parallel to the rider's line of vision on either side of the experimental set-up from the edges of the projection screen to the back of the simulator. SimPiste software (Persival Industrie, Saumur, France) was used to create a computer-generated movie projected on the screen. The resulting 3D animated scene represented a classic situation of a ride in a show jumping arena from the rider's viewpoint and was synchronized with the simulator's movements. The visual environment included several fences around which the horse-rider pair moved at a gallop. Thus, the visual scene simulated displacement around the fences and the mechanical movements of the simulator maintained a gallop pace with no jumps.

Procedure and Experimental Design

The experimental session began with the assessment of the participants' visual field dependence using a portable Rod and Frame Test (RFT; Oltman, 1968). In this test, participants are required to adjust a rod enclosed within a square frame on the physical vertical. The frame and the rod were tilted 18° clockwise or counterclockwise from the vertical, where the frame effect has been found to be maximal (Zoccolotti et al., 1993). Each of the four resulting conditions was presented five times, resulting in 20 randomized trials. Clear and stable differences have been found among subjects' scores on the RFT and have led to the establishment of the well-known dimension of "field dependence–independence" (Oltman, 1968; Gueguen et al., 2012): Field Dependent participants (FD) align the rod on the framework, whereas Field Independent participants (FI) align the rod on the gravitational vertical.

Next, the participants were invited to mount the riding simulator and were equipped with the Fastrack receivers. After a short period of familiarization (30 s) with the simulator, four visual conditions were presented in a randomized order as separate 50-s trials. The mechanical horse's movements were similar in every visual condition and reproduced a gallop gait. The participants were instructed to "look straight ahead and to stabilize their posture as in real practice" for each of these conditions.

– In the *no simulated scene condition* (No scene), the virtual scene was not projected and the participants faced the white projection screen under normal lighting. In this condition, continuous visual information was available from the fixed

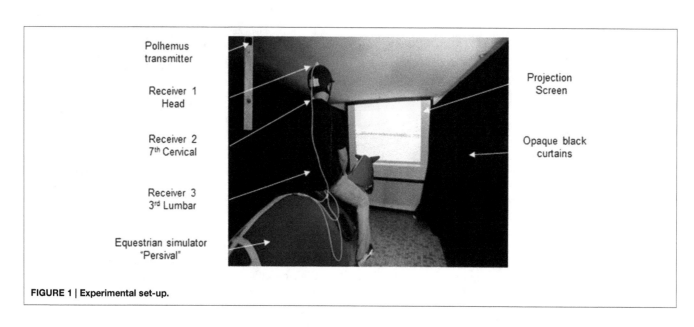

FIGURE 1 | Experimental set-up.

surroundings, constituting a stable reference frame for postural control.

– In the *continuous simulated scene condition* (Cont scene), the animated virtual scene from SimPiste was projected on the screen with normal lighting. In this condition, the visual scene reproduced what a rider sees in the real context of a ride in a show jumping arena, with forward displacements and turns in the virtual environment.

– In the *stroboscopic simulated scene condition* (Strob scene), the animated virtual scene was projected on the screen but its dynamic visual cues were eliminated by stroboscopic illumination (2.8 flash/s). In this condition, visual information was reduced to static visual cues in order to evaluate the various contributions of static visual cues vs. dynamic visual cues, available in normal lighting, to postural stability (Amblard and Crémieux, 1976; Amblard et al., 1985).

– In the *No vision condition* (No vision), the participants wore opaque glasses (swimming goggles covered with opaque adhesive tape) that prevented access to environmental information. This condition assessed the general contribution of vision to the riders' postural stability.

The Strob scene and No vision conditions corresponded to visually altered conditions in which the availability of dynamic visual cues (Strob scene) or the totality of the visual scene (No vision) was suppressed. The No scene condition was used as a reference condition in which postural control was expected to be facilitated by the presence of fixed surroundings (e.g., Lee and Lishman, 1975; Guerraz et al., 2001).

The participants were given a few minutes' break between conditions. The experiment took about 40 min to complete from the RFT to the last vision condition on the simulator.

Data Analysis

The raw position data collected by the magnetic tracking system were processed and analyzed using Matlab software (R2009b, The MathWorks Inc., Natick, MA, USA). In order to eliminate the

initiation of the simulator's motion and participants' adaptation phase to it, we considered position data from the fifth second to the end of each trial. Two types of dependent variables were computed from the position data. First, the variability of the displacement of each segment (head, C7, L3) was quantified by computing the standard deviation of the position along the anteroposterior (SD_{AP}), mediolateral (SD_{ML}), and vertical (SD_V) axes. These measurements were used to quantify the degree of stability of the head, the cervical segment (upper trunk) and the lumbar segment (lower trunk) in space (the lower the standard deviation of position, the more stable the segment is in space).

Second, we evaluated the coordination modes the riders used to stabilize their posture. Because the control of the hips, trunk and neck impacts mainly the displacements of the upper body in the AP axis, we analyzed postural coordination along this axis. Coordination modes were computed from position data in the AP axis using the mean relative phases ϕ_{L-C}, ϕ_{L-H}, and ϕ_{C-H} between the lumbar and the cervical segments, the lumbar segment and the head, and the cervical segment and the head, respectively (**Figure 2A**). The standard deviations of the mean relative phases ($SD\phi_{L-C}$, $SD\phi_{L-H}$, $SD\phi_{C-H}$) were computed as measurements of the within-participants dispersion around the mean relative phase.

Prior to relative phase computation, position data were filtered with a recursive second-order Butterworth filter with a cutoff frequency of 2 Hz. For each pair of segments, we computed the point estimate of relative phase (e.g., Zanone and Kelso, 1992) using the maximum position of each segment in the AP axis for every movement cycle:

$$\phi_{rel} = \frac{(t_1 - t_2)}{(t_1 - t_0)} \times 360° \tag{1}$$

where t_0 and t_1 are the time of occurrence of two successive maximum positions along the AP axis for the reference segment, and t_2 is the time of occurrence of maximum position of the

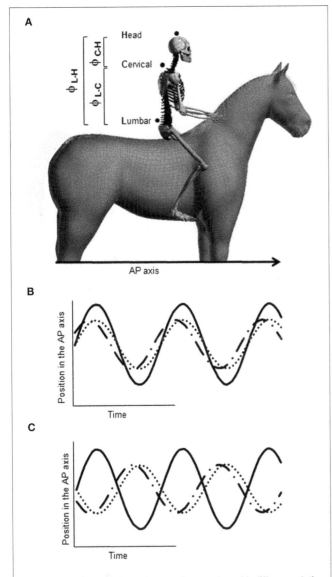

A

Head

Cervical

ϕ_{CH}

ϕ_{L-H}

ϕ_{C-H}

ϕ_{L-C}

Lumbar

AP axis

B

Position in the AP axis

Time

C

Position in the AP axis

Time

FIGURE 2 | Illustration of the coordination modes with different relative phase values. (A) Illustration of the relative phases computed (ϕ_{L-C}, ϕ_{L-H}, ϕ_{C-H}). **(B)** In-phase coordination between the referent segment (bold line) and the segment represented by the dotted line (the segments move synchronously in the same direction resulting in a relative phase of 0°); relative phase of −30° (=330°) between the referent segment (bold line) and the segment represented by the dash-dotted line. **(C)** Anti-phase coordination (the segments move synchronously in opposite directions, resulting in a relative phase of 180°) between the referent segment (bold line) and the segment represented by the dotted line; relative phase of 150° between the referent segment (bold line) and the segment represented by the dash-dotted line.

second segment. In other words, the time difference between the position peaks of the two segments is expressed in degrees relative to the period of the reference segment.

Each trial (corresponding to one visual condition) comprised about 65 movement cycles. Mean relative phases and their standard deviations were computed in a circular fashion (Batschelet, 1981) over the 65 resulting discrete relative phase values. **Figures 2B,C** illustrates different relative phase values in

the temporal domain. A mean relative phase of 0° (corresponding to an in-phase coordination mode) indicates that the two segments were moving synchronously forward and backward. A relative phase of 180° (corresponding to an anti-phase coordination mode) indicates that the two segments were moving in opposite directions. Other relative phase values indicate a lead or a lag of one segment with respect to the other: for ϕ_{L-C} and ϕ_{L-H}, values between 0 and 180° indicate that the movement peak of the lumbar segment preceded the movement peak of the cervical segment and the movement peak of the head, respectively; for ϕ_{C-H}, values between 0 and 180° indicate that the movement peak of the cervical segment preceded the movement peak of the head.

Finally, RFT perceptual scores revealing errors in the gravitational vertical estimation due to the tilted frame were computed using Nyborg and Isaksen's method 1974.

Statistical Analysis

Levene's tests were conducted on SD_{AP}, SD_{ML}, and SD_V to assess the homogeneity of variance between the Professional and Club riders for each vision condition (No scene, Cont scene, Strob scene, No vision) and each segment (head, C7, L3). Of the 36 resulting comparisons, only two were significant (at an uncorrected significance level of 0.05) with the standard deviation of the head being higher for the Club riders than for the Professional riders in the AP axis in the No Vision condition (uncorrected $p = 0.028$) and in the ML axis in the Cont scene condition (uncorrected $p = 0.034$). Since the variances of the groups were homogenous overall, we conducted separate Expertise (Professional riders, Club riders) × Segment (Head, Cervical, Lumbar) × Vision (No scene, Cont scene, Strob scene, No vision) ANOVAs with repeated measures on the two last factors on SD_{AP}, SD_{ML}, and SD_V. In order to address our second hypothesis, planned comparisons of least-squares means were used to compare specifically head variability between the Professional and Club riders in the different conditions of vision.

Rayleigh Uniformity Tests conducted on ϕ_{L-C}, ϕ_{L-H}, and ϕ_{C-H} for each trial and each participant revealed that relative phase distributions were significantly directional (i.e., not uniform), $ps < 0.05$. One of the Club riders presented a distribution that did not differ from a uniform distribution in several trials ($ps > 0.05$) and was thus removed from the analyses on coordination modes. Levene's tests conducted on ϕ_{L-C}, ϕ_{L-H}, and ϕ_{C-H} for each vision condition revealed no significant difference between the variance of the Professional and Club riders (uncorrected $ps \geq 0.063$). These results, plus the fact that the range of mean relative phase values over participants did not exceed 180° in every experimental condition, allowed us to conduct analyses of variance[2] on ϕ_{L-C}, ϕ_{L-H}, ϕ_{C-H}, and on their standard deviations. For each variable, we conducted an Expertise (Professional riders, Club riders) × Vision (No scene, Cont scene, Strob scene,

---

[2]When the range of distribution does not exceed 180°, circular statistics (Batschelet, 1981; Mardia and Jupp, 2000) and regular linear statistics result in virtually identical outcomes.

No vision) ANOVA with repeated measures on the second factor.

For each significant effect, we conducted *post-hoc* comparisons with corrected *p*-values according to the Holm-Bonferroni procedure. The results were considered significant at the level of 5% and the effect size was estimated using partial eta squared (η_p^2).

RESULTS

Postural Stability

In order to address our main hypotheses with conciseness, we describe the results of the three separate ANOVAs conducted on SD_{AP}, SD_{ML}, and SD_V together for each main effect and each interaction in the following paragraphs (**Table 2**).

The ANOVAs revealed a significant main effect of Expertise on SD_{AP} [$F_{(1, 23)} = 5.64$, $p = 0.026$] showing that anteroposterior motion was greater for the Club riders (mean ± SE: 2.58 cm ± 0.09) than for the Professional riders (mean ± SE: 2.27 cm ± 0.10). The main effect of Expertise was not significant for SD_{ML} [$F_{(1, 23)} = 3.76$, $p = 0.065$] and SD_V [$F_{(1, 23)} = 1.37$, $p = 0.254$].

The main effect of Segment did not reach significance for SD_{AP} [$F_{(2, 46)} = 2.89$, $p = 0.066$] but was significant for SD_{ML} [$F_{(2, 46)} = 23.56$, $p < 0.001$] and SD_V [$F_{(2, 46)} = 18.68$, $p < 0.001$]. Holm-Bonferroni *post-hoc* tests showed that for both axes, head variability (mean ± SE: $SD_{ML} = 1.37$ cm, ± 0.11; $SD_Z = 5.17$ cm, ± 0.09) was greater, $ps < 0.001$, than the variability of the cervical segment (mean ± SE: $SD_{ML} = 0.86$ cm, ± 0.04; $SD_V = 4.76$ cm, ± 0.05) and the lumbar segment (mean ± SE: $SD_{ML} = 0.73$ cm, ± 0.04; $SD_Z = 4.71$ cm, ± 0.06), which did not differ from each other, $ps > 0.20$.

The Expertise × Segment interaction was significant for SD_V [$F_{(2, 46)} = 3.95$, $p = 0.026$], revealing that the head was more stable along the vertical axis for the Professional riders (mean ± SE: 4.97 cm ± 0.13) than for the Club riders (mean ± SE: 5.34 cm ± 0.12), $p = 0.047$. No influence of expertise was found for the cervical segment and the lumbar segment, $ps > 0.95$ (**Figure 3**). The Expertise × Segment interactions were not significant for SD_{AP} [$F_{(2, 46)} = 0.14$, $p = 0.867$] and SD_{ML} [$F_{(2, 46)} = 2.76$, $p = 0.074$].

The ANOVAs also revealed main effects of Vision on SD_{AP} [$F_{(3, 69)} = 5.07$, $p = 0.003$] and SD_{ML} [$F_{(3, 69)} = 7.75$, $p < 0.001$], but not on SD_V [$F_{(3, 69)} = 0.76$, $p = 0.522$]. Holm-Bonferroni *post-hoc* tests showed that SD_{AP} was significantly lower in the No scene condition than in the No vision condition, $p = 0.010$, and that SD_{ML} was significantly greater in the Cont Scene condition than in the No scene and the No vision conditions, $ps \leq 0.007$.

The main effects of Vision can be further specified by the significant Segment × Vision interactions observed on SD_{AP} and SD_{ML} (**Figure 4**). For SD_{AP}, the Segment × Vision interaction [$F_{(6, 138)} = 4.86$, $p < 0.001$] indicated that the vision condition influenced the anteroposterior variability of the head and cervical segment, but had no effect on the lumbar segment (**Figure 4A**). More precisely, Holm-Bonferroni *post-hoc* tests showed that the No scene condition led to lower anteroposterior variability of head movements than the No vision condition ($p < 0.001$) and that the variability of C7 in the anteroposterior axis was significantly lower in the No scene condition than in all other vision conditions ($ps \leq 0.002$). There was no other significant difference in segment variability between vision conditions for the AP axis.

For SD_{ML}, the Segment × Vision interaction [$F_{(6, 138)} = 2.73$, $p = 0.015$] also indicated that lumbar segment variability was not influenced by the vision condition unlike variability of the head and cervical segment (**Figure 4B**). Holm-Bonferroni *post-hoc* tests conducted on SD_{ML} showed that both the Cont scene condition and the Strob scene condition led to greater mediolateral variability of head movements than the No vision and No scene conditions ($ps \leq 0.012$). Mediolateral variability of the cervical segment was significantly greater in the Cont scene condition than in the No scene condition ($p = 0.001$). There was no other significant difference in segment variability between vision conditions for the ML axis.

Finally, the ANOVA conducted on SD_{ML} indicated that the Expertise × Segment × Vision interaction was close to significance [$F_{(6, 138)} = 2.16$, $p = 0.051$]. The Expertise × Segment × Vision interactions were not significant for SD_{AP} and SD_V [$Fs_{(6, 138)} \leq 1.21$, $ps \geq 0.302$], and there were no significant Vision × Expertise interactions in any axis of movement [$Fs_{(3, 69)} \leq 2.00$, $ps \geq 0.122$].

TABLE 2 | Results of the Expertise × Segment × Vision ANOVAs conducted on SD$_{AP}$, SD$_{ML}$, and SD$_V$.

	SD$_{AP}$			SD$_{ML}$			SD$_V$		
	F	*p*	η_p^2	*F*	*p*	η_p^2	*F*	*p*	η_p^2
Expertise	**5.64**	**0.026**	**0.197**	3.77	0.065	0.141	1.37	0.254	0.056
Segment	2.89	0.066	0.112	**23.56**	**0.000**	**0.506**	**18.68**	**0.000**	**0.448**
Vision	**5.07**	**0.003**	**0.181**	**7.75**	**0.000**	**0.252**	0.76	0.522	0.032
Segment × Expertise	0.14	0.867	0.006	2.76	0.074	0.107	**3.95**	**0.026**	**0.147**
Vision × Expertise	1.76	0.163	0.071	2.00	0.122	0.080	0.91	0.438	0.038
Segment × Vision	**4.86**	**0.000**	**0.175**	**2.73**	**0.015**	**0.106**	0.96	0.453	0.040
Segment × Vision × Expertise	0.46	0.837	0.020	2.16	0.051	0.086	1.21	0.302	0.050

Significant differences are indicated in bold. η_p^2 = Partial Eta Squared.

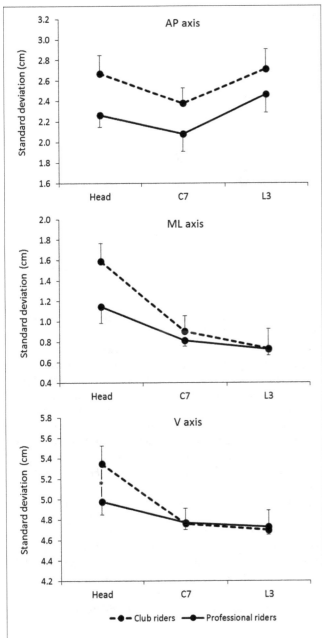

FIGURE 3 | Mean standard deviation of segment position for the Club riders and the Professional riders in the three axes of movement. The Expertise × Segment interaction was significant for SD_V and not significant for SD_{AP} and SD_{ML}. See the text for details. *$p < 0.05$. The error bars represent standard error.

Contribution of Visual Information to Head Stability Depending on Expertise
Effect of Expertise on Head Stability
The ANOVAs presented in the previous section revealed a main effect of Expertise on SD_{AP} and some interactions involving Expertise for SD_{ML} and SD_V. In order to specifically address our second hypothesis that head variability would be lower for the Professional riders compared to the Club riders under visually

altered conditions, we conducted planned comparisons of least-squares means on SD_{AP}, SD_{ML}, and SD_V for the head only for each vision condition (**Figure 5**).

We found that the position of the head was significantly less variable for the Professional riders than for the Club riders in the anteroposterior axis (SD_{AP}) in the Strob scene [$F_{(23)} = 7.37, p = 0.012$] and in the No Vision [$F_{(23)} = 4.93, p = 0.036$] conditions. In the mediolateral axis, the position of the head was significantly less variable for the Professional riders than for the Club riders in the Cont scene [$F_{(23)} = 5.09, p = 0.033$] and in the Strob scene [$F_{(23)} = 5.60, p = 0.026$] conditions. In the vertical axis, the difference between Professional and Club riders was close to significance in the Strob scene condition [$F_{(23)} = 3.93, p = 0.059$], in the No Vision condition [$F_{(23)} = 3.62, p = 0.070$] and in the Cont scene condition [$F_{(23)} = 3.57, p = 0.072$]. Other differences were not significant, $ps \geq 0.186$.

Visual Field Dependence-Independence and Head Stability
A t-test comparing the RFT perceptual scores of the Professional and Club riders revealed a significant difference between the two groups [$t_{(23)} = 4.53, p = 0.044$]. The 13 Club riders achieved a mean error of $7.30°$ (SE $± 1.35°$) and the 12 Professional riders a mean error of $4.13°$ (SE $± 0.49°$). These results indicated that the Professional riders were less dependent on the visual field than were the Club riders.

To evaluate the relation between perceptual style and postural stability, we performed Pearson's correlation analyses between RFT scores and head variability. We found significant positive correlations between the standard deviations of the head in the ML axis and the RFT scores in all conditions of vision: Cont scene [$r_{(24)} = 0.54, p < 0.001$], Strob scene [$r_{(24)} = 0.55, p < 0.001$], No scene [$r_{(24)} = 0.39, p < 0.001$], and No vision [$r_{(24)} = 0.23, p = 0.014$]. We also found a significant positive correlation between head stability along the V axis and RFT scores in the Cont scene [$r_{(24)} = 0.15, p = 0.048$] and No vision [$r_{(24)} = 0.23, p = 0.013$] conditions. Finally, no significant correlation was found between head displacements along the AP axis and RFT scores.

Coordination Modes
Analyses of the variability of segment position revealed significant differences between the Professional and Club riders. In particular, the Professional riders were found to stabilize their head better in the anteroposterior axis than the Club riders. The following analyses were conducted to assess whether this better stabilization was associated with specific postural coordination modes in the anteroposterior axis. For each variable, we conducted an Expertise × Vision ANOVA with repeated measures on the second factor. The results of these analyses are reported in **Table 3**. **Figure 6** presents the mean relative phases for the Club and Professional riders in the four vision conditions.

Coordination between the Lumbar and Cervical Segments (ϕ_{L-C} and $SD\phi_{L-C}$)
The ANOVA conducted on ϕ_{L-C} revealed a main effect of Expertise [$F_{(1, 22)} = 8.20, p = 0.009$] with a mean relative phase

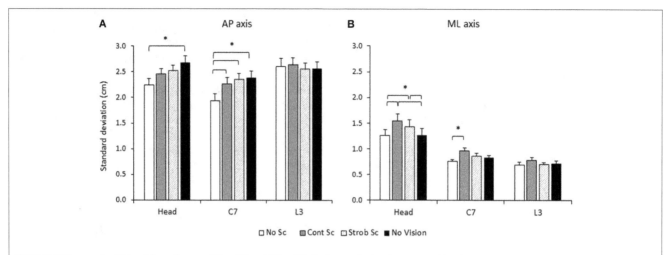

FIGURE 4 | Segment × Vision interactions on SD$_{AP}$ (A) and SD$_{ML}$ (B). No Sc, no simulated scene condition; Cont Sc, continuous simulated scene condition; Strob Sc, stroboscopic simulated scene condition; No vision, No vision condition. *p < 0.05. See the text for details. The error bars represent standard error.

of 188.27° ($SD\phi_{L-C}$ = 24.24°) for the Club riders and of 153.99° ($SD\phi_{L-C}$ = 22.67°) for the Professional riders. This result shows that unlike the Club riders who exhibited an anti-phase pattern between the lower and the upper trunk, the movement cycle of the upper trunk appeared sooner after the movement cycle of the lower trunk in the Professional riders. The main effect of Vision [$F_{(3, 66)}$ = 1.77, p = 0.161] and the Expertise × Vision interaction [$F_{(3, 66)}$ < 0.99, p = 0.043] were not significant.

The ANOVA conducted on $SD\phi_{L-C}$ revealed a main effect of Vision on the within-participants dispersion around the mean relative phase [$F_{(1, 66)}$ = 3.26, p = 0.027]. However, Holm-Bonferroni *post-hoc* tests revealed no significant difference between vision conditions from pairwise comparisons, p ≥ 0.18. The main effect of Expertise [$F_{(1, 22)}$ < 0.15, p = 0.694] and the Expertise × Vision interaction were not significant [$F_{(3, 66)}$ < 0.19, p = 0.898].

Coordination between the Lumbar Segment and the Head (ϕ_{L-H} and $SD\phi_{L-H}$)

The ANOVA conducted on ϕ_{L-H} revealed a main effect of Vision [$F_{(3, 66)}$ = 4.59, p = 0.006]. Holm-Bonferroni *post-hoc* tests showed a significant difference between the coordination modes in the No vision condition (ϕ_{L-H} = 152.4 ± 47.16°) and the Strob scene and No scene conditions, ps ≤ 0.050, with mean relative phases of 172.16° (± 42.59°) and 168.01° (± 44.36°) for the Strob scene and the No scene conditions, respectively. No other difference between vision conditions was significant. The main effect of Expertise [$F_{(1, 22)}$ = 2.66, p = 0.117] and the Expertise × Vision interaction were not significant [$F_{(3, 66)}$ = 2.24, p = 0.092].

The ANOVA conducted on $SD\phi_{L-H}$ showed no main effect of Expertise [$F_{(1, 22)}$ < 1, p = 0.77] and Vision [$F_{(3, 66)}$ = 1.33, p = 0.27], but revealed a significant Expertise × Vision interaction [$F_{(3, 66)}$ = 4.95, p = 0.004]. However, Holm-Bonferroni *post-hoc* tests revealed no significant difference from pairwise comparisons (ps ≥ 0.156).

Coordination between the Cervical Segment and the Head (ϕ_{C-H} and $SD\phi_{C-H}$)

The ANOVA conducted on ϕ_{C-H} revealed a main effect of Vision [$F_{(3, 66)}$ = 3.09, p = 0.033] and a significant Vision × Expertise interaction [$F_{(3, 66)}$ = 3.18, p = 0.030]. Holm-Bonferroni *post-hoc* tests showed that ϕ_{C-H} differed between the No vision (mean ϕ_{C-H} = −10.30°, SD ± 24.66°) and the Cont scene (mean ϕ_{C-H} = 14.74°, SD ± 34.13°) conditions for the Professional riders only (p = 0.037), and that no other difference between vision conditions was significant for either group of participants. The main effect of Expertise was not significant [$F_{(1, 22)}$ < 0.66, p = 0.427].

The ANOVA conducted on $SD\phi_{C-H}$ showed no main effect of Expertise [$F_{(1, 22)}$ < 1, p = 0.52] or Vision [$F_{(3, 66)}$ = 2.53, p = 0.064]. However, the Vision × Expertise interaction was significant [$F_{(3, 66)}$ = 7.08, p < 0.001]. Holm-Bonferroni *post-hoc* tests specified that the within-participants dispersion around the mean relative phase was lower in the No vision condition than in the Cont scene condition (p = 0.033) and in the No scene condition (p = 0.036) for the Professional riders only.

DISCUSSION

The purpose of this study was to evaluate the relative contribution of visual information to head and trunk stability in Club and Professional horseback riders and the coordination modes adopted to regulate balance according to expertise. Modes of spatial referencing were taken into account to determine the riders' perceptual typology and its possible relation to postural stability.

Before addressing our main hypotheses, it should be noted that overall expertise levels and vision conditions, the head exhibited larger displacements than the upper trunk and the lower trunk in the mediolateral and vertical axes. We did not find such an effect of body segment along the anteroposterior axis: the displacements of the head, the upper trunk and the lower

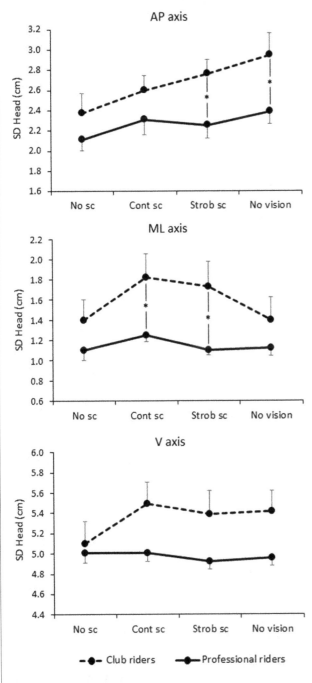

FIGURE 5 | Head variability depending on vision condition and expertise for the three axes of movement. No sc, no simulated scene condition; Cont sc, continuous simulated scene condition; Strob sc, stroboscopic simulated scene condition; No vision, No vision condition. *$p < 0.05$. See the text for details. The error bars represent standard error.

take place to maintain balance in response to the perturbations induced by the simulator's movements.

We can also note several general results independent of expertise regarding the influence of vision condition on the stability of the different levels of the spine. First, we observed no influence of the vision condition on the variability of the lumbar segment. This result suggests, unsurprisingly, that the stability of the lower trunk is influenced mainly by the mechanical perturbations of the support surface and not by the visual information available. Second, the head and the cervical segments were significantly more stable in the AP axis when the riders faced the white projection screen (No scene condition) than in the other vision conditions. This result is in accordance with previous research that showed the stabilizing effect of fixed surroundings (e.g., Lee and Lishman, 1975; Guerraz et al., 2001). Third, we found no influence of the vision condition on postural stability along the V axis. A likely explanation is that the magnitude of the mechanical perturbations induced by the movements of the riding simulator along the vertical axis has much more influence on postural stability than the visual information available.

Postural Stability and Horseback Riding Expertise

Our first hypothesis was that Professional riders would produce lower postural displacements and deploy more efficient postural control from the top of the head to the lower trunk, leading them to better stabilize their head. Our findings support this hypothesis. First, riding expertise appears to be characterized by the ability to minimize postural displacements in the anteroposterior axis. Overall body segments (i.e., head, upper trunk, and lower trunk) and vision conditions, the Professional riders exhibited greater postural stability in the anteroposterior axis than the Club riders. Overall vision conditions, the Professional riders also exhibited greater head stability in the V axis than the Club riders, while there was no significant difference in the stability of the upper trunk and the lower trunk based on the level of expertise. These findings suggest that postural stability of the overall upper body in the AP axis and more specifically of the head in the V axis is a signature of expertise in horseback riding. However, a closer look at the results according to vision conditions is needed to specify the influence of expertise on postural stability.

Relative Contribution of Sensory Information to Riders' Postural Stability Depending on Expertise

Our second hypothesis was that the contribution of visual information to riders' postural stability is reduced among expert riders in favor of vestibular and somesthetic reliance, leading the experts to maintain head stability better in visually altered conditions. Based on our hypothesis, we expected the selective or total suppression of static and dynamic visual cues to induce greater displacements of the head in the Club riders than in the Professionals.

We found no difference in head stability between the Professional and the Club riders in the two unrestricted visual

trunk remained in the same range of motion in the AP axis. This suggests that the inverted pendulum model of balance often used to describe quiet standing (e.g., Winter et al., 1997; Peterka, 2002) does not apply to postural regulation in horseback riding. This is a first indication that more complex coordination patterns

TABLE 3 | Results of the Expertise × Vision ANOVAs conducted on the mean relative phases and their standard deviations.

	Lumbar-Cervical (ϕ_{L-C})			Lumbar-Head (ϕ_{L-H})			Cervical-Head (ϕ_{C-H})		
Mean (ϕ)	**F**	**p**	**η_p^2**	**F**	**p**	**η_p^2**	**F**	**p**	**η_p^2**
Expertise	**8.20**	**0.009**	**0.271**	2.66	0.117	0.108	0.66	0.427	0.029
Vision	1.77	0.161	0.074	**4.59**	**0.006**	**0.173**	**3.09**	**0.033**	**0.123**
Expertise × Vision	0.99	0.401	0.043	2.24	0.092	0.092	**3.18**	**0.030**	**0.126**
Standard deviation ($SD\phi$)									
Expertise	0.15	0.694	0.007	0.08	0.775	0.004	0.42	0.522	0.019
Vision	**3.26**	**0.027**	**0.129**	1.33	0.271	0.057	2.53	0.064	0.103
Expertise × Vision	0.19	0.898	0.009	**4.95**	**0.004**	**0.184**	**7.08**	**0.000**	**0.243**

Significant differences are indicated in bold. η_p^2 = Partial Eta Squared.

conditions (Cont scene and No scene) for the different axes of movement (AP, ML, V). The only exception was head variability in the ML axis in the Cont scene condition, with the Club riders exhibiting greater head displacements than the Professional riders. One possible explanation for this result might be that Club and Professional riders use different strategies during the turns simulated by the visual scene. Indeed, the riding simulator reproduces the perturbation of the chosen pace (gallop in our case) with a fixed orientation of the mechanical horse. Thus, unlike a real ride, the back of the mechanical horse does not turn in the horizontal plane when the visual scene indicates a curved trajectory of the route. The riders might have dealt with this discrepancy differently depending on their level of expertise. It is also possible that the Club riders did not use the visual information provided by the simulated scene with sufficient efficiency to stabilize their head in the ML axis as well as the Professional riders. Solving this question would necessitate a coupling between movement measures and data from the simulated visual scene that is not currently available with the Persival simulator. This coupling would represent a major evolution of the apparatus for research purposes.

The results obtained under stroboscopic illumination were in accordance with our hypothesis. In this condition, the Club riders exhibited greater head displacements compared to the Professionals. The difference was significant in the AP and ML axes, and close to significance in the vertical axis. Dynamic visual cues have been shown to play a major role in postural stabilization during upright stance (e.g., Amblard and Crémieux, 1976; Amblard and Carblanc, 1980; Amblard et al., 1985). In particular, postural stability was found to be severely impaired under stroboscopic illumination (Amblard and Crémieux, 1976; Paulus et al., 1984; Amblard et al., 1985; Assländer et al., 2015), though with some interindividual differences (Crémieux and Mesure, 1994; Isableu et al., 2010, 2011). The present findings highlight these interindividual differences in relation to sports expertise. Suppressing dynamic visual cues differently affected head stability depending on the level of expertise in horseback riding: the Club riders appear to rely more on dynamic visual cues than the Professionals in order to control head stability.

The results obtained in the absence of visual information also agreed with our hypothesis. The position of the head along the AP axis was less variable for the Professional riders than for the Club riders in the No vision condition. However, we found no significant difference along the ML and V axes. These findings reveal that experts handle the absence of visual information better than less experienced riders to maintain head stability in the AP axis.

In order to complete our analysis on the relative contribution of sensory information to postural stability, we examined the relations between perceptual typologies, postural stability and expertise in horseback riding. The perceptual scores obtained with the RFT revealed that the Professional riders were less dependent on the visual field than the Club riders. This predominant perceptual typology in experts agrees with previous findings in other physical activities (e.g., Golomer et al., 1999; Liu, 2003; Guillot and Collet, 2004; Rousseu and Crémieux, 2005) and, in line with our second hypothesis, suggests that expert horseback riders rely more on vestibular and somesthetic information than less experienced riders. This enhanced reliance on non-visual information likely explains the greater head stabilization observed in the Professional riders in visually altered conditions (i.e., No vision and Strob scene conditions) compared to the Club riders (Isableu et al., 2003, 2010; Brady et al., 2012). Correlation analyses showed that field dependence–independence scores measured with the RFT were positively correlated with the variability of the head along the ML and V axes. This result provides an additional demonstration of the effect of perceptual typology on postural control (e.g., Isableu et al., 2010, 2011).

The joint analysis of postural stability and perceptual typology highlights a major result of the present study. Except for the mediolateral variability of the head in the Cont scene condition discussed above, the Club riders managed to maintain a level of head stability similar to the Professional riders when visual information was available, whether the visual environment was fixed (No scene condition) or simulated displacements corresponding to a ride (Cont scene condition). In fact, in these unrestricted visual conditions, the Club riders could rely on visual information to stabilize their head in space. Given that the Club riders tended to be field-dependent, the postural task was considerably harder in visually altered conditions. The Club riders appeared unable to reweight the sensory information to respond to the lack of visual cues. In contrast,

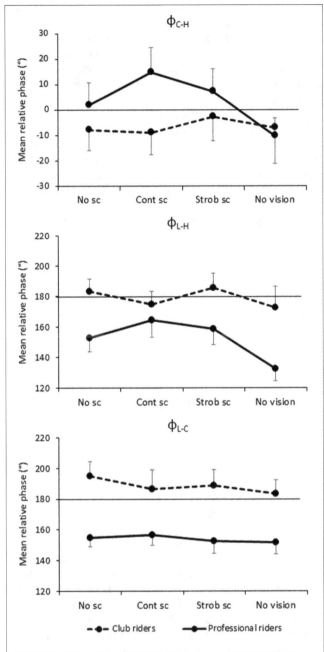

FIGURE 6 | Mean relative phases in degrees between the cervical segment and the head (ϕ_{C-H}), between the lumbar segment and the head (ϕ_{L-H}), and between the lumbar and the cervical segments (ϕ_{L-C}) according to visual condition and expertise. No sc, no simulated scene condition; Cont sc, continuous simulated scene condition; Strob sc, stroboscopic simulated scene condition; No vision, No vision condition. See the text for statistical significance. The error bars represent standard error.

than the rider's postural stability in unrestricted visual conditions. However, this conclusion does not tell us if there are different sensorimotor processes involved in expert and non-expert riders to reach the same level of head stability in unrestricted conditions of vision. The experts' ability to use vestibular and somesthetic information in altered visual conditions does not necessarily mean that they do not use visual information when it is available. Also, the fact that head stability was equivalent in experts and non-experts does not necessarily mean that they adopted similar motor behaviors to achieve this level of stability. Fully addressing these questions would necessitate a complete specific design (e.g., Oie et al., 2001; Peterka, 2002). Nevertheless, the present results on postural coordination modes do provide initial insights.

Postural Coordination Modes

Our third hypothesis was that horseback riding experts would exhibit specific coordination modes to maintain a high level of postural stability. Research has shown that when two joints oscillate together, they are strongly attracted toward in-phase (relative phase close to 0°) or anti-phase (relative phase close to 180°) patterns. These two attractive states have been identified in numerous joint pairings, including bimanual (e.g., Yamanishi et al., 1980; Kelso, 1984), arm-leg (e.g., Kelso and Jeka, 1992), elbow-wrist (e.g., Kelso et al., 1991), ankle-wrist (e.g., Carson et al., 1995), and ankle-hip (e.g., Bardy et al., 1999; Faugloire et al., 2005). The execution of patterns differing from in-phase and anti-phase often requires intensive practice (e.g., Zanone and Kelso, 1992; Faugloire et al., 2006, 2009). The results of the present study demonstrate that these spontaneous modes found in many effector systems are also found in the postural coordination of horseback riders in the anteroposterior axis: The Club riders exhibited an anti-phase coordination mode (segments moving synchronously in opposite directions) both between the lower trunk and the upper trunk and between the lower trunk and the head, and an in-phase coordination mode (segments moving synchronously forward and backward) between the upper trunk and the head.

Interestingly, the Professional riders adopted coordination modes that departed from pure in-phase and anti-phase patterns. In particular, they exhibited a mean relative phase of 154° between the lower and the upper trunk (ϕ_{L-C}) in every vision condition, while the Club riders adopted an anti-phase pattern (mean $\phi_{L-C} = 188°$). In other words, the Professional riders anticipated the anteroposterior movements of the upper trunk compared to the Club riders: the maximal position of the cervical segment occurred sooner in the Professional riders than in the Club riders, for whom the maximal position of the cervical segment (forward) was almost perfectly synchronized with the minimal position of the lumbar segment (backward).

Another interesting result is that, unlike the Club riders, the Professional riders exhibited changes in coordination modes between the cervical segment and the head depending on available visual information. The Club riders exhibited a close to in-phase coordination mode with a slight lag of the cervical segment with respect to the movement of the head (indicated by the negative values of the relative phases) in every vision condition (mean ϕ_{C-H} ranging from −8.83° in the Cont

the Professional riders, who were more field-independent, were able to maintain a high level of head stability regardless of the availability of visual information. These results strongly suggest that the capacity to reweight the relative contribution of different sensory information depending on environmental conditions is a more prominent indicator of expertise in horseback riding scene condition to $-2.75°$ in the Strob scene condition). By contrast, the Professional riders adopted coordination patterns ranging from $+14.74°$ in the Cont scene condition to $-10.30°$ in the No vision condition (**Figure 6**). When the simulated scene was projected on the screen, the Professional riders anticipated the cervical segment's movements with respect to the head's movements (positive ϕ_{C-H} of $+14.74°$ in the Cont scene condition). When no visual information was available, the Professional riders adopted a coordination pattern similar to the Club riders with the movement of the cervical segment following the head movement with a slight delay (negative ϕ_{C-H} of $-10.30°$ in the No vision condition). Again, it is interesting to note that this cervical-head coordination mode observed when no visual information was available was also adopted by the Club riders in every other vision condition. This result reveals that, although the Professional riders were able to stabilize their head better than the Club riders in visually altered conditions, they did not rely only on vestibular and somesthetic information in unrestricted visual conditions. The specific relative phase between the cervical segment and the head exhibited by the Professional riders in the Cont scene conditions suggests that the experts did use visual information in this condition to adapt their postural coordination modes to environmental conditions. This interesting result is difficult to discuss further and would have to be connected to other dependent variables such as the flexion-extension of the neck and the visual search behavior of the participants.

Finally, we found that the coordination between the lumbar segment and the head (ϕ_{L-H}) depended on the vision condition over the two levels of expertise, with a significant difference between the No vision condition ($\phi_{L-H} = 152.42°$) and every other vision condition (ϕ_{L-H} ranging from $168.01°$ in the No scene condition to $172.16°$ in the Strob scene condition). **Figure 6** (middle panel) strongly suggests that this effect of vision is due mainly to a change in the coordination mode of the Professional riders who exhibited relative phases between the lumbar segment and the head ranging from $164.33°$ in the Cont scene condition to $132.42°$ in the No vision condition, while the Club riders maintained an anti-phase coordination mode in every vision condition. This result is likely to be the direct consequence of the behavior observed on the two underlying levels of lumbar-head coordination, namely lumbar-cervical and cervical-head coordination.

Limitations and Perspectives

The present study is the first to investigate the contribution of visual information to postural stability and the postural coordination modes in horseback riding depending on expertise. As such, several experimental features can potentially be enhanced in future work. Using an equestrian simulator enabled us to overcome difficulties encountered in studies on horseback riding such as controlling and reproducing the horses' movements, facilitating data collection, and manipulating vision conditions. However, while the projected visual scene simulated the horizontal displacements corresponding to a ride, including turns, the mechanical horse's orientation was fixed. Therefore, while the riding simulator faithfully reproduced the vertical

and pitch perturbations of the chosen pace, it did not produce any horizontal movements, either in yaw or in translation. Consequently, the mechanical perturbations were only partially similar to a real ride. In addition, there was a discrepancy between the visual information provided by the projected visual scene and the mechanical horse's motion. Given the current technical constraints of riding simulators, it seems that only a study in the field could overcome these limitations, though with all the other difficulties that this method would entail. A related issue concerns the possibility to match precisely the data from the projected visual scene and movement measures. This coupling would help understand more finely how riders react to the different events simulated in the visual scene, such as the aforementioned turns. This might have helped interpret the difference in head stability in the mediolateral axis between the Professional and Club riders that we observed only when the simulated visual scene was projected.

Another limitation concerns the size of the visual field occupied by the projected scene. The simulated scene used in the present study was limited to the participants' central visual field, thereby reducing the possibility of using peripheral vision which is known to play an important role in postural control (e.g., Pavard et al., 1976; Amblard et al., 1985). A multi-sided immersive environment would make it possible to strengthen and extend the conclusions of the present study. Another, non-exclusive, perspective would be to collect and combine additional data about pelvis orientation, angular displacements (of the hips, neck and knees), and/or horse-rider interactions, for example. Indeed, the new insights we have gained through the study of horseback riders' postural control encourage further investigations to better understand the highly complex task that is horseback riding.

CONCLUSIONS

The present study demonstrates a differential contribution of visual information to postural stability in horseback riding depending on expertise. First, compared to the Club riders, the Professional riders exhibited greater head stability in the anteroposterior axis when vision conditions were altered. Second, RFT perceptual scores revealed that the Professional riders were less dependent on the visual field than the Club riders. Third, we found that the more dependent the riders were on the visual field, the greater their head variability. These results suggest that expert horseback riders rely more on vestibular and somesthetic information to stabilize their head in space than less experienced riders. Our assessment of the coordination modes between the different levels of the spine completes and specifies this conclusion. Unlike the Club riders, who exhibited similar in-phase or anti-phase patterns in the different vision conditions, the Professional riders exhibited changes in coordination modes depending on the visual information available. Thus, even though the expert riders proved to be less dependent on visual information to stabilize their head than the non-expert riders, they appeared to make use of visual information when it was available to adapt their postural coordination modes. The combination of stability, perceptual typology and postural coordination measures therefore strongly suggests that expert riders are better able to reweight sensory information in order to control their posture according to task constraints.

AUTHOR CONTRIBUTIONS

AO, LL, and EF designed the study. AO and SB performed the experiments. AO and EF analyzed the data and AO, EF, LL, and BI wrote the manuscript.

FUNDING

Part of data analysis and the writing of this paper was supported by the "Institut Français du Cheval et de l'Equitation" (IFCE) and the "Fonds Eperon" as part of the "RiderFeel" proposals.

ACKNOWLEDGMENTS

We sincerely thank the Saumur National Riding School (ENE) for their welcome and all of the riders for their participation.

REFERENCES

Amblard, B., Assaiante, C., Vaugoyeau, M., Baroni, G., Ferrigno, G., and Pedotti, A. (2001). Voluntary head stabilisation in space during oscillatory trunk movements in the frontal plane performed before, during and after a prolonged period of weightlessness. *Exp. Brain Res.* 137, 170–179. doi: 10.1007/s002210000621

Amblard, B., and Carblanc, A. (1980). Role of foveal and peripheral visual information in maintenance of postural equilibrium in man. *Percept. Mot. Skills* 51, 903–912. doi: 10.2466/pms.1980.51.3.903

Amblard, B., and Crémieux, J. (1976). Rôle de l'information visuelle du mouvement dans le maintien de l'eÌÂquilibre postural chez l'homme. *Agressologie* 17, 26–36.

Amblard, B., Crémieux, J., Marchand, A. R., and Carblanc, A. (1985). Lateral orientation and stabilization of human stance: static versus dynamic visual cues. *Exp. Brain Res.* 61, 21–37. doi: 10.1007/bf00235617

Assaiante, C., and Amblard, B. (1993). Ontogenesis of head stabilization in space during locomotion in children: influence of visual cues. *Exp. Brain Res.* 93, 499–515. doi: 10.1007/bf00229365

Assaiante, C., and Amblard, B. (1995). An ontogenetic model for the sensorimotor organization of balance control in humans. *Hum. Mov. Sci.* 14, 13–43. doi: 10.1016/0167-9457(94)00048-J

Assländer, L., Hettich, G., and Mergner, T. (2015). Visual contribution to human standing balance during support surface tilts. *Hum. Mov. Sci.* 41, 147–164. doi: 10.1016/j.humov.2015.02.010

Bardy, B. G., Marin, L., Stoffregen, T. A., and Bootsma, R. J. (1999). Postural coordination modes considered as emergent phenomena. *J. Exp. Psychol.* 25, 1284–1301. doi: 10.1037/0096-1523.25.5.1284

Batschelet, E. (1981). *Circular Statistics in Biology*. New-York, NY: Academic Press.

Baumberger, B., Isableu, B., and Flückiger, M. (2004). The visual control of stability in children and adults: postural readjustments in a ground optical flow. *Exp. Brain Res.* 159, 33–46. doi: 10.1007/s00221-004-1930-1

Berencsi, A., Ishihara, M., and Imanaka, K. (2005). The functional role of central and peripheral vision in the control of posture. *Hum. Mov. Sci.* 24, 689–709. doi: 10.1016/j.humov.2005.10.014

Bizid, R., and Paillard, T. (2006). Les activités posturales de footballeurs de niveau national diffèrent-elles entre les attaquants et les défenseurs? *Sci. Sports* 21, 23–25. doi: 10.1016/j.scispo.2005.12.003

Brady, R. A., Peters, B. T., Batson, C. D., Ploutz-Snyder, R., Mulavara, A. P., and Bloomberg, J. J. (2012). Gait adaptability training is affected by visual dependency. *Exp. Brain Res.* 220, 1–9. doi: 10.1007/s00221-012-3109-5

Bringoux, L., Marin, L., Nougier, V., Barraud, P. A., and Raphel, C. (2000). Effects of gymnastics expertise on the perception of body orientation in the pitch dimension. *J. Vestib. Res.* 10, 251–258.

Bringoux, L., Scotto Di Cesare, C., Borel, L., Macaluso, T., and Sarlegna, F. R. (2016). Do visual and vestibular inputs compensate for somatosensory loss in the perception of spatial orientation? Insights from a deafferented patient. *Front. Hum. Neurosci.* 10:181. doi: 10.3389/fnhum.2016.00181

Byström, A., Rhodin, M., Peinen, K., Weishaupt, M. A., and Roepstorff, L. (2009). Basic kinematics of the saddle and rider in high-level dressage horses trotting on a treadmill. *Equine Vet. J.* 41, 280–284. doi: 10.2746/042516409x394454

Byström, A., Roepstroff, L., Geser-von Peinen, K., Weishaupt, M. A., and Rhodin, M. (2015). Differences in rider movement pattern between different degrees of

collection at the trot in high-level dressage horses ridden on a treadmill. *Hum. Mov. Sci.* 41, 1–8. doi: 10.1016/j.humov.2015.01.016

Callier, J., Oysel, S., Hausmann, I., and Tordi, N. (2001). "Equilibre statique bipodal sous deux conditions visuelles en fonction du sexe chez des gymnasts de 9-10 ans," in *Nouveauté Conceptuelles Instrumentales et Clinique*, ed M. Lacour (Paris: Solal De Boeck), 65–69.

Carson, R. G., Goodman, D., Elliott, D., and Kelso, J. A. S. (1995). Asymmetries in the dynamics of interlimb coordination. *Adv. Psychol.* 111, 255–288. doi: 10.1016/s0166-4115(06)80013-0

Clément, G., Pozzo, T., and Berthoz, A. (1988). Contribution of eye positioning to control of the upside-down standing posture. *Exp. Brain Res.* 73, 569–576. doi: 10.1007/bf00406615

Collins, J. J., and De Luca, C. J. (1995). The effects of visual input on open-loop and closed-loop postural control mechanisms. *Exp. Brain Res.* 103, 151–163. doi: 10.1007/bf00241972

Crémieux, J., and Mesure, S. (1994). Differential sensitivity to static visual cues in the control of postural equilibrium in man. *Percept. Mot. Skills* 78, 67–74. doi: 10.2466/pms.1994.78.1.67

Eckardt, F., and Witte, K. (2016). Kinematic analysis of the rider according to different skill levels in sitting trot and canter. *J. Equine Vet. Sci.* 39, 51–57. doi: 10.1016/j.jevs.2015.07.022

Engell, M. T., Clayton, H. M., Egenvall, A., Weishaupt, M. A., and Roepstorff, L. (2016). Postural changes and their effects in elite riders when actively influencing the horse versus sitting passively at trot. *Comp. Exerc. Physiol.* 12, 27–33. doi: 10.3920/cep150035

Era, P., Konttinenf, N., Mehto, P., Saarela, P., and Lyytinent, H. (1996). Postural stability and skilled performance-a study on top-level and naive rifle shooters. *J. Biomech.* 29, 301–306. doi: 10.1016/0021-9290(95)00066-6

Ericsson, K. A., Krampe, R. T., and Tesch-Römer, C. (1993). The role of deliberate practice in the acquisition of expert performance. *Psychol. Rev.* 100, 363–406. doi: 10.1037/0033-295x.100.3.363

Ericsson, K. A., and Lehmann, A. C. (1996). Expert and exceptional performance: evidence of maximal adaptation to task constraints. *Annu. Rev. Psychol.* 47, 273–305. doi: 10.1146/annurev.psych.47.1.273

Faugloire, E., Bardy, B. G., Merhi, O., and Stoffregen, T. A. (2005). Exploring coordination dynamics of the postural system with real-time visual feedback. *Neurosci. Lett.* 374, 136–141. doi: 10.1016/j.neulet.2004.10.043

Faugloire, E., Bardy, B. G., and Stoffregen, T. A. (2006). The dynamics of learning new postural patterns. *J. Mot. Behav.* 38, 299–312. doi: 10.3200/jmbr.38.4.299-312

Faugloire, E., Bardy, B. G., and Stoffregen, T. A. (2009). (De)Stabilization of required and spontaneous postural dynamics with learning. *J. Exp. Psychol.* 35, 170–187. doi: 10.1037/0096-1523.35.1.170

Forssberg, H., and Hirschfeld, H. (1994). Postural adjustments in sitting humans following external perturbations: muscle activity and kinematics. *Exp. Brain Res.* 97, 515–527. doi: 10.1007/bf00241545

Galloux, P., Richard, N., Dronka, T., Leard, M., Perrot, A., Jouffroy, J. L., et al. (1994). Analysis of equine gait using three-dimensional accelerometers fixed on the saddle. *Equine Vet. J.* (Suppl. 26), 44–47. doi: 10.1111/j.2042-3306.1994.tb04872.x

Gautier, G., Marin, L., Leroy, D., and Thouvarecq, R. (2009). Dynamics of expertise level: coordination in handstand. *Hum. Mov. Sci.* 28, 129–140. doi: 10.1016/j.humov.2008.05.003

Gautier, G., Thouvarecq, R., and Vuillerme, N. (2008). Postural control and perceptive configuration: influence of expertise in gymnastics. *Gait Posture* 28, 46–51. doi: 10.1016/j.gaitpost.2007.09.007

Golomer, E., Crémieux, J., Dupui, P., Isableu, B., and Ohlmann, T. (1999). Visual contribution to self-induced body sway frequencies and visual perception of male professional dancers. *Neurosci. Lett.* 267, 189–192. doi: 10.1016/s0304-3940(99)00356-0

Gresty, M. A., and Bronstein, A. M. (1992). Visually controlled spatial stabilisation of the human head: compensation for the eye's limited ability to roll. *Neurosci. Lett.* 140, 63–66. doi: 10.1016/0304-3940(92)90682-W

Gueguen, M., Vuillerme, N., and Isableu, B. (2012). Does the integration of haptic and visual cues reduce the effect of a biased visual reference frame on the subjective head orientation? *PLoS ONE* 7:e34380. doi: 10.1371/journal.pone.0034380

Guerraz, M., Gianna, C. C., Burchill, P. M., Gresty, M. A., and Bronstein, A. M. (2001). Effect of visual surrounding motion on body sway in a three-dimensional environment. *Percept. Psychophys.* 63, 47–58. doi: 10.3758/bf03200502

Guillot, A., and Collet, C. (2004). Field dependence–independence in complex motor skills. *Percept. Mot. Skills* 98, 575–583. doi: 10.2466/pms.98.2.575-583

Hosseinimehr, S. H., Norasteh, A. A., Abbasi, A., Tazji, M. K., and Hosseinimehr, S. H. (2009). The comparision of dependency on vision and proprioception in gymnastic, wrestling and soccer. *Braz. J. Biomotr.* 3, 332–338.

Isableu, B., Fourre, B., Vuillerme, N., Giraudet, G., and Amorim, M. A. (2011). Differential integration of visual and kinaesthetic signals to upright stance. *Exp. Brain Res.* 212, 33–46. doi: 10.1007/s00221-011-2693-0

Isableu, B., Ohlmann, T., Crémieux, J., and Amblard, B. (1997). Selection of spatial frame of reference and postural control variability. *Exp. Brain Res.* 114, 584–589. doi: 10.1007/pl00005667

Isableu, B., Ohlmann, T., Crémieux, J., and Amblard, B. (2003). Differential approach to strategies of segmental stabilisation in postural control. *Exp. Brain Res.* 150, 208–221. doi: 10.1007/s00221-003-1446-0

Isableu, B., Ohlmann, T., Cremieux, J., Vuillerme, N., Amblard, B., and Gresty, M. A. (2010). Individual differences in the ability to identify, select and use appropriate frames of reference for perceptuo-motor control. *Neuroscience* 169, 1199–1215. doi: 10.1016/j.neuroscience.2010.05.072

Janura, M., Svoboda, Z., Cabell, L., Dvořáková, T., and Jelen, K. (2015). Effect of repeated therapeutic horse riding sessions on the trunk movement of the rider. *Neuroendocrinol. Lett.* 36, 481–489. doi: 10.1016/j.gaitpost.2011.10.305

Kang, O.-D., Ryu, Y.-C., Ryew, C.-C., Oh, W.-Y., Lee, C.-E., and Kang, M.-S. (2010). Comparative analyses of rider position according to skill levels during walk and trot in Jeju horse. *Hum. Mov. Sci.* 29, 956–963. doi: 10.1016/j.humov.2010.05.010

Kelso, J. A., and Jeka, J. J. (1992). Symmetry breaking dynamics of human multilimb coordination. *J. Exp. Psychol.* 18, 645–668. doi: 10.1037/0096-1523.18.3.645

Kelso, J. A. S. (1984). Phase transitions and critical behavior in human bimanual coordination. *Am. J. Physiol.* 15, R1000–R1004.

Kelso, J. A. S., Buchanan, J. J., and Wallace, S. A. (1991). Order parameters for the neural organization of single, multijoint limb movement patterns. *Exp. Brain Res.* 85, 432–444. doi: 10.1007/bf00229420

Keshner, E. A. (2003). Head-trunk coordination during linear anterior-posterior translations. *J. Neurophysiol.* 89, 1891–1901. doi: 10.1007/s00221-004-1893-2

Keshner, E. A. (2004). Head-trunk coordination in elderly subjects during linear anterior-posterior translations. *Exp. Brain Res.* 158, 213–222. doi: 10.1007/s00221-004-1893-2

Kluzik, J., Horak, F. B., and Peterka, R. J. (2005). Differences in preferred reference frames for postural orientation shown by after-effects of stance on an inclined surface. *Exp. Brain Res.* 162, 474–489. doi: 10.1007/s00221-004-2124-6

Lagarde, J., Peham, C., Licka, T., and Kelso, J. A. S. (2005). Coordination dynamics of the horse-rider system. *J. Mot. Behav.* 37, 418–424. doi: 10.3200/jmbr.37.6.418-424

Laurent, M., and Pailhous, J. (1982). Contribution à l'étude de pointage locomoteur, Application au saut en longueur et au saut d'obstacles en équitation. *STAPS* 5, 1–13.

Laurent, M., Phung, R. D., and Ripoll, H. (1989). What visual information is used by riders in jumping? *Hum. Mov. Sci.* 8, 481–501. doi: 10.1016/0167-9457(89)90032-8

Lee, D. N., and Lishman, J. R. (1975). Visual and proprioceptive control of stance. *J. Hum. Mov. Stud.* 1, 87–95. doi: 10.3758/bf03199297

Liu, W. (2003). Field dependence-independence and sports with a preponderance of closed or open skill. *J. Sport Behav.* 26, 285–297.

Luyat, M., Olhmann, T., and Barraud, P. A. (1997). Subjective vertical and postural activity. *Acta Psychol. (Amst.)* 95, 181–193. doi: 10.1016/s0001-6918(96)00015-7

Mardia, K. V., and Jupp, P. E. (2000). *Directional Statistics*. Chichester: Wiley. doi: 10.1002/9780470316979

Marin, L., Bardy, B. G., and Bootsma, R. J. (1999). Level of gymnastic skill as an intrinsic constraint on postural coordination. *J. Sports Sci.* 17, 615–626. doi: 10.1080/026404199365641

Münz, A., Eckardt, F., Heipertz-Hengst, C., Peham, C., and Witte, K. (2013). A preliminary study of an inertial sensor-based method for the assessment of human pelvis kinematics in dressage riding. *J. Equine Vet. Sci.* 33, 950–955. doi: 10.1016/j.jevs.2013.02.002

Münz, A., Eckardt, F., and Witte, K. (2014). Horse–rider interaction in dressage riding. *Hum. Mov. Sci.* 33, 227–237. doi: 10.1016/j.humov.2013.09.003

Nashner, L. M., and McCollum, G. (1985). The organization of human postural movements: a formal basis and experimental synthesis. *Behav. Brain Sci.* 8, 135–150. doi: 10.1017/s0140525x00020008

Newell, K. M., van Emmerik, R. E., Lee, D., and Sprague, R. L. (1993). On postural stability and variability. *Gait Posture* 1, 225–230. doi: 10.1016/0966-6362(93)90050-b

Nyborg, H., and Isaksen, B. O. (1974). A method for analysing performance in the rod-and-frame test. II Test of the Statistical Model. *Scand. J. Psychol.* 15, 124–126. doi: 10.1111/j.1467-9450.1974.tb00564.x

Oie, K. S., Kiemel, T., and Jeka, J. J. (2001). Human multisensory fusion of vision and touch: detecting non-linearity with small changes in the sensory environment. *Neurosci. Lett.* 315, 113–116. doi: 10.1016/s0304-3940(01)02348-5

Olivier, A., Faugloire, E., Biau, S., Lejeune, L., and Isableu, B. (2012). "Sensibilité proprioceptive et stabilité de la tête: marqueur d'expertise chez les cavaliers," in *Institut Français du Cheval et de l'équitation*, ed Actes de la 38ème Journée de la Recherche Équine: Sport de haut niveau (Paris. Saumur: IFCE), 119–127.

Oltman, P. (1968). A portable rod and frame apparatus. *Percept. Mot. Skills* 26, 503–506. doi: 10.2466/pms.1968.26.2.503

Paillard, J. (1971). Les déterminants moteurs de l'organisation spatiale. *Cahiers Psychol.* 14, 261–316.

Paillard, T., Margnes, E., Portet, M., and Breucq, A. (2011). Postural ability reflects the athletic skill level of surfers. *Eur. J. Appl. Physiol.* 111, 1619–1623. doi: 10.1007/s00421-010-1782-2

Paillard, T., Noé, F., Riviere, T., and Vincent, M. (2006). Postural performance and strategy in the unipedal stance of soccer players at different levels of competition. *J. Athl. Train.* 41, 172–176.

Paulus, W. M., Straube, A., and Brandt, T. H. (1984). Visual stabilization of posture. *Brain* 107, 1143–1163. doi: 10.1093/brain/107.4.1143

Pavard, B., Berthoz, A., and Lestienne, F. (1976). Rôle de la vision périphérique dans l'évaluation du mouvement linéaire interaction visuo-vestibulaire et effets posturaux. *Le Travail Humain*, 39, 115–138.

Peham, C., Licka, T., Schobesberger, H., and Meschan, E. (2004). Influence of the rider on the variability of the equine gait. *Hum. Mov. Sci.* 23, 663–671. doi: 10.1016/j.humov.2004.10.006

Perrin, P., Schneider, D., Deviterne, D., Perrot, C., and Constantinescu, L. (1998). Training improves the adaptation to changing visual conditions in maintaining human posture control in a test of sinusoidal oscillation of the support. *Neurosci. Lett.* 245, 155–158. doi: 10.1016/s0304-3940(98)00208-0

Perrot, C., Moes, R., Deviterne, D., and Perrin, P. (1998). Adaptation posturales lors de gestuelle spécifiques aux sports de combat. *Sci. Sports* 13, 64–74. doi: 10.1016/s0765-1597(97)86902-x

Peterka, R. J. (2002). Sensorimotor integration in human postural control. *J. Neurophysiol.* 88, 1097–1118. doi: 10.1152/jn.00516.2003

Pozzo, T., Berthoz, A., and Lefort, L. (1990). Head stabilization during various locomotor tasks in humans. *Exp. Brain Res.* 82, 97–106. doi: 10.1007/bf00230842

Ripoll, H., Bard, C., and Paillard, J. (1986). Stabilization of head and eyes on target as a factor in successful basketball shooting. *Hum. Mov. Sci.* 5, 47–58. doi: 10.1016/0167-9457(86)90005-9

Robert, G., Gueguen, N., Avogadro, P., and Mouchnino, L. (2004). Anticipatory balance control is affected by loadless training experiences. *Hum. Mov. Sci.* 23, 169–183. doi: 10.1016/j.humov.2004.08.001

Rougier, P., Zanders, E., and Borlet, E. (2003). Influence of visual cues on upright postural control: differentiated effects of eyelids closure. *Rev. Neurol. (Paris).* 159, 180–188.

Rousseu, C., and Crémieux, J. (2005). Perception de l'orientation visuelle chez des experts en taekwondo. *STAPS* 65, 79–96. doi: 10.3917/sta.065.0079

Schmid, M., Casabianca, L., Bottaro, A., and Schieppati, M. (2008). Graded changes in balancing behavior as a function of visual acuity. *Neuroscience* 153, 1079–1091. doi: 10.1016/j.neuroscience.2008.03.024

Silva e Borges, M. B., Werneck, M. J., da, S., Silva, M. de L. da, Gandolfi, L., and Pratesi, R. (2011). Therapeutic effects of a horse riding simulator in children with cerebral palsy. *Arq. Neuropsiquiatr.* 69, 799–804. doi: 10.1590/s0004-282x 2011000600014

Slaboda, J. C., Lauer, R. T., and Keshner, E. A. (2011). Continuous visual field motion impacts the postural responses of older and younger women during and after support surface tilt. *Exp. Brain Res.* 211, 87–96. doi: 10.1007/s00221-011-2655-6

Stambolieva, K., Diafas, V., Bachev, V., Christova, L., and Gatev, P. (2011). Postural stability of canoeing and kayaking young male athletes during quiet stance. *Eur. J. Appl. Physiol.* 112, 1807–1815. doi: 10.1007/s00421-011-2151-5

Strogatz, S. H. (1994). *Nonlinear dynamics and chaos*. Reading, MA: Addison-Wesley.

Terada, K. (2000). Comparison of head movement and EMG activity of muscles between advanced and novice horseback riders at different gaits. *J. Equine Sci.* 11, 83–90. doi: 10.1294/jes.11.83

Terada, K., Mullineaux, D. R., Lanovaz, J., Kato, K., and Clayton, H. M. (2004). Electromyographic analysis of the rider's muscles at trot. *Equine Comp. Exerc. Physiol.* 1, 193–198. doi: 10.1079/ecp200420

Vereijken, B., Van Emmerik, R. E. A., Bongaardt, R., Beek, W. J., and Newell, K. M. (1997). Changing coordinative structures in complex skill acquisition. *Hum. Mov. Sci.* 16, 823–844. doi: 10.1016/S0167-9457(97)00021-3

Vibert, N., MacDougall, H. G., de Waele, C., Gilchrist, D. P., Burgess, A. M., Sidis, A., et al. (2001). Variability in the control of head movements in seated humans: a link with whiplash injuries? *J. Physiol. (Lond).* 532, 851–868. doi: 10.1111/j.1469-7793.2001.0851e.x

Vitte, E., Pozzo, T., and Soulie, D. (1995). Equilibre et équilibration. *Méd. Sport* 69, 177–180. doi: 10.1016/s1246-7391(98)85009-4

Vuillerme, N., Danion, F., Marin, L., Boyadjian, A., Prieur, J. M., Weise, I., et al. (2001a). The effect of expertise in gymnastics on postural control. *Neurosci. Lett.* 303, 83–86. doi: 10.1016/s0304-3940(01)01722-0

Vuillerme, N., Teasdale, N., and Nougier, V. (2001b). The effect of expertise in gymnastics on proprioceptive sensory integration in human subjects. *Neurosci. Lett.* 311, 73–76. doi: 10.1016/s0304-3940(01)02147-4

Winter, D. A., Prince, F., and Patla, A. (1997). Validity of the inverted pendulum model of balance in quiet standing. *Gait Post.* 5, 153–154. doi: 10.1016/s0966-6362(97)83376-0

Witkin, H. A. (1950). Individual differences in ease of perception of embedded figures. *J. Pers.* 19, 1–15. doi: 10.1111/j.1467-6494.1950.tb01084.x

Wolframm, I. A., Bosga, J., and Meulenbroek, R. G. J. (2013). Coordination dynamics in horse-rider dyads. *Hum. Mov. Sci.* 32, 157–170. doi: 10.1016/j.humov.2012.11.002

Yamanishi, J. I., Kawato, M., and Suzuki, R. (1980). Two coupled oscillators as a model for the coordinated finger tapping by both hands. *Biol. Cybern.* 37, 219–225. doi: 10.1007/bf00337040

Zanone, P. G., and Kelso, J. A. (1992). Evolution of behavioral attractors with learning: nonequilibrium phase transitions. *J. Exp. Psychol.* 18:403. doi: 10.1037/0096-1523.18.2.403

Zoccolotti, P., Antonucci, G., and Spinelli, D. (1993). The gap between rod and frame influences the rod-and-frame effect with small and large inducing displays. *Percept. Psychophys.* 54, 14–19. doi: 10.3758/bf03206933

11

Electromyographic Pattern during Gait Initiation Differentiates Yoga Practitioners among Physically Active Older Subjects

Thierry Lelard[1]*, Pierre-Louis Doutrellot[1,2], Abdou Temfemo[1,3] and Said Ahmaidi[1]

[1]EA-3300: Adaptations Physiologiques à l'Exercice et Réadaptation à l'Effort, Faculté des Sciences du Sport, Université de Picardie Jules Verne, Amiens, France, [2]Service Medecine Physique et Rééducation, Centre Hospitalier Universitaire, Amiens, France, [3]Department of Biological Sciences, Faculty of Medicine and Pharmaceutical Sciences, University of Douala, Douala, Cameroon

*Correspondence:
Thierry Lelard
thierry.lelard@u-picardie.fr

During gait initiation, postural adjustments are needed to deal with balance and movement. With aging, gait initiation changes and reflects functional degradation of frailty individuals. However, physical activities have demonstrated beneficial effects of daily motor tasks. The aim of our study was to compare center of pressure (COP) displacement and ankle muscle co-activation during gait initiation in two physically active groups: a group of walkers ($n = 12$; mean age $\pm$ SD 72.6 ± 3.2 years) and a yoga group ($n = 11$; 71.5 ± 3.8 years). COP trajectory and electromyography of leg muscles were recorded simultaneously during five successive trials of gait initiation. Our main finding was that yoga practitioners had slower COP displacements ($p < 0.01$) and lower leg muscles % of coactivation ($p < 0.01$) in comparison with walkers. These parameters which characterized gait initiation control were correlated ($r = 0.76$; $p < 0.01$). Our results emphasize that lengthy ankle muscle co-activation and COP path in gait initiation differentiate yoga practitioners among physically active subjects.

Keywords: anticipatory postural adjustments, gait, aged, yoga, electromyography

INTRODUCTION

In older adults, physiological changes and physical inactivity are associated with a decrease in personal independence in general and in walking ability in particular. Indeed, older subjects with impaired gait are scared of falls and thus limit their physical activity and activities of daily living (Alexander, 1994; Maki and McIlroy, 1996). For example, individuals adopt a more conservative, basic gait pattern (Menz et al., 2003). Because of socio-economics impact of falling, several studies were lead to determine predictive factors of falling in older population. Gait initiation parameters (as described below) may be sensitive indicators of balance dysfunction and the risk of falls in older adults (Chang and Krebs, 1999). Indeed, gait initiation is a transient phase during which postural control and balance maintenance systems are highly active. Specifically, gait initiation consists in creating forward momentum from a quiet stance. Muscle activity creates internal forces that dissociate the center of pressure (COP) from the center of gravity (COG), in order to produce the initiation step (Mann et al., 1979; Brunt et al., 1991). While momentum creation disturbs balance, anticipatory postural adjustments (APA) are needed to deal with balance and allow efficient step initiation.

Several studies have evidenced the degradation of gait initiation with age. The older people show a decrease in the peak moment arm between the body's COG and the COP (Brunt et al., 1991; Polcyn et al., 1998; Chang and Krebs, 1999). The decrease in this forward momentum is associated with lower COG velocity and lower first step amplitude (Patchay et al., 1997, 2002; Halliday et al., 1998). It has been suggested that this change in kinetic gait initiation parameters occurs because older subjects do not tolerate a deviation of the body as a whole (COG) from the ground reaction forces (COP). In order to initiate gait and compensate for impairments in the moment arm, older subjects have to perform additional trunk movements (Martin et al., 2002).

The observed changes in kinetic parameters have also been explained in terms of impaired muscle activation patterns. The role of muscle activity is to create internal forces in order to dissociate the COP from the COG (Mann et al., 1979; Brunt et al., 1991). For that reason, the electromyographic (EMG) sequence recorded during gait initiation can be considered as "a motor program that adjusts the configuration of external forces, which acts directly on the position of the COP and joint position" (Crenna and Frigo, 1991). Several studies described a stereotypical pattern of muscle activation in healthy, younger adults: (i) starting from a postural quiet stance, postural muscles are activated in order to maintain postural alignment; and (ii) in order to initiate gait *per se*, postural muscle activity is inhibited and motor muscles are then activated (Mann et al., 1979; Brunt et al., 1991, 1999). Difficulties in inhibiting antigravity muscles prior to movement are correlated with the age-related loss of Betz cells in the motor cortex (Scheibel et al., 1977; Scheibel, 1985). Higher levels of muscle coactivation have been reported in older subjects during activities of daily living–such as bipedal stance (Laughton et al., 2003; Nagai et al., 2011) and dynamic balance (Hortobágyi and DeVita, 2000; Larsen et al., 2008; Schmitz et al., 2009; Pereira and Goncalves, 2011). During gait initiation, the duration of postural and motor muscle coactivation increases with age. Indeed, it appears that the degradation of central mechanisms in gait initiation translates into a decrease in the ankle muscle antagonist coordination pattern (Polcyn et al., 1998; Henriksson and Hirschfeld, 2005), i.e., coactivation of the tibialis anterior (TA) and triceps surae muscles. The difference between young adults and older adults is more obvious for the swing limb (SWL), which shows greater degradation than the stance limb (STL) does (Polcyn et al., 1998).

It has often been suggested that physical activity improves functional ability in older people (Lord and Castell, 1994; Maki and McIlroy, 1996; Lelard and Ahmaidi, 2015). As an indicator of functional status, physically active olders show higher walking velocity compared to aged-matched sedentary adults. However, it seems that the characteristics of the physical activity, duration and frequency of training sessions induce differentiated effects on motor ability. Tai Chi training also showed an enhancement of gait initiation control (Hass et al., 2004; Vallabhajosula et al., 2014). These studies focused on CoP-CoG displacements during APA. These findings demonstrated that proprioceptive physical activity could help to improve gait initiation control via

better COP displacement. Gait initiation is a pre-programmed task (Fiolkowski et al., 2002) which need APA controlled by an open-loop mechanism (Massion, 1992). As neuromuscular activity reflects motor program, previous results may explain this improvement by enhanced neuromuscular coordination after proprioceptive training (Chen et al., 2012a,b). Indeed, Nagai et al. (2012) have demonstrated significant changes in muscle coactivation after balance training (relative to an untrained group). Most of these studies reported beneficial effects of proprioceptive practice on postural control, however, differential effects depending on the type of practice were described on postural control (Gauchard et al., 2003). As described by these authors, proprioceptive activities such as yoga consist to produce a sequence of postures that need to deal with balance and movements improving body schema knowledge. To our knowledge, no study was performed to compare the effects of different types of physical activity on gait initiation.

Since differentiated effects on postural control were previously reported according the type of training program, we hypothesize that practicing different type of physical activity would show differences in APA during gait initiation. To initiate the first step, the central nervous system has to deal with the antigravity function of the posture and production of movements. Motor program has to switch from postural activity (Triceps Surae) to focal movements (TA). A time course analysis of co-activation and COP displacement might then be an effective indicator of efficiency of gait initiation. The aim of the present study was thus to investigate potentially differentiating patterns of leg muscle co-activation and COP displacements during gait initiation in yoga practitioners and physically active group (regular walkers).

MATERIALS AND METHODS

Subjects

Twenty-three volunteers healthy subjects aged from 68 years to 78 years took part in the study. Regular yoga practitioners ($n = 11$; 71.5 ± 3.8 years old; 1.59 ± 0.08 m height; 66.8 ± 9.3 kg weight) and walkers subjects ($n = 12$; 72.6 ± 3.2 years old; 1.61 ± 0.03 m height; 64.3 ± 8.6 kg weight) were recruited from community dwelling. The group of yoga practitioners was standardized in terms of time (more than 1 year) weekly sessions (1) and sessions duration (1 h) of practice. The physically active group was selected on the basis of a questionnaire. Their physical activity level was equal or higher than 1 h of walking per week. All subjects signed prior the study an informed consent which was accepted by the local ethical committee (Comité de protection des Personnes Nord Ouest 2, Amiens, France) in accordance with Helsinki Declaration of 1975. Prior to taking part in the study, all participants reported their medical history. Clinical examination and questioning was conducted in order to exclude subjects showing any possible causes of balance alteration (medication or disease). Subjects were free from any disease which could influence postural maintaining and were able to walk without external help. Subjects did not show cognitive impairments with a score superior to 24 points in Mini-Mental State Evaluation (Folstein et al., 1975). The participants were independent as revealed by a maximal score in the Activities of Daily Living (Katz et al., 1963).

Experimental Devices

A Piezoelectric force plate (Kistler type 9281 B11, Kistler AG, Winterthur, Switzerland) associated with a calculator was used to assess the temporal time-course of the COP displacements in antero-posterior (AP) and medio-lateral (ML) from the ground reaction forces and their moments in the three planes. The analogic signal was digitized at a sampling frequency of 1000 Hz.

Electromyograms (EMG) of leg muscles were collected using bipolar Ag/AgCl surface electrodes (Beckmann, 8-mm diameter) on the first leg that leaves the floor (initial SW limb). Before the electrode positioning, the skin was slightly abraded and cleaned with an alcohol solution in order to reduce the interelectrode resistance to below 5 kΩ. An electrolytic gel was placed between the skin and the electrodes to insure electrical contact. The electrodes were fixed (2 cm apart center to center) over the muscle bellies for TA and lateral gastrocnemius (LG) muscles. The EMG signals were amplified and filtered using a bandwidth of 10–1000 Hz (Gould 6600), and then addressed to an analog-digital converter piloted by the Turbolab software (SM2I, France) for their digitization at a sampling rate of 1000 Hz.

Procedure

After two learning trials, the subjects performed five gait initiation trials. In order to standardize the starting conditions, the subjects placed their bare feet on foot marks drawn on the platform. They had to keep their arms by their sides, relax their jaw and fix a spot on a wall 10 m in front. The experiments took place in a quiet room with no visual perturbations.

In each test, the experimenter triggered the acquisition of the COP displacement and EMG signals. The order to initiate gait was given by the experimenter after at least 2 s of steady-state postural recording (judged by visual inspection of the EMG signal).

Data Analysis

Usually, based on COP displacement, three gait initiation phases were described (Halliday et al., 1998; Martin et al., 2002; Hass et al., 2004), the first phase represents the backward COP displacements that create the forward momentum thanks to COP-COG dissociation, the second the weight bearing transfer from SWL to STL, and the third the forward COP displacement.

These phases were identified in our study thanks to the gait initiation events using landmarks on the COP trajectory (**Figure 1**). Landmark 1 (L1) represents the mean position of COP during quiet stance. Landmark 2 (L2) represents the most posterior and lateral position toward the SWL of COP location. Landmark 3 (L3) represents the most posterior and lateral position toward the STL of COP location. The end of the recording of COP displacement represents the outgoing of

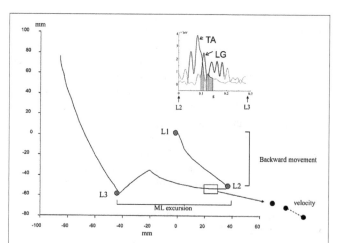

FIGURE 1 | Kinetic and electromyographic (EMG) data used to describe gait initiation. Center of pressure (COP) displacement during gait initiation. L1 represents the position of the COP in normal quiet standing. L2 represents the backward of COP. L3 represents the COP displacement toward the stance limb (STL). Parameters used were the backward COP position during the phase 1 (L1–L2), the medio-lateral (ML) excursion, the velocity (path reported to phase duration). Insert represents tibialis anterior (TA) and lateral gastrocnemius (LG) vs. time during the weight bearing transfer from swing limb (SWL) to STL (From L2 to L3). The bold lines represent when muscle are activated (>25 ms consecutive above the threshold corresponding to the mean ± 3 standard deviation). Gray area represents the phase of coactivation of LG and TA muscles.

COP from the force plate. The identification of these landmarks was conducted with an application of Matlab Program (The Mathworks, Inc., Natick, MA, USA), under visual control. In order to characterize the COP displacement, we calculated the excursion separating two landmarks, the average velocity (sum of distance separating two points of acquisition related to time elapsed in the phase (**Figure 1**).

For EMG data, we have analyzed the period corresponding to weight bearing transfer from STL to SWL during which an inhibition of postural muscle and activation of motor muscles were reported. From an algorithm developed with Matlab program, we determined phasic activation of LG and TA of the SWL under visual control. The Matlab application was developed using previous methodological studies (Mickelborough et al., 2004). EMG data were smoothed with low-pass filter cut off frequency of 20 Hz. The threshold for EMG activation detection was defined as mean added with 3 standard deviations of reference phase. The muscle was considered as active after 25 ms of consecutive above the threshold. Then, we calculated relative time of coactivation of LG and TA muscles during weight bearing transfer from SWL to STL (ratio of time of coactivation with time elapse in the phase).

Statistics

Statistical analysis was carried out with Statview software (SAS Institute, Cary, NC, USA). Given that the data were normally distributed (according to a Kolmogorov-Smirnov test) and the equality of variance Levene median test) was confirmed, an unpaired t-test was used to compare the physically active group and yoga group in terms of kinetic and EMG values. The threshold for statistical significance was set to $p < 0.05$.

We also assessed the relationship between kinetic COP displacement parameters and muscle coactivation by applying Pearson's correlation test.

RESULTS

COP Movements

The yoga and physically active groups do not differ significantly in terms of displacements during the first phase of gait initiation (**Figure 2A**). The mean $\pm$ SD backward movement of COP position shows non-significant lower values in the yoga group than in the group of walkers (-27.8 ± 5.3 vs. -31.1 ± 13.6 mm respectively).

For the second phase of gait initiation, we characterized the excursion and velocity of COP displacement from the SWL to the STL. We did not find significant differences in COP excursion during this phase (110.8 ± 12.1 vs. 102.5 ± 19.7 mm for the yoga and physically active groups, respectively; **Figure 2B**). The COP velocity was significantly lower in yoga practitioners than in the walkers (555.2 ± 32.5 vs. 624.0 ± 50.3 mm.s^{-1}, respectively; $p < 0.01$; **Figure 2C**).

Leg Muscle Co-Activation

During gait initiation, we found significant differences in leg muscle co-activation between the two physically active groups (**Figure 2D**). In fact, leg muscle co-activation is lower in yoga practitioners than in the walkers ($3.9 \pm 6.0\%$ vs. $10.5 \pm 5.1\%$, respectively; $p < 0.01$).

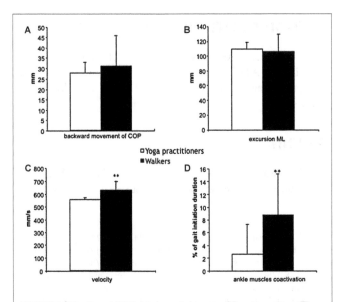

FIGURE 2 | Kinetic and EMG data recorded in yoga (□) and in walkers (■) subjects (mean and standard deviation). **(A)** The backward movement of COP during the phase 1 of gait initiation. **(B)** The excursion of COP displacement (in mm) during phase 2 of gait initiation. **(C)** Velocity of COP displacement (in mm) during phase 2 of gait initiation. **(D)** Percent of time during which LG and TA are coactivated during phase 2 of gait initiation. Significant differences were expressed as **$p < 0.01$.

The relationships between kinetic variables and leg muscle co-activation reveal that muscle co-activation is correlated with the velocity measured during the SWL-to-STL phase ($r = 0.76$; $p < 0.01$).

DISCUSSION

The objective of the present study was to assess the effect of regular yoga practice in gait initiation control in the elderly. This was characterized in terms of COP excursion, COP velocity and muscle co-activation. We hypothesized that Yoga practitioners present differences in APA during gait initiation compared to physically active older adults. Indeed, Gauchard et al. (2003) demonstrated that proprioceptive activities enhance sensory inputs and improve the subject's knowledge of the body scheme and gravity effects. Significant results were reported during the SWL to STL transfer for the COP velocity and % of leg muscle coactivation between the two groups. Lastly, the observed link between COP path and muscle co-activation duration confirmed the interaction between muscle co-activation and the COP trajectory during gait initiation.

During gait initiation, the central postural control system has two main functions: (i) maintenance of balance; and (ii) creation of the anteroposterior moment needed to produce the first step (via a stereotyped pattern of leg muscle activation). In the present study, we did not observe any significant intergroup differences in the rearward COP excursion during the first phase of gait initiation. Previous studies have found that older and disabled subjects exhibit a lower arm peak moment (i.e., a smaller COP-COG distance; Polcyn et al., 1998; Chang and Krebs, 1999; Martin et al., 2002). Based on COP displacements, the present study does not allow to demonstrate differentiated effect between type of physical activity practiced on COP rearward during the first phase of APA.

The second phase of gait initiation consisted in transferring body weight from the initial SWL to initial STL. In the present study, we reported higher average velocity of the COP in the physically active group as compared to the yoga group for a similar ML excursion. In previous studies, smoother COP displacement during gait initiation was seen after 48 weeks of tai chi practice (Hass et al., 2004) and was also described in healthy older subjects (relative to disabled subjects; Martin et al., 2002). The reason for this significant difference remains unclear: the lower COP velocity in the yoga group might be related to the specific, slow movements performed during this activity. Then, it might be the consequence of a behavioral change in yoga practitioners.

However, our results might also be related to adaptations of the central nervous system in the yoga group (relative to the physically active group). To our knowledge, the present study is the first investigation conducted to explore differentiated coactivation of the leg muscles during gait initiation in two types of physical activity practitioners. The time course analysis of EMG data assessed the time during which muscles were involved in postural maintaining (LG) and movement (TA) (Polcyn et al., 1998; Henriksson and Hirschfeld, 2005). The duration of coactivation (expressed as a % of APA duration) might be an indicator of CNS adaptation to deal with postural constraints induced by gravity and movement production during the preparation phase of gait. This muscle pattern (inhibition of postural muscle) was described in healthy young adults (Mann et al., 1979; Brunt et al., 1991, 1999) and seem to be altered with aging and/or disability (Scheibel et al., 1977; Scheibel, 1985; Polcyn et al., 1998; Henriksson and Hirschfeld, 2005). In the present study, Yoga practitioners present lower TA/LG muscles coactivation than the physically active group. The result should be related to a previous study that demonstrated that muscle activation during gait initiation can reflect different behavior in counteracting and using gravity (Honeine et al., 2014).

One specific feature of the present study was the observed association between COP displacement and the EMG motor program. As previously described, the EMG sequence recorded during gait initiation can be considered as a motor program that acts on the COP's position (Crenna and Frigo, 1991). APA are pre-programmed by an open-loop mechanism, then their improvements need better body scheme knowledge. In our study, we reported a significant correlation ($r = 0.76$; $p < 0.01$) between TA/LG coactivation and COP displacement. The relationship obtained between muscle co-activation (time of coactivation/time) and velocity (path/time), demonstrates that the path length is greater when the duration of muscle co-activation is longer. Leg muscle coactivation previously reported in frailty adults might also reflect hesitation or difficulties in initiating gait (i.e., pain, motor impairment, fear of falls, etc.). Several studies have shown that changes in ankle control occur with age and may be associated with an increased risk of falling. A previous study has shown that ankle dorsiflexion was significantly delayed and its amplitude was lower for fallers during gait (Kemoun et al., 2002). Simoneau et al. (2007) explained the decrease in dorsiflexion maximal voluntary contraction torque with aging by neural factor (Simoneau et al., 2007). The question of the benefit of reducing muscle co-activation in frailty adults should then be explored.

Our results suggest that the neuro-adaptation related to yoga performance can modify leg muscle pattern during gait initiation.

This result should also be related to the reduction in muscle coactivation during other dynamic tasks after practice (Chu et al., 2009; Chen et al., 2012a,b; Nagai et al., 2012).

However, the present study may have some limitations inherent to cross-sectional studies. Even if our inclusion criteria allow us to select a healthy elderly population in this cross-sectional study, the two groups might not present similar health conditions. Comparison with other groups should help to understand the effects of physical activity on gait initiation by comparing our results with groups of young adults, sedentary older adults or with other type of physical activity (exercises at a fast pace way requiring balance). We can also note that due to the absence of kinematic data, we could not determine the position of the COG. Therefore, the COP-COG dissociation could not be assessed in the present study.

CONCLUSION

The actual results obtained did not accurately demonstrated that gait initiation is more efficient (in terms of COP-COG dissociation and in term of amplitude of the first step) in yoga practitioners than in regular walkers. However, Yoga practitioners showed slower COP displacement associated with lower leg muscle coactivation. This last point result might be a marker of the use of a different strategy to prepare the first step. Further studies are needed to explore the clinical interests of proprioceptive activities on muscle coactivation during gait initiation and the relationship between gait initiation efficiency (COP-COG, step length) and leg muscle coactivation.

AUTHOR CONTRIBUTIONS

TL, P-LD and SA: project creation. TL: data collection. TL, P-LD and AT: data analysis. TL, P-LD, AT and SA: discussed the results; revised the manuscript. TL and AT: drafted the manuscript.

FUNDING

This work was funded by Université de Picardie Jules Verne and Centre hospitalier Universitaire d'Amiens.

REFERENCES

Alexander, N. B. (1994). Postural control in older adults. *J. Am. Geriatr. Soc.* 42, 93–108. doi: 10.1111/j.1532-5415.1994.tb06081.x

Brunt, D., Lafferty, M. J., McKeon, A., Goode, B., Mulhausen, C., and Polk, P. (1991). Invariant characteristics of gait initiation. *Am. J. Phys. Med. Rehabil.* 70, 206–212. doi: 10.1097/00002060-199108000-00009

Brunt, D., Liu, S. M., Trimble, M., Bauer, J., and Short, M. (1999). Principles underlying the organization of movement initiation from quiet stance. *Gait Posture* 10, 121–128. doi: 10.1016/s0966-6362(99)00020-x

Chang, H., and Krebs, D. E. (1999). Dynamic balance control in elders: gait initiation assessment as a screening tool. *Arch. Phys. Med. Rehabil.* 80, 490–494. doi: 10.1016/s0003-9993(99)90187-9

Chen, Y. -S., Crowley, Z., Zhou, S., and Cartwright, C. (2012a). Effects of 12-week Tai Chi training on soleus H-reflex and muscle strength in older adults: a pilot study. *Eur. J. Appl. Physiol.* 112, 2363–2368. doi: 10.1007/s00421-011-2182-y

Chen, Y. -S., Zhou, S., and Cartwright, C. (2012b). Effect of 12 weeks of Tai Chi training on soleus Hoffmann reflex and control of static posture in older adults. *Arch. Phys. Med. Rehabil.* 92, 886–891. doi: 10.1016/j.apmr.2010.12.043

Chu, Y. H., Tang, P. F., Chen, H. Y., and Cheng, C. H. (2009). Altered muscle activation characteristics associated with single volitional forward stepping in middle-aged adults. *Clin. Biomech.* 24, 735–743. doi: 10.1016/j.clinbiomech.2009.06.012

Crenna, P., and Frigo, C. (1991). A motor programme for the initiation of forward-oriented movements in humans. *J. Physiol.* 437, 635–653. doi: 10.1113/jphysiol.1991.sp018616

Fiolkowski, P., Brunt, D., Bishop, M., and Woo, R. (2002). Does postural instability affect the initiation of human gait? *Neurosci. Lett.* 323, 167–170. doi: 10.1016/s0304-3940(02)00158-1

Folstein, M. F., Folstein, S. E., and McHugh, P. R. (1975). "Mini-mental state". A practical method for grading the cognitive state of patients for the clinician. *J. Psychiatr. Res.* 12, 189–198. doi: 10.1016/0022-3956(75)90026-6

Gauchard, G. C., Tessier, A., Jeandel, C., and Perrin, P. P. (2003). Improved muscle strength and power in elderly exercising regularly. *Int. J. Sports Med.* 24, 71–74. doi: 10.1055/s-2003-37203

Halliday, S. E., Winter, D. A., Frank, J. S., Patla, A. E., and Prince, F. (1998). The initiation of gait in young, elderly, and Parkinson's disease subjects. *Gait Posture* 8, 8–14. doi: 10.1016/s0966-6362(98)00020-4

Hass, C. J., Gregor, R. J., Waddell, D. E., Oliver, A., Smith, D. W., Fleming, R. P., et al. (2004). The influence of Tai Chi training on the center of pressure trajectory during gait initiation in older adults. *Arch. Phys. Med. Rehabil.* 85, 1593–1598. doi: 10.1016/j.apmr.2004.01.020

Henriksson, M., and Hirschfeld, H. (2005). Physically active older adults display alterations in gait initiation. *Gait Posture* 21, 289–296. doi: 10.1016/j.gaitpost.2004.03.001

Honeine, J. -L., Schieppati, M., Gagey, O., and Do, M. -C. (2014). By counteracting gravity, triceps surae sets both kinematics and kinetics of gait. *Physiol. Rep.* 2:e00229. doi: 10.1002/phy2.229

Hortobágyi, T., and DeVita, P. (2000). Muscle pre- and coactivity during downward stepping are associated with leg stiffness in aging. *J. Electromyogr. Kinesiol.* 10, 117–126. doi: 10.1016/s1050-6411(99)00026-7

Katz, S., Ford, A. B., Boskowitz, R. W., Jackson, B. A., and Jaffe, M. W. (1963). Studies of illness in the aged. The index of adl: a standardized measure of biological and psychosocial function. *JAMA* 185, 914–919. doi: 10.1001/jama.1963.03060120024016

Kemoun, G., Thoumie, P., Boisson, D., and Guieu, J. D. (2002). Ankle dorsiflexion delay can predict falls in the elderly. *J. Rehabil. Med.* 34, 278–283. doi: 10.1080/165019702760390374

Larsen, A. H., Puggaard, L., Hämäläinen, U., and Aagaard, P. (2008). Comparison of ground reaction forces and antagonist muscle coactivation during stair walking with ageing. *J. Electromyogr. Kinesiol.* 18, 568–580. doi: 10.1016/j.jelekin.2006.12.008

Laughton, C. A., Slavin, M., Katdare, K., Nolan, L., Bean, J. F., Kerrigan, D. C., et al. (2003). Aging, muscle activity, and balance control: physiologic changes associated with balance impairment. *Gait Posture* 18, 101–108. doi: 10.1016/s0966-6362(02)00200-x

Lelard, T., and Ahmaidi, A. (2015). Effects of physical training on age-related balance and postural control. *Neurophysiol. Clin.* 45, 357–369. doi: 10.1016/j.neucli.2015.09.008

Lord, S. R., and Castell, S. (1994). Physical activity program for older persons: effect on balance, strength, neuromuscular control, and reaction time. *Arch. Phys. Med. Rehabil.* 75, 648–652. doi: 10.1016/0003-9993(94)90187-2

Maki, B. E., and McIlroy, W. E. (1996). Postural control in the older adult. *Clin. Geriatr. Med.* 12, 635–658.

Mann, R. A., Hagy, J. L., White, V., and Liddell, D. (1979). The initiation of gait. *J. Bone Joint Surg. Am.* 61, 232–239. doi: 10.2106/00004623-197961020-00011

Martin, M., Shinberg, M., Kuchibhatla, M., Ray, L., Carollo, J. J., and Schenkman, M. L. (2002). Gait initiation in community-dwelling adults with Parkinson disease: comparison with older and younger adults without the disease. *Phys. Ther.* 82, 566–577. doi: 10.1093/ptj/82.6.566

Massion, J. (1992). Movement, posture and equilibrium: interaction and coordination. *Prog. Neurobiol.* 38, 35–56. doi: 10.1016/0301-0082(92)90034-c

Menz, H. B., Lord, S. R., and Fitzpatrick, R. C. (2003). Age-related differences in walking stability. *Age Ageing* 32, 137–142. doi: 10.1093/ageing/32.2.137

Mickelborough, J., van der Linden, M. L., Tallis, R. C., and Ennos, A. R. (2004). Muscle activity during gait initiation in normal elderly people. *Gait Posture* 19, 50–57. doi: 10.1016/s0966-6362(03)00016-x

Nagai, K., Yamada, M., Mori, S., Tanaka, B., Uemura, K., Aoyama, T., et al. (2011). Effect of the muscle coactivation during quiet standing on dynamic postural control in older adults. *Arch. Gerontol. Geriatr.* 56, 129–133. doi: 10.1016/j.archger.2012.08.009

Nagai, K., Yamada, M., Tanaka, B., Uemura, K., Mori, S., Aoyama, T., et al. (2012). Effects of balance training on muscle coactivation during postural control in older adults: a randomized controlled trial. *J. Gerontol. A Biol. Sci. Med. Sci.* 67, 882–889. doi: 10.1093/gerona/glr252

Patchay, S., Gahery, Y., and Serratrice, G. (1997). Gait initiation and impairments of ground reaction forces as illustrated in old age by 'La marche a petits pas'. *Neurosci. Lett.* 236, 143–146. doi: 10.1016/s0304-3940(97)00781-7

Patchay, S., Gahery, Y., and Serratrice, G. (2002). Early postural adjustments associated with gait initiation and age-related walking difficulties. *Mov. Disord.* 17, 317–326. doi: 10.1002/mds.10074

Pereira, M. P., and Goncalves, M. (2011). Muscular coactivation (CA) around the knee reduces power production in elderly women. *Arch. Gerontol. Geriatr.* 52, 317–321. doi: 10.1016/j.archger.2010.04.024

Polcyn, A. F., Lipsitz, L. A., Kerrigan, D. C., and Collins, J. J. (1998). Age-related changes in the initiation of gait: degradation of central mechanisms for momentum generation. *Arch. Phys. Med. Rehabil.* 79, 1582–1589. doi: 10.1016/s0003-9993(98)90425-7

Scheibel, A. B. (1985). Falls, motor dysfunction, and correlative neurohistologic changes in the elderly. *Clin. Geriatr. Med.* 1, 671–677.

Scheibel, M. E., Tomiyasu, U., and Scheibel, A. B. (1977). The aging human Betz cell. *Exp. Neurol.* 56, 598–609. doi: 10.1016/0014-4886(77)90323-5

Schmitz, A., Silder, A., Heiderscheit, B., Mahoney, J., and Thelen, D. G. (2009). Differences in lower-extremity muscular activation during walking between healthy older and young adults. *J. Electromyogr. Kinesiol.* 19, 1085–1091. doi: 10.1016/j.jelekin.2008.10.008

Simoneau, E., Martin, A., and Van Hoecke, J. (2007). Effects of joint angle and age on ankle dorsi- and plantar-flexor strength. *J. Electromyogr. Kinesiol.* 17, 307–316. doi: 10.1016/j.jelekin.2006.04.005

Vallabhajosula, S., Roberts, B. L., and Hass, C. J. (2014). Tai chi intervention improves dynamic postural control during gait initiation in older adults: a pilot study. *J. Appl. Biomech.* 30, 697–706. doi: 10.1123/jab.2013-0256

12

Influence of the Plantar Cutaneous Information in Postural Regulation Depending on the Age and the Physical Activity Status

Julien Maitre *and* Thierry P. Paillard *

Laboratoire Mouvement Equilibre, Performance et Santé, EA 4445, Département Sciences et Techniques des Activités Physiques et Sportives (STAPS), Université de Pau et des Pays de l'Adour, Tarbes, France

Correspondence:
Thierry P. Paillard
thierry.paillard@univ-pau.fr

The aim was to compare the balance control adaptation to different supporting surfaces depending on the age and the physical activity status. The balance control of two groups of young ($n = 17$) and old ($n = 17$) participants who practiced regular physical activity (active groups) and two groups of young ($n = 17$) and old ($n = 17$) participants who did not practice physical activity (non-active groups) was compared on a firm surface and on a foam surface. The parameters of the center of foot pressure (COP) displacement were compared between the groups. The two older groups were more disturbed than the two younger groups when they stood on a foam surface and there was no difference between active and non-active groups. This result may be linked to the structural and functional involutions of the plantar cutaneous sole and foot that occur with age advancement. The participants' physical activity practice might be not specific enough to generate a more efficient postural adaption to the foam condition for the active groups than the non-active groups within their respective age groups.

Keywords: balance, aging, physical activity, foam, cutaneous, postural control

INTRODUCTION

The skin is a highly complex interface, innervated by a wide array of specialized sensory neurons sensitive to heat, cold, pressure, irritation, itch and pain (McGlone and Reilly, 2010). Tactile information provides feedback about the environment that contributes to balance control (Massion, 1994; Palluel et al., 2008). Indeed, as the feet interface directly with the ground, the cutaneous afferents, emanating from the soles of the feet, provide sensory information on force distribution during upright stance. Thereby, the plantar sole may be considered as a "dynamometric map" (Kavounoudias et al., 1998). To maintain an upright stance, the central nervous system (CNS) integrates cutaneous afferents with other sensory afferents emanating from visual, vestibular and proprioceptive systems (Massion, 1994). An efficient balance control requires availability and accuracy of the sensory afferents (Maitre et al., 2013a). In the context of exogenous perturbation that alters postural segment positions and compromise upright stance, the CNS triggers compensatory postural strategies (Horak and Nashner, 1986) and sensory reweighting (Oie et al., 2002) to preserve balance. Nevertheless, with increasing age, individuals undergo involutions, which result in balance disorder and reduce the ability to compensate for unreliable or discordant sensory input (Sturnieks et al., 2008). These involutions may decrease the efficiency of the central processing mechanisms (Hay et al., 1996) and the neuromuscular function (Aagaard et al., 2010). Moreover, the functional ability of the sensory systems may be reduced with increasing age (Sturnieks et al., 2008).

Although aging has deleterious effects on balance control, the iterative stimulations of the visual, vestibular and proprioceptive systems, induced by the regular practice of physical activity, are known to preserve their functional abilities (Gauchard et al., 2001, 2003; Ribeiro and Oliveira, 2007) and can even improve their contribution in the postural regulation (Quarck and Denise, 2005; Jafarzadehpur et al., 2007; Aman et al., 2015). Moreover, the beneficial effects of the physical activity can also contribute to enhance the ability to detect the plantar pressure distributions (Schlee et al., 2007; Li and Manor, 2010).

It is known that foot problems may occur with aging and are associated with impaired balance and functional ability and increased risk of falls (Menz et al., 2006). With increasing age, the foot undergoes structural and functional involutions, which may result in flatter feet, reduced range of motion of the ankle joint, a higher prevalence of hallux valgus, toe deformities and toe plantarflexor weakness, and reduced plantar tactile sensitivity (Scott et al., 2007). Since the physical activity appears to have opposite effects to the age-related involutions in terms of balance control, it would be interesting to clarify the resultant between the benefits induced by the physical activity and the involutions induced by aging in an ecological context. The use of a foam-supporting surface appears to be a relevant tool to challenge balance control and produces a substantial and multi-directional balance perturbation (Patel et al., 2008a,b) to detect age-related changes (Choy et al., 2003) and exercise (Hue et al., 2004) effects on the postural function. Static standing on a foam surface would change the multiple biomechanical variables in the foot, resulting in an alteration of the distribution of the plantar pressures (Chiang and Wu, 1997). Consequently, the aim of this study was to compare the balance control adaptation to different characteristics of the supporting surface (i.e., firm surface and foam surface) between young and old participants in relation to their physical activity status (i.e., active and non-active). We hypothesized that physically active participants would demonstrate better postural control in context of an altered support surface (i.e., foam surface) than non-active participants whatever the age considered.

MATERIALS AND METHODS

Participants

Recruitment for this study involved the participation of 68 women who gave their informed consent. The experiments received the approval of the local committee for the protection of human participants. All the participants were free from any disorder after medical examination (i.e., neurological, motor and metabolic disorders). The cutaneous sensations under the feet were screened with a pencil and participants were free from any foot disorders and lesion of the foot skin support surface. Four groups were made up according to the age (i.e., young and old) and the physical activity status (i.e., active and non-active). The inclusion criteria in each group were previously described

(Maitre et al., 2013b). The young active group ($n = 17$; age: 20.5 ± 1.1 years; height: 164.8 ± 5.7 cm; weight: 60.5 ± 7.1 Kg; foot size: 26.0 ± 0.9 cm) was formed with sports science students who have practiced sports (for 3 h or more each week, at least at regional level; i.e., swimming, gymnastics, handball, basketball, athletics). The young non-active group ($n = 17$; age: 20.0 ± 1.3 years; height: 162.3 ± 5.4 cm; weight: 56.2 ± 9.2 Kg; foot size: 25.5 ± 0.8 cm) was formed with students who have not practiced physical activities for at least 3 years. The old active group ($n = 17$, age: 74.0 ± 3.8 years; height: 156.6 ± 4.2 cm; weight: 63.2 ± 6.9 Kg; foot size: 25.6 ± 0.8 cm) was formed with healthy older women who practice (for 3 h or more each week) and have regularly practiced (for at least 3 years) physical activity in a sports club (i.e., gymnastics, walking, dancing, aquarobics). The old non-active group ($n = 17$, age: 74.7 ± 6.3 years; height: 155.8 ± 5.7 cm; weight: 62.4 ± 9.0 Kg; foot size: 25.3 ± 0.7 cm) was formed with healthy older women who have not practiced any physical activity (for at least 3 years) except for daily tasks.

Measurements

The participants were tested on a force platform with three strain gauges (Techno Concept^{TM} Mane, France; 40 Hz frequency, 12 bit A/D conversion) in two bipodal conditions with eyes open (i.e., eyes fixed straight ahead on a target at 1.5 m). They were asked to take an upright stance (i.e., barefoot, 30° of feet angle, inter-malleolar distance of 9 cm), as still as possible, with their arms at their side in a "reference condition" (REF condition, i.e., stance on a firm surface) and in a "Foam condition". During the Foam condition, the participants were asked to take an upright stance on a foam surface (15 mm, 70 kg.m^{-3}; TG700, Domyos$^\circledR$, Villeneuve d'Ascq, France) fitted on the force platform to modify the contribution of plantar cutaneous information in postural regulation (Chiang and Wu, 1997). The main objective of the foam condition was to alter plantar cutaneous sensory information in order to determine the reliance attributed to this input in postural regulation. Each condition lasted 20 s. Before the two condition tests, participants benefited from at least 2 min of familiarization with the force platform (as still as possible with eyes open and eyes closed).

The acquisition of the center of foot pressure (COP) displacements was done using Posturowin software (Techno Concept^{TM}, Mane, France) to calculate the parameters that give features of the balance control: the postural stability (i.e., COP surface, mm^2; Caron et al., 2000) and the postural control (i.e., the COP velocity, mm.s^{-1}; Caron et al., 2000). The COP velocity may be calculated for the frontal (COP$_X$ velocity, mm.s^{-1}) and the sagittal (COP$_Y$ velocity, mm.s^{-1}) directions. The smaller these parameters (i.e., velocity and surface) the better the balance control.

Statistical Analysis

Statistical treatment of data was achieved using Statistica software. The one-factor analysis of variance (ANOVA) was used to test the mean differences among the four groups for the anthropometrical data and for the COP displacement parameters in the reference condition. A three factor ANOVA with repeated measures was used to test the condition (reference and foam condition), the age (young and old) and the activity (active and non-active) effects. The differences among means were tested using the Newman-Keuls *post hoc* analysis when significant main effect was found. The results were considered significant at the level of 5%.

RESULTS

Age and Anthropometrical Data

The results indicated significant age differences between the younger and older groups ($F = 1158.7$, $p < 0.001$). The young active and non-active groups were respectively younger than the old active ($p < 0.001$ and $p < 0.001$) and non-active ($p < 0.001$ and $p < 0.001$). Furthermore, there were significant height differences between the younger participant groups and the older participant groups ($F = 11.8$, $p < 0.001$). The young active and non-active groups were respectively taller than the old active ($p < 0.001$ and $p < 0.01$) and non-active ($p < 0.001$ and $p < 0.01$).

Center of Foot Pressure Displacement Parameters

The COP displacement parameters for the reference and the foam condition is presented in the **Figures 1–3**.

Reference Condition

The results concerning the reference condition comparisons indicated that the COP surface ($F = 4.6$, $p < 0.01$) and the COP$_Y$ velocity ($F = 9.3$, $p < 0.001$) differed significantly between the four groups. The *post hoc* analyses indicate that the COP surface (**Figure 1**) and the COP$_Y$ velocity (**Figure 3**) were lower for the young active group than for the two older groups (i.e., the active and non-active groups) in the reference condition. Furthermore,

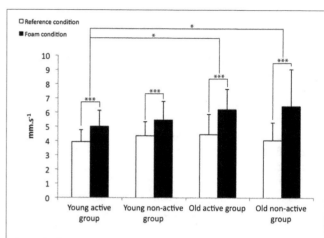

FIGURE 2 | Means and standard deviations for the COP$_X$ velocity for the reference and the foam conditions. $^*p < 0.05$, $^{***}p < 0.001$.

the COP$_Y$ velocity (**Figure 3**) was lower for the young non-active group than the two older groups (i.e., the active and non-active groups).

Differences Between the Firm and Foam Condition

All the COP displacement parameters presented significant condition effects for the COP surface ($F = 82.4$, $p < 0.001$), the COP$_X$ velocity ($F = 77.5$, $p < 0.001$) and the COP$_Y$ velocity ($F = 110.4$, $p < 0.001$). These results indicate that the COP displacement parameters increased for all the groups (**Figures 1–3**). Otherwise, there is a significant condition × age interaction for the COP surface ($F = 7.5$, $p < 0.01$), the COP$_X$ velocity ($F = 7.5$, $p < 0.01$) and the COP$_Y$ velocity ($F = 25.0$, $p < 0.001$). These results indicate that the balance control was more altered for the older participants than for the younger participants, particularly on the Y-axis. The COP surface and the COP$_Y$ velocity increased less for the two younger groups (i.e., the active and non-active) than for the two older groups

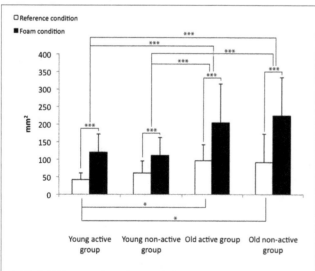

FIGURE 1 | Means and standard deviations for the center of foot pressure (COP) surface for the reference and the foam conditions. $^*p < 0.05$, $^{***}p < 0.001$.

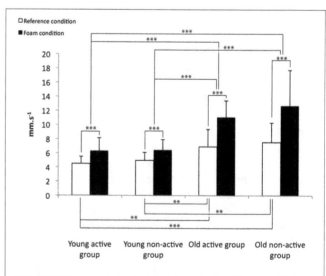

FIGURE 3 | Means and standard deviations for the COP$_Y$ velocity for the reference and the foam conditions. $^{**}p < 0.01$, $^{***}p < 0.001$.

(i.e., the active and non-active; **Figures 1**, **3**). In addition, the COP_X velocity increased less for the young active group than the two older groups (i.e., the active and non-active groups; **Figure 2**).

DISCUSSION

The aim of this study was to compare the balance control adaptation to different characteristics of the supporting surface (i.e., firm surface and foam surface) between young and old participants in relation to their physical activity status (i.e., active and non-active). We did not find support for our hypothesis. The main result of this study indicated that there is no difference between active and non-active participants within their respective age groups for the reference and the foam conditions. The older participants demonstrated less efficient balance control on the firm surface (i.e., reference condition) than the younger participants. Moreover, balance control was disturbed for all the participants when they stood on a foam surface, but the older participants were more disturbed than the younger participants.

As suggested by previous results, aging alters balance control even for a simple postural task (i.e., bipedal stance with eyes open on a firm surface; Choy et al., 2003). In the present study, the COP_Y velocity differences between the younger and older groups indicated that older participants demonstrated a poorer postural control than the younger participants, in the anteroposterior direction. This result is supported by the literature (Du Pasquier et al., 2003) and may be due to the unavoidable involutions of the postural function (i.e., alteration of the sensory, central processing, and muscular functions; Sturnieks et al., 2008). Furthermore, the postural differences between younger and older individuals may be more highlighted in the context of challenged postural task (Maitre et al., 2013a,b).

In the present study, when participants stood on the foam surface the COP surface and the COP velocities on the X and Y axes increase significantly as compared to the firm surface. The disturbing effects of standing on a foam surface have been investigated previously in several studies (Chiang and Wu, 1997; Patel et al., 2008a,b). Static standing on a foam surface would change the multiple biomechanical variables in the foot, resulting in an alteration of the distribution of the plantar pressures (Chiang and Wu, 1997). Foam condition would affect the input of both joint and cutaneous mechanoreceptors. The foam condition would alter the spatial configuration of the cutaneous mechanoreceptors in the foot, thereby reducing the ability to sense pressure distribution and body orientation (Chiang and Wu, 1997). Moreover, the mechanical properties of the compliant surface may also alter the postural behavior. The elastic characteristics of the foam enable smaller opposing mechanical resistance than a firm surface that could cushion the foot movements produced by the ankle musculature, which reduces the motor output generated for postural stabilization (Horak and Hlavacka, 2001; Patel et al., 2008b). Consequently, the balance control is altered on a foam-supporting surface.

Relative to the reference condition, the COP surface and the COP_Y velocity increased significantly more for the older groups than the younger groups while standing on the foam. This result corroborates previous work (Choy et al., 2003), which indicated that older participants demonstrated poorer balance control on a foam-supporting surface than younger participants. The poorer postural control achieved by the older groups compared to the younger groups could be explained in two ways. Firstly, it could be linked to a plantar tactile sensitivity malfunction in the older groups in comparison with the younger groups. Although participants of this study were free from any foot disorders and lesion of the foot skin support surface, we cannot exclude that the plantar tactile sensitivity differs between the younger and older groups. Indeed, it is known that foot and ankle undergo involutions with aging that may alter balance function (Menz et al., 2006). Older individuals may exhibit flatter feet, reduced range of motion of the ankle joint, a higher prevalence of hallux valgus, toe deformities and toe plantarflexor weakness, and reduced plantar tactile sensitivity (Perry, 2006; Scott et al., 2007). Cutaneous mechanoreceptors decrease in number and have a progressive structural deterioration with ageing (Shaffer and Harrison, 2007; Decorps et al., 2014). These elements may contribute to decrease the ability of the older groups to accurately detect foot pressure distribution and correctly regulate posture (Menz et al., 2006). Indeed, several authors (Simmons et al., 1997; Horak and Hlavacka, 2001) showed that when somatosensory information is reduced postural control might be altered. Secondly, the poorer postural control achieved by the older groups compared to the younger groups could be linked to the inability of the older groups to take advantage of the non-altered sensory information as effectively as the younger groups. Indeed, in a context of a sensory alteration, the balance control mechanism requires the availability as well as the accuracy of information emanating from the non-altered sensory systems to enable the CNS to integrate the information and to initiate a compensatory motor strategy limiting the postural disturbance related to the foam surface (Massion, 1994; Peterka, 2002). When cutaneous information is reduced, individuals are compelled to rely more on other sensory systems (i.e., visual, vestibular and proprioceptive systems) to maintain their stability (Lord and Menz, 2000; Horak and Hlavacka, 2001; Paillard et al., 2007). Although, Meyer et al. (2004) suggested that, in a context of plantar cutaneous anesthesia, plantar sensation is of moderate importance for the maintenance of normal standing balance, the impact of reduced plantar sensitivity on postural control increases with the loss of additional sensory modalities. With increased age, there is a progressive loss of functioning of visual, vestibular and proprioceptive systems, which can contribute to balance deficits (Sturnieks et al., 2008). In addition, the ability to correctly reweight sensory information may be altered with aging (Horak et al., 1989). Thereby, in the present study, the older participants may be less able to counteract postural disruption due to the foam-supporting surface than the younger groups.

The main result indicated that there is no difference between active and non-active participants within their respective age groups for the reference and foam conditions, yet, previous studies have demonstrated that regular practice of physical activity may enhance balance control for young (Kiers et al., 2013) and old (Howe et al., 2007) individuals. In the present study, several elements could explain this lack of significant results. Firstly, as suggested by Kiers et al. (2013), the reference condition (i.e., bipedal stance with eyes open on a firm surface) probably constitutes a too simple postural task to produce evidence of differences between active and non-active participants. Secondly, the active participants might have improved their ability to maintain dynamic balance more than static balance with their physical practice. Indeed, the ability to maintain balance is likely to be specific to the training tasks (Hrysomallis, 2011). In this study, the postural tasks were statics and the active participants mainly practiced dynamic physical activities. Thirdly, the rubber of foam used in the foam condition was probably too thin to sufficiently challenge the balance control in order to demonstrate difference in relation to the physical activity status. Patel et al. (2008a,b) have suggested that thin rubber of foam enables closer contact with the rigid surface beneath the foam, which allows plantar tactile sensory feedback and ankle movements to be more effective. In addition, the deformation properties of the foam surface matched to the participants' weight (Gosselin and Fagan, 2015). The heavier participants might be in closer contact with surface beneath the foam. In the present study, the foam characteristics were relevant to highlight differences in relation to the age, but probably not appropriate to highlight difference in relation to the physical activity status. Caution should be taken when using foam pads on force platforms during balance assessments. To evidence a postural control difference in relation to the physical activity status, the postural task difficulty has to be accurately calibrated, since the foam properties (Patel et al., 2008a,b) and the anthropometric characteristics of the participant (Gosselin and Fagan, 2015) may alter posturographic data.

This study suggests that the ability to detect the distribution of the plantar pressure contributes to the balance control. Although foot problems may occur with increasing age (Menz et al., 2006), previous studies have demonstrated that augmenting tactile sensory information from the sole of the foot may improve balance in older people (Palluel et al., 2008). Furthermore, the regular practice of physical activity may improve the tactile sensitivity (Schlee et al., 2007; Kerr et al., 2008; Li and Manor, 2010; Kattenstroth et al., 2013). Nevertheless, in the present study, the effect of the regular practice of physical activity appeared to be not strong enough and/or appropriate to generate postural difference between active and non-active participants within their respective age groups. It is known that physical activity induces specific postural adaptation (Hrysomallis, 2011). In the present study, it could be construed that the characteristics of the physical activities practiced by the participants might not be specific enough to generate a more efficient postural adaption to the foam condition for the active groups than the non-active groups within their respective age groups (Paillard et al.,

2010). Most of the participants in the active groups do not practice barefoot physical activities that specifically stimulate cutaneous mechanoreceptors. Specific training that stimulates plantar cutaneous sensory mechanoreceptors improves postural function (Morioka et al., 2011). Practiced barefoot, physical activity could enhance plantar cutaneous sensitivity (Schlee et al., 2007). Hence, the data of the present study suggest that the practice of barefoot exercises could be recommended to improve efficiency of the postural function on altered support surface.

CONCLUSION

This study corroborates that, with increased age, there is an alteration of the contribution of plantar cutaneous information. This loss of functioning was present for a simple postural task (i.e., upright stance with eyes open on a firm surface) and for a more complex postural task (i.e., upright stance with eyes open on a foam surface). Relative to the reference condition, when the cutaneous sensory information was altered by the use of a foam-supporting surface, the balance control was more disrupted for the older participants than the younger participants. The inability to counteract this sensory alteration might be linked to the unavoidable structural and functional involutions of the plantar cutaneous sole and foot that occur with age advancement. The main result of this study suggests that there is no difference between active and non-active participants within their respective age groups in the foam conditions. Physical activity traditionally practiced with shoes might not sufficiently stimulate the cutaneous mechanoreceptor to counteract the effects of aging on the plantar skin sensitivity. In order to extend the analysis of the effects of physical activity on the cutaneous sensitivity in relation to the age and the physical activity status, participants should be compared according to the type of sports (i.e., with shoes or barefoot) and the cutaneous sensitivity should be analyzed by the use of specific tests (e.g., vibrotactile or monofilament sensitivity). Identifying influence of barefoot physical activity would enable clinician to prevent loss of plantar skin sensitivity and so improve postural control in older people.

AUTHOR CONTRIBUTIONS

JM and TPP contributed to the conception and design of the work; and the acquisition, analysis, and interpretation of data.

FUNDING

The investigation was supported by grants from the Association Nationale de la Recherche et de la Technologie and the Conseil Général des Hautes Pyrénées.

ACKNOWLEDGMENTS

The authors thank all the participants for their helpful cooperation.

REFERENCES

Aagaard, P., Suetta, C., Caserotti, P., Magnusson, S. P., and Kjær, M. (2010). Role of the nervous system in sarcopenia and muscle atrophy with aging: strength training as a countermeasure. *Scand. J. Med. Sci. Sports* 20, 49–64. doi: 10. 1111/j.1600-0838.2009.01084.x

Aman, J. E., Elangovan, N., Yeh, I. L., and Konczak, J. (2015). The effectiveness of proprioceptive training for improving motor function: a systematic review. *Front. Hum. Neurosci.* 8:1075. doi: 10.3389/fnhum.2014. 01075

Caron, O., Gelat, T., Rougier, P., and Blanchi, J. P. (2000). A comparative analysis of the center of gravity and center of pressure trajectory path lengths in standing posture: an estimation of active stiffness. *J. Appl. Biomech* 16, 234–247.

Chiang, J. H., and Wu, G. (1997). The influence of foam surfaces on biomechanical variables contributing to postural control. *Gait Posture* 5, 239–245. doi: 10. 1016/s0966-6362(96)01091-0

Choy, N. L., Brauer, S., and Nitz, J. (2003). Changes in postural stability in women aged 20 to 80 years. *J. Gerontol. A Biol. Sci. Med. Sci.* 58, 525–530. doi: 10. 1093/gerona/58.6.m525

Decorps, J., Saumet, J. L., Sommer, P., Sigaudo-Roussel, D., and Fromy, B. (2014). Effect of ageing on tactile transduction processes. *Ageing Res. Rev.* 13, 90–99. doi: 10.1016/j.arr.2013.12.003

Du Pasquier, R. A., Blanc, Y., Sinnreich, M., Landis, T., Burkhard, P., and Vingerhoets, F. J. (2003). The effect of aging on postural stability: a cross sectional and longitudinal study. *Neurophysiol. Clin.* 33, 213–218. doi: 10. 1016/j.neucli.2003.09.001

Gauchard, G. C., Gangloff, P., Jeandel, C., and Perrin, P. P. (2003). Physical activity improves gaze and posture control in the elderly. *Neurosci. Res.* 45, 409–417. doi: 10.1016/s0168-0102(03)00008-7

Gauchard, G. C., Jeandel, C., and Perrin, P. P. (2001). Physical and sporting activities improve vestibular afferent usage and balance in elderly human subjects. *Gerontology* 47, 263–270. doi: 10.1159/000052810

Gosselin, G., and Fagan, M. (2015). Foam pads properties and their effects on posturography in participants of different weight. *Chirop. Man. Therap* 23:2. doi: 10.1186/s12998-014-0045-4

Hay, L., Bard, C., Fleury, M., and Teasdale, N. (1996). Availability of visual and proprioceptive afferent messages and postural control in elderly adults. *Exp. Brain Res.* 108, 129–139. doi: 10.1007/bf00242910

Horak, F. B., and Hlavacka, F. (2001). Somatosensory loss increases vestibulospinal sensitivity. *J. Neurophysiol.* 86, 575–585.

Horak, F. B., and Nashner, L. M. (1986). Central programming of postural movements: adaptation to altered support-surface configurations. *J. Neurophysiol.* 55, 1369–1381.

Horak, F. B., Shupert, C. L., and Mirka, A. (1989). Components of postural dyscontrol in the elderly: a review. *Neurobiol. Aging* 10, 727–738. doi: 10. 1016/0197-4580(89)90010-9

Howe, T. E., Rochester, L., Jackson, A., Banks, P. M., and Blair, V. A. (2007). Exercise for improving balance in older people. *Cochrane Database Syst. Rev.* 4:CD004963. doi: 10.1002/14651858.cd004963

Hrysomallis, C. (2011). Balance ability and athletic performance. *Sports Med.* 41, 221–232. doi: 10.2165/11538560-000000000-00000

Hue, O. A., Seynnes, O., Ledrole, D., Colson, S. S., and Bernard, P. L. (2004). Effects of a physical activity program on postural stability in older people. *Aging Clin. Exp. Res.* 16, 356–362. doi: 10.1007/bf03324564

Jafarzadehpur, E., Aazami, N., and Bolouri, B. (2007). Comparison of saccadic eye movements and facility of ocular accommodation in female volleyball players and non-players. *Scand. J. Med. Sci. Sports* 17, 186–190. doi: 10.1111/j.1600-0838.2005.00535.x

Kattensroth, J. C., Kalisch, T., Holt, S., Tegenthoff, M., and Dinse, H. R. (2013). Six months of dance intervention enhances postural, sensorimotor and cognitive performance in elderly without affecting cardio-respiratory functions. *Front. Aging Neurosci.* 5:5. doi: 10.3389/fnagi.2013.00005

Kavounoudias, A., Roll, R., and Roll, J. P. (1998). The plantar sole is a 'dynamometric map' for human balance control. *Neuroreport* 9, 3247–3252. doi: 10.1097/00001756-199810050-00021

Kerr, C., Shaw, J., Wasserman, R., Chen, V., Kanojia, A., Bayer, T., et al. (2008). Tactile acuity in experienced Tai Chi practitioners: evidence for use dependent plasticity as an effect of sensory-attentional training. *Exp. Brain Res.* 188, 317–322. doi: 10.1007/s00221-008-1409-6

Kiers, H., Van Dieën, J., Dekkers, H., Wittink, H., and Vanhees, L. (2013). A systematic review of the relationship between physical activities in sports or daily life and postural sway in upright stance. *Sports Med.* 43, 1171–1189. doi: 10.1007/s40279-013-0082-5

Li, L., and Manor, B. (2010). Long term tai chi exercise improves physical performance among people with peripheral neuropathy. *Am. J. Chin. Med.* 38, 449–459. doi: 10.1142/s0192415x1000797x

Lord, S. R., and Menz, H. B. (2000). Visual contributions to postural stability in older adults. *Gerontology* 46, 306–310. doi: 10.1159/0000 22182

Maitre, J., Gasnier, Y., Bru, N., Jully, J. L., and Paillard, T. (2013a). Discrepancy in the involution of the different neural loops with age. *Eur. J. Appl. Physiol.* 113, 1821–1831. doi: 10.1007/s00421-013-2608-9

Maitre, J., Jully, J. L., Gasnier, Y., and Paillard, T. (2013b). Chronic physical activity preserves efficiency of proprioception in postural control in older women. *J. Rehab. Res. Dev.* 50, 811–820. doi: 10.1682/JRRD.2012.08.0141

Massion, J. (1994). Postural control system. *Curr. Opin. Neurobiol.* 4, 877–887. doi: 10.1016/0959-4388(94)90137-6

McGlone, F., and Reilly, D. (2010). The cutaneous sensory system. *Neurosci. Biobehav. Rev.* 34, 148–159. doi: 10.1016/j.neubiorev.2009.08.004

Menz, H. B., Morris, M. E., and Lord, S. R. (2006). Foot and ankle risk factors for falls in older people: a prospective study. *J. Gerontol. A Biol. Sci. Med. Sci.* 61, 866–870. doi: 10.1093/gerona/61.8.866

Meyer, P. F., Oddsson, L. I., and De Luca, C. J. (2004). The role of plantar cutaneous sensation in unperturbed stance. *Exp. Brain Res.* 156, 505–512. doi: 10.1007/s00221-003-1804-y

Morioka, S., Fujita, H., Hiyamizu, M., Maeoka, H., and Matsuo, A. (2011). Effects of plantar perception training on standing posture balance in the old old and the very old living in nursing facilities: a randomized controlled trial. *Clin. Rehabil.* 25, 1011–1020. doi: 10.1177/0269215510 395792

Oie, K. S., Kiemel, T., and Jeka, J. J. (2002). Multisensory fusion: simultaneous re-weighting of vision and touch for the control of human posture. *Brain Res. Cogn. Brain Res.* 14, 164–176. doi: 10.1016/s0926-6410(02)00071-x

Paillard, T., Bizid, R., and Dupui, P. (2007). Do sensorial manipulations affect subjects differently depending on their postural abilities? *Br. J. Sports Med.* 41, 435–438. doi: 10.1136/bjsm.2006.032904

Paillard, T., Margnes, E., Portet, M., and Breucq, A. (2010). Postural ability reflects the athletic skill level of surfers. *Eur. J. Appl. Physiol.* 111, 1619–1623. doi: 10.1007/s00421-010-1782-2

Palluel, E., Nougier, V., and Olivier, I. (2008). Do spike insoles enhance postural stability and plantar-surface cutaneous sensitivity in the elderly? *Age (Dordr)* 30, 53–61. doi: 10.1007/s11357-008-9047-2

Patel, M., Fransson, P. A., Lush, D., and Gomez, S. (2008a). The effect of foam surface properties on postural stability assessment while standing. *Gait Posture* 28, 649–656. doi: 10.1016/j.gaitpost.2008.04.018

Patel, M., Fransson, P. A., Lush, D., Petersen, H., Magnusson, M., Johansson, R., et al. (2008b). The effects of foam surface properties on standing body movement. *Acta Otolaryngol* 128, 952–960. doi: 10.1080/00016480701827517

Perry, S. D. (2006). Evaluation of age-related plantar-surface insensitivity and onset age of advanced insensitivity in older adults using vibratory and touch sensation tests. *Neurosci. Lett.* 392, 62–67. doi: 10.1016/j.neulet.2005.08.060

Peterka, R. J. (2002). Sensorimotor integration in human postural control. *J. Neurophysiol.* 88, 1097–1118.

Quarck, G., and Denise, P. (2005). Vestibulo-ocular reflex characteristics in gymnasts. *Sci. Mot.* 55, 101–112.

Ribeiro, F., and Oliveira, J. (2007). Aging effects on joint proprioception: the role of physical activity in proprioception preservation. *Eur. Rev. Aging Phys. Act.* 4, 71–76. doi: 10.1007/s11556-007-0026-x

Schlee, S. T., Sterzing, T., and Milani, T. L. (2007). "Infuence of footwear on foot sensitivity: a comparison between barefoot and shod sports," in *XXV International Symposium on Biomechanics in Sports* (Ouro Preto, Brazil), 285–288.

Scott, G., Menz, H. B., and Newcombe, L. (2007). Age-related differences in foot structure and function. *Gait Posture* 26, 68–75. doi: 10.1016/j.gaitpost.2006. 07.009

Shaffer, S. W., and Harrison, A. L. (2007). Aging of the somatosensory system: a translational perspective. *Phys. Ther.* 87, 193–207. doi: 10.2522/ptj.200 60083

Simmons, R. W., Richardson, C., and Pozos, R. (1997). Postural stability of diabetic patients with and without cutaneous sensory deficit in the foot. *Diabetes Res. Clin. Pract.* 36, 153–160. doi: 10.1016/s0168-8227(97)0 0044-2

Sturnieks, D. L., St George, R., and Lord, S. R. (2008). Balance disorders in the elderly. *Neurophysiol. Clin.* 38, 467–478. doi: 10.1016/j.neucli.2008. 09.001

13

An Increase in Postural Load Facilitates an Anterior Shift of Processing Resources to Frontal Executive Function in a Postural-Suprapostural Task

Cheng-Ya Huang[1,2], Gwo-Ching Chang[3], Yi-Ying Tsai[4] and Ing-Shiou Hwang[4,5]*

[1] School and Graduate Institute of Physical Therapy, College of Medicine, National Taiwan University, Taipei City, Taiwan,
[2] Physical Therapy Center, National Taiwan University Hospital, Taipei, Taiwan, [3] Department of Information Engineering,
I-Shou University, Kaohsiung City, Taiwan, [4] Institute of Allied Health Sciences, College of Medicine, National Cheng Kung
University, Tainan City, Taiwan, [5] Department of Physical Therapy, College of Medicine, National Cheng Kung University,
Tainan City, Taiwan

*Correspondence:
Ing-Shiou Hwang
ishwang@mail.ncku.edu.tw

Increase in postural-demand resources does not necessarily degrade a concurrent motor task, according to the adaptive resource-sharing hypothesis of postural-suprapostural dual-tasking. This study investigated how brain networks are organized to optimize a suprapostural motor task when the postural load increases and shifts postural control into a less automatic process. Fourteen volunteers executed a designated force-matching task from a level surface (a relative automatic process in posture) and from a stabilometer board while maintaining balance at a target angle (a relatively controlled process in posture). Task performance of the postural and suprapostural tasks, synchronization likelihood (SL) of scalp EEG, and graph-theoretical metrics were assessed. Behavioral results showed that the accuracy and reaction time of force-matching from a stabilometer board were not affected, despite a significant increase in postural sway. However, force-matching in the stabilometer condition showed greater local and global efficiencies of the brain networks than force-matching in the level-surface condition. Force-matching from a stabilometer board was also associated with greater frontal cluster coefficients, greater mean SL of the frontal and sensorimotor areas, and smaller mean SL of the parietal-occipital cortex than force-matching from a level surface. The contrast of supra-threshold links in the upper alpha and beta bands between the two stance conditions validated load-induced facilitation of inter-regional connections between the frontal and sensorimotor areas, but that contrast also indicated connection suppression between the right frontal-temporal and the parietal-occipital areas for the stabilometer stance condition. In conclusion, an increase in stance difficulty alters the neurocognitive processes in executing a postural-suprapostural task. Suprapostural performance is not degraded by increase in postural load, due to (1) increased effectiveness of information transfer, (2) an anterior shift of processing resources toward frontal executive function, and (3) cortical dissociation of control hubs in the parietal-occipital cortex for neural economy.

Keywords: dual-task, graph analysis, functional connectivity, event-related potential, network-based statistics

INTRODUCTION

Postural control is a continuum raging from "controlled to automatic" processing, depending on the level of postural demand and the capacity of attentional resources (Stins et al., 2009; Boisgontier et al., 2013). Maintenance of posture with bilateral stance on a stable surface is an automatic process that requires minimal attentional resources to stabilize the center of gravity of the postural system within the limits of the sway range. When stance difficulty increases, the postural task shifts to a controlled process, manifested with an enhanced postural regularity (Donker et al., 2007; Sarabon et al., 2013). Parallel loading of two component tasks, posture and supraposture tasks, results in an intricate trade-off for central resource allocation (Temprado et al., 2001), depending on the task priority (Levy and Pashler, 2001), response compatibility (Stelzel et al., 2006), relative task difficulty of the two concurrent tasks (Huang and Hwang, 2013), and so on. For some postural-suprapostural dual-tasking, such as golf putting and surgery, withdrawing attention from postural control could help to maximize the precision of the added motor task (Balasubramaniam et al., 2000; Stoffregen et al., 2007). Postural sway is less regular in the dual-task condition than in a single postural task (Donker et al., 2007; Kuczyński et al., 2011). In this context, at least two critical issues with the limited central resource arise. The first issue is that relative cost of postural-suprapostural performance varies with stance difficulty, as differently predicted by the resource-competition model (Woollacott and Shumway-Cook, 2002) and the adaptive resource-sharing model (Mitra, 2004; Mitra and Fraizer, 2004). However, direct neural mechanism regarding to how the brain reorganizes functional networks is largely unknown. Second, most research designed to investigate the neural control of a postural-suprapostural task has employed a concurrent cognitive task as part of the dual-task configuration. Traditional dual-task setups and a postural-suprapostural task with a suprapostural motor goal are very likely to produce different types of resource competition. The reason is that the task quality of a suprapostural motor task must take kinematical advantages of stance stability (Wulf et al., 2004; Stoffregen et al., 2007; Huang and Hwang, 2013), whereas a postural-suprapostural task with a cognitive goal typically has low response compatibility between the two component tasks (Weeks et al., 2003).

The fronto-parietal brain network is a flexible hub of dual-task control (Cole et al., 2013), although the role of the frontal and parietal areas in a dual-task is still debatable. Some neuroimaging studies have reported greater activation of the frontal or prefrontal areas during dual-task trials than during single-task trials (D'Esposito et al., 1995; Collette et al., 2005), whereas others have revealed no specific frontal or prefrontal activation in the dual-task condition (Klingberg, 1998; Adcock et al., 2000; Bunge et al., 2000). In other studies, dual-tasking, as compared to both individual visual and auditory single tasks, activated a predominantly parietal network in the right hemisphere (Deprez et al., 2013), whereas simultaneous car driving and language

comprehension suppressed parietal activation in reference to two single tasks (Just et al., 2008). In addition to a paradigm-specific interaction between component tasks (Salo et al., 2015), one of the most appealing explanations to reconcile those seemingly paradoxical results is that a dual-task may not necessarily recruit additional cortical areas; it may instead alter the interactions of the frontal/prefrontal areas with other cortical regions [such as parietal (Gontier et al., 2007) and premotor areas (Marois et al., 2006)]. Consequently, it is more important to examine changes in the inter-regional connectivity than to investigate changes in regional excitability of a dual-task by referencing the baseline activity of a single task.

Recently, graph theoretical analysis has been developed to characterize the topology of inter-regional connectivity and the efficacy of information transmission in brain networks, with important implications for adaptive or pathological changes in brain function (Reijneveld et al., 2007; Bullmore and Sporns, 2012). As postural-suprapostural behaviors involve information mastery potentially contingent upon the fronto-parietal network (Huang and Hwang, 2013), challenging postural sets could affect network connectivity for static stance, compromising the wiring-cost minimization, and postural load increment to achieve a suprapostural goal. Within the brain connectome context, this study aimed to extend the limited previous work by exploring the brain connectome in a particular postural-suprapostural task, when stance difficulty increases. This increase in stance difficulty must be associated with resource allocation of the brain, especially that of the fronto-parietal network, so that suprapostural motor performance and stance stability are jointly optimized. This exploratory study hypothesized that concurrent force-matching from a stabilometer stance would lead to changes in the inter-regional connectivity and the efficacy of information transfer, as compared to force-matching from a level-surface stance.

MATERIALS AND METHODS

Subjects

The study was conducted with 14 healthy right-handed volunteers (7 males, 7 females; mean age: 23.8 ± 3.8 years) from a university campus. All subjects were asked to abstain from stimulants (such as cigarettes, alcohol, and caffeine) for 24 h before the experiment. All subjects were volunteers naive to the purpose of the experiments and received no reimbursement. The experiment was conducted in accordance with the Declaration of Helsinki and with the approval of the local ethics committee (National Taiwan University Hospital Research Ethics Committee; no. 201312077RINC), and the subjects took part after signing personal consent forms.

Procedures

Before the experiment, the maximum voluntary contraction (MVC) of the right thumb-index precision grip and the maximal anterior tilt angle during stabilometer stance of each participant were determined respectively. For each participant, there were two experimental conditions for concurrent postural and motor tasks with different postural challenges (level-surface stance vs.

Abbreviations: SampEn, sample entropy; SL, synchronization likelihood; C_w, clustering coefficient; E_{glob}, global coefficient; E_{loc}, local coefficient.

stabilometer stance). The participants were required to conduct a thumb-index precision grip to couple a target line of 50% MVC force in response to auditory cues (force-matching task) while standing on a level surface or a tilted stabilometer. The two conditions were varied in a random order. For the level-surface condition, the participants were instructed to execute the force-matching task as accurately as possible while standing on a level surface. Therefore, the participants focused the majority of their attention on the force-matching task and maintained the upright posture automatically. For the stabilometer condition, the participants performed the force-matching task while standing on a stabilometer [a wooden platform (50 × 58 cm) with a curved base (height: 25 cm)]. They were instructed to execute the force-matching task as accurately as possible while maintaining the stabilometer at 50% of the maximal anterior tilt with minimal ankle movement (**Figure 1A**). Therefore, the participants had to pay attention simultaneously to both the force-matching task and postural maintenance. In the stabilometer condition, the subjects were provided with on-line visual feedback regarding the ankle displacement and force output on a computer screen 60 cm in front of them at the participants' eye-level. The target signals for force-matching and posture were presented at the same vertical position of the monitor to reduce the visual load during the concurrent tasking. With visual feedback, the participants could minimize fluctuations of the ankle and force-error in reference to the target angle at all times. In the level-surface condition, only the force-matching related visual feedback was provided. We understood that relative task difficulty could affect the reciprocal effect and task outcome of a postural-suprapostural task. Therefore, the target force for the concurrent motor task and target angle for the postural task were empirically selected based on our previous experiment (Hwang and Huang, 2016; Hung et al., in press). A high target force for force-matching of over 50% MVC and a tilting angle of the stabilometer plate >50% of the maximal anterior tilt were not suitable for repeated measures of event-related potential because of the potential fatigue effect. Moreover, the present combination of tasks was intended to provide a unique dual-task situation that would prevent a marked reduction in force-matching performance due to stabilometer stance for the majority of young healthy adults in the laboratory.

The force-matching act was guided by warning and executive tones, with a total of 14 warning-executive signal pairs in an experimental trial. A warning tone (an 800 Hz tone lasting for 100 ms) was randomly presented at different intervals of 1.5, 1.75, 2, 2.25, 2.5, 2.75, or 3 s before an executive tone (a 500 Hz tone lasting for 100 ms). The interval between the end of the executive tone and the beginning of the next warning tone was 3.5 s. Upon hearing the executive tone, the participants started a quick thumb-index precision grip (force impulse duration <0.5 s) to quickly couple the peak precision-grip force with the force target on the monitor. There were six trials of the postural-suprapostural dual-task for each stance condition, and each trial was composed of 14 precision grips.

Experimental Setting

An electrogoniometer (Model SG110, Biometrics Ltd, UK) was used to record the angular motion of the right (dominant) ankle joint. The electrogoniometer consisted of a 12-bit analog-to-digital converter box and 2 sensors for measuring their relative positions in space. One sensor was placed on the dorsum of the right foot between the second and third metatarsal heads, and the other sensor was fastened along the midline of the middle third of the anterior aspect of the lower leg. The level of force-matching was recorded with a load cell (15-mm diameter × 10-mm thickness, net weight = 7 grams; Model: LCS, Nippon Tokushu Sokki Co., Japan) mounted on the right thumb. The load cell was connected to a distribution box by a thin wire that could not provide stable mechanical support for the postural stance via the grip force apparatus. The auditory stimuli and target signals for conducting the force-matching and postural subtasks were generated with LabVIEW software (National Instruments, Austin, TX, USA). Thirty-two Ag-AgCl scalp electrodes (Fp$_{1/2}$, F$_z$, F$_{3/4}$, F$_{7/8}$, FT$_{7/8}$, FC$_z$, FC$_{3/4}$, C$_z$, C$_{3/4}$, CP$_z$, CP$_{3/4}$, P$_z$, P$_{3/4}$, T$_{3/4}$, T$_{5/6}$, TP$_{7/8}$, O$_z$, O$_{1/2}$, and A$_{1/2}$) with a NuAmps amplifier (NeuroScan Inc., El Paso, TX, USA) were used to register scalp voltage fluctuations in accordance with the extended 10–20 system. The ground electrode was placed along the midline ahead of F$_z$. Electrodes placed above the arch of the left eyebrow and below the eye were used to monitor eye movements and blinks. The impedances of all the electrodes were below 5 kΩ and were referenced to linked mastoids of both sides. All physiological data were synchronized and digitized at a sample rate of 1 kHz.

Data Analyses
Behavior Data

Reaction time (RT) and force error of force-matching was used to represent suprapostural performance in the present study. The RT of force-matching was denoted as the timing interval between the executive tone and the onset of grip force. The onset of grip force was defined as the force impulse profile exceeding the mean plus 3 times the standard deviation of the baseline activity of the force profile (500 ms before and after each warning tone). The RT of each force-matching trial was averaged across trials for each participant in the level-surface and stabilometer conditions. Force error of each force impulse was determined by normalized force-matching error (NFE), denoted as $\frac{|PGF - TF|}{TF} \times 100\%$ (where PGF: peak grip force; TF: target force; **Figure 1B**). The NFEs of all force-matching events were also averaged across trials for each participant in the level-surface and stabilometer conditions. On the other hand, the kinematic properties of ankle movement fluctuations during the interval between the executive tone and the onset of the force impulse profile were used to represent postural performance. The amplitude and regularity of the ankle movement fluctuations were assessed with root mean square and sample entropy (SampEn) after down-sampling of the kinematic data to 125 Hz. SampEn is a popular entropy measure used to characterize the temporal aspects of the variability of biological data, with high consistency and less sensitivity to short data length (Richman and Moorman, 2000; Yentes et al., 2013). A SampEn close to 0 represents greater regularity, while a value near 2 represents higher irregularity. A higher postural irregularity indicates less attentional resources allocated to postural control and thus more autonomous processing (Donker et al., 2007; Kuczyński et al.,

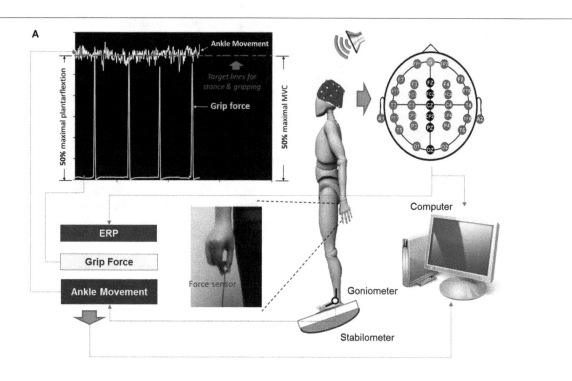

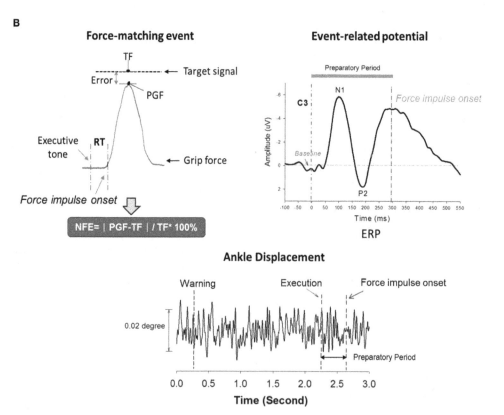

FIGURE 1 | Schematic illustration of experimental setup (A) and physiological data (B). Real-time display of precision grip force, ankle displacement, and target signals for concurrent force-matching and postural tasks. By separate scale-tuning of the manual force target and postural target, the target signals of both postural and force-matching tasks could be displayed in an identical position on the monitor. Suprapostural performance was assessed with the reaction time (RT) and normalized force error (NFE) of a force-matching act. The event-related potential (ERP) of the force-matching act was recorded with scalp electroencephalography. ERP between the executive tone and onset of the force-impulse profile was denoted as preparatory ERP, composed of N1 and P2 components. TF, target force; PGF, peak grip force.

2011). The mathematical formula for *SampEn* was

$$SampEn(m, r, N) = \ln\left(\frac{\sum\limits_{i=1}^{N-m} n_i^m}{\sum\limits_{i=1}^{N-m-1} n_i^{m+1}}\right) = \ln\left(\frac{n_n}{n_d}\right)$$

where N is the total data point number. In this study, m equaled 3 and the tolerance range of r was $0.15 \times$ the standard deviation of the standardized ankle movement fluctuations. For the level-surface condition, the data of the absolute ankle joint angle were used for amplitude and *SampEn* measurement; for the stabilometer condition, the data of the mismatch between the absolute ankle joint angle and the target line were used for amplitude and *SampEn* measurement.

Functional Connectivity Assessment

The DC shift and artifacts of electrical noise of each channel were conditioned with third-order trend correction and a low pass filter (40 Hz/48 dB roll-off) over the entire set of recorded data in off-line analysis. The conditioned EEG data were then segmented into epochs of 700 ms, including 100 ms before the onset of each execution signal. Each epoch was corrected with the NeuroScan 4.3 software program (NeuroScan Inc., EI Paso, TX, USA) to remove artifacts (such as excessive drift, eye movements, or blinks) in reference to baseline activities at the pre-stimulus interval. Poor epochs were also discarded by visual inspection (rejection rate of inappropriate trials: <10%). The remaining artifact-free epochs were averaged for an experimental trial in the level-surface and stabilometer conditions.

Since brain networks can be coupled in a highly non-linear manner (Pijnenburg et al., 2008), the synchronization likelihood (SL) was used to assess the degrees of linear and non-linear dimensions of EEG coupling within cortical networks (Leistedt et al., 2009; Boersma et al., 2011). Theoretically, SL takes into account the recurrences of state space vectors occurring at the same moment that are converted from two time series of interest (Boersma et al., 2011). An SL close to 0 indicates no coupling, whereas an SL of 1 indicates complete coupling. For brevity, detailed descriptions of SL calculation (Stam and van Dijk, 2002; Stam et al., 2003) and parameter settings (Montez et al., 2006) can be found in previous works. Because we were interested in cortical modulation during preparation process for a postural-suprapostural task, we selected the duration of averaged epochs between the executive tone and force-matching onset for SL analysis. A square 30×30 SL adjacent matrix was obtained by computing the SL of ERP data from all pairwise combinations of channels in the preparatory period (**Figures 1B, 2**). In the **Figure 1B**, the 0 of ERP plot represents the onset of the executive signal. Each entry in the SL adjacent matrix represented the connectivity strength within the functional networks. For each participant, the overall SL adjacent matrix from 6 experimental trials in the level-surface or stabilometer condition was averaged. As the choice of the threshold is fairly arbitrary in the literature, we built functional connectomes across various SL thresholds from 0.1 to 0.9. The SL adjacent matrix was rescaled with the proportion of strongest weights, such that all other weights below

a given threshold (including SL on the main diagonal) were set to 0. For instance, when the threshold value was 0.1, only the top 10% of the strongest weights in the SL adjacent matrix were considered to determine the network properties of the functional connectome. The mean SL of all the 32 recording sites, frontal (F_z, F_3, F_4, F_7, and F_8), sensorimotor (C_3, C_z, C_4, CP_3, CP_z, and CP_4), and parietal-occipital areas (P_3, P_z, P_4, O_1, O_z, and O_2), were determined for the level-surface and stabilometer conditions.

Using a causal finite impulse response (FIR) filter (24 dB/octave roll-off), we digitally filtered the ERP signal into the classic frequency bands in the theta (4–8 Hz), upper alpha (10–13 Hz), and beta (13–35 Hz) ranges. Spectral connectivity analysis was performed following the construction of theta and beta SL adjacent matrices with the conditioned ERP signal of both specific bands in the preparatory period. As action monitoring and planning for visuomotor tasks are reported to be linked to the mid-frontal theta rhythm (4–8 Hz; Luu et al., 2004; Armbrecht et al., 2012), the SL in the theta band that connected the mid-frontal areas (F_z and FC_z) and other scalp electrodes was used to examine stance-related differences in central executive function (Tanaka et al., 2009). Another research interest was the SL in the upper alpha (10–13 Hz) and beta bands (13–35 Hz) that connected sensorimotor (C_3, C_z, C_4, CP_3, CP_z, and CP_4) or parietal-occipital areas (P_3, P_z, P_4, O_1, O_z, and O_2), as oscillatory changes in these areas are related to preparation for fine motor/postural control (MacKay and Mendonca, 1995; Brovelli et al., 2004; Babiloni et al., 2008) and early perception information processing (Nierhaus et al., 2015). Especially, upper alpha power is more associated with movement performance than low alpha power is (Babiloni et al., 2008). The calculation of SL was accomplished with functions of HERMES for Matlab (Niso et al., 2013).

Graph Theoretical Analysis

Graph theoretical analysis was conducted with weighted network measures to best utilize the weight information. In terms of SL adjacent matrixes at various threshold values, the mean clustering coefficient (C_w), local coefficient (E_{loc}), global coefficient (E_{glob}), and small-world index (*sigma*, σ) of the resulting graphs were determined. Functionally, C_w, E_{loc}, and E_{glob} are metrics of information flow in a brain network. The clustering coefficient (C_w^i) for a vertex i quantifies the proportion of its neighboring vertices j that are connected to each other. The clustering coefficient C_w^i of vertex i was denoted as $C_w^i = \frac{\sum_{j \neq i} \sum_{k \neq i,j} w_{ij} w_{ik} w_{jk}}{\sum_{j \neq i} \sum_{k \neq i,j} w_{ij} w_{ik}}$. Topological mapping of the clustering coefficient was constructed with the clustering coefficients of all nodes. Another network metric, E_{loc} can be defined as $E_{loc} = \frac{1}{N} \sum_{i \in G} E(G_i)$, where G_i is the subgraph of the neighbors of a node i and $E(G_i)$ indicates the efficiency of the subgraph G_i. E_{glob} was calculated with $E_{glob} = \frac{1}{N(N-1)} \sum_{i \neq j \in G} \frac{1}{L_{i,j}}$, where $L_{i,j}$ is the shortest path length from node i to node j. Presuming that cortical regions under different electrodes exchange packets of information concurrently, E_{glob} is a quantitative measure of the efficiency of a parallel information transfer, with greater E_{glob} indicating

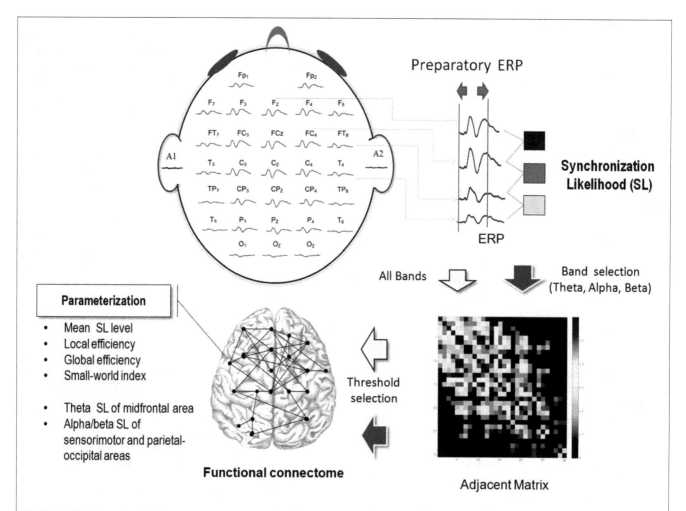

FIGURE 2 | Workflow of cortical network construction with ERP in the preparatory period. Functional connectivity was characterized with the synchronization likelihood (SL) of the paired preparatory ERP of different recording electrodes. The adjacent matrix represents the strengths of inter-electrode synchronization likelihood following appropriate threshold selection. With the adjacent matrix, connectomes in the preparatory period in the level-surface, and stabilometer conditions were established.

better functional integration of brain networks. In contrast to E_{glob}, which indexes a network property of functional integration (Rubinov and Sporns, 2010; Yu et al., 2013), C_w and E_{loc} reflect a network property of functional segregation (Rubinov and Sporns, 2010; Yu et al., 2013). By contrasting the random and regular networks of the same numbers of nodes and edges (Watts and Strogatz, 1998), the small-world index (σ) can provide the network's small-worldness regarding the balance of information flow between local segregation and global integration in a network (Watts and Strogatz, 1998). When σ is >1, the network exhibits small-world properties (Humphries et al., 2006; Stam et al., 2007a). The small-world index (σ) is mathematically formulated as $\sigma = \gamma/\lambda$. Here, $\gamma = C_w/C_{w\_rand}$ and $\lambda = L_p/L_{p\_rand}$. The C_w and L_p are the clustering coefficient and the characteristic path length of the functional network. The characteristic path length is formulated as $L_p = \frac{1}{n}\sum_{i \in N} L_i = \frac{1}{n}\sum_{i \in N} \frac{\sum_{j \in N, j \neq i, \wedge d_{i,j}}}{n-1}$, where L_i is the average distance between mode i and all other nodes. Both C_{w_rand} and L_{p_rand} were obtained by averaging 50 populations of

random networks. The parameterization of network properties was accomplished with functions of the Brain Connectivity Toolbox (Rubinov and Sporns, 2010).

Statistical Analysis

For behavior data, paired t-test was used to examine the significance of differences between the level-surface and stabilometer conditions in normalized force-matching error (NFE), reaction time (RT), amplitude of ankle movement fluctuations (AMF_RMS), and sample entropy of ankle movement fluctuations (AMF_SampEn). Since these resemble behavior variables, paired t-test was used to contrast all the network parameters [mean SL of all electrode pairs (SL_all), in the frontal (SL_F), sensorimotor (SL_SM), parietal-occipital (SL_PO) areas, E_{glob}, E_{loc}, and small-world index (σ)] of the level-surface and stabilometer conditions across different threshold values. The significance of the stance effect on modulation of clustering coefficients and the mean SL of all electrode pairs was displayed with t-values on the basis of a paired difference

TABLE 1 | Means and standard errors of force-matching and postural variables for the concurrent force-matching and postural tasks in the level-surface and stabilometer conditions.

Mean ± SE	Level-surface	Stabilometer	Statistics
NFE (%)	9.89 ± 0.78	10.01 ± 0.79	$t_{(13)} = -0.328, p = 0.748$
RT (ms)	304.8 ± 9.6	310.7 ± 9.8	$t_{(13)} = -1.720, p = 0.109$
AMF_RMS (degree)	0.012 ± 0.001	0.151 ± 0.023[†††]	$t_{(13)} = -6.138, p < 0.001$
AMF_SampEn	0.514 ± 0.013	0.382 ± 0.006[†††]	$t_{(13)} = 8.049, p < 0.001$

NFE, normalized force-matching error; RT, reaction time for force-matching; AMF_RMS, root mean square value of ankle movement fluctuations; AMF_SampEn, sample entropy of ankle movement fluctuations; [†††], stabilometer > level-surface, p < 0.001.

test. The level of significance of the above-mentioned statistical analyses was set at $p = 0.05$. Network-based statistics were performed to identify spectral connectivity in the theta, upper alpha, and beta bands of the node pairs that significantly changed with variations in stance configuration. For this purpose, paired t-tests were independently performed at each synchronization value of the spectral bands of interest, and t-statistics larger than an uncorrected threshold of $t_{(13)} = 3.012$ ($p = 0.005$) were extracted into a set of supra-threshold connections. Then we identified all connected components in the adjacency matrix of the supra-threshold links and saved the number of links. A permutation test was performed 5000 times to estimate the null distribution of maximal component size, and the corrected p-value was calculated as the proportion of permutations for which the most connected components consisted of two or more links. Methodological details of network-based statistics are documented in Zalesky et al. (2010). Statistical analyses were performed in Matlab (Mathworks Inc. Natick, MA, USA) and SPSS v.19.0 (SPSS Inc. Chicago, IL, USA). All data are represented as mean ± standard error.

RESULTS

Force-Matching and Stance Performance

For the suprapostural task, the paired t-test revealed that the force-matching error (NFE: level-surface = 9.89 ± 0.78%; stabilometer = 10.01 ± 0.79%) and reaction time (RT: level-surface = 304.8 ± 9.6 ms; stabilometer = 310.7 ± 9.8 ms) of the force-matching task did not change with stance configuration ($p > 0.05$; **Table 1**). For the postural task, the magnitude of ankle movement fluctuations (AMF_RMS) was stance-dependent, for AMF_RMS of the stabilometer condition (0.151 ± 0.023) was greater than that of the level-surface condition (0.012 ± 0.001; $p < 0.001$). The sample entropy of ankle movement fluctuations (AMF_SampEn) was subject to postural load, for AMF_SampEn (0.382 ± 0.006) was lower in the stabilometer condition than in the level-surface condition (0.514 ± 0.013; $p < 0.001$).

Global Network Metrics and Inter-Regional Connectivity

Figure 3 contrasts different network metrics as a function of threshold value between the level-surface and stabilometer

conditions. For the majority of the threshold values, the global coefficient (E_{glob}) and the local coefficient (E_{loc}) in the stabilometer condition were significantly larger than those in the level-surface condition ($p < 0.05$), especially for the higher threshold values. However, the small-world index (σ) was stance-invariant for all threshold values ($p > 0.05$). In terms of synchronization likelihood, we found significant stance effects on inter-regional coupling of ERP in the preparatory stage. The mean values of the SL of all the electrode pairs in the frontal and sensorimotor areas (SL_F and SL_SM) were larger in the stabilometer condition than in the level-surface condition ($p < 0.05$). Mean SL in the parietal-occipital area (SL_PO) showed the reverse trend, with lower SL_PO in the stabilometer condition at lower threshold values (threshold = 0.1, 0.2, 0.3, and 0.4; $p < 0.05$). Overall, the mean SL of all the electrode pairs (SL_all) was enhanced in the stabilometer condition ($p < 0.05$). Except for the small-world index, the network parameters were stance-dependent when the threshold was set to 0.3 or 0.4. **Figure 4** displays the population means of adjacent SL matrices in the two different stance conditions (threshold value = 0.3), as well as t-values for the examination of the stance effects on the adjacent matrices. In line with the patterned change in the mean level of SL, adjacent SL matrices in the frontal and sensorimotor areas were enhanced, whereas adjacent SL matrices in the parietal-occipital area were suppressed in the stabilometer condition. **Figure 5A** presents the pooled topology of the clustering coefficients (C_w) for the level-surface and stabilometer conditions (threshold value = 0.3), which suggested different functional segregations between the two stance conditions from the standpoint of information flow. The concurrent postural and force-matching tasks in the level-surface condition exhibited a high probability of node connection to neighbors in the parietal lobes and the right fronto-temporal area, in contrast to high frontal C_w in the stabilometer condition. **Figure 5B** is a topological plot of t-values for contrasting the spatial distribution of C_w between the level-surface and stabilometer conditions. The stabilometer condition produced a higher C_w in the mid-frontal area but a lower C_w in the parietal area as compared to those in the level-surface condition ($p < 0.05$).

Network-Based Statistics of Spectral Connectivity

Based on the supra-threshold connectivity and permutation test, network-based statistics revealed localized networks (i.e., connected and clustered components) with significantly stance-dependent SL-values in the theta, upper alpha, and beta bands ($p = 0.0002$, corrected). The contrast of stance-related average values of the spectral connectivity in the pairwise connections of interest is displayed in **Figure 6**. Theta connectivity (4–8 Hz) to the mid-frontal area (F_z, FC_z) was stronger in the stabilometer condition than in the level-surface condition (**Figure 6A**). On the other hand, there was a neat dichotomy of stance-related differences in upper alpha (10–13 Hz) and beta (13–35 Hz) connectivity to the sensorimotor (C_3, C_z, C_4, CP_3, CP_z, and

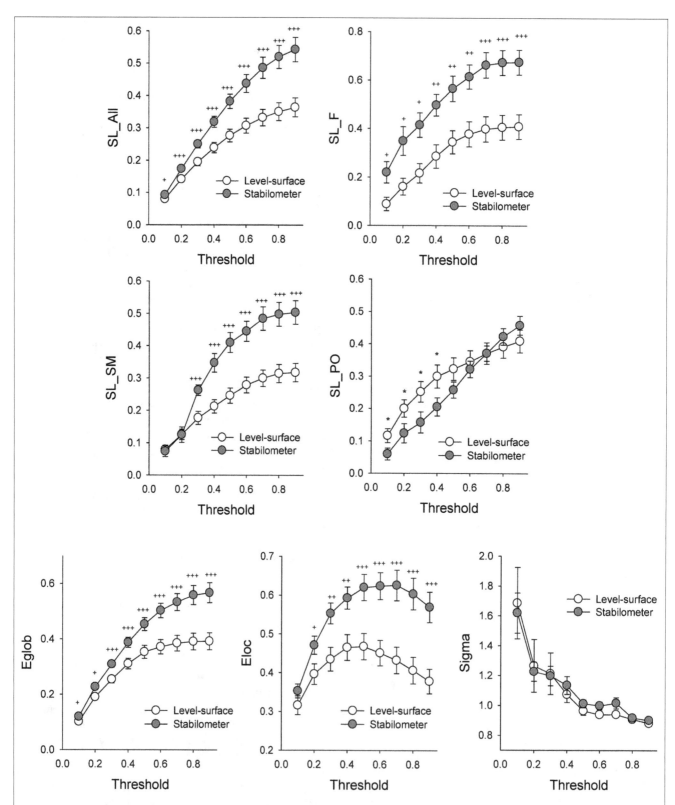

FIGURE 3 | The contrast of network parameters between the concurrent force-matching and postural tasks in the level-surface and stabilometer conditions at different threshold values. E_{glob}, global efficiency; E_{loc}, local efficiency; *Sigma*, small-world index; *, level-surface > stabilometer, $p < 0.05$; †, stabilometer > level-surface, $p < 0.05$; ††, stabilometer > level-surface, $p < 0.01$; †††, stabilometer > level-surface, $p < 0.001$.

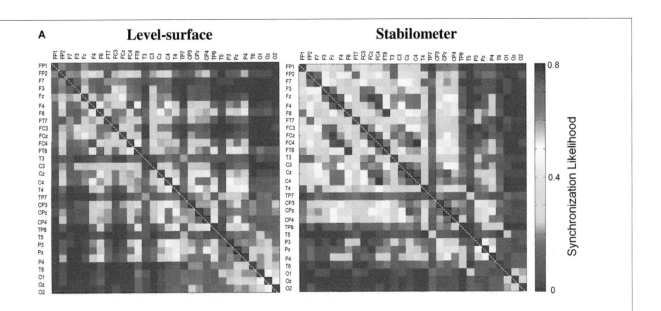

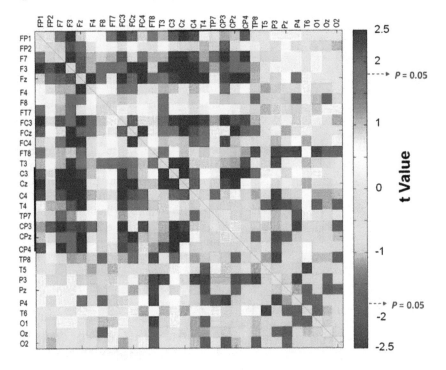

FIGURE 4 | The pooled adjacent matrix of synchronization likelihood (SL) of preparatory ERP for the concurrent force-matching and postural tasks in the level-surface and stabilometer conditions (threshold value = 0.3). (A) Population means of SL adjacent matrix in the surface (left) and stabilometer (right) conditions. **(B)** The adjacent matrix of t-values for contrasting SL between the level-surface and stabilometer conditions ($t > 1.771$, stabilometer SL > level-surface SL, $p < 0.05$; $t < -1.771$, level-surface SL > stabilometer SL, $p < 0.05$).

CP_4) and parietal-occipital cortex (P_3, P_z, P_4, O_1, O_z, and O_2; **Figure 6B**). In comparison with the level-surface stance, the upper alpha and beta connectivity to the parietal-occipital cortex, especially the supra-threshold linkages from the right frontal-temporal (FT_8), temporal (TP_8, T_4), and sensorimotor areas (CP_3, CP_z, and CP_4; $p < 0.005$), was significantly suppressed with stabilometer stance ($p < 0.05$). However, the long-distance connectivity of the upper alpha and beta bands to the sensorimotor area (C_3, C_z, C_4, CP_3, CP_z, and CP_4), especially the supra-threshold linkages from the prefrontal and

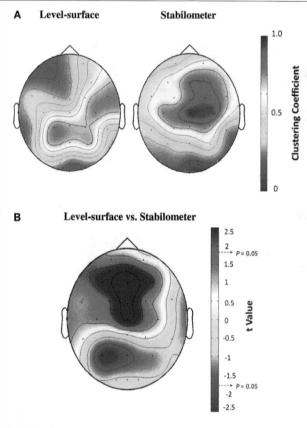

FIGURE 5 | (A) The pooled topological mapping of clustering coefficients (C_W) between concurrent force-matching and postural tasks in the level-surface and stabilometer conditions (threshold value = 0.3). **(B)** The stance-dependent difference in the distribution of clustering coefficients, in terms of the topography of t-values plotted on the scalp ($t > 1.771$, stabilometer C_W > level-surface C_W, $p < 0.05$; $t < -1.771$, level-surface C_W > stabilometer C_W, $p < 0.05$).

frontal areas ($p < 0.005$), was enhanced in the stabilometer condition.

DISCUSSION

As expected, the brain adopted a more controlled process for stabilometer stance in respond to increases in the magnitude and regularity of ankle movement. However, the accuracy and reaction time of suprapostural force-matching from stabilometer stance were not significantly affected by increases in postural threats. Our data did not support the facilitation of suprapostural performance by attention withdrawal from the postural task under the framework of resource competition (Cavanaugh et al., 2007; Donker et al., 2007; Derlich et al., 2011; Kuczyński et al., 2011). In fact, the combination of postural and suprapostural tasks of different task loads could result in a variety of performance outcomes, which are not always explainable with behavior contexts. The adaptive resource-sharing hypothesis (Mitra, 2004; Mitra and Fraizer, 2004) seems to be more appropriate for explaining the present observations,

for concurrent force-matching was not affected by increasing attentional focus on the postural task. This preliminary study first revealed that brain reorganization under this particular circumstance involved (1) increased efficacy of information transmission, (2) anterior shift of processing resources, and (3) superior network economy in the preparatory period of force-matching.

Enhanced Efficacy of Information Transfer for the Increased Postural Challenge

In light of the global and local efficiencies (E_{loc} and E_{glob}; **Figure 3**, the third row), the information transfer in the brain network was significantly enhanced in the stabilometer condition. Analogous to difficult manipulation of a mathematical task (Klados et al., 2013), the information transfer in brain networks for a postural-suprapostural task consistently increased with stance difficulty for all SL thresholds. The stance-related increase in E_{loc} reflects more short-range connections between neighboring brain regions (particularly in the frontal and premotor areas), by virtue of the high clustering coefficients during concurrent force-matching from stabilometer stance (**Figure 5**). This increasing nodal organization was compelling evidence of context-dependent recruitment of the local frontal area with high postural demands (Mihara et al., 2008; Huang et al., 2014; Mirelman et al., 2014), which allowed the participants to effectively resolve behavioral interference between the component tasks and to plan the timing of force-matching (Pfurtscheller and Berghold, 1989) under the critical posture condition. On the other hand, an enhanced E_{glob} indicates a more optimal network architecture for direct information transfer among distributed regions, commonly seen in skill advancement following motor learning (Sami and Miall, 2013). In the stabilometer condition, the long-distance connectivity between the prefrontal/frontal area and the sensorimotor area (**Figures 4B, 6B**) facilitates the integration of posture-stabilizing information by selectively gating sensory inputs from multiple sources from the sensorimotor area with the central executive function. However, the small-world property (*sigma*) did not vary with stance configuration (**Figure 3**), indicating a stance-independent balance between local processing specialization and global information propagation.

Anterior Shift in Processing Resources in the Stabilometer Condition

The second major finding of this study was that the increase in stance difficulty caused an anterior shift in processing resources for force-matching from stabilometer stance, in support of several lines of evidence, including increasing frontal emphasis of the SL adjacent matrix (**Figures 3, 4**), potentiation of frontal clustering coefficients (**Figure 5B**), enhancement of mid-frontal theta connectivity (**Figure 6A**), and increases in inter-regional coupling from frontal to sensorimotor networks in the upper alpha and beta bands (**Figure 6B**). These scenarios jointly suggested a transition of the postural-suprapostural task, which is typically regulated by the frontal-parietal executive

A

Level-surface vs. Stabilometer

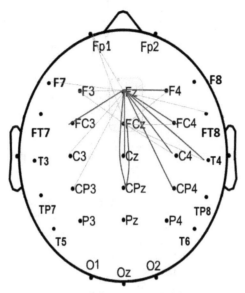

Theta band (4-8 Hz)

Threshold=0.3, p = 0.0002 (corrected)

B

Level-surface vs. Stabilometer

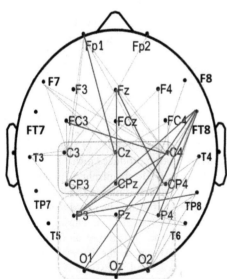

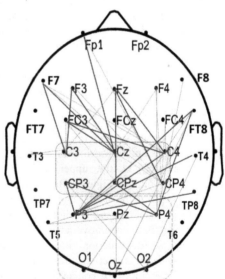

Upper alpha band (10-13 Hz)

Threshold=0.3, p = 0.0002 (corrected)

Beta band (13-35 Hz)

Threshold=0.3, p = 0.0002 (corrected)

FIGURE 6 | Spectral connectivity analysis for contrasting wiring diagrams between the concurrent force-matching and postural tasks in the level-surface and stabilometer conditions (threshold value = 0.3). (A) Synchronization likelihood in the theta band (4–8 Hz) that connects to the mid-frontal area (F_z and FC_z). **(B)** Synchronization likelihood in the upper alpha (10–13 Hz) and beta band (13–35 Hz) of recording electrodes that connect to the sensorimotor (C_3, C_z, C_4, CP_3, CP_z, and CP_4) and parietal-occipital (P_3, P_z, P_4, P_3, O_1, O_z, and O_2) areas (thin red line, stabilometer connectivity > level-surface connectivity, $p < 0.05$; bold red line, stabilometer connectivity of supra-threshold > level-surface connectivity of supra-threshold, $p < 0.005$; thin blue line, level-surface connectivity > stabilometer connectivity, $p < 0.05$; bold blue line, level-surface connectivity of supra-threshold > stabilometer connectivity of supra-threshold, $p < 0.005$).

system in the level-surface condition, to a state in which the frontal strategic control prevails for concurrent force-matching from the stabilometer stance (Slobounov et al., 2009; Ferraye et al., 2014; Karim et al., 2014). The stabilometer stance altered brain resource reallocation in at least three different aspects: recruitment of resources necessary for dealing with the postural instability, target detection for force-matching, and task-switching associated with the increase in postural load. First, the additional recruitment of frontal executive resources was partly attributable to the attentional focus being shifted to postural destabilization due to variations in stabilometer movement (Dault et al., 2001), as previous studies have found from recording cortical activation in the prefrontal cortex, frontal cortex, and supplementary motor area following posture perturbation (Mihara et al., 2008; Fujimoto et al., 2014). Next, stabilometer movement aggravated externally-induced retinal image motion, adding difficulty to the action monitoring and error detection with visual feedback for force-matching (Sipp et al., 2013; Hülsdünker et al., 2015). Therefore, the enhanced mid-frontal theta activity could also reflect heightened selective attention to improve gaze stability for the detection and prediction of target movements (Mihara et al., 2008). Third, for a postural-suprapostural setup with a suprapostural motor goal, the amplitudes of the N1 and P2 components in the preparation period are related to variations in the task-load of the postural and suprapostural tasks, respectively (Huang and Hwang, 2013). This fact clearly suggests that tasks are scheduled in a sequential order to execute a force-matching act with postural prioritization. Since switch costs are greater when switching from a more difficult task to an easier task (Schneider and Anderson, 2010; Barutchu et al., 2013), the switch cost from the postural task to force-matching in the stabilometer condition was multiplied, entailing an extra computational load on frontal executive function (Liefooghe et al., 2008) in the preparatory period. In addition to increases in the SL_F and frontal clustering coefficients, it was of great significance to observe the increases in the connectivity of functionally specialized regions between the left prefrontal area (Fp$_1$) and sensorimotor cortex (C$_3$, C$_4$, C$_z$, CP$_3$, CP$_4$, and CP$_z$) in the upper alpha (10–13 Hz) and beta (13–35 Hz) bands (**Figure 6B**). Such long-distance connectivity well explains the greater global coefficient (E_{glob}) for concurrent force-matching and stabilometer stance (**Figure 3**), suggesting underlying cooperative activities within the dorsolateral prefrontal cortex, anterior cingulate cortex, and supplementary motor area (Kondo et al., 2004; Hashimoto et al., 2011). Taxing frontal resources for concurrent postural-suprapostural tasks under high postural threats conceptually supports the previous thinking that the prefrontal or frontal network could be a common bottleneck for dual-tasks (Dux et al., 2006). In addition, the overall increase in functional connectivity (SL_all) with a frontal emphasis is direct neurophysiological evidence of increasing stance-related attentional control over a postural-suprapostural task with increasing postural difficulty, hypothetically indexed with entropy measures of the posture component task (**Table 1**) and previous work (Donker et al., 2007; Stins et al., 2009).

Brain Network Economy for Postural-Suprapostural Task with Increased Postural Challenge

The most interesting finding was a strategic trade-off to avoid a resource ceiling by reducing reliance on the temporal-parietal-occipital network, when the stance difficulty increased for a postural-suprapostural dual-task. In a challenging posture such as the stabilometer condition, stronger inter-dependencies among the temporal-parietal junction (Tachibana et al., 2011; Karim et al., 2013) and parietal-occipital areas (Slobounov et al., 2005, 2009; Pellijeff et al., 2006) are expected, as the subjects needed to depend on an enhanced vestibule-ocular response, visual-proprioceptive control, and motion vision to establish dynamic representations of body schema due to postural destabilization. However, in view of the lower SL_PO (**Figures 3, 4**) and parietal clustering coefficients (**Figure 5**), the present study conversely exhibited desynchronization of the parietal-occipital network. Moreover, the spectral connectivity of the upper alpha and beta bands in the temporal-parietal-occipital regions (particularly in the right hemisphere) was suppressed during concurrent force-matching from a stabilometer (**Figure 6B**). These facts suggest neural economy to prevent excessive consumption of brain resources, affected by restricting the division of attentional resources toward multisensory information before the force-matching act from the stabilometer stance. It seems that the visuospatial attention to postural control to detect enhanced postural fluctuations could be temporarily disengaged during preparation to execute a force-matching task. We argue that the information inhibition is potentially advantageous in that it increases the resources allocated to frontal executive function, empowering conflict detection, task switching, and facilitation of the suprapostural goal. Due to the flexible resource allocation, the accuracy and responsiveness of force-matching were not affected by postural destabilization (**Table 1**). Supporting the notion of a domain-specific idling of dorsal networks to prevent a resource ceiling, previous neuroimaging studies also reported a comparable neural economy under the condition of relatively high postural threats. Imaged locomotion produced lower activity in the vestibular and somatosensory (right hemisphere preponderance) areas than that during imagined standing (Jahn et al., 2004; Zwergal et al., 2012). However, it should be noted that resource allocation for a dual-task is context dependent. During the concurrent execution of two verbal tasks, Mizuno et al. (2012) found no significant connectivity changes in the parietal and temporal areas with increases in task load. Classic dual task setups (cognitive or verbal tasks) might have very different task compatibilities and reciprocal effects from a postural-suprapostural task (Huang and Hwang, 2013), since a postural subtask is always prioritized naturally, consuming a variety of brain resources.

Methodology Issue

The execution of postural-suprapostural tasks must rely on coordination interactions of neuronal sources across distributed brain regions. Among the several quantitative approaches,

SL was used to characterize the inter-dependences between two cortical activities because it is the most popular index for estimating functional connectivity for neurophysiological data. SL has been widely been used to assess connectivity strength in the graphic based studies using either low-density (Pijnenburg et al., 2004; Smit et al., 2012; Boersma et al., 2013; Liu et al., 2015; Herrera-Díaz et al., 2016) or high-density EEG (Polanía et al., 2011; Cao et al., 2014), because SL is able to account for the repertoire of network states, considering linear and nonlinear interactions between multiple synchronized neural sources in the brain (Stam and van Dijk, 2002). Also, SL can sensitively detect slight and complex variations in the coupling strength (Koenis et al., 2013) and resolve synchronization patterns on a fine time scale (Stam and van Dijk, 2002; Betzel et al., 2012). These advantages were especially helpful in highlighting stance-related differences in rapid dynamic of the ERP with low-frequency oscillations (such frontal theta synchronization and long-stance upper alpha desynchronization; **Figures 6A,B**). However, a few researchers based on stimulation studies to argue that SL is not immune to a volume conduction effect that might cause spurious coupling from common diploe sources (Stam et al., 2005; Tognoli and Kelso, 2009). If the physical synchronization did exist during the experiment, we could not conclusively deny overestimation of the observed differences in local clustering schema, since correlations generated from single diploes tend to be strongest within neighboring electrodes. Despite a potential volume conduction effect, physical synchronization did not rationally explain the patterned changes in network connectivity of the frontal, sensorimotor, and parietal-occipital networks (**Figures 4B, 5B**), as a global rise or fall of state transition was not influenced by intermittent activity of a single common source. In addition, the stance-dependent changes in network properties of spatially distributed communities was observed across the threshold values (**Figure 3**), which are hard to reconcile with known spatial influences due to volume conduction. To date, there is no perfect mathematical tool to assess inter-regional connectivity. Although some measures of inter-regional connectivity have been proposed to counter common sources like phase lag index (Stam et al., 2007b), yet these phase-based approaches actually measures different inter-dependence properties of regional EEG signals as the SL. In fact, phase-based approaches can be more susceptible to small perturbations (Vinck et al., 2011), raising another validity issue to identify ERP connectivity in the presence of noise and non-stationarities (Cohen, 2015). Therefore, a further study may consider EEG recordings simultaneously with BLOD activation patterns for methodological exactness. However, it is beyond the scope in this study to utterly preclude hypothetical common source with the present setup.

Next, in addition to stimulus-locked ERP used in this study, an alternative analysis is to lock EEG activity with force-matching event (response-locked ERP). The selection of time-lock depends on the experimental design to highlight different information processing underlying response preparation. The response-lock approach is recommended, if the experiment does not change premotor processing (Mordkoff and Gianaros, 2000). When response preparation varies with experimental manipulation, information processing in the time domain is stretched or compressed with the use of response-locked ERP. As reaction time of force-matching was hypothesized to vary with the effect of stance configuration, we favored stimulus-locked ERP to assess dual-task effects in this study. Analysis using response-locked ERP seems to be more popular in those single motor task experiments.

CONCLUSIONS

With brain connectivity analysis, the present work highlights the availability of adaptive resource allocation to explain concurrent suprapostural performance that is insusceptible to increasing postural load. Theoretical graphic analysis validated the hypothesis that brain reorganization would lead to a functional network with superior efficacy and global information transfer to cope with increasing stance difficulty for a postural-suprapostural task. In addition, we have identified fine-grained details regarding cost-effective mechanisms for this particular dual-task condition, involving an anterior shift to frontal processing resources and dorsal idling of the parietal-occipital networks.

AUTHOR CONTRIBUTIONS

Substantial contributions to the conception or design of the work; or the acquisition, analysis, or interpretation of data for the work: Conception or design of the work, CH, IH; Acquisition, YT; Analysis, GC, IH; Interpretation of data, CH, IH. Drafting the work or revising it critically for important intellectual content: CH, GC, YT, IH. Final approval of the version to be published: CH, GC, YT, IH. Agreement to be accountable for all aspects of the work in ensuring that questions related to the accuracy or integrity of any part of the work are appropriately investigated and resolved: CH, GC, YT, IH.

FUNDING

This research was supported by grants from the Ministry of Science and Technology, R.O.C. Taiwan, under grant no. MOST 103-2314-B-002 -007 -MY3 and MOST 104-2314-B-006 -016 -MY3.

REFERENCES

Adcock, R. A., Constable, R. T., Gore, J. C., and Goldman-Rakic, P. S. (2000). Functional neuroanatomy of executive processes involved in dual-task performance. *Proc. Natl. Acad. Sci. U.S.A.* 97, 3567–3572. doi: 10.1073/pnas.97.7.3567

Armbrecht, A. S., Gibbons, H., and Stahl, J. (2012). Monitoring force errors: medial-frontal negativity in a unimanual force-production task. *Psychophysiology* 49, 56–72. doi: 10.1111/j.1469-8986.2011. 01282.x

Babiloni, C., Del Percio, C., Iacoboni, M., Infarinato, F., Lizio, R., Marzano, N., et al. (2008). Golf putt outcomes are predicted by sensorimotor cerebral EEG rhythms. *J. Physiol.* 586, 131–139. doi: 10.1113/jphysiol.2007. 141630

Balasubramaniam, R., Riley, M. A., and Turvey, M. T. (2000). Specificity of postural sway to the demands of a precision task. *Gait Posture* 11, 12–24. doi: 10.1016/S0966-6362(99)00051-X

Barutchu, A., Becker, S. I., Carter, O., Hester, R., and Levy, N. L. (2013). The role of task-related learned representations in explaining asymmetries in task switching. *PLoS ONE* 8:e61729. doi: 10.1371/journal.pone.0061729

Betzel, R. F., Erickson, M. A., Abell, M., O'Donnell, B. F., Hetrick, W. P., and Sporns, O. (2012). Synchronization dynamics and evidence for a repertoire of network states in resting EEG. *Front. Comput. Neurosci.* 6:74. doi: 10.3389/fncom.2012.00074

Boersma, M., Smit, D. J., Boomsma, D. I., De Geus, E. J., Delemarre-van de Waal, H. A., and Stam, C. J. (2013). Growing trees in child brains: graph theoretical analysis of electroencephalography-derived minimum spanning tree in 5- and 7-year-old children reflects brain maturation. *Brain Connect.* 3, 50–60. doi: 10.1089/brain.2012.0106

Boersma, M., Smit, D. J., de Bie, H. M., Van Baal, G. C., Boomsma, D. I., de Geus, E. J., et al. (2011). Network analysis of resting state EEG in the developing young brain: structure comes with maturation. *Hum. Brain Mapp.* 32, 413–425. doi: 10.1002/hbm.21030

Boisgontier, M. P., Beets, I. A., Duysens, J., Nieuwboer, A., Krampe, R. T., and Swinnen, S. P. (2013). Age-related differences in attentional cost associated with postural dual tasks: increased recruitment of generic cognitive resources in older adults. *Neurosci. Biobehav. Rev.* 37, 1824–1837. doi: 10.1016/j.neubiorev.2013.07.014

Brovelli, A., Ding, M., Ledberg, A., Chen, Y., Nakamura, R., and Bressler, S. L. (2004). Beta oscillations in a large-scale sensorimotor cortical network: directional influences revealed by Granger causality. *Proc. Natl. Acad. Sci. U.S.A.* 101, 9849–9854. doi: 10.1073/pnas.0308538101

Bullmore, E., and Sporns, O. (2012). The economy of brain network organization. *Nat. Rev. Neurosci.* 13, 336–349. doi: 10.1038/nrn3214

Bunge, S. A., Klingberg, T., Jacobsen, R. B., and Gabrieli, J. D. (2000). A resource model of the neural basis of executive working memory. *Proc. Natl. Acad. Sci. U.S.A.* 97, 3573–3578. doi: 10.1073/pnas.97.7.3573

Cao, R., Wu, Z., Li, H., Xiang, J., and Chen, J. (2014). Disturbed connectivity of EEG functional networks in alcoholism: a graph-theoretic analysis. *Biomed. Mater. Eng.* 24, 2927–2936. doi: 10.3233/BME-141112

Cavanaugh, J. T., Mercer, V. S., and Stergiou, N. (2007). Approximate entropy detects the effect of a secondary cognitive task on postural control in healthy young adults: a methodological report. *J. Neuroeng. Rehabil.* 4:42. doi: 10.1186/1743-0003-4-42

Cohen, M. X. (2015). Effects of time lag and frequency matching on phase-based connectivity. *J. Neurosci. Methods* 250, 137–146. doi: 10.1016/j.jneumeth.2014.09.005

Cole, M. W., Reynolds, J. R., Power, J. D., Repovs, G., Anticevic, A., and Braver, T. S. (2013). Multi-task connectivity reveals flexible hubs for adaptive task control. *Nat. Neurosci.* 16, 1348–1355. doi: 10.1038/nn.3470

Collette, F., Olivier, L., Van der Linden, M., Laureys, S., Delfiore, G., Luxen, A., et al. (2005). Involvement of both prefrontal and inferior parietal cortex in dual-task performance. *Brain Res. Cogn. Brain Res.* 24, 237–251. doi: 10.1016/j.cogbrainres.2005.01.023

Dault, M. C., Geurts, A. C., Mulder, T. W., and Duysens, J. (2001). Postural control and cognitive task performance in healthy participants while balancing on different support-surface configurations. *Gait Posture* 14, 248–255. doi: 10.1016/S0966-6362(01)00130-8

Deprez, S., Vandenbulcke, M., Peeters, R., Emsell, L., Amant, F., and Sunaert, S. (2013). The functional neuroanatomy of multitasking: combining dual tasking with a short term memory task. *Neuropsychologia* 51, 2251–2260. doi: 10.1016/j.neuropsychologia.2013.07.024

Derlich, M., Krêcisz, K., and Kuczyński, M. (2011). Attention demand and postural control in children with hearing deficit. *Res. Dev. Disabil.* 32, 1808–1813. doi: 10.1016/j.ridd.2011.03.009

D'Esposito, M., Detre, J. A., Alsop, D. C., Shin, R. K., Atlas, S., and Grossman, M. (1995). The neural basis of the central executive system of working memory. *Nature* 378, 279–281. doi: 10.1038/378279a0

Donker, S. F., Roerdink, M., Greven, A. J., and Beek, P. J. (2007). Regularity of center-of-pressure trajectories depends on the amount of attention invested in postural control. *Exp. Brain Res.* 181, 1–11. doi: 10.1007/s00221-007-0905-4

Dux, P. E., Ivanoff, J., Asplund, C. L., and Marois, R. (2006). Isolation of a central bottleneck of information processing with time-resolved FMRI. *Neuron* 52, 1109–1120. doi: 10.1016/j.neuron.2006.11.009

Ferraye, M. U., Debû, B., Heil, L., Carpenter, M., Bloem, B. R., and Toni, I. (2014). Using motor imagery to study the neural substrates of dynamic balance. *PLoS ONE* 9:e91183. doi: 10.1371/journal.pone.0091183

Fujimoto, H., Mihara, M., Hattori, N., Hatakenaka, M., Kawano, T., Yagura, H., et al. (2014). Cortical changes underlying balance recovery in patients with hemiplegic stroke. *Neuroimage* 85(Pt 1), 547–554. doi: 10.1016/j.neuroimage.2013.05.014

Gontier, E., Le Dantec, C., Leleu, A., Paul, I., Charvin, H., Bernard, C., et al. (2007). Frontal and parietal ERPs associated with duration discriminations with or without task interference. *Brain Res.* 1170, 79–89. doi: 10.1016/j.brainres.2007.07.022

Hashimoto, T., Umeda, S., and Kojima, S. (2011). Neural substrates of implicit cueing effect on prospective memory. *Neuroimage* 54, 645–652. doi: 10.1016/j.neuroimage.2010.07.047

Herrera-Díaz, A., Mendoza-Quiñones, R., Melie-Garcia, L., Martínez-Montes, E., Sanabria-Diaz, G., Romero-Quintana, Y., et al. (2016). Functional connectivity and quantitative Eeg in women with alcohol use disorders: a resting-state study. *Brain Topogr.* 29, 368–381. doi: 10.1007/s10548-015-0467-x

Huang, C. Y., and Hwang, I. S. (2013). Behavioral data and neural correlates for postural prioritization and flexible resource allocation in concurrent postural and motor tasks. *Hum. Brain Mapp.* 34, 635–650. doi: 10.1002/hbm.21460

Huang, C. Y., Zhao, C. G., and Hwang, I. S. (2014). Neural basis of postural focus effect on concurrent postural and motor tasks: phase-locked electroencephalogram responses. *Behav. Brain Res.* 274, 95–107. doi: 10.1016/j.bbr.2014.07.054

Hülsdünker, T., Mierau, A., Neeb, C., Kleinöder, H., and Strüder, H. K. (2015). Cortical processes associated with continuous balance control as revealed by EEG spectral power. *Neurosci. Lett.* 592, 1–5. doi: 10.1016/j.neulet.2015. 02.049

Humphries, M. D., Gurney, K., and Prescott, T. J. (2006). The brainstem reticular formation is a small-world, not scale-free, network. *Proc. Biol. Sci.* 273, 503–511. doi: 10.1098/rspb.2005.3354

Hung, Y. T., Yu, S. H., Fang, J. H., and Huang, C. Y. (in press). Effects of precision-grip force on postural-suprapostural task. *Formosan J. Phys. Ther.*

Hwang, I. S., and Huang, C. Y. (2016). Neural correlates of task cost for stance control with an additional motor task: phase-locked electroencephalogram responses. *PLoS ONE* 11:e0151906. doi: 10.1371/journal.pone.0151906

Jahn, K., Deutschländer, A., Stephan, T., Strupp, M., Wiesmann, M., and Brandt, T. (2004). Brain activation patterns during imagined stance and locomotion in functional magnetic resonance imaging. *Neuroimage* 22, 1722–1731. doi: 10.1016/j.neuroimage.2004.05.017

Just, M. A., Keller, T. A., and Cynkar, J. (2008). A decrease in brain activation associated with driving when listening to someone speak. *Brain Res.* 1205, 70–80. doi: 10.1016/j.brainres.2007.12.075

Karim, H., Fuhrman, S. I., Sparto, P., Furman, J., and Huppert, T. (2013). Functional brain imaging of multi-sensory vestibular processing during computerized dynamic posturography using near-infrared spectroscopy. *Neuroimage* 74, 318–325. doi: 10.1016/j.neuroimage.2013.02.010

Karim, H. T., Sparto, P. J., Aizenstein, H. J., Furman, J. M., Huppert, T. J., Erickson, K. I., et al. (2014). Functional MR imaging of a simulated balance task. *Brain Res.* 1555, 20–27. doi: 10.1016/j.brainres.2014.01.033

Klados, M. A., Kanatsouli, K., Antoniou, I., Babiloni, F., Tsirka, V., Bamidis, P. D., et al. (2013). A Graph theoretical approach to study the organization of the cortical networks during different mathematical tasks. *PLoS ONE* 8:e71800. doi: 10.1371/journal.pone.0071800

Klingberg, T. (1998). Concurrent performance of two working memory tasks: potential mechanisms of interference. *Cereb. Cortex* 8, 593–601. doi: 10.1093/cercor/8.7.593

Koenis, M. M., Romeijn, N., Piantoni, G., Verweij, I., Van der Werf, Y. D., Van Someren, E. J., et al. (2013). Does sleep restore the topology of functional brain networks? *Hum. Brain. Mapp.* 34, 487–500. doi: 10.1002/hbm.21455

Kondo, H., Osaka, N., and Osaka, M. (2004). Cooperation of the anterior cingulate cortex and dorsolateral prefrontal cortex for attention shifting. *Neuroimage* 23, 670–679. doi: 10.1016/j.neuroimage.2004.06.014

Kuczyński, M., Szymańska, M., and Bieć, E. (2011). Dual-task effect on postural control in high-level competitive dancers. *J. Sports Sci.* 29, 539–545. doi: 10.1080/02640414.2010.544046

Leistedt, S. J., Coumans, N., Dumont, M., Lanquart, J. P., Stam, C. J., and Linkowski, P. (2009). Altered sleep brain functional connectivity in acutely depressed patients. *Hum. Brain. Mapp.* 30, 2207–2219. doi: 10.1002/hbm.20662

Levy, J., and Pashler, H. (2001). Is dual-task slowing instruction dependent? *J. Exp. Psychol. Hum. Percept. Perform.* 27, 862–869. doi: 10.1037/0096-1523.27.4.862

Liefooghe, B., Barrouillet, P., Vandierendonck, A., and Camos, V. (2008). Working memory costs of task switching. *J. Exp. Psychol. Learn. Mem. Cogn.* 34, 478–494. doi: 10.1037/0278-7393.34.3.478

Liu, T., Chen, Y., Lin, P., and Wang, J. (2015). Small-world brain functional networks in children with attention-deficit/hyperactivity disorder revealed by EEG synchrony. *Clin. EEG Neurosci.* 46, 183–191. doi: 10.1177/1550059414523959

Luu, P., Tucker, D. M., and Makeig, S. (2004). Frontal midline theta and the error-related negativity: neurophysiological mechanisms of action regulation. *Clin. Neurophysiol.* 115, 1821–1835. doi: 10.1016/j.clinph.2004.03.031

MacKay, W. A., and Mendonca, A. J. (1995). Field potential oscillatory bursts in parietal cortex before and during reach. *Brain Res.* 704, 167–174. doi: 10.1016/0006-8993(95)01109-9

Marois, R., Larson, J. M., Chun, M. M., and Shima, D. (2006). Response-specific sources of dual-task interference in human pre-motor cortex. *Psychol. Res.* 70, 436–447. doi: 10.1007/s00426-005-0022-6

Mihara, M., Miyai, I., Hatakenaka, M., Kubota, K., and Sakoda, S. (2008). Role of the prefrontal cortex in human balance control. *Neuroimage* 43, 329–336. doi: 10.1016/j.neuroimage.2008.07.029

Mirelman, A., Maidan, I., Bernad-Elazari, H., Nieuwhof, F., Reelick, M., Giladi, N., et al. (2014). Increased frontal brain activation during walking while dual tasking: an fNIRS study in healthy young adults. *J. Neuroeng. Rehabil.* 11:85. doi: 10.1186/1743-0003-11-85

Mitra, S. (2004). Adaptive utilization of optical variables during postural and suprapostural dual-task performance: comment on Stoffregen, Smart, Bardy, and Pagulayan (1999). *J. Exp. Psychol. Hum. Percept. Perform.* 30, 28–38. doi: 10.1037/0096-1523.30.1.28

Mitra, S., and Fraizer, E. V. (2004). Effects of explicit sway-minimization on postural–suprapostural dual-task performance. *Hum. Mov. Sci.* 23, 1–20. doi: 10.1016/j.humov.2004.03.003

Mizuno, K., Tanaka, M., Tanabe, H. C., Sadato, N., and Watanabe, Y. (2012). The neural substrates associated with attentional resources and difficulty of concurrent processing of the two verbal tasks. *Neuropsychologia* 50, 1998–2009. doi: 10.1016/j.neuropsychologia.2012.04.025

Montez, T., Linkenkaer-Hansen, K., van Dijk, B. W., and Stam, C. J. (2006). Synchronization likelihood with explicit time-frequency priors. *Neuroimage* 33, 1117–1125. doi: 10.1016/j.neuroimage.2006.06.066

Mordkoff, J. T., and Gianaros, P. J. (2000). Detecting the onset of the lateralized readiness potential: a comparison of available methods and procedures. *Psychophysiology* 37, 347–360. doi: 10.1111/1469-8986.3730347

Nierhaus, T., Forschack, N., Piper, S. K., Holtze, S., Krause, T., Taskin, B., et al. (2015). Imperceptible somatosensory stimulation alters sensorimotor background rhythm and connectivity. *J. Neurosci.* 35, 5917–5925. doi: 10.1523/JNEUROSCI.3806-14.2015

Niso, G., Bruña, R., Pereda, E., Gutiérrez, R., Bajo, R., Maestú, F., et al. (2013). HERMES: towards an integrated toolbox to characterize functional and effective brain connectivity. *Neuroinformatics* 11, 405–434. doi: 10.1007/s12021-013-9186-1

Pellijeff, A., Bonilha, L., Morgan, P. S., McKenzie, K., and Jackson, S. R. (2006). Parietal updating of limb posture: an event-related fMRI study. *Neuropsychologia* 44, 2685–2690. doi: 10.1016/j.neuropsychologia.2006.01.009

Pfurtscheller, G., and Berghold, A. (1989). Patterns of cortical activation during planning of voluntary movement. *Electroencephalogr. Clin. Neurophysiol.* 72, 250–258. doi: 10.1016/0013-4694(89)90250-2

Pijnenburg, Y. A., v d Made, Y., van Cappellen van Walsum, A. M., Knol, D. L., Scheltens, P., and Stam, C. J. (2004). EEG synchronization likelihood in mild cognitive impairment and Alzheimer's disease during a working memory task. *Clin. Neurophysiol.* 115, 1332–1339. doi: 10.1016/j.clinph.2003.12.029

Pijnenburg, Y. A., Strijers, R. L., Made, Y. V., van der Flier, W. M., Scheltens, P., and Stam, C. J. (2008). Investigation of resting-state EEG functional connectivity in frontotemporal lobar degeneration. *Clin. Neurophysiol.* 119, 1732–1738. doi: 10.1016/j.clinph.2008.02.024

Polanía, R., Nitsche, M. A., and Paulus, W. (2011). Modulating functional connectivity patterns and topological functional organization of the human brain with transcranial direct current stimulation. *Hum. Brain Mapp.* 32, 1236–1249. doi: 10.1002/hbm.21104

Reijneveld, J. C., Ponten, S. C., Berendse, H. W., and Stam, C. J. (2007). The application of graph theoretical analysis to complex networks in the brain. *Clin. Neurophysiol.* 118, 2317–2331. doi: 10.1016/j.clinph.2007.08.010

Richman, J. S., and Moorman, J. R. (2000). Physiological time-series analysis using approximate entropy and sample entropy. *Am. J. Physiol. Heart Circ. Physiol.* 278, H2039–H2049.

Rubinov, M., and Sporns, O. (2010). Complex network measures of brain connectivity: uses and interpretations. *Neuroimage* 52, 1059–1069. doi: 10.1016/j.neuroimage.2009.10.003

Salo, E., Rinne, T., Salonen, O., and Alho, K. (2015). Brain activations during bimodal dual tasks depend on the nature and combination of component tasks. *Front. Hum. Neurosci.* 9:102. doi: 10.3389/fnhum.2015.00102

Sami, S., and Miall, R. C. (2013). Graph network analysis of immediate motor-learning induced changes in resting state BOLD. *Front. Hum. Neurosci.* 7:166. doi: 10.3389/fnhum.2013.00166

Sarabon, N., Rosker, J., Loefler, S., and Kern, H. (2013). The effect of vision elimination during quiet stance tasks with different feet positions. *Gait Posture* 38, 708–711. doi: 10.1016/j.gaitpost.2013.03.005

Schneider, D. W., and Anderson, J. R. (2010). Asymmetric switch costs as sequential difficulty effects. *Q. J. Exp. Psychol. (Hove)* 63, 1873–1894. doi: 10.1080/17470211003624010

Sipp, A. R., Gwin, J. T., Makeig, S., and Ferris, D. P. (2013). Loss of balance during balance beam walking elicits a multifocal theta band electrocortical response. *J. Neurophysiol.* 110, 2050–2060. doi: 10.1152/jn.00744.2012

Slobounov, S., Cao, C., Jaiswal, N., and Newell, K. M. (2009). Neural basis of postural instability identified by VTC and EEG. *Exp. Brain Res.* 199, 1–16. doi: 10.1007/s00221-009-1956-5

Slobounov, S., Hallett, M., Stanhope, S., and Shibasaki, H. (2005). Role of cerebral cortex in human postural control: an EEG study. *Clin. Neurophysiol.* 116, 315–323. doi: 10.1016/j.clinph.2004.09.007

Smit, D. J., Boersma, M., Schnack, H. G., Micheloyannis, S., Boomsma, D. I., Hulshoff Pol, H. E., et al. (2012). The brain matures with stronger functional connectivity and decreased randomness of its network. *PLoS ONE* 7:e36896. doi: 10.1371/journal.pone.0036896

Stam, C. J., Breakspear, M., van Cappellen van Walsum, A. M., and van Dijk, B. W. (2003). Nonlinear synchronization in EEG and whole-head MEG recordings of healthy subjects. *Hum. Brain Mapp.* 19, 63–78. doi: 10.1002/hbm.10106

Stam, C. J., Jones, B. F., Nolte, G., Breakspear, M., and Scheltens, P. (2007a). Small-world networks and functional connectivity in Alzheimer's disease. *Cereb. Cortex* 17, 92–99. doi: 10.1093/cercor/bhj127

Stam, C. J., Montez, T., Jones, B. F., Rombouts, S. A., van der Made, Y., Pijnenburg, Y. A., et al. (2005). Disturbed fluctuations of resting state EEG synchronization in Alzheimer's disease. *Clin. Neurophysiol.* 116, 708–715. doi: 10.1016/j.clinph.2004.09.022

Stam, C. J., Nolte, G., and Daffertshofer, A. (2007b). Phase lag index: assessment of functional connectivity from multi channel EEG and MEG with diminished bias from common sources. *Hum. Brain Mapp.* 28, 1178–1193. doi: 10.1002/hbm.20346

Stam, C. J., and van Dijk, B. W. (2002). Synchronization likelihood: an unbiased measure of generalized synchronization in multivariate data sets. *Physica D* 163, 236–251. doi: 10.1016/S0167-2789(01)00386-4

Stelzel, C., Schumacher, E. H., Schubert, T., and D'Esposito, M. (2006). The neural effect of stimulus-response modality compatibility on dual-task performance: an fMRI study. *Psychol. Res.* 70, 514–525. doi: 10.1007/s00426-005-0013-7

Stins, J. F., Michielsen, M. E., Roerdink, M., and Beek, P. J. (2009). Sway regularity reflects attentional involvement in postural control: effects of expertise, vision and cognition. *Gait Posture* 30, 106–109. doi: 10.1016/j.gaitpost.2009. 04.001

Stoffregen, T. A., Hove, P., Bardy, B. G., Riley, M., and Bonnet, C. T. (2007). Postural stabilization of perceptual but not cognitive performance. *J. Mot. Behav.* 39, 126–138. doi: 10.3200/JMBR.39.2.126-138

Tachibana, A., Noah, J. A., Bronner, S., Ono, Y., and Onozuka, M. (2011). Parietal and temporal activity during a multimodal dance video game: an fNIRS study. *Neurosci. Lett.* 503, 125–130. doi: 10.1016/j.neulet.2011.08.023

Tanaka, Y., Fujimura, N., Tsuji, T., Maruishi, M., Muranaka, H., and Kasai, T. (2009). Functional interactions between the cerebellum and the premotor cortex for error correction during the slow rate force production task: an fMRI study. *Exp. Brain Res.* 193, 143–150. doi: 10.1007/s00221-008-1682-4

Temprado, J. J., Monno, A., Laurent, M., and Zanone, P. G. (2001). A dynamical framework to understand performance trade-offs and interference in dual tasks. *J. Exp. Psychol. Hum. Percept. Perform.* 27, 1303–1313. doi: 10.1037/0096-1523.27.6.1303

Tognoli, E., and Kelso, J. A. (2009). Brain coordination dynamics: true and false faces of phase synchrony and metastability. *Prog. Neurobiol.* 87, 31–40. doi: 10.1016/j.pneurobio.2008.09.014

Vinck, M., Oostenveld, R., van Wingerden, M., Battaglia, F., and Pennartz, C. M. (2011). An improved index of phase-synchronization for electrophysiological data in the presence of volume-conduction, noise and sample-size bias. *Neuroimage* 55, 1548–1565. doi: 10.1016/j.neuroimage.2011.01.055

Watts, D. J., and Strogatz, S. H. (1998). Collective dynamics of 'small-world' networks. *Nature* 393, 440–442. doi: 10.1038/30918

Weeks, D., Forget, R., Mouchnino, L., Gravel, D., and Bourbonnais, D. (2003). Interaction between attention demanding motor and cognitive tasks and static postural stability. *Gerontology* 49, 225–232. doi: 10.1159/0000 70402

Woollacott, M., and Shumway-Cook, A. (2002). Attention and the control of posture and gait: a review of an emerging area of research. *Gait Posture* 16, 1–14. doi: 10.1016/S0966-6362(01)00156-4

Wulf, G., Mercer, J., McNevin, N., and Guadagnoli, M. A. (2004). Reciprocal influences of attentional focus on postural and suprapostural task performance. *J. Mot. Behav.* 36, 189–199. doi: 10.3200/JMBR.36.2.189-199

Yentes, J. M., Hunt, N., Schmid, K. K., Kaipust, J. P., McGrath, D., and Stergiou, N. (2013). The appropriate use of approximate entropy and sample entropy with short data sets. *Ann. Biomed. Eng.* 41, 349–365. doi: 10.1007/s10439-012-0668-3

Yu, Q., Sui, J., Kiehl, K. A., Pearlson, G., and Calhoun, V. D. (2013). State-related functional integration and functional segregation brain networks in schizophrenia. *Schizophr. Res.* 150, 450–458. doi: 10.1016/j.schres.2013.09.016

Zalesky, A., Fornito, A., and Bullmore, E. T. (2010). Network-based statistic: identifying differences in brain networks. *Neuroimage* 53, 1197–1207. doi: 10.1016/j.neuroimage.2010.06.041

Zwergal, A., Linn, J., Xiong, G., Brandt, T., Strupp, M., and Jahn, K. (2012). Aging of human supraspinal locomotor and postural control in fMRI. *Neurobiol. Aging* 33, 1073–1084. doi: 10.1016/j.neurobiolaging.2010.09.022

14

Holding a Handle for Balance during Continuous Postural Perturbations—Immediate and Transitionary Effects on Whole Body Posture

Jernej Čamernik [1,2], Zrinka Potocanac [1], Luka Peternel [1,3] and Jan Babič [1]*

[1] Department for Automation, Biocybernetics and Robotics, Jožef Stefan Institute, Ljubljana, Slovenia, [2] Jožef Stefan International Postgraduate School, Ljubljana, Slovenia, [3] HRI2 Laboratory, Department of Advanced Robotics, Istituto Italiano di Tecnologia, Genoa, Italy

Correspondence:
Jan Babič
jan.babic@ijs.si

When balance is exposed to perturbations, hand contacts are often used to assist postural control. We investigated the immediate and the transitionary effects of supportive hand contacts during continuous anteroposterior perturbations of stance by automated waist-pulls. Ten young adults were perturbed for 5 min and required to maintain balance by holding to a stationary, shoulder-high handle and following its removal. Center of pressure (COP) displacement, hip, knee and ankle angles, leg and trunk muscle activity and handle contact forces were acquired. The analysis of results show that COP excursions are significantly smaller when the subjects utilize supportive hand contact and that the displacement of COP is strongly correlated to the perturbation force and significantly larger in the anterior than posterior direction. Regression analysis of hand forces revealed that subjects utilized the hand support significantly more during the posterior than anterior perturbations. Moreover, kinematical analysis showed that utilization of supportive hand contacts alter posture of the whole body and that postural readjustments after the release of the handle, occur at different time scales in the hip, knee and ankle joints. Overall, our findings show that supportive hand contacts are efficiently used for balance control during continuous postural perturbations and that utilization of a handle has significant immediate and transitionary effects on whole body posture.

Keywords: falls, handle, grasping, postural balance, balance recovery

INTRODUCTION

With aging society, falls are becoming an increasingly large problem. A large proportion of falls occur due to the improper weight shifts (Robinovitch et al., 2013) and impaired postural control is a landmark of aging (Maki and McIlroy, 2006; Mansfield and Maki, 2009). When postural control is impaired, handrails, canes and handles are often used to assist maintaining balance by providing additional supportive contacts with the environment. This indicates that holding onto a physical aid is beneficial for postural control.

With respect to the use of hand contacts for postural control, one of the widely investigated phenomena is "light touch" (Jeka, 1997; Krishnamoorthy et al., 2002). These light, fingertip contacts with stationary objects can extend the base of support (Bateni and Maki, 2005) and provide an additional sensory input, which helps individuals to better position them in space (Jeka, 1997). Such sensory information improves postural control in quiet standing by reducing the amplitude of center of pressure (COP) movement (Jeka, 1997; Johannsen et al., 2007; Kouzaki and Masani, 2008; Wing et al., 2011).

On the other hand, in case of perturbed balance reaching arm movements with the aim to grasp for a nearby object is a widely utilized change-in-support strategy (Maki and McIlroy, 2006). Such hand contacts provide mechanical support in addition to the sensory augmentation of the light touch and thus offer a better stabilizing potential in the presence of perturbations (Maki and McIlroy, 1997). Specifically, holding onto a handle increases the base of support of a standing individual and enables a person to generate necessary hand forces to better counteract the perturbations (Babič et al., 2014; Sarraf et al., 2014). A recent study by Babič et al. (2014) showed that the location of the supporting hand contact is important to maximize its stabilizing potential and that the peak forces exerted at the handle during the support surface perturbations are related to the location of the handle.

Aforementioned studies were based on the discrete perturbations of balance which predominantly evoke feedback postural responses. A major component of such responses is comprised of motor actions that are related to various sensorimotor reflexes and to a lesser extent to the feed-forward components of the postural control (Mergner, 2010). Moreover, the discrete perturbations evoke reach-to-grasp arm movements even when the perturbations are so light that they do not physically disturb postural balance (McIlroy and Maki, 1995; Corbeil et al., 2013). In contrast to the discrete perturbations of balance, perturbations that continuously disturb postural balance evoke both feedback and feed-forward components of motor action and in this sense offer a complementary insight into the postural control (Dietz et al., 1993; Schmid et al., 2011).

The remaining question is what is the role of hand contact during continuous perturbations? Therefore, the aim of this article is to study situations where balance of an individual is challenged by continuous postural perturbations and to investigate the role of supportive hand contact in counteracting postural perturbations. Specifically, our goal was to investigate the immediate and the transitionary effects of a supportive hand contact on postural control of an individual whose balance is challenged by continuous anteroposterior perturbations of stance.

Our hypothesis is that a supportive hand contact has a significant influence on postural balance by reducing the COP excursion during the perturbation and that the utilization of the hand contact is more prominent for postural perturbations in the backward direction which are more threatening than the perturbations in the forward direction. Moreover, we hypothesize that utilization of the additional hand support not only alters posture of the human body while the hand is in

contact with the environment but also after the release of the handle. To effectively address these hypotheses, we developed an experimental framework where we continuously perturbed postural balance and investigated the relationships between the perturbation force and the COP displacement, kinematical parameters of the human body, and the forces exerted by the supportive hand.

MATERIALS AND METHODS

Participants
Thirteen healthy right-handed young adults participated in this study after giving their written consent. Data of three subjects were excluded from the analyses due to technical problems during acquisition, therefore we used the data of ten subjects (average age = 22.3 years, SD = 2.2 years, average height 179.2 cm, SD = 5.9 cm and average weight = 76.9 kg, SD = 8.2 kg). The experimental procedures conformed to the latest revision of the Declaration of Helsinki and were approved by the Slovenian National Medical Ethics Committee (No. 112/06/13).

Measurement Protocol
Subjects were asked to step on a force plate, stand straight with the feet placed at hip width and look straight ahead. They were required to keep upright posture and maintain balance without making any unnecessary corrective steps while their balance was continuously perturbed in anteroposterior direction by a motorized waist-pull system (Peternel and Babič, 2013) as depicted in **Figure 1**. During the experiment, the subjects were not allowed to change their base of support. We marked their individual standing position on the force plate prior to the start of the experiment which was used as a reference for foot position during the experiment. This ensured that the different stance width would not affect subjects' balance since it has been shown by Bingham and Ting (2013) that active torque at ankle and hip joints scale with stance width. To emulate mild, daily life perturbations such as those during riding on buses, subways and trains (Graaf and van Weperen, 1997) the motorized waist-pull system perturbed the subjects using a band-pass filtered white noise signal (0.25–1.00 Hz) with the maximal perturbation force of 11% of the subjects' body weight (**Figure 2**).

The experiment consisted of two consecutive 5 min trials of different standing conditions: balancing while holding to a handle [*with-handle (WH)*] and without holding to a handle [*no-handle (NH)*]. First, the subjects were exposed to 5 min of perturbations in the *WH* trial. In the *WH* trial, subjects held onto a stationary handle (diameter = 3.2 cm, length = 12 cm) positioned at shoulder height with their right hand. After 5 min the perturbation stopped, subjects released the handle and folded their arms across their chest. Then, on average less than 60 s later, the second trial of 5 min of perturbation started (*NH* trial). In the *NH* trial, subjects were standing with their arms folded across their chest. In both trials, subjects were instructed to look straight ahead at all times at a fixed point positioned at the subject's eyelevel and 3 m in front of the experimental setup.

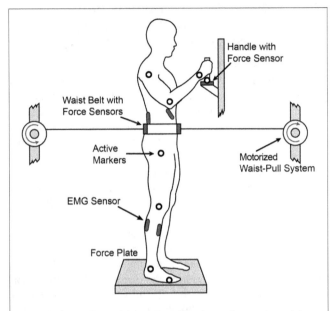

FIGURE 1 | **Experimental setup.** The subject is standing on a force plate, wearing a waist belt connected to the motorized waist-pull system which generated translational force perturbations in the anterior-posterior direction using a band-filtered white noise signal constructed to emulate mild, daily life perturbations.

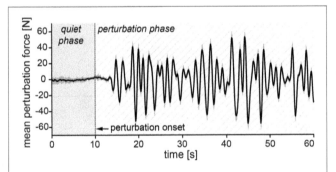

FIGURE 2 | **Perturbation signal sample.** Solid black curve represents first 60 s of mean perturbation signal from all 10 subjects with ±1 standard error of the mean (gray shade around the curve). In the first 10 s of each trial the perturbation value was at 0 N—quiet phase. After 10 s (perturbation onset), the perturbation gradually increased with alternated direction and amplitude—perturbation phase. Positive values of mean perturbation force represent forces in anterior direction and negative values represent forces in posterior direction. The perturbation signal was identical in both trials.

To induce response adaptations (Van Ooteghem et al., 2008; Schmid et al., 2011), the subjects were allowed to familiarize with the experimental procedures prior to the main experimental trials.

Kinetic data were collected using a force plate (9281CA, Kistler Instrumente AG, Winterthur, Switzerland) under the subjects' feet and a 3-axis force sensor (45E15A, JR3, Woodland, CA, USA) on the handle, both at 1000 samples/s.

Kinematic data were collected at a sampling rate of 100 samples/s using a contactless motion capture system (3D Investigator, Northern Digital Inc., Waterloo, ON, Canada) consisting of a 3 × 3 camera array. Nine active markers

were placed at the apparent axis of rotation of the fifth metatarsophalangeal, ankle, knee, hip, shoulder, elbow and wrist joints on the subject's right side as well as at the base of the platform and the handle.

Anteroposterior displacement of the subject's COP was derived from the force plate data. In the first 10 s of each trial, the subjects stood quietly (holding a handle with right hand in the first trial, or both arms folded across their chest in the second trial) and no perturbation was applied at the waist (see **Figure 2** for reference regarding perturbation signal). The mean COP position from this time period (we refer to this as *quiet phase*) served as a baseline for calculation of COP excursions in the anterior and posterior direction in the following perturbations (*perturbation phase*).

Handle forces were calculated by considering the torques of the lever (distance from force sensor to the middle of the subject's hand on the handle). Kinematic data were low pass filtered (zero lag, 2nd order Butterworth filter with a cut-off frequency 20 Hz). Ankle angle was calculated as the angle between the foot (line connecting the fifth metatarsal and ankle) and the shank (line connecting the ankle and the knee), knee angle as the angle between the shank and thigh (line connecting the knee and the hip), and hip as the angle between the thigh and torso (line connecting the hip and the shoulder). To evaluate the adaptation effects of releasing the handle in the *NH* trial, an exponential fit of group average joint angles was calculated (Franklin et al., 2003). Adaptation was considered as final once the given joint angle reached the plateau defined by three time constants of the fitted exponential decay function, i.e., once the fitted exponential decay function fell to 5% of its starting value (Honeine et al., 2015; Assländer and Peterka, 2016).

Electromyographical (EMG) electrodes were placed on the right leg (TA, Tibialis Anterior; GA, Gastrocnemius Lateralis; and trunk (MF, Multifidus; OE, Obliques Externus) muscles and their activity was measured using Biometrics DataLOG MW8X at a sampling rate of 1000 samples/s. Preparation of the skin and positioning of the electrodes was performed according to the SENIAM protocol (Hermens et al., 2000). Before the start of the experiment, subjects performed three maximal voluntary contractions (MVC) against resistance of each of the measured muscles. MVC's were used in EMG post-processing for normalization, to establish a common ground when comparing data between subjects. All EMG signals were band-pass filtered (zero lag, 2nd order Butterworth filter with cut-off frequencies of 20 and 450 Hz), full-wave rectified and low pass filtered (zero lag, 2nd order Butterworth algorithm, 10 Hz cut-off frequency). Finally, EMG signals were normalized with respect to the MVCs and integrated over time (iEMG) to express the magnitude of muscle activity.

We divided COP excursions and contact forces exerted on the handle in two data sets based on their direction—anterior and posterior. For each data set, average values from all 10 subjects were calculated and used in the statistical analysis.

Average hip, knee and ankle angles over the 5 min for each subject were calculated and used for statistical analysis.

Differences between COP displacement in the anterior and posterior directions and subject average joint angles were analyzed using paired samples t-tests. Differences between the *WH* and *NH* trials in subject average COP displacements were analyzed for the anterior and posterior directions separately, using a paired samples t-test. The relationship between group average COP excursion and the magnitude of the perturbation and between group average perturbation magnitude and the exerted handle contact force was analyzed using separate linear correlations for anterior and posterior directions. All statistical analyses were performed using SPSS 21 Inc., Chicago, IL, USA at $\alpha = 0.05$. Effect size (d) was calculated using standard Cohen's equation (Cohen, 1988).

RESULTS

Supportive Hand Contact has Significant Influence on Postural Balance by Reducing COP Excursion during Perturbation

The diagram in **Figure 3** shows the comparison of mean COP excursion between the conditions when the subjects counteracted postural perturbations without using the additional hand contact (NH) and when they did use the handle (WH). Paired samples t-test showed significant effect in reducing the mean COP excursion when the subjects were holding to the handle compared to when they did not hold to the handle. The differences of COP excursion were significantly larger both in the anterior direction (difference of 20.3 mm, $t_{(9)} = 7.78, p = 0.001$, $d = -4.15$) and posterior direction (difference of 23.9 mm, $t_{(9)} = -11.09, p = 0.001, d = -3.8$).

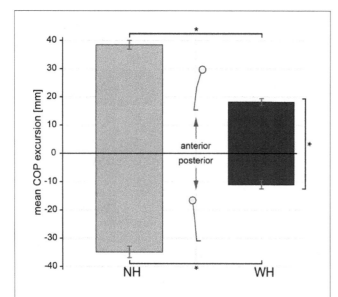

FIGURE 3 | Comparison of center of pressure (COP) excursion between trials when subjects either used additional hand contact or not. Bars represent mean COP excursion during no-handle (NH) and with-handle (WH) trials for the anterior (positive) and posterior (negative) directions. Error bars indicate ±1 standard error of the mean. Statistically significant differences are indicated (*$p \leq 0.02$).

Utilization of Hand Contact is more Prominent for Postural Perturbations in Backward Direction than for Perturbations in Forward Direction

In both, *NH* and *WH* trials, the COP excursion was larger in the anterior direction (mean ± SE: *NH* 38.5 ± 1.6 mm, *WH* 18.2 ± 1.2 mm) compared to the posterior (mean ± SE: *NH* −34.9 ± 2 mm, *WH* −11.0 ± 1.5 mm), but this difference was significant only for the *WH* trial ($t_{(9)} = 2.81, p = 0.02$, $d = 1.52$).

We further assessed the effects of utilizing the additional hand contact, and the direction and intensity of perturbation on the maximal COP displacement. The diagrams in **Figure 4** show correlations between the perturbation force and the group average COP excursion during *NH* and *WH* trials. Additionally, the correlation between the perturbation force and the handle force is shown for the *WH* trials. The group average COP excursion was strongly correlated with perturbation force in both posterior ($r_p = 0.77$ and $r_p = 0.67$) and anterior ($r_a = 0.82$ and $r_a = 0.89$) directions in the *NH* and *WH* trials, respectively (all $p < 0.001$). Similarly, the forces that

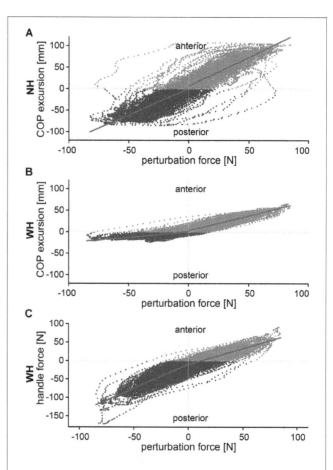

FIGURE 4 | Correlations between perturbation force and (A) COP excursion in NH trial, (B) COP excursion in WH trial and (C) handle force in the WH trial. Correlations were calculated separately for the anterior (positive) and posterior (negative) direction.

subjects applied on the handle was also strongly correlated with the perturbation force (**Figure 4C**) in both anterior ($r_p = 0.85$, $p < 0.001$) and posterior directions ($r_a = 0.81$, $p < 0.001$). Moreover, the slope of the regression line is significantly larger for perturbations in the posterior direction ($k_p = 1.3$), compared to the perturbations in the anterior direction ($k_a = 0.86$).

Supportive Hand Contact Affects Whole Body Posture

To investigate how the additional hand contact affects the body posture during the perturbations, we compared the mean values of ankle, knee and hip joint angles between the conditions when the subjects counteracted perturbations without the additional hand contact (NH) and when they did use the handle (WH). The comparison is shown in the diagram in **Figure 5**.

Multiple paired samples t-tests showed significant effect of the hand contact on all three observed joint angles. Specifically, mean joint angles were significantly lower during the *NH* trials compared to the *WH* trials. Differences were the largest in the knee (mean ± SE: 165.1 ± 1.9° for NH, 173.2 ± 1.5° for WH, $t_{(9)} = -6.70, p < 0.001, d = 1.4$), followed by the hip (mean ± SE: 171.4 ± 2.8° for NH, 181.5 ± 1.6° WH, $t_{(9)} = -6.68, p < 0.001$, $d = 1.1$) and the ankle (mean ± SE: 108 ± 1.2° for NH, 112 ± 1.1° WH, $t_{(9)} = -5.67, p < 0.001, d = 1.1$).

Utilization of Hand Contact has Non-Uniform Transitionary Effect on Whole Body Posture after Release of Handle

To investigate the effect of supportive hand contact on the body posture, an exponential curve was fitted to the group average ankle, knee and hip joint angles calculated during the *NH* trial that immediately followed the *WH* trial (**Figure 6**).

Exponential fits revealed that postural readjustments after the release of the handle did not occur simultaneously throughout the body. Instead, the readjustments occurred at different time scales in the hip, knee and ankle joints. Specifically, joint angles stabilized first in the ankle (mean ± SE: 133 ± 103.5 s after

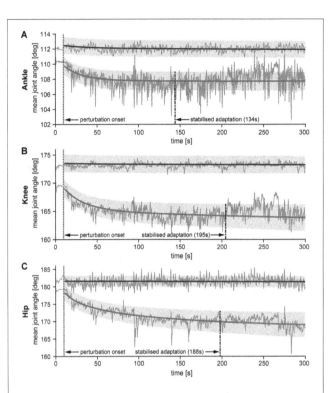

FIGURE 6 | Ankle (A) knee (B) and hip (C) angles over the time course of the perturbation. Thin solid lines represent mean joint angles from all 10 subjects during NH and WH trials. Thick solid lines represent exponential curve fit denoting adaptation of joint angles in the NH (red color) and WH trials (gray color), while shaded areas represent ±1 standard error of the mean of the exponential decay curve. Mean R^2 value for the exponential decay curves for ankle joint in the NH trial was mean ± SE: 0.27 ± 0.06, for the knee joint mean ± SE: 0.31 ± 0.08 and for the hip joint mean ± SE: 0.61 ± 0.08. The dotted vertical lines represent perturbation onset while the dashed vertical lines indicate the mean time of stabilized changes in the joint angles after perturbation onset.

perturbation onset), followed by the hip (mean ± SE: 188 ± 90.8 s after the perturbation onset) and finally in the knee (mean ± SE: 195 ± 92.5 s after the perturbation onset). However, a paired-samples t-test did not show statistically significant difference between any of the compared pairs due to the high variability of data.

Analysis of Muscle Activity

Muscle activity was significantly lower during the WH trial than during the NH condition both for the leg muscles (GA $t_{(9)} = 3.57, p = 0.04, d = -0.89$; TA $t_{(9)} = 6.41, p = 0.002$, $d = -23\ 1.85$) and one of the trunk muscles (MF $t_{(9)} = 6.5$, $p = 0.001, d = -1.01$), as can be seen in **Figure 7**. Leg muscle activity was 18.4 ± 4.9% lower in the GA (mean ± SE: NH: 28.9 ± 6.5% MVC, WH: 10.6 ± 2.3% MVC) and for 23.7 ± 3.5% in the TA (mean ± SE: NH: 27.2 ± 4% MVC, WH: 3.47 ± 1.88% MVC), while the trunk muscle activity was 14.3 ± 2.1% lower in the MF (mean ± SE: NH: 36.2 ± 4.5% MVC, WH: 21.8 ± 3.7% MVC), but no significant change was observed in the OE (mean ± SE: NH: 10.4 ± 7.4% MVC, WH: 8.97 ± 4.63% MVC).

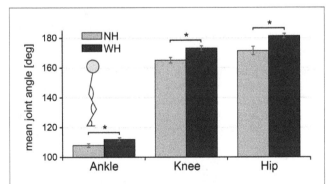

FIGURE 5 | Comparison of body posture between trials when subjects either used additional hand contact or not. Bars represent mean ankle, knee and hip joint angles during NH and WH trials. Error bars indicate ±1 standard error of the mean. Statistically significant differences are indicated (*$p \leq 0.02$).

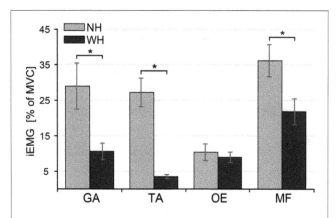

FIGURE 7 | Comparison of integrated Electromyographical (EMG) between trials when subjects either used additional hand contact or not. Bars represent iEMG of four muscles (GA, Gastrocnemius Lateralis; TA, Tibialis Anterior; OE, Obliques Externus; MF, Multifidus) during NH and WH trials. Error bars indicate ±1 standard error of the mean. Statistically significant differences are indicated ($*p \leq 0.02$).

DISCUSSION

We investigated how subjects used an additional hand support (handle) to maintain upright posture when exposed to mild and continuous perturbations elicited by waist-pull apparatus in the anteroposterior directions. The use of handle reduced the destabilizing effect of the applied perturbation by reducing the excursions of COP. These results are in line with previous studies that investigated light-touch contacts. Those studies found a reduction of COP excursions during bipedal stance with (Johannsen et al., 2007; Hausbeck et al., 2009) and without externally applied perturbations (Jeka, 1997; Krishnamoorthy et al., 2002; Kouzaki and Masani, 2008). However, in our case the handle compensated for a significant load and served more than just a light-touch contact. The mean force in the handle was over 24 N (mean ± SE: 24.5 ± 7.9 N) where in other light-touch studies, contact forces usually did not exceed 3 N (Krishnamoorthy et al., 2002; Johannsen et al., 2007; Kouzaki and Masani, 2008). Comparison between measured mean handle force and mean perturbation force, which was ~20 N (mean ± SE: 19.5 ± 1.7 N), indicates that a significant portion of perturbation on postural stability was counterbalanced by the hand.

COP excursions were strongly correlated with the perturbation force in both directions, indicating the perturbations were effective, albeit mild. When holding a handle, the excursions of the COP were larger in the anterior than in posterior direction and less correlated with the perturbation force. Due to the specifics of our design, i.e., the use of a continuous perturbation, it was impossible to investigate pure feedback postural responses to the specific direction of the perturbation. However, asymmetry in COP excursion might to be due to a differential use of the handle, indicated by a steeper slope of the regression line between the perturbation force and the forces exerted on the handle for the posterior direction.

This indicates that subjects have utilized the handle more when they counteracted the posterior COP excursions. This may be related to a more threatening situation due to the inability of the subjects to see (look) behind them, as the directions to the subjects were to look straight ahead at all times, and due to smaller stability margin in the posterior direction (Pai and Patton, 1997; Hof et al., 2005). This finding is in line with our previous study using a similar handle location and discrete perturbations caused by support platform translations, in which COP excursions were larger in the anterior direction (Babič et al., 2014).

Using a handle for balance support was beneficial, since it resulted in less displacement of COP and a smaller deviation from the neutral posture, as evident by the average joint angles. Measured joint angles in WH condition stayed closer to the neutral anatomic position than joint angles in the NH condition. Additionally, leg and trunk muscle activity was also significantly lower during the WH trial compared to the NH trial. This is consistent with the decreased leg muscle activity reported previously, when subjects had to hold (Cordo and Nashner, 1982) or touch (Sozzi et al., 2012) a surrounding object. Unlike other muscles, we found no decrease of muscle activity in the OE, which controls the rotation of the torso (Ng et al., 2001). The unilateral hand support might have caused a rotation of the trunk, which the subjects had to counteract by the OE activity. Prior to experiments we instructed subjects to use the handle in any way they prefer. Overall reduced muscle activity in legs and trunk and increased activity in arm muscles in case of using handle indicate that a portion of significant perturbation load was shifted from legs/trunk to arms. The same can be confirmed by high measured handle forces and lesser COP excursions in case of WH trial. The use of hand contact to compensate a significant portion of perturbation, even though it could be counteracted solely by legs/trunk, might be preferred since legs in a stance already have to compensate the load of the body mass (Bateni and Maki, 2005; Mergner, 2010).

Finally, when subjects had to release the handle for balance control they prepared for the more difficult NH condition even before the perturbation onset, as evident from differences in the starting joint angles. When the perturbation began this preparation was even more pronounced and joint angles changed further. These postural readjustments appear to occur at different time scales in the hip, knee and ankle joints, however that was not statistically confirmed. The subjects bended their ankle, knee and hip joints which resulted in a more flexed leg and lower hip position. Hip position can serve as an indication of the COM position and lowering of the COM could facilitate balance control (Rosker et al., 2011). Hence, these changes indicate feed-forward preparation to ease control of balance when expecting more challenging conditions, i.e., in the absence of handle. Along the same line, anticipation of the upcoming perturbations was also reported to cause changes in kinematics during quiet stance (Santos et al., 2010), walking (Pijnappels et al., 2001), recovery stepping (Pater et al., 2015) and tripping (Potocanac et al., 2014).

AUTHOR CONTRIBUTIONS

JC, LP and JB designed the study. JC and LP performed the experiments. JC, LP, ZP and JB analyzed the data and wrote the manuscript.

FUNDING

The work presented in this article was supported by the European Community Framework Programme 7 through the CoDyCo project, contract no. 600716.

REFERENCES

Assländer, L., and Peterka, R. J. (2016). Sensory reweighting dynamics following removal and addition of visual and proprioceptive cues. *J. Neurophysiol.* 116, 272–285. doi: 10.1152/jn.01145.2015

Babič, J., Petrič, T., Peternel, L., and Šarabon, N. (2014). Effects of supportive hand contact on reactive postural control during support perturbations. *Gait Posture* 40, 441–446. doi: 10.1016/j.gaitpost.2014.05.012

Bateni, H., and Maki, B. E. (2005). Assistive devices for balance and mobility: benefits, demands and adverse consequences. *Arch. Phys. Med. Rehabil.* 86, 134–145. doi: 10.1016/j.apmr.2004.04.023

Bingham, J. T., and Ting, L. H. (2013). Stability radius as a method for comparing the dynamics of neuromechanical systems. *IEEE Trans. Neural Syst. Rehabil. Eng.* 21, 840–848. doi: 10.1109/TNSRE.2013.2264920

Cohen, J. (1988). *Statistical Power Analysis for the Behavioral Sciences.* 2nd Edn. Mahwah, NJ: Lawrence Erlbaum Associates.

Corbeil, P., Bloem, B. R., van Meel, M., and Maki, B. E. (2013). Arm reactions evoked by the initial exposure to a small balance perturbation: a pilot study. *Gait Posture* 37, 300–303. doi: 10.1016/j.gaitpost.2012.07.017

Cordo, P. J., and Nashner, L. M. (1982). Properties of postural adjustments associated with rapid arm movements. *J. Neurophysiol.* 47, 287–302.

Dietz, V., Trippel, M., Ibrahim, I. K., and Berger, W. (1993). Human stance on a sinusoidally translating platform: balance control by feedforward and feedback mechanisms. *Exp. Brain Res.* 93, 352–362. doi: 10.1007/bf00228405

Franklin, D. W., Osu, R., Burdet, E., Kawato, M., and Milner, T. E. (2003). Adaptation to stable and unstable dynamics achieved by combined impedance control and inverse dynamics model. *J. Neurophysiol.* 90, 3270–3282. doi: 10.1152/jn.01112.2002

Graaf, B. D., and van Weperen, W. (1997). The retention of balance: an exploratory study into the limits of acceleration the human body can withstand without losing equilibrium. *Hum. Factors* 39, 111–118. doi: 10.1518/001872097778940614

Hausbeck, C. J., Strong, M. J., Tamkei, L. S., Leonard, W. A., and Ustinova, K. I. (2009). The effect of additional hand contact on postural stability perturbed by a moving environment. *Gait Posture* 29, 509–513. doi: 10.1016/j.gaitpost.2008.11.014

Hermens, H. J., Freriks, B., Disselhorst-Klug, C., and Rau, G. (2000). Development of recommendations for SEMG sensors and sensor placement procedures. *J. Electromyogr. Kinesiol.* 10, 361–374. doi: 10.1016/s1050-6411(00)00027-4

Hof, A. L., Gazendam, M. G. J., and Sinke, W. E. (2005). The condition for dynamic stability. *J. Biomech.* 38, 1–8. doi: 10.1016/j.jbiomech.2004.03.025

Honeine, J.-L., Crisafulli, O., Sozzi, S., and Schieppati, M. (2015). Processing time of addition or withdrawal of single or combined balance-stabilizing haptic and visual information. *J. Neurophysiol.* 114, 3097–3110. doi: 10.1152/jn.00618.2015

Jeka, J. J. (1997). Light touch contact as a balance aid. *Phys. Ther.* 77, 476–487.

Johannsen, L., Wing, A. M., and Hatzitaki, V. (2007). Effects of maintaining touch contact on predictive and reactive balance. *J. Neurophysiol.* 97, 2686–2695. doi: 10.1152/jn.00038.2007

Kouzaki, M., and Masani, K. (2008). Reduced postural sway during quiet standing by light touch is due to finger tactile feedback but not mechanical support. *Exp. Brain Res.* 188, 153–158. doi: 10.1007/s00221-008-1426-5

Krishnamoorthy, V., Slijper, H., and Latash, M. L. (2002). Effects of different types of light touch on postural sway. *Exp. Brain Res.* 147, 71–79. doi: 10.1007/s00221-002-1206-6

Maki, B. E., and McIlroy, W. E. (1997). The role of limb movements in maintaining upright stance: the "change-in-support" strategy. *Phys. Ther.* 77, 488–507.

Maki, B. E., and McIlroy, W. E. (2006). Control of rapid limb movements for balance recovery: age-related changes and implications for fall prevention. *Age Ageing* 35, ii12–ii18. doi: 10.1093/ageing/afl078

Mansfield, A., and Maki, B. E. (2009). Are age-related impairments in change-in-support balance reactions dependent on the method of balance perturbation? *J. Biomech.* 42, 1023–1031. doi: 10.1016/j.jbiomech.2009.02.007

McIlroy, W. E., and Maki, B. E. (1995). Early activation of arm muscles follows external perturbation of upright stance. *Neurosci. Lett.* 184, 177–180. doi: 10.1016/0304-3940(94)11200-3

Mergner, T. (2010). A neurological view on reactive human stance control. *Annu. Rev. Control* 34, 177–198. doi: 10.1016/j.arcontrol.2010.08.001

Ng, J. K.-F., Parnianpour, M., Richardson, C. A., and Kippers, V. (2001). Functional roles of abdominal and back muscles during isometric axial rotation of the trunk. *J. Orthop. Res.* 19, 463–471. doi: 10.1016/s0736-0266(00)90027-5

Pai, Y. C., and Patton, J. (1997). Center of mass velocity-position predictions for balance control. *J. Biomech.* 30, 347–354. doi: 10.1016/s0021-9290(96)00165-0

Pater, M. L., Rosenblatt, N. J., and Grabiner, M. D. (2015). Expectation of an upcoming large postural perturbation influences the recovery stepping response and outcome. *Gait Posture* 41, 335–337. doi: 10.1016/j.gaitpost.2014.10.026

Peternel, L., and Babič, J. (2013). Learning of compliant human-robot interaction using full-body haptic interface. *Adv. Robot.* 27, 1003–1012. doi: 10.1080/01691864.2013.808305

Pijnappels, M., Bobbert, M. F., and van Dieën, J. H. (2001). Changes in walking pattern caused by the possibility of a tripping reaction. *Gait Posture* 14, 11–18. doi: 10.1016/s0966-6362(01)00110-2

Potocanac, Z., de Bruin, J., van der Veen, S., Verschueren, S., van Dieën, J., Duysens, J., et al. (2014). Fast online corrections of tripping responses. *Exp. Brain Res.* 232, 3579–3590. doi: 10.1007/s00221-014-4038-2

Robinovitch, S. N., Feldman, F., Yang, Y., Schonnop, R., Leung, P. M., Sarraf, T., et al. (2013). Video capture of the circumstances of falls in elderly people residing in long-term care: an observational study. *Lancet* 381, 47–54. doi: 10.1016/S0140-6736(12)61263-X

Rosker, J., Markovic, G., and Sarabon, N. (2011). Effects of vertical center of mass redistribution on body sway parameters during quiet standing. *Gait Posture* 33, 452–456. doi: 10.1016/j.gaitpost.2010.12.023

Santos, M. J., Kanekar, N., and Aruin, A. S. (2010). The role of anticipatory postural adjustments in compensatory control of posture: 2. Biomechanical analysis. *J. Electromyogr. Kinesiol.* 20, 398–405. doi: 10.1016/j.jelekin.2010.01.002

Sarraf, T. A., Marigold, D. S., and Robinovitch, S. N. (2014). Maintaining standing balance by handrail grasping. *Gait Posture* 39, 258–264. doi: 10.1016/j.gaitpost.2013.07.117

Schmid, M., Bottaro, A., Sozzi, S., and Schieppati, M. (2011). Adaptation to continuous perturbation of balance: progressive reduction of postural muscle activity with invariant or increasing oscillations of the center of mass depending on perturbation frequency and vision conditions. *Hum. Mov. Sci.* 30, 262–278. doi: 10.1016/j.humov.2011.02.002

Sozzi, S., Do, M. C., Monti, A., and Schieppati, M. (2012). Sensorimotor integration during stance: processing time of active or passive addition or

withdrawal of visual or haptic information. *Neuroscience* 212, 59–76. doi: 10.
1016/j.neuroscience.2012.03.044

Van Ooteghem, K., Frank, J. S., Allard, F., Buchanan, J. J., Oates, A. R., and
Horak, F. B. (2008). Compensatory postural adaptations during continuous,
variable amplitude perturbations reveal generalized rather than sequence-
specific learning. *Exp. Brain Res.* 187, 603–611. doi: 10.1007/s00221-008-
1329-5

Wing, A. M., Johannsen, L., and Endo, S. (2011). Light touch for balance: influence
of a time-varying external driving signal. *Philos. Trans. R. Soc. Lond. B Biol. Sci.*
366, 3133–3141. doi: 10.1098/rstb.2011.0169

15

Plantar Sole Unweighting Alters the Sensory Transmission to the Cortical Areas

Laurence Mouchnino[1]*, Olivia Lhomond[1], Clément Morant[1,2] and Pascale Chavet[2]

[1]*Aix-Marseille Université, CNRS, Laboratoire de Neurosciences Cognitives, FR 3C, Marseille, France,* [2]*Aix-Marseille Université, CNRS, Institut des Sciences du Mouvement, Marseille, France*

*Correspondence:
Laurence Mouchnino
laurence.mouchnino@univ-amu.fr

It is well established that somatosensory inputs to the cortex undergo an early and a later stage of processing. The later has been shown to be enhanced when the earlier transmission decreased. In this framework, mechanical factors such as the mechanical stress to which sensors are subjected when wearing a loaded vest are associated with a decrease in sensory transmission. This decrease is in turn associated with an increase in the late sensory processes originating from cortical areas. We hypothesized that unweighting the plantar sole should lead to a facilitation of the sensory transmission. To test this hypothesis, we recorded cortical somatosensory evoked potentials (SEPs) of individuals following cutaneous stimulation (by mean of an electrical stimulation of the foot sole) in different conditions of unweighting when standing still with eyes closed. To this end, the effective bodyweight (BW) was reduced from 100% BW to 40% BW. Contrary to what was expected, we found an attenuation of sensory information when the BW was unweighted to 41% which was not compensated by an increase of the late SEP component. Overall these results suggested that the attenuation of sensory transmission observed in 40 BW condition was not solely due to the absence of forces acting on the sole of the feet but rather to the current relevance of the afferent signals related to the balance constraints of the task.

Keywords: plantar sole afferents, unweighting, EEG, standing balance

INTRODUCTION

Somatosensory processes have been accorded an important role in triggering and shaping rapid postural responses to unexpected perturbation of the support surface while standing. Indeed, when removing somatosensory inputs in cats with Pirydoxine, Stapley et al. (2002) showed delayed postural responses. The importance of cutaneous inputs in the setting of forces exerted on the ground is supported by a deficit in weight-bearing during locomotion in cats after cutaneous nerve section (Bouyer and Rossignol, 2003). Equally in humans, the significance of cutaneous inputs for controlling postural adjustments has been evidenced by studies of anesthetized foot plantar soles (Do et al., 1990). In addition, in vestibular-loss animals after bilateral labyrinthectomy (Inglis and Macpherson, 1995), the latencies of the postural responses were normal ($\sim$375 ms) or even earlier ($\sim$325 ms) suggesting a critical role of somatosensory inputs in balance control during perturbation rather than a vestibular-based control. However, when balance control is not challenged (i.e., due to a perturbation or voluntary movements) during the maintenance of normal standing, Meyer et al. (2004) showed that the reduced plantar sensitivity after anesthesia did not alter the postural sway.

These studies and others (Ruget et al., 2008; Mouchnino and Blouin, 2013) have highlighted the role of cutaneous afferents when relevant for the task (i.e., challenged balance control). Remarkably, modulation of the excitability of somatosensory areas can be observed in tasks requiring high somatosensory control (Staines et al., 1997; McIlroy et al., 2003). Indeed, cortical responsiveness to sensory stimuli can be increased in challenging balance situations while standing still (Bolton et al., 2011). For instance, using the somatosensory-evoked potential (SEP) technique, Bolton et al. (2011) found an increased sensitivity to somatosensory inputs of the hand when participants, who were standing with one foot in front of the other (i.e., Romberg's challenging balance task), lightly touched a fixed support surface with their hand. Importantly, this sensory facilitation was associated with improved balance control (i.e., less postural oscillations) compared to a condition with the same light touch on a support attached to the participant's wrist (i.e., not referenced to the external environment). Bolton et al. (2011) concluded that the external-referenced touch enhanced the perception of self-generated postural oscillations relative to the external world. Therefore, enhancing the transmission of relevant somatosensory input from the foot sole during challenging balance control, would allow participants to control body sway relative to the external gravity and balance constraints.

However, compensatory postural regulations and functional consequences are load-dependent changes. Carrying extra weight on the body translates into a decreased of the SEP likely indicating a depressed transmission of cutaneous input (Lhomond et al., 2016). Indeed, such variations were observed by Desmedt and Robertson (1977) as early as 55 ms after a tactile electrical stimulation. This early component was interpreted as reflecting the activity of the primary somatosensory cortex (SI; Hari et al., 1984; Hämäläinen et al., 1990). For example, Salinas et al. (2000) showed that the majority of SI neurons in monkeys were phase-locked with the vibratory stimulus. These neurons encoded the stimulus frequency, suggesting a high relationship of SI activity with the incoming sensory inputs. The decrease in the transmission of the afferent cutaneous inflow arising from the periphery to SI could originate from foot deformation resulting from the extra loading. Indeed, it has been reported that obese individuals (Hills et al., 2001) showed higher pressures under the heel, mid-foot and metatarsal regions of the foot compared to normal-weight individuals. Subsequently other studies have observed a greater total plantar force and a greater total contact area (Gravante et al., 2003; Birtane and Tuna, 2004) in obese individuals. A related study by Vela et al. (1998) showed similar observations when normal-weight individuals were loaded with external weights to simulate obesity. Therefore, skin compression where the tactile receptors were embedded could be at the origin of sensory transmission attenuation. For example, under foot loading, the height of the arch of the foot decreases (Bandholm et al., 2008; McPoil et al., 2009) and almost 50% of this change could be accounted for by skin compression (Wright et al., 2012). These behavioral studies together with Lhomond et al.'s (2016) electrophysiological study

suggest that the attenuation of the sensory transmission of cutaneous inputs comes from a mechanical origin due to foot sole loading. This phenomenon may be explained by refractoriness in the peripheral nerves themselves (skin receptors firing is already saturated due to load), by depression of synaptic transmission (slowly adapting receptors reduce their input due to adaptation from the foot sole loading), or by alteration of the transmission anywhere along the ascending sensory pathway and within the cortex itself. Therefore if the mechanoreceptors are even partly silenced by the additional weight compressing the skin of the foot sole, the transmission to S1 should be altered.

On the basis of the behavioral and electrophysiological findings reported above, we hypothesized that unweighting the plantar sole should lead to a facilitation of the sensory transmission. To this end, we recorded cortical SEPs following cutaneous stimulation (by mean of an electrical stimulation of the foot sole) in different conditions of unweighting.

MATERIALS AND METHODS

Ten participants (6 males and 4 females) performed a bipedal balance task (mean age: 32 ± 13 years; mean height: 173 ± 9 cm; mean weight: 65 ± 4 kg). All participants were free of neurological and musculoskeletal disorders that could influence postural control and had a good fitness base (for review see Paillard, 2017). Informed consent was obtained from all participants, and all procedures were in accord with the ethical standards set out in the Declaration of Helsinki and ethic committee Sud Méditerranée (ID RCB:2010-A00074-35). A Lower Body Positive Pressure (LBPP) treadmill (M310 Anti-gravity Treadmill®, AlterG Inc., Fremont, CA, USA) enables an individual's bodyweight (BW) to be varied. LBPP technology applies a consistent and substantial lifting force opposite to BW. The AlterG® treadmill includes an airtight flexible chamber applied distally to the subject's iliac crest. This creates local unweighing of the lower limbs while the upper body and all gravity-receptors still experience earth gravity (Sainton et al., 2015; **Figure 1A**). The electrical signal of the differential pressure (Patmospheric $-$ Pchamber) was recorded with the vertical ground reaction force obtained from four dynamical load cells (XA-shear beam load cell, Sentran®, Ontario, CA, USA) located under the frame of the AlterG® treadmill. The ground reaction forces were summed to compute the real BW of the participants.

Participants wore neoprene shorts and stood barefoot on the AlterG® treadmill. Initially, they remained stationary, with their arms alongside their bodies (**Figure 1A**). The neoprene shorts were sealed to the inflatable chamber. The seal height was adjusted to be level with each participant's iliac crest, so that the seal itself exerted little or no vertical force. In addition, the compliance properties of the chamber were such that participants' body was free to move in all directions and participants were even able to walk and run comfortably as shown by Cutuk et al. (2006).

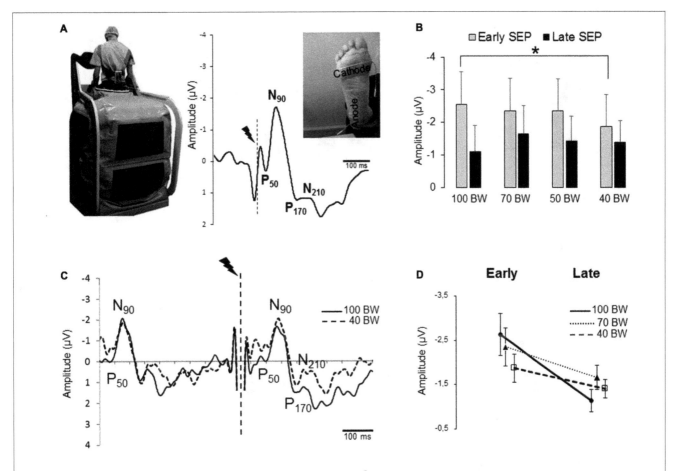

FIGURE 1 | (A) Image displaying the position of participants in the Anti-gravity Treadmill®. Grand-average EPs for 10 participants recorded over Cz electrode during quiet standing which exhibits an early somatosensory evoked potential (SEP; P_{50}-N_{90}) followed by a later component (P_{170}-N_{210}). The vertical dotted lines indicate the stimulation onset. **(B)** Mean for the 80 stimulations of the Early P_{50}-N_{90} and late P_{170}-N_{210} SEPs amplitudes for all participants (error bars are standard deviation across participants). (*$p < 0.05$). **(C)** The traces corresponds to the average SEP in 100 bodyweight (BW) and 40 BW conditions for one participant. The break in the curves corresponds to the electrical stimulation artifact. Note that the presence of a first P_{50}-N_{90} SEP is due to the time-window shown in the figure that encompasses two stimulations interspace of 500 ms. **(D)** Interaction between the early and late SEPs for 100 BW, 70 and 40 BW conditions. The error bars are standard error of the mean.

Participants were requested to self-select a side-by-side foot position (approximately feet shoulder-width apart, wide stance) and to keep their eyes closed. Here, particular attention was paid to maintaining the self-selected foot position (i.e., feet shoulder-width apart before each trial) because of the effect of stance width on both postural control and the use of sensory feedback. As shown by Jacobs et al. (2015), the corticomuscular coupling of the bêta frequency band known to represent both afferent and efferent coupling between sensorimotor regions of cerebral cortex and muscle, is sensitive to changes in biomechanical conditions (i.e., wide- or narrow-stance) but not to sensory conditions (foam surface or eyes closed).

The participants were then submitted to different unweighting conditions without changing this initial wide-stance. Four different weighting conditions were applied: 100% of BW, 70 BW, 50 BW and 30 BW. These target values set in the AlterG were held constant for a while (2–3 mn) during the recording session. The changes in BW were applied in a descending sequence (D) from 100D to 30D and then upwards

from (U) 50U, 70U and 100U. The participants were blind to the weight conditions and to the sequence. Instead, they were instructed that the BW could be modulated randomly either by increasing or decreasing the weight.

At every stage of unweighting, the participants were asked to estimate the percentage of BW they were experiencing. In order to avoid any prediction of the percentage of the unweighting, the target weight was not reached directly but only after exploring other weighting. In a control task, participants adopted a semi-supine position (Supine, **Figures 1C, 2A**) seated in a reclining chair with their plantar soles without a contact with a support surface. The order of the Supine and the Standing task on the treadmill were counterbalanced across participants.

Stimulation Procedure

While standing the plantar sole of the left foot was stimulated four times with a constant 500 ms interval between each electrical stimulus. This was designed to avoid the "interference phenomenon" (Burke and Gandevia, 1988; i.e., depressed

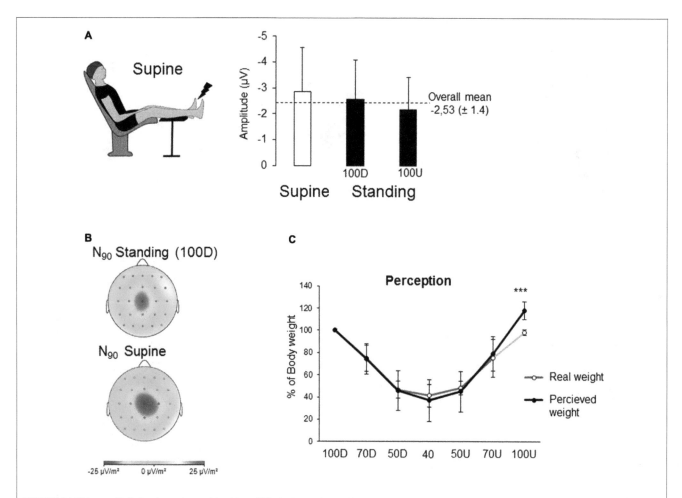

FIGURE 2 | (A) Image displaying the supine position. Mean SEPs for the supine position and both 100% of BW conditions. (B) To enhance the spatial resolution of the recordings, topographical current source density (CSD) maps were computed using Laplacian transformation with Brain Vision Analyzer. The signal was interpolated with a spherical spline interpolation procedure in order to compute the second order derivatives in two dimensions of space (order of splines: 3; maximal degree of Legendre polynomials: 15). CSDs are independent of the reference electrode site and are much less affected by far-field generators than monopolar recordings. The cortical maps are shown at the latency of the peak negativity (i.e., N90). (C) Comparison between the perception of BW given by the participants and the real weight computed by the vertical forces recorded by the treadmill. Each dot corresponds to the mean of 10 participants for all the weighting conditions (error bars are standard deviation across participants; ***$p < 0.001$).

SEPs when stimulations are too close in time, i.e., less than 300 ms according to Morita et al., 1998). The electrical stimulus was delivered by a DS5 isolated bipolar constant current stimulator (Digitimer, Welwyn Garden City, UK). The cathode was located under the metatarsal region and the anode was positioned underneath the heel of the supporting foot (**Figure 1A**, 5 × 9 cm electrodes, Platinum Foam Electrodes). The stimulation consisted of a single rectangular 10 ms pulse applied under the supporting foot. Taking into account the signature of the cutaneous reflexes reported in Sayenko et al.'s (2009) study, we carefully selected both the position of the electrodes to stimulate the plantar sole as a whole without targeting a specific portion of the foot, and the amplitude of the stimulation to avoid cutaneous reflexes. The stimulation intensity was set as in our previous studies (Mouchnino et al., 2015; Lhomond et al., 2016). For each participant, and while standing, we first found the minimum intensity which gave a constant perception of the stimulations (mean amplitude

6.2 ± 0.1 mA). This stimulation was determined as the baseline value. The stimulation intensity for each participant was set at 25% higher than the baseline value (i.e., well below the motor threshold). Each condition of weighting was divided into 20 standing trials of 5 s. During each trial 4 electrical stimuli were triggered (80 stimulations per condition).

Electroencephalography and Behavioral Recordings and Analyses

Electroencephalographic (EEG) activity was recorded continuously from 64 Ag/AgCl surface electrodes embedded on an elastic cap (ActiveTwo system, BioSemi, Netherlands). According to the specification of the BioSemi system, "ground" electrodes were replaced by Common Mode Sense active and Driven Right Leg passive electrodes. These two electrodes, located near Pz and POz electrodes, form a feedback loop, which drives the average potential of the participant (the Common

Mode voltage) as close as possible to the anolog-digital converter (ADC) reference voltage in the AD-box. The signals were pre-amplified at the electrode sites and post-amplified with DC amplifiers and digitized at a sampling rate of 1024 Hz (24-bit resolution). Signals from each channel were referenced using the average of the 64 scalp electrodes. The signals were further filtered off-line with 35 Hz (high cut-off) filters (digital filters, 48 dB/octave) and 0.1 Hz (low cut-off) filters (digital filters, 12 dB/octave; BrainVision Analyzer 2, Brain Products, Germany).

SEPs, (**Figure 1A**) were obtained by averaging, for each participant and condition, all synchronized epochs (i.e., 80) relative to the electrical stimulus. The average amplitude of the (-100; -50 ms) pre-stimulus epoch served as baseline. The -50 ms relative to the stimulation was chosen to avoid any artifact related to the stimulation procedure. We examined the SEPs over the Cz electrode as this electrode overlays the sensorimotor cortices on the homunculus, the feet are located on the inner surface of the longitudinal fissure. The earliest discernible positive (P_{50}) and negative (N_{90}) peaks after each stimulus were identified. Such peaks latencies are comparable to latencies observed by Altenmüller et al. (1995) and Duysens et al. (1995) evoked by stimulating the sural nerve. The fact that the sural nerve is a primarily/exclusively cutaneous nerve (Burke et al., 1981) lends argument for the P_{50}-N_{90} originating from cutaneous input. The amplitude of the P_{50}-N_{90} waveform was measured peak-to-peak., a late SEP component (P_{170}-N_{210}) was observed at a latency similar to latencies observed in Lhomond et al.'s (2016) study.

Head acceleration was measured by using a triaxial accelerometer (Model 4630: Measurement Specialties, Virginia, VA, USA) placed on the chin. The rationale for using head acceleration as an index for whole body stability relative to space is that for balance and posture the whole body can be assumed to act as a rigid segment (inverted pendulum model) about the subtalar joint of the feet (MacKinnon and Winter, 1993). For example, Jeka et al. (1997) showed that during a light finger touch on a stationary bar, the lateral displacements of head and center of pressure were in phase and superimposable. For each trial, after applying a 4th order *Butterworth* filter with 3 Hz cut-off frequency on the raw data over time, de-biasing and rectifying the signal, we computed the integral of a 1600 ms time-window which encompassed the four stimulations periods including the $P_{50}N_{90}$ component following the last stimulation (**Figure 3A**).

We analyzed the ground reaction force from one gauge (located on the right non-stimulated side). After applying a 4th order *Butterworth* filter with 3 Hz cut-off frequency on the raw data over time, the data were rectified, integrated and normalized relative to the body mass index of each participant.

Bipolar surface electromyography (EMG; Bortec AMT-8 system; Bortec Biomedical, Calgary, Canada) was used to record bilaterally the activity of the tibialis anterior (TA) and gastrocnemius medialis (GM) muscle. EMG signals were preamplified at the skin site ($\times 1000$), analog filtered with a preset bandpass (20–250 Hz) and sampled at 1000 Hz, then rectified.

These recordings were performed to evaluate the level of muscle activation during the standing task. To quantify these activations, we computed the integral of the EMG activity (iEMG) for each muscle during five 400 ms time-windows. The first time-window was computed before the stimulation (i.e., baseline [-450; -50]). The other time-windows were computed after each stimulation (i.e., [50; 450], [550; 950], [1050; 1450], [1550; 1950]). As no differences were observed between the four iEMG-windows during the stimulation period we computed the mean iEMG from the four time-windows. One of the participants had no available recordings for the 100D condition and was discarded from the analyses.

Statistical Analyses

The amplitudes and latencies of the SEPs were submitted to repeated-measures analysis of variance (ANOVA) designed with conditions of weighting (100D, 70D, 50D and 30). Significant effects were further analyzed with Newman-Keuls *post hoc* tests. For the size effect calculation we used the η^2 (Eta squared), and to work out effect size we used the Cohen's (1988) guidelines (Fritz et al., 2012). We also conducted paired *t*-tests when necessary. The level of significance was set at 5% for all analyses. All dependent variables (EEG and behavioral data) showed normal distributions (i.e., $p > 0.05$, Kolmogorov-Smirnov test).

RESULTS

The assessment of the precision of the BW level was performed a posteriori; 70 BW corresponded to $75 \pm 10\%$, 50 BW was $47 \pm 5\%$ and 30 BW was $41 \pm 10\%$ for all participants. In order to determine if the real unweighting experienced by each participant corresponded to the target unweighting set in the AlterG, the real unweighting was compared to a standard value (i.e., target unweighting) for each condition. These analyses revealed that the real weight for the 70 and 50 BW conditions were not different from their standard values ($t_9 = 1.32$; $p = 0.21$ and $t_9 = -1.48$; $p = 0.17$, respectively). In the 30 BW condition the real weight is increased relative to the standard value set in the AlterG ($t_9 = 3.81$; $p = 0.004$). We therefore chose a new and more appropriate standard value of 40 ($t_9 = 0.72$; $p = 0.48$). For clarity of purpose, we replaced the 30 BW condition by 40 BW below in the results section to denote each unweighting levels.

Somatosensory Evoked Potentials

During quiet standing, the foot stimulation evoked typical EEG signals. **Figure 1A** shows the grand average at electrode Cz for all participants. Both an early and a late sensory processes were identified. The early SEP consisted in a small positive component (P_{50}) followed by a prominent negative deflection (N_{90}). First of all, to assess that decreasing and increasing the weight on the feet (i.e., order effect) did not change the amplitude of the SEP, we compared the 100, 70, 50 Down with the 50, 70, 100 Up. SEP amplitudes were submitted to 2 modes (decreasing, increasing) $\times$ 3 BW (100, 70, 50 BW) repeated measures ANOVAs. The results showed that the amplitude of the P_{50}-N_{90} SEP did not depend on the order (i.e., Down or

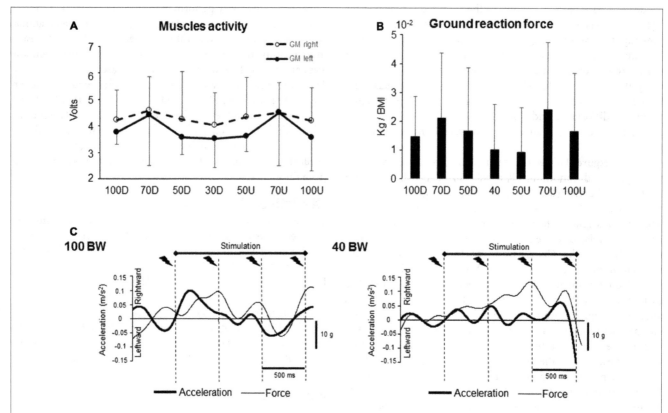

FIGURE 3 | (A) Integrals of both right and left gastrocnemius medialis (GM) muscles activity recorded during a 450 ms duration period. **(B)** Integrals of the vertical ground reaction force during a 2100 ms duration period that encompassed the whole stimulation procedure. **(C)** Mean head lateral acceleration and ground reaction force non-rectified traces for one participants (100 BW and 40 BW).

Up) of the unweighting ($F_{(1,9)} = 0.34$; $p = 0.57$) nor on the BW ($F_{(2,18)} = 0.14$; $p = 0.86$). Therefore we will use the descending order to compare the 100D, 70D, 50D and 40 BW conditions.

SEP data (amplitude and latencies) were submitted to repeated measures ANOVA with different condition of BW (100D, 70D, 50D and 40) as the main factor. The results showed a BW main effect on the P_{50}-N_{90} SEP amplitude ($F_{(3,27)} = 3.41$; $p = 0.031$) with a large size effect of 0.27. As the decrease at 40% BW is relatively small with large standard deviation, we used the Tukey's HSD test (i.e., less liberal test than the Newman-Keul's *post hoc* test) and found that the SEP had a smaller amplitude in the 40 BW condition (-1.86 ± 1 μV) compared to the 100 BW conditions (-2.56 ± 1.5 μV; $p = 0.02$; **Figure 1B**). In addition, no BW effect was observed for the latencies of P_{50} ($F_{(3,27)} = 0.93$; $p = 0.43$; overall mean of 64 ± 17 ms) and of N_{90} ($F_{(3,27)} = 0.59$; $p = 0.62$; overall mean of 96 ± 19 ms). It was noticed that the ANOVA did not show a general BW effect (100, 70, 50 and 40 BW) on the late SEP component (**Figure 1B**, $F_{(2,27)} = 1.60$; $p = 0.21$).

To assess whether the decreased SEP observed in 40 BW was due to an altered use of mechanoreceptors provoked by the unloading of BW, a supine position (i.e., weightless) was compared to both Standing conditions (i.e., 100D and 100U, **Figures 2A,B**). The results did not show a condition effect on the early SEP amplitude (overall mean: -2.53 ± 1.4; $F_{(2,18)} = 2.94$;

$p = 0.07$) or on the P_{50} and N_{90} latencies (P_{50} overall mean: 62 ms ± 13; $F_{(2,18)} = 0.60$; $p = 0.55$ and N_{90} overall mean: 92 ms ± 15; $F_{(2,18)} = 0.42$; $p = 0.66$).

To further test whether the attenuated transmission of sensory inputs (P_{50}-N_{90} SEP) in the 40 BW condition was associated with an altered late potential (P_{170}-N_{210} SEP), SEP data were submitted to repeated measures ANOVA with conditions (100 BW, 70 BW and 40 BW) and SEPs components (early P_{50}-N_{90} and late P_{170}-N_{210} components) as the main factor (**Figures 1C,D**). We have discarded the 50 BW condition from the analyses to lessen the variability. The results revealed a main component effect ($F_{(1,9)} = 7.17$; $p = 0.02$ with an interaction SEP (early and late components) × BW ($F_{(2,18)} = 5.09$; $p = 0.17$). Post hoc analyses showed that the early components were greater than the late components in 100 BW and 70 BW conditions ($p < 0.05$) and of approximately equal amplitudes in 40 BW condition ($p = 0.12$). In addition *post hoc* analyses confirmed that the early SEP recorded in the 100 BW condition was greater than the early SEP of the 40 BW condition ($p = 0.016$) but not different from the 70 BW condition ($p = 0.35$). What is informative (Hsu, 1996) is that the late SEP in the 70 BW condition was greater than in the 100 BW although this statistical value fell short of the conventional 0.05 cut-off value for statistical significance ($p = 0.07$). No difference was observed between the late SEP in 100 BW and in 40 BW ($p = 0.23$).

Perception and Behavior

Due to the difference between target value and real weight, it was considered more pertinent to compare the perception of the weight to the real weight. In addition, the 100D condition was excluded as it started the experiment in the AlterG and all participants were aware of the 100% BW condition. With regard to perception (**Figure 2C**), results showed a significant interaction between conscious perception of the BW and real conditions of weighting ($F_{(5,45)} = 2.58$; $p = 0.038$) with a large size effect of 0.22; *post hoc* analyses confirmed that the participants' own BW was perceived heavier in the 100 Up (117 ± 8% of BW) than the real BW (i.e., 98 ± 2 of BW; $p < 0.001$).

The behavioral data (activity of ankle musculature, vertical ground reaction force, and head acceleration) were submitted to repeated measures ANOVA with different condition of BW (100D, 70D, 50D 40, 50U, 70U, 100U) as the main factor during the stimulation procedure (i.e., stimulation).

To verify if the difference in the SEPs amplitude was not due to a difference in the motor activity, we compared the iEMG of TA and GM muscles of both legs computed in the different conditions. The muscle activity did not change across the unweighting condition; however, the activity of the left GM showed a slight rise in activity for both 70D and 70U BW conditions without reaching the significant level (**Figure 3A**, $F_{(6,48)} = 2.09$; $p = 0.07$). No condition effect was observed for the other ankle muscles ($F_{(6,48)} = 0.38$; $p = 0.88$; $F_{(6,48)} = 1.36$; $p = 0.24$; $F_{(6,48)} = 0.51$; $p = 0.79$ for the right GM and right and left TA, respectively). Overall, these results suggest that the depression of the early SEP in 40 BW condition was not related to an increase in muscular activity which indeed could have induced a sensory suppression (Cohen and Starr, 1987; Seki and Fetz, 2012).

After normalization to the body mass index (including participant's weight and height), ground reaction force and head acceleration data were analyzed (**Figure 3C**). No difference was observed neither for the forces (**Figure 3B**, $F_{(6,54)} = 1.68$; $p = 0.14$, for the main condition effect) or for the head acceleration ($F_{(6,54)} = 1.45$; $p = 0.21$, $F_{(6,54)} = 1.63$; $p = 0.15$, in the mediolateral and anteroposterior direction, respectively).

DISCUSSION

The aim of this study was to identify whether the sensory transmission from the plantar sole tactile receptors in a bipedal standing position is modulated relative to the force acting on the foot sole. A facilitation of the sensory transmission was expected in the unweighting condition.

Surprisingly our results did not show an increase in transmission as expected but rather a decreased early activity over SI in the unweighting 40 BW condition compared to full BW (i.e., 100 BW). One possible explanation for these findings is that the unweighting 40 BW condition with reduced loading of the feet could have induced a change in sensory noise (i.e., background sensory traffic). Indeed, mechanoreceptors adaptation to the static pressure due to normal BW could not take place under such unloading and may give raise to a sensorial

"noise" (Weerakkody et al., 2007). This sensorial "noise" or interference phenomenon (Burke and Gandevia, 1988) could be at the origin of a low perception. For example Mildren and Bent (2016) have shown that cutaneous stimulation at different skin regions across the foot can influence proprioception at the ankle joint (i.e., perception of feet orientation). The authors concluded that inputs from cutaneous mechanoreceptors had an influence on ankle proprioception and this error of perception could be due to an inhibition of cutaneous or spindle proprioceptive feedback, causing the perception of smaller movement magnitudes. This sensorial "noise" could be also observed when wearing a loaded vest (i.e., low SEP, Lhomond et al., 2016) or when comparing standing to sitting (Mildren et al., 2016). However, the perception of participants' weight in the 40 BW condition was preserved (i.e., no difference between the real, 41% and the perceived weight, 37%) despite the decrease sensory transmission (i.e., lower early SEP). The accurate perception of BW in the 40 BW condition could not dismiss the sensory "noise" hypothesis. Indeed, Bays and Wolpert (2007) suggested that the noise in the sensory system could lead to a reweighting of the available sensory sources. Therefore, the integration of other modalities could compensate for the sensory "noise" and preserve an accurate perception of the BW.

While in most previous studies an increase in sensory transmission has been shown to be related to an increased perception of tactile stimuli when relevant to the motor task (Duysens et al., 1995; Cybulska-Klosowicz et al., 2011), our results suggest a less straightforward causal relationship between transmission and perception. In the current study, the perception was altered (i.e., overestimated, about 120%) with the presence of a full amplitude SEP (i.e., 100Up BW) and, conversely perception was preserved with a decreases SEP amplitude (i.e., in 40 BW). Therefore perception does not depend solely on early sensory transmission but rather relies predominantly on processing signals originating from sensorimotor-related neural mechanisms. Among these sensorimotor mechanisms were those involved in the prediction of the sensory consequence of our own action even if this action consists in preserving body equilibrium (Blakemore et al., 1998, 1999a,b; Voisin et al., 2011; Cullen and Brooks, 2015; Benazet et al., 2016).

Evidence for task-specific gating of the cortical transmission in the 40 BW condition observed in the current study parallels that seen in McIlroy et al.'s (2003) study. For instance, these authors showed that the SEPs evoked by tibial nerve stimuli in a seated task while the participants were to relax (i.e., Supine condition here, in our study) were similar to those of a task (termed "Threatened balance") in which the seated participants were maintaining the position of an inverted pendulum with threat of external perturbation by balancing a platform under their feet (i.e., Standing 100% BW here, in our study). In addition, in a third sitting task without a threat to the stability of the pendulum (i.e., No balance constraints) but with the same forces exerted on the foot sole (i.e., muscle contraction or ankle angle), the SEP was depressed by 28%. This study (McIlroy et al., 2003) together with the depressed SEP in the 40 BW condition (i.e., low balance constraints) may support the idea that the central nervous system decreases sensory transmission according to the decrease in the balance constraints of the task. Indeed, the 40 BW condition did not endanger the equilibrium as it was reported by Ritzmann et al. (2015) in underloading situations during parabolic flight (i.e., 0.16 and 0.38 g). These authors showed that the center of gravity is suitably adjusted above the base of support and that was achieved by a slow body motion control resulting from the noticeably reduced ankle joint torque.

Our results suggest that the brain exerts a dynamic control over the transmission of the afferent signal (i.e., attenuation) according to their current relevance to the task. The idea that the attenuation probably occurs at a cortical level has been previously suggested by Applegate et al. (1988). This study suggests that the attenuation of short latency cerebral potentials during standing relative to voluntary isometric plantarflexion while sitting may not be explicable entirely by the change in background muscle activity and by non-specific effects exerted on relay nuclei by standing because the subcortical component (P_{32}-N_{38}) was not reduced by stance. Additional support suggesting that the altered transmission of afferent inputs is centrally-driven comes from the late SEP analyses. Remarkably, the decrease of the early SEP in 40 BW condition was not associated with an increase in the late sensory processes (i.e., same amplitude of late SEP in 40 BW and in 100 BW) contrary to what was observed in overloading condition (Lhomond et al., 2016). In this previous study, the enhancement of the late-stage sensory integration was interpreted as a mechanism aimed at compensating for decreased early sensory transmission in order to control whole body stability which was decreased with additional loading. Even though the transmission of cutaneous input is depressed and the late integrative process remained unchanged in the current study, both head acceleration and vertical force exerted onto the ground were similar to the normal weight condition. These results suggested that there was no need for further compensation (i.e., increase late sensory process) as body balance was not endangered by the unweighting 40 BW condition.

In addition, the late SEP was greater and associated with an increased lateral head acceleration during the first unweighting change experienced by the participants (i.e., 70D

condition). This condition separates for the first time the gravitational somatosensory information (i.e., altered) provided by the contact forces of the feet with the supporting surface from the vestibular cues provided by the gravity acceleration (i.e., unchanged). The late sensory upregulation together with the decreased whole body stability observed here most likely reflects an enhancement of the integration of somatosensory and vestibular inputs from the head acceleration, to reset an internal model of gravity (Papaxanthis et al., 2003; Indovina et al., 2005; Herold et al., 2017). A similar increased activation has been reported by Miyai et al. (2006) in healthy participants during gait on a treadmill with unusual partial BW support (10%).

In conclusion, our study is the first to examine the unweighting effects on the transmission of afferent inputs from the periphery to the cortical areas during upright standing. We observed a suppression of sensory transmission in particular within a threshold range from 47% to 41% of BW (i.e., respectively, 50 BW and 40 BW conditions) experienced by the healthy participants. This is partly because the tactile information from the foot sole is less relevant in terms of balance constraints with underloading. In this context, as the AlterG® treadmill can be considered as a safety device for loading and unloading lower extremities in patients with lower limb injuries and disorders, the efficacy of the rehabilitation programs should consider the sensory mechanisms together with the motor aspects of standing, walking and running.

AUTHOR CONTRIBUTIONS

LM, OL and PC contributed to the conception and design of the work. LM, OL, CM and PC contributed to the acquisition, analysis, or interpretation of data for the work, contributed to the writting of the work or revising it critically.

ACKNOWLEDGMENTS

This study was funded by the Scientific Research and Innovation program of the DGA (2014600051).

REFERENCES

Altenmüller, E., Berger, W., Prokop, T., Trippel, M., and Dietz, V. (1995). Modulation of sural nerve somatosensory evoked potentials during stance and different phases of the step-cycle. *Electroencephalogr. Clin. Neurophysiol.* 96, 516–525. doi: 10.1016/0013-4694(95)00093-e

Applegate, C., Gandevia, S. C., and Burke, D. (1988). Changes in muscle and cutaneous cerebral potentials during standing. *Exp. Brain Res.* 71, 183–188. doi: 10.1007/bf00247533

Bandholm, T., Boysen, L., Haugaard, S., Zebis, M. K., and Bencke, J. (2008). Foot medial longitudinal-arch deformation during quiet standing and gait in subjects with medial tibial stress syndrome. *J. Foot Ankle Surg.* 47, 89–95. doi: 10.1053/j.jfas.2007.10.015

Bays, P. M., and Wolpert, D. M. (2007). Computational principles of sensorimotor control that minimize uncertainty and variability. *J. Physiol.* 578, 387–396. doi: 10.1113/jphysiol.2006.120121

Benazet, M., Thénault, F., Whittingstall, K., and Bernier, P. M. (2016). Attenuation of visual reafferent signals in the parietal cortex during voluntary movement. *J. Neurophysiol.* 116, 1831–1839. doi: 10.1152/jn.00231.2016

Birtane, M., and Tuna, H. (2004). The evaluation of plantar pressure distribution in obese and non-obese adults. *Clin. Biomech.* 19, 1055–1059. doi: 10.1016/j.clinbiomech.2004.07.008

Blakemore, S. J., Frith, C. D., and Wolpert, D. M. (1999a). Spatio-temporal prediction modulates the perception of self-produced stimuli. *J. Cogn. Neurosci.* 11, 551–559. doi: 10.1162/089892999563607

Blakemore, S. J., Wolpert, D. M., and Frith, C. D. (1999b). The cerebellum contributes to somatosensory cortical activity during self-produced tactile stimulation. *Neuroimage* 10, 448–459. doi: 10.1006/nimg.1999.0478

Blakemore, S. J., Wolpert, D. M., and Frith, C. D. (1998). Central cancellation of self-produced tickle sensation. *Nat. Neurosci.* 1, 635–640. doi: 10.1038/2870

Bolton, D. A. E., McIlroy, W. E., and Staines, W. R. (2011). The impact of light fingertip touch on haptic cortical processing during a standing balance task. *Exp. Brain Res.* 212, 279–291. doi: 10.1007/s00221-011-2728-6

Bouyer, L. J., and Rossignol, S. (2003). Contribution of cutaneous inputs from the hindpaw to the control of locomotion. II. Spinal cats. *J. Neurophysiol.* 90, 3640–3653. doi: 10.1152/jn.00497.2003

Burke, D., and Gandevia, S. C. (1988). Interfering cutaneous stimuli and the muscle afferent contribution to cortical potentials. *Electroencephalogr. Clin. Neurophysiol.* 70, 118–125. doi: 10.1016/0013-4694(88)90112-5

Burke, D., Skuse, N. F., and Lethlean, A. K. (1981). Cutaneous and muscle afferent components of the cerebral potential evoked by electrical stimulation of human peripheral nerves. *Electroenceph. Clin. Neurophysiol.* 51, 579–588. doi: 10.1016/0013-4694(81)90202-9

Cohen, J. (1988). *Statistical Power Analysis for the Behavioral Sciences.* 2nd Edn. Hillsdale, NJ: Erlbaum.

Cohen, L. G., and Starr, A. (1987). Localization, timing and specificity of gating of somatosensory evoked potentials during active movement in man. *Brain* 110, 451–467. doi: 10.1093/brain/110.2.451

Cullen, K. E., and Brooks, J. X. (2015). Neural correlates of sensory prediction errors in monkeys: evidence for internal models of voluntary self-motion in the cerebellum. *Cerebellum* 14, 31–34. doi: 10.1007/s12311-014-0608-x

Cutuk, A., Groppo, E. R., Quigley, E. J., White, K. W., Pedowitz, R. A., and Hargens, A. R. (2006). Ambulation in simulated fractional gravity using lower body positive pressure: cardiovascular safety and gait analyses. *J. Appl. Physiol.* 101, 771–777. doi: 10.1152/japplphysiol.00644.2005

Cybulska-Klosowicz, A., Meftah, El-M., Raby, M., Lemieux, M. L., and Chapman, C. E. (2011). A critical speed for gating of tactile detection during voluntary movement. *Exp. Brain Res.* 210, 291–301. doi: 10.1007/s00221-011-2632-0

Desmedt, J. E., and Robertson, D. (1977). Differential enhancement of early and late components of the cerebral somatosensory evoked potentials during forced-paced cognitive tasks in man. *J. Physiol.* 271, 761–782. doi: 10.1113/jphysiol.1977.sp012025

Do, M. C., Bussel, B., and Breniere, Y. (1990). Influence of plantar cutaneous afferents on early compensatory reactions to forward fall. *Exp. Brain Res.* 79, 319–324. doi: 10.1007/bf00608241

Duysens, J., Tax, A. A., Nawijn, s., Berger, W., Prokop, T., and Altenmüller, E. (1995). Gating of sensation and evoked potentials following foot stimulation during human gait. *Exp. Brain Res.* 105, 423–431. doi: 10.1007/bf00233042

Fritz, C. O., Morris, P. E., and Richler, J. J. (2012). Effect size estimates. Current use, calculations and interpretation. *J. Exp. Psychol. Gen.* 141, 2–18. doi: 10.1037/a0024338

Gravante, G., Russo, G., Pomara, F., and Ridola, C. (2003). Comparison of ground reaction forces between obese and control young adults during quiet standing on a baropodometric platform. *Clin. Biomech. (Bristol Avon)* 18, 780–782. doi: 10.1016/s0268-0033(03)00123-2

Hämäläinen, H., Kekoni, J., Sams, M., Reinikainen, K., and Näätänen, R. (1990). Human somatosensory evoked potentials to mechanical pulses and vibration: contributions of SI and SII somatosensory cortices to P50 and P100 components. *Electroencephalogr. Clin. Neurophysiol.* 75, 13–21. doi: 10.1016/0013-4694(90)90148-d

Hari, R., Reinikainen, K., Kaukoranta, E., Hämäläinen, M., Ilmoniemi, R., Penttinen, A., et al. (1984). Somatosensory evoked cerebral magnetic fields from SI and SII in man. *Electroencephalogr. Clin. Neurophysiol.* 57, 254–263. doi: 10.1016/0013-4694(84)90126-3

Herold, F., Orlowski, K., Börmel, S., and Müller, N. G. (2017). Cortical activation during balancing on a balance board. *Hum. Mov. Sci.* 51, 51–58. doi: 10.1016/j.humov.2016.11.002

Hills, A. P., Hennig, E. M., McDonald, M., and Bar-Or, O. (2001). Plantar pressure differences between obese and non-obese adults: a biomechanical analysis. *Int. J. Obes. Relat. Metab. Disord.* 25, 1674–1679. doi: 10.1038/sj.ijo.0801785

Hsu, J. C. (Ed.) (1996). "Abuses and misconceptions in multiple comparisons," in *Multiple Comparisons: Theory and Methods*, New York, NY: Chapman & Hall. 175–180

Indovina, I., Maffei, V., Bosco, G., Zago, M., Macaluso, E., and Lacquaniti, F. (2005). Representation of visual gravitational motion in the human vestibular cortex. *Science* 308, 416–419. doi: 10.1126/science.1107961

Inglis, J. T., and Macpherson, J. M. (1995). Bilateral labyrinthectomy in the cat: effects on the postural response to translation. *J. Neurophysiol.* 73, 1181–1191.

Jacobs, J. V., Wu, G., and Kelly, K. M. (2015). Evidence for beta corticomuscular coherence during human standing balance: effects of stance width, vision, and support surface. *Neuroscience* 298, 1–11. doi: 10.1016/j.neuroscience.2015.04.009

Jeka, J. J., Schöner, G., Dijkstra, T., Ribeiro, P., and Lackner, J. R. (1997). Coupling of fingertip somatosensory information to head and body sway. *Exp. Brain Res.* 113, 475–483. doi: 10.1007/pl00005600

Lhomond, O., Teasdale, N., Simoneau, M., and Mouchnino, L. (2016). Neural consequences of increasing body weight: evidence from somatosensory evoked potentials and the frequency-specificity of brain oscillations. *Front. Hum. Neurosci.* 10:318. doi: 10.3389/fnhum.2016.00318

MacKinnon, C. D., and Winter, D. A. (1993). Control of whole body balance in the frontal plane during human walking. *J. Biomech.* 26, 633–644. doi: 10.1016/0021-9290(93)90027-c

McIlroy, W. E., Bishop, D. C., Staines, W. R., Nelson, A. J., Maki, B. E., and Brooke, J. D. (2003). Modulation of afferent inflow during the control of balancing tasks using the lower limbs. *Brain Res.* 961, 73–80. doi: 10.1016/s0006-8993(02)03845-3

McPoil, T. G., Cornwall, M. W., Medoff, L., Vicenzino, B., Fosberg, K. K., and Hilz, D. (2009). Arch height change during sit-to-stand: an alternative for the navicular drop test. *J. Foot Ankle Res.* 1:3. doi: 10.1186/1757-1146-2-17

Meyer, P. F., Oddsson, L. I., and De Luca, C. J. (2004). Reduced plantar sensitivity alters postural responses to lateral perturbations of balance. *Exp. Brain Res.* 157, 526–536. doi: 10.1007/s00221-004-1868-3

Mildren, R. L., and Bent, L. R. (2016). Vibrotactile stimulation of fast-adapting cutaneous afferents from the foot modulates proprioception at the ankle joint. *J. Appl. Physiol.* 120, 855–864. doi: 10.3410/f.726107715.793519295

Mildren, R. L., Strzalkowski, N. D., and Bent, L. R. (2016). Foot sole skin vibration perceptual thresholds are elevated in a standing posture compared to sitting. *Gait Posture* 43, 87–92. doi: 10.1016/j.gaitpost.2015.10.027

Miyai, I., Suzuki, M., Hatakenaka, M., and Kubota, K. (2006). Effect of body weight support on cortical activation during gait in patients with stroke. *Exp. Brain Res.* 169, 85–91. doi: 10.1007/s00221-005-0123-x

Morita, H., Petersen, N., and Nielsen, J. (1998). Gating of somatosensory evoked potentials during voluntary movement of the lower limb in man. *Exp. Brain Res.* 120, 143–152. doi: 10.1007/s002210050388

Mouchnino, L., and Blouin, J. (2013). When standing on a moving support, cutaneous inputs provide sufficient information to plan the anticipatory postural adjustments for gait initiation. *PLoS One* 8:e55081. doi: 10.1371/journal.pone.0055081

Mouchnino, L., Fontan, A., Tandonnet, C., Perrier, J., Saradjian, A., Blouin, J., et al. (2015). Facilitation of cutaneous inputs during the planning phase of gait initiation. *J. Neurophysiol.* 114, 301–308. doi: 10.1152/jn.00668.2014

Paillard, T. (2017). Plasticity of the postural function to sport and/or motor experience. *Neurosci. Biobehav. Rev.* 72, 129–152. doi: 10.1016/j.neubiorev.2016.11.015

Papaxanthis, C., Pozzo, T., Kasprinski, R., and Berthoz, A. (2003). Comparison of actual and imagined execution of whole-body movements after a long exposure to microgravity. *Neurosci. Lett.* 339, 41–44. doi: 10.1016/s0304-3940(02)01472-6

Ritzmann, R., Freyler, K., Weltin, E., Krause, A., and Gollhofer, A. (2015). Load dependency of postural control-kinematic and neuromuscular changes in response to over and under load conditions. *PLoS One* 10:e0128400. doi: 10.1371/journal.pone.0128400

Ruget, H., Blouin, J., Teasdale, N., and Mouchnino, L. (2008). Can prepared anticipatory postural adjustments be updated by proprioception? *Neuroscience* 155, 640–648. doi: 10.1016/j.neuroscience.2008.06.021

Sainton, P., Nicol, C., Cabri, J., Barthelemy-Montfort, J., Berton, E., and Chavet, P. (2015). Influence of short-term unweighting and reloading on running kinetics and muscle activity. *Eur. J. Appl. Physiol* 115, 1135–1145. doi: 10.1007/s00421-014-3095-3

Salinas, E., Hernandez, A., Zainos, A., and Romo, R. (2000). Periodicity and firing rate as candidate neural codes for the frequency of vibrotactile stimuli. *J. Neurosci.* 20, 5503–5515.

Sayenko, D. G., Vette, A. H., Obata, H., Alekhina, M. I., Akai, M., and Nakazawa, K. (2009). Differential effects of plantar cutaneous afferent excitation on soleus stretch and H-reflex. *Muscle Nerve* 39, 761–769. doi: 10.1002/mus.21254

Seki, K., and Fetz, E. E. (2012). Gating of sensory input at spinal and cortical levels during preparation and execution of voluntary movement. *J. Neurosci.* 32, 890–902. doi: 10.1523/JNEUROSCI.4958-11.2012

Staines, W. R., Brooke, J. D., Cheng, J., Misiaszek, J. E., and MacKay, W. A. (1997). Movement-induced gain modulation of somatosensory potentials and soleus H-reflexes evoked from the leg. I. Kinaesthetic task demands. *Exp. Brain Res.* 115, 147–155. doi: 10.1007/pl00005674

Stapley, P. J., Ting, L. H., Hulliger, M., and Macpherson, J. M. (2002). Automatic postural responses are delayed by pyridoxine-induced somatosensory loss. *J. Neurosci.* 22, 5803–5807.

Vela, S. A., Lavery, L. A., Armstrong, D. G., and Anaim, A. A. (1998). The effect of increased weight on peak pressures: implications for obesity and diabetic foot pathology. *J. Foot Ankle Surg.* 37, 416–420; discussion 448–449. doi: 10.1016/s1067-2516(98)80051-3

Voisin, J. I., Mercier, C., Jackson, P. L., Richards, C. L., and Malouin, F. (2011). Is somatosensory excitability more affected by the perspective or modality content of motor imagery? *Neurosci. Lett.* 493, 33–37. doi: 10.1016/j.neulet.2011.02.015

Weerakkody, N. S., Mahns, D. A., Taylor, J. L., and Gandevia, S. C. (2007). Impairment of human proprioception by high-frequency cutaneous vibration. *J. Physiol.* 581, 971–980. doi: 10.1113/jphysiol.2006.126854

Wright, W. G., Ivanenko, Y. P., and Gurfinkel, V. S. (2012). Foot aatomy specialization for postural sensation and control. *J. Neurophysiol.* 107, 1513–1521. doi: 10.1152/jn.00256.2011

16

Influence of Lumbar Muscle Fatigue on Trunk Adaptations during Sudden External Perturbations

Jacques Abboud [1]*, François Nougarou [2], Arnaud Lardon [3,4], Claude Dugas [4]
and Martin Descarreaux [4]

[1] Département d'Anatomie, Université du Québec à Trois-Rivières, Trois-Rivières, QC, Canada, [2] Département de Génie Électrique, Université du Québec à Trois-Rivières, Trois-Rivières, QC, Canada, [3] Institut Franco-Européen de Chiropraxie, Ivry-Sur-Seine, France, [4] Département des Sciences de l'Activité Physique, Université du Québec à Trois-Rivières, Trois-Rivières, QC, Canada

*Correspondence:
Jacques Abboud
jacques.abboud@uqtr.ca

Introduction: When the spine is subjected to perturbations, neuromuscular responses such as reflex muscle contractions contribute to the overall balance control and spinal stabilization mechanisms. These responses are influenced by muscle fatigue, which has been shown to trigger changes in muscle recruitment patterns. Neuromuscular adaptations, e.g., attenuation of reflex activation and/or postural oscillations following repeated unexpected external perturbations, have also been described. However, the characterization of these adaptations still remains unclear. Using high-density electromyography (EMG) may help understand how the nervous system chooses to deal with an unknown perturbation in different physiological and/or mechanical perturbation environments.

Aim: To characterize trunk neuromuscular adaptations following repeated sudden external perturbations after a back muscle fatigue task using high-density EMG.

Methods: Twenty-five healthy participants experienced a series of 15 sudden external perturbations before and after back muscle fatigue. Erector spinae muscle activity was recorded using high-density EMG. Trunk kinematics during perturbation trials were collected using a 3-D motion analysis system. A two-way repeated measure ANOVA was conducted to assess: (1) the adaptation effect across trials; (2) the fatigue effect; and (3) the interaction effect (fatigue × adaptation) for the baseline activity, the reflex latency, the reflex peak and trunk kinematic variables (flexion angle, velocity and time to peak velocity). Muscle activity spatial distribution before and following the fatigue task was also compared using *t*-tests for dependent samples.

Results: An attenuation of muscle reflex peak was observed across perturbation trials before the fatigue task, but not after. The spatial distribution of muscle activity was significantly higher before the fatigue task compared to post-fatigue trials. Baseline activity showed a trend to higher values after muscle fatigue, as well as reduction through perturbation trials. Main effects of fatigue and adaptation were found for time to peak velocity. No adaptation nor fatigue effect were identified for reflex latency, flexion angle or trunk velocity.

Conclusion: The results show that muscle fatigue leads to reduced spatial distribution of back muscle activity and suggest a limited ability to use across-trial redundancy to adapt EMG reflex peak and optimize spinal stabilization using retroactive control.

Keywords: high-density electromyography, spinal stability, muscle fatigue, reflex, habituation

INTRODUCTION

Over the past years, several studies have shown that neuromuscular adaptations are observed under the influence of back muscle fatigue (Allison and Henry, 2001; Boyas and Guével, 2011; Monjo et al., 2015). Indeed, some authors have reported that a reorganization of motor strategies is used to prevent the onset of muscle fatigue (Fuller et al., 2011) and that such adaptations in muscle activity recruitment patterns are present, such as co-contraction phenomena (Allison and Henry, 2001), or within muscle changes in recruitment patterns, suggesting a spatial dependency in the control of motor units in the erector spinae (Tucker et al., 2009; Abboud et al., 2014). These neuromuscular adaptations have been also reported when participants are asked to perform a voluntary perturbation, such as goal-directed movements. Previous studies have shown that, in the presence of muscle fatigue, compensatory neuromuscular adaptations occur in order to maintain the task requirement (Côté et al., 2002; Missenard et al., 2009). Such neuromuscular strategies are part of the feedforward control, which allows the central nervous system to predict the muscle activation needed to achieve a desired motor task (Shadmehr and Mussa-Ivaldi, 1994). On the other hand, when subjected to unpredictable perturbations, neither feedback, nor anticipation strategies are sufficient to adjust movement on-line. Determining the influence of muscle fatigue during an unpredictable perturbation is therefore of great interest.

More specifically, this study focusses on understanding neuromuscular adaptations to unexpected trunk perturbation, which are believed to affect spinal stability. In everyday life, the human body is constantly under the influence of mechanical forces applied in different directions, sometimes unexpected and continuously triggering postural adjustments. Examples of such spinal perturbations can be drawn from various common activities such as sport contacts, tripping, slipping, weight lifting, etc. Panjabi (1992) described spinal stability as a complex mechanism involving three essential components: spinal muscles, passive spinal tissues and neuromuscular control (Panjabi, 1992). Alterations, such as physiological and/or mechanical ones, of one or more of these components have been shown to be a direct or indirect manifestation of spinal instability.

Despite the number of studies that have investigated fatigue and unexpected loading effects on spinal stability, results vary from one study to the other (Granata et al., 2001, 2004; Chow et al., 2004; Herrmann et al., 2006; Mawston et al., 2007; Grondin and Potvin, 2009; Dupeyron et al., 2010; Sánchez-Zuriaga et al., 2010). Such differences could be partly due to methodological choices in trunk perturbation experimental protocols, such as participant positions (standing vs. sitting), familiarization

of the external perturbation, perturbation magnitudes, etc. Furthermore, variables selected to assess neuromuscular responses to a sudden trunk perturbation are far from consistent across studies. The most common variables used to assess the effect of unexpected trunk loading under muscle fatigue are baseline muscle activity, reflex latency and reflex amplitude. In a context of unexpected trunk perturbation, current evidence shows inconsistencies in baseline activity responses under the influence of muscle fatigue (Granata et al., 2001, 2004; Herrmann et al., 2006; Mawston et al., 2007; Grondin and Potvin, 2009; Dupeyron et al., 2010) with studies showing no adaptation after a back fatigue task (Herrmann et al., 2006; Mawston et al., 2007; Dupeyron et al., 2010), while other ones reveal an increase in baseline activity with muscle fatigue (Granata et al., 2001, 2004; Grondin and Potvin, 2009). On the other hand, most studies investigating neuromuscular responses following an unexpected trunk perturbation showed that reflex latency is not affected by the presence of low back muscle fatigue (Granata et al., 2004; Herrmann et al., 2006; Dupeyron et al., 2010; Sánchez-Zuriaga et al., 2010). As for the reflex amplitude of low back muscles, it was found not to be affected by muscle fatigue in several studies (Granata et al., 2004; Grondin and Potvin, 2009; Sánchez-Zuriaga et al., 2010), whereas few studies found a higher back reflex amplitude following a fatigue protocol (Herrmann et al., 2006; Dupeyron et al., 2010). Overall, the effect of muscle fatigue on neuromuscular adaptations during unexpected loading remains unclear.

Inconsistencies reported in the literature regarding neuromuscular responses under muscle fatigue during unexpected perturbation could also be explained by the fact that most of the studies have been limited by the amplitude and frequency behavior because of the use of classic bipolar electromyography (EMG), which covers only a small portion of the explored muscle. Recent technologies, such as high-density surface EMG (sEMG), because it can cover a large surface area, offer a unique perspective on muscle activity spatial distribution (Zwarts and Stegeman, 2003; Merletti et al., 2008; Holobar et al., 2009; Martinez-Valdes et al., 2016). Indeed, data extracted from high-density sEMG have enabled the mapping of muscle activity recruitment distribution in the low back region during a voluntary contraction. Results have revealed a shift in muscle activity spatial distribution to the lateral-caudal direction in the low back region during muscle fatigue (Tucker et al., 2009). This migration in muscle activity distribution could be associated with changes in muscle fiber recruitment to avoid overloading of the same fibers (Rantanen et al., 1994). Adopting non-uniform muscle activity recruitment may help participants develop motor strategies and facilitate adaptation to different physiological and/or mechanical perturbations of the spine. Low back muscle activity measured by high-density sEMG has also been shown to discriminate patients with chronic low back pain from healthy individuals through different motor tasks (Abboud et al., 2014; Falla et al., 2014). To our knowledge, no study has investigated muscle activity reflex variables with high-density sEMG.

Reflex muscle activity has also been studied following a series of unexpected external perturbations. The first research exploring this question was conducted by Nashner (1976), who showed that neuromuscular adaptations, such as the attenuation of lower limb muscle reflex activation, occur following repeated ankle dorsiflexion to improve postural balance. More recently, similar results have been reported in presence of several unexpected external perturbations of the cervical region (Blouin et al., 2003; Siegmund et al., 2003). A reduction of neck muscle activity was observed across perturbation trials (Blouin et al., 2003; Siegmund et al., 2003). Back muscles seem to follow a similar response pattern during unexpected forward perturbation. Skotte et al. (2004) showed a reduction of the average erector spinae EMG amplitude from the first trial to the next one. A more recent study reported similar results in paraspinal muscle responses to a series of unexpected tilts from a surface platform (Oude Nijhuis et al., 2010). The authors observed that EMG amplitude responses adapted rapidly between the first two trials, whereas adaptation was more gradual over the next trials (Oude Nijhuis et al., 2010). Based on these results, it could be suggested that, whenever possible, the central nervous system attempts to minimize unnecessary or excessive responses to perturbation.

Moreover, adaptations throughout repetitions of the same perturbation have been previously shown to compensate for the effect of muscle fatigue (Takahashi et al., 2006; Kennedy et al., 2012). Such compensations were indeed observed following upper limb and ankle muscle fatigue when movement accuracy and postural stability were respectively maintained (Takahashi et al., 2006; Kennedy et al., 2012). However, in the study of Kennedy et al. (2012), the authors did not assess adaptation across repeated perturbation trials. Participants had to perform few perturbation trials to allow habituation to perturbations, to limit changes caused by habituation to the motor task. On the other hand, Takahashi et al. (2006) studied adaptation across perturbation trials. The unexpected perturbation was applied while participants reached to a target and results showed that even when participants were in a state of fatigue, they were still able to reach the target and adapt to perturbations.

The assessment of neuromuscular adaptations when the patients are submitted to the same perturbation during a rehabilitation protocols could be used to monitor progress and adaptations. As suggested by Hodges and Tucker (2011), adaptations to pain have immediate and short term benefit for the spinal system. They may, however, have detrimental long-term consequences and should therefore be monitored and perhaps treated in rehabilitation. The aim of the present study was to characterize trunk neuromuscular adaptations in response to a sudden external perturbation after a back fatigue task. Its second aim was to identify if trunk neuromuscular

control can be modulated by a previous instability experience in the presence of back muscle fatigue using high-density sEMG. Based on current evidence, it was hypothesized that back muscle fatigue would alter trial-to-trial neuromuscular adaptions during a series of repeated sudden external perturbations. Moreover, it was hypothesized that trial-to-trial neuromuscular adaptations would lead to a migration of muscle activity within the erector spinae, and that this spatial muscle activity migration would be limited in the presence of muscle fatigue.

MATERIALS AND METHODS

Recruitment
Twenty-five healthy adult participants (22 men and 3 women) were recruited from the university community. Participants with one of the following criteria were excluded: history of acute/chronic thoracic or low back pain in the past 6 months, ankylosing spondylitis, trunk neuromuscular disease, inflammatory arthritis, scoliosis ($\geq 15°$), and previous spinal surgery. Participant mean (M) age, height, weight and BMI were respectively 26.8 (standard deviation (SD) = 5.5) years, $M = 1.76$ ($SD = 0.7$) m, $M = 76.6$ ($SD = 12.1$) kg and $M = 24.5$ ($SD = 3.1$) kg/m^2. The project received approval from the university's ethics committee for research with humans (Comité d'éthique de la recherche avec des êtres humains). All participants gave their written informed consent prior to their participation in this study.

Experimental Protocol
First, EMG electrodes and light-emitting diodes from the 3-D motion analysis system were installed over the participants. The experimentation protocol was divided in three phases: pre-fatigue perturbations, fatigue protocol and post-fatigue perturbations. Before the first phase, two or three isometric trunk flexion maximal voluntary contractions (MVC) were performed, as well as two or three isometric maximal contractions in trunk extension. The third trial of MVC was only performed if the participants' second MVC was superior to the first one. MVC was assessed in a semi-seated position on a modified ergonomic back chair custom-built for the study (**Figure 1**). For the trunk flexion MVC, participants were asked to pull anteriorly against a cable. Their trunk was attached at T8 level to a load cell (Model LSB350; Futek Advanced Sensor Technology Inc., Irvine, CA, USA) with a cable using a pulley system. As for trunk extension MVC, participants were asked to pull posteriorly against the cable. Since no warm up exercise was provided, participants were invited to perform some trunk extension and flexion contractions before the MVC protocol. The goal of these contractions was to help participants familiarize with the MVC protocol.

The first phase of the protocol, pre-fatigue perturbations, consisted in a series of 15 sudden external perturbations. Participants were asked to adopt the same position as the one used during the MVC protocol (**Figure 1**). Their trunk was attached to a perturbation trigger with a cable using a pulley

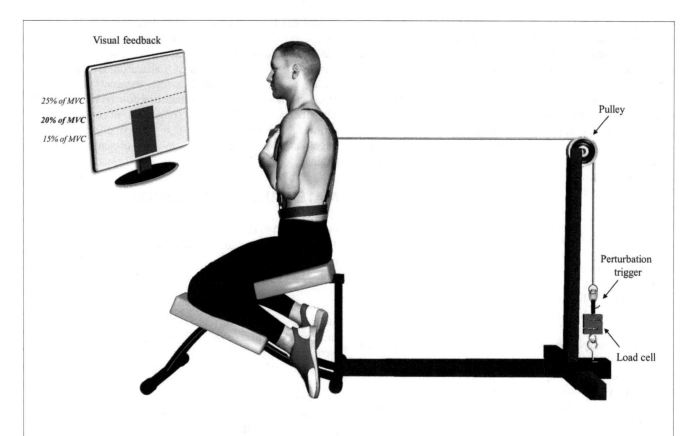

FIGURE 1 | Illustration of the perturbation protocol. Participants were positioned in a semi-seated position with their trunk attached to a manual trigger by a cable using a pulley system. A visual feedback was provided using a screen indicating the target of 20% of their trunk flexion maximal voluntary contraction.

system. This set-up was designed to generate a posterior to anterior perturbation of the trunk. The trigger was connected to a load cell (Model LSB350; Futek Advanced Sensor Technology Inc., Irvine, CA, USA) to objectively measure the pulling trunk flexion force exerted by participants. Participants were asked to maintain a pulling force corresponding to 20% of their trunk flexion MVC and to return to the neutral equilibrium position as quickly as possible after the perturbation. The perturbation magnitude corresponded on average to 55N, ranging from 37N to 76N across participants, which is similar to the perturbation magnitude used in similar perturbation protocols (Radebold et al., 2000; Reeves et al., 2005). The higher value of trunk flexion MVC was used to determine the target force for the perturbation protocol. To help participants reach and stabilize their pulling target force, a visual feedback was provided using a screen indicating real time traction (**Figure 1**). Once the force was stabilized, one of the assessors triggered the perturbation after 1, 3 or 5 s according to a random sequence. The perturbation sequences were different for each participant and each condition (pre- and post-fatigue) to avoid any anticipation of the perturbation onset.

Following the first phase, the fatigue task consisted of a modified version of the Sorensen endurance test (Champagne et al., 2009). Participants were asked to lay in a prone position on a 45° Roman chair, with the iliac crests aligned with the chair cushion edge. In order to quickly induce muscular fatigue, participants had to lift a 12.5-kg weight plate during the task, and hold it as close as possible to their chest. The participants' trunk was maintained unsupported in a horizontal position relative to the ground for as long as possible. The investigators gave similar verbal encouragement to all subjects. Perceived effort scale (6–20; Borg, 1982), measuring the intensity of the fatigue task, was rated by each participant at the end of the fatigue test. Before and after the fatigue protocol, an MVC protocol was performed in the same position as the fatigue task; a belt was fixed to the ground and installed over the participants' shoulders and they were asked to perform a maximal trunk extension contraction against the belt.

The last phase of the experimentation, post-fatigue perturbations, was performed immediately after the fatigue protocol. To avoid the attenuation of muscle fatigue effects, the transition between the fatigue protocol and the second series of perturbation was made as quickly as possible. The time needed between the end of the fatigue protocol and the acquisition of the data ranged from 2 min to 4 min. In this last phase, participants were submitted to 15 more perturbations, identical to the ones received before the fatigue protocol. This part of the experiment lasted no more than 8 min. The total duration of the last phase of the experimentation ranged from 10 min to 12 min.

Data Acquisition

Two different EMG acquisition systems were used to record trunk muscle activity. sEMG of the right and left erector spinae muscles was recorded using two adhesive matrices of 64 electrodes (model ELSCH064; LISiN-OT Bioelettronica; Torino, Italy). The array grid consisted of 64 electrodes placed in an 8 × 8 matrix (10 mm inter-electrode distance). The center of each grid was located at L3 level, and one bracelet ground electrode was placed on the right wrist. The bipolar EMG signals were amplified (64-channel sEMG amplifier, SEA 64, LISiN-OT Bioelettronica; Torino, Italy; −3 dB bandwidths 10–500 Hz) by a factor of 5000 during the perturbations' protocol, while a 2000 factor was applied during the fatigue protocol. The signal was sampled at 2048 Hz and converted to digital form by a 12-bit A/D converter. Rectus abdominis and external obliquus abdominis muscle activity were recorded using a differential Ag sEMG sensor with a common mode rejection ratio of 92 dB at 60 Hz, a noise level of 1.2 µV, a gain of 10 V/V ± 1%, a bandwidth of 20–450 ± 10% (Model DE2.1, Delsys Inc., Boston, MA, USA), amplified by a factor 10,000 and sampled at 2048 Hz with a 12-bit A/D converter (PCI 6024E, National Instruments, Austin, TX, USA). Each bipolar signal was digitally band-pass filtered in the frequency bandwidth-30-450 Hz (2nd order Butterworth filter). Notch filters were also applied to eliminate the 60 Hz and 100 Hz power line interference and its harmonics. To avoid inter-rater variability, anatomical structures palpation and placement of electrodes were assessed by the same investigator for all participants. The electrode position for rectus abdominis and external obliquus was located over the midsection of the muscle and parallel to the fibers orientation, as described by Criswell and Cram (2011). Before the application of an electrode, skin impedance was reduced by shaving body hair, gently exfoliating the skin with fine-grade sandpaper (Red DotTrace Prep, 3 M; St. Paul, MN, USA) and wiping the skin with alcohol swabs. The data from both EMG acquisition systems were collected using the OT Bioelettronica custom software and processed by Matlab (MathWorks; Natick, MA, USA). Trunk extensor and trunk flexor myoelectric signals from EMG were normalized with respect to the trunk extension and flexion MVC values.

Finally, trunk kinematics during perturbation trials was collected using a 3-D motion analysis system (Optotrak Certus, Northern Digital, Waterloo, ON, Canada). Light-emitting diodes were positioned on the left side of the participants over two anatomical landmarks: (1) L1, (2) T11. A third light-emitting diode was placed on the trigger perturbation. Data were sampled at 100 Hz and low-pass filtered by a dual-pass, fourth-order Butterworth filter with a cut-off frequency of 5 Hz. EMG data and kinematic data were synchronized through a signal triggered by OT Bioelettronica software and Matlab (MathWorks). Both EMG and kinematics were recorded for 10 s.

Data Analysis

From high-density sEMG signals, in order to confirm the presence of erector spinae muscle fatigue, the mean normalized slope of the median frequency (MDF; mean of the 64 electrodes of each matrix) was calculated from adjacent non-overlapping signal epochs of 0.5 s. Moreover, the percentage of EMG amplitude root mean square (RMS) diminution between the MVC pre-fatigue and MVC post-fatigue was calculated. Finally, four variables were extracted: the baseline activity, the reflex latency, the reflex peak and the area of muscle activity spatial distribution. Left and right erector spinae muscles were analyzed separately. From abdominal EMG signals, reflex activity was also computed. For all variables, reflex responses latencies superior to 300-ms from the perturbation onset were not analyzed to avoid inclusion of any voluntary responses.

Baseline Activity

Erector spinae baseline activity was quantified as the mean EMG amplitude RMS using a 500-ms window prior to the onset of the perturbation. The mean of all electrodes for each high-density sEMG (left and right) was calculated.

Reflex Latency

Reflex latency of erector spinae muscles was defined as the time delay from the perturbation onset to the EMG reflex onset. To calculate the reflex onset, EMG signals were Butterworth filtered (sixth-order, 50 Hz cut-off frequency) and assessed using a sliding window of 25-ms (Larivière et al., 2010). Muscle activity onset was then determined when the EMG signals exceeded three SD (Hodges and Bui, 1996) above the mean baseline EMG amplitude, which was calculated from a 1-s window before the perturbation onset (**Figure 2**). Reflex latency was also identified by a visual inspection of the EMG recordings by the same investigator. The reflex onset was defined as the beginning of the first peak EMG post perturbation that exceeded approximately two times the mean baseline activity. Due to the high number of electrodes, visual detection technique was only applied on four electrodes by trials. Mean of these four reflex latencies were used during subsequent statistical analyses.

Reflex Peak

The reflex peak corresponded to the highest RMS value following perturbation onset. Reflex peak had to be present in a 300-ms window following the perturbation onset to be considered a reflex response (**Figure 2**).

Area of Reflex Activity Spatial Distribution

To characterize reflex activity, spatial distribution of the dispersion variable representing the muscle activity range of displacement (centroid) was extracted from the bipolar EMG signals. As described in our previous study (Abboud et al., 2014), the centroid was defined as the mean RMS of all 64 electrodes of each high-density EMG. Specifically, the centroid value from each EMG signal was obtained by calculating the mean of RMS value from a window of 100-ms, divided equally (50-ms) on either side of the reflex peak. This operation was repeated through the 15 sudden perturbation trials pre- and post-fatigue protocol to produce dispersion values (see **Figure 3** for more details). The dispersion of erector spinae muscles has been shown to be highly reliable (Abboud et al., 2015).

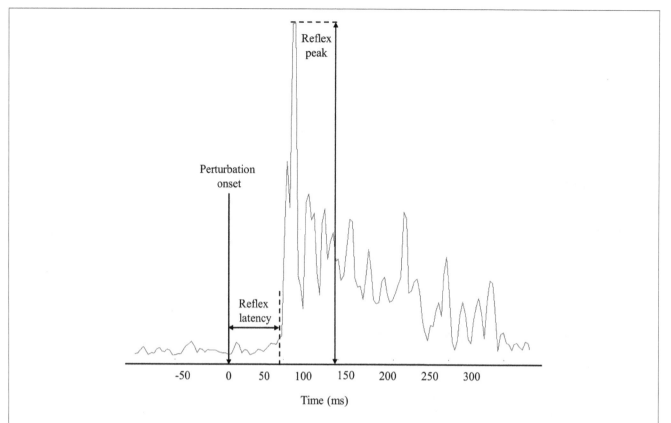

FIGURE 2 | Representation of muscle reflex variables extracted from one high-density electromyography (EMG) electrode during one perturbation trial.

Abdominal Reflex Activity

Since reflex activity in the rectus abdominis and external obliquus rarely occurred after the perturbation, mean RMS values of the abdominal muscles were computed based on the same window of 100-ms used for erector spinae signal analyses. Since no difference was identified between left and right sides, mean values of left and right rectus abdominis as well as mean values of left and right external obliquus were used for the analyses.

Trunk Kinematic

Trunk kinematics were analyzed using the two adjacent LED to create a vector. Lumbar spine motion was obtained by calculating the trunk flexion angle between the T11-L1 vector and a horizontal vector relative to the ground. The angle values corresponded to the range of motion between the starting position before the perturbation, and the maximal trunk flexion following perturbation onset. From the trunk flexion angle, peak velocity and time to peak velocity were calculated. The third kinematic LED was used to determine the exact moment when the perturbation started.

Statistical Analysis

Normality of distribution for every dependent variable was assessed using the Kolmogorov—Smirnov test, in addition to visual inspection of the data. Student t-tests for dependent samples used to compare EMG amplitude RMS between

MVC pre- and post-fatigue. Student t-tests for dependent samples were also used to compare muscle activity spatial distribution before and following the fatigue task. The first trial pre-fatigue was also compared to the first trial post-fatigue for each dependent variables using t-tests for dependent samples. A mixed model two-way repeated measure ANOVA was conducted to assess: (1) the adaptation effect across trials; (2) the fatigue effect; and (3) the interaction effect (fatigue × adaptation) for each dependent variable (baseline activity, reflex latency, reflex peak, abdominal reflex activity and trunk kinematic). For the variables: baseline, reflex latency, reflex peak and kinematic variables, the means of the first and last five perturbation trials before and after fatigue were considered for the two-way repeated measures ANOVA. When necessary, the Tukey *post hoc* test was performed for pair-wise comparisons. Repeated measures ANOVA followed by quadratic polynomial contrast trend analyses were also conducted for reflex peak values to assess adaptation across perturbation trials before and after muscle fatigue. The reliability of the reflex latency values were estimated by the intraclass correlation (ICC, type 3,1). $ICC_{3,1}$ evaluated inter-rater reliability, using the Matlab software (MathWorks; Natick, MA, USA) representing one rater and visual detection the other one. The standard error of measurement (SEM) was also assessed using the formula $SEM = SD * \sqrt{1 - ICC}$. For all statistical analyses, $p < 0.05$ was considered to be statistically significant.

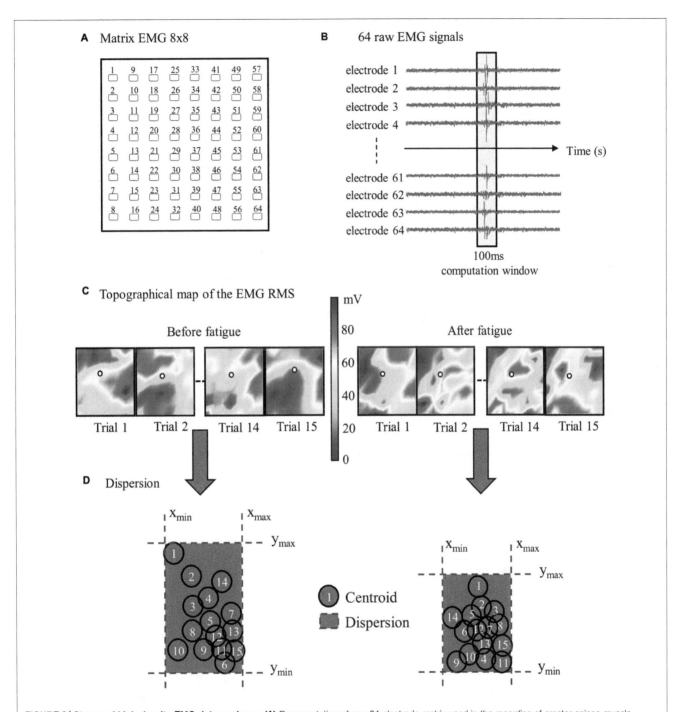

FIGURE 3 | Stages of high-density EMG data analyses. (A) Representation of one 64-electrode matrix used in the recording of erector spinae muscle activity. **(B)** Myoelectric signals from 64 electrodes of one matrix in a random healthy participant during one perturbation trial. **(C)** Centroid migration from topographical representation of root mean square (RMS) reflex values computed within 100 ms windows at each trial. Note the difference between muscle activity recruitment pattern (color variation) between pre- and post-fatigue. **(D)** Dispersion representation from the 15 centroid position before and after the fatigue protocol.

RESULTS

From the 25 original participants, one participant was excluded from all analyses due to the impossibility of identifying the beginning of the perturbation. Moreover, 2% of all perturbation trials from high-density sEMG were not considered for the analyses due to the absence of a reflex response. As for abdominal muscle reflex activity analyses, three participants were excluded due to the poor quality of EMG signals.

Presence of Low Back Muscle Fatigue

The mean endurance time of the fatigue protocol was 125 s ($SD = 39.4$). During the fatigue protocol, a negative slope of MDF values was observed. MDF slope values were -0.184 ($SD = 0.09$) on the right side and -0.165 ($SD = 0.09$) on the left side of the erector spinae. As expected, a significant reduction of EMG amplitude RMS was found between MVC pre- and post-fatigue on the right side of the erector spinae ($p \leq 0.001$) and on the left side ($p \leq 0.001$). Moreover, reductions of EMG amplitude RMS of 28% and 24% on the right and left side, respectively, were found. The perceived effort mean score was 17.6 ($SD = 1.7$), which corresponds to the "very hard" level of perceived effort on the Borg scale. Such level is described as the highest level of activity you can sustain (Borg, 1982).

First Perturbation Trial

In most of cases, the first perturbation trial response pre- and post-fatigue was not affected by the presence of muscle fatigue. Dependent t-tests revealed no significant difference between the first perturbation trial before fatigue and the first perturbation trial after fatigue on both sides of the erector spinae muscles for the baseline activity (right side, $p = 0.55$; left side, $p = 0.14$), the reflex latency (right side, $p = 0.84$; left side, $p = 0.49$), the reflex peak (right side, $p = 0.91$; left side, $p = 0.29$), as well as for the rectus abdominis ($p = 0.41$) and external obliquus ($p = 0.05$) reflex amplitudes. As for the kinematic variables, dependent t-tests revealed no significant difference between the first perturbation trial before fatigue and the first perturbation trial after fatigue for the trunk flexion angle ($p = 0.78$) and the peak velocity ($p = 0.46$), while a significant decrease between the first perturbation trial before fatigue and the first perturbation trial after fatigue was found for time to peak velocity ($p = 0.007$).

Trunk Kinematic

Most of the trunk kinematic variables did not change with the presence of muscle fatigue and did not adapt over perturbation trials. Only the time to peak velocity were found to be altered. The mixed model repeated measure ANOVA revealed no significant adaptation effect across trials ($F_{(1,23)} = 1.06$, $p = 0.31$) nor a main effect of fatigue ($F_{(1,23)} = 0.22$, $p = 0.64$) for the trunk flexion angle. As for peak velocity, the analyses showed no main effect of fatigue ($F_{(1,23)} = 0.72$, $p = 0.41$) and no adaptation effect ($F_{(1,23)} = 3.56$, $p = 0.07$). Results from the mixed model repeated measure ANOVA also showed a main effect of fatigue for time to peak velocity, with a longer time to peak velocity before the fatigue task ($F_{(1,23)} = 27.25$, $p \leq 0.001$). Additionally, a significant reduction of time to peak velocity was found, representing a main effect of adaptation across trials ($F_{(1,23)} = 7.01$, $p = 0.01$; see **Table 1** for mean and SD values).

Baseline Activity

Small changes were observed in baseline activity after the muscle fatigue protocol as well as over the perturbation trials. The analyses yielded a main effect of fatigue for baseline activity with a higher baseline value after the fatigue task on the left side ($F_{(1,23)} = 5.18$, $p = 0.03$), but not on the right side ($F_{(1,23)} = 1.90$, $p = 0.18$). Similarly, a significant main effect of adaptation, represented by a reduction of baseline activity through the perturbation trials, was observed on the left side ($F_{(1,23)} = 6.63$, $p = 0.02$), but not on the right side ($F_{(1,23)} = 0.33$, $p = 0.57$; see **Table 1** for mean and SD values).

Reflex Latency

Erector spinae reflex latency remained unchanged with or without muscle fatigue and over the perturbation trials. The mixed model repeated measure ANOVA showed no significant

TABLE 1 | Mean values SD of the first and last five perturbation trials before and after the fatigue protocol (maximal voluntary contraction, MVC; L, left side of the erector spinae; R, right side of the erector spinae).

			First five trials mean	Last five trials mean	p*	
					Fatigue	Adaptation
Flexion angle (°)		Pre-fatigue	6.2 (4.0)	5.9 (4.1)	$p = 0.64$	$p = 0.31$
		Post-fatigue	6.0 (3.9)	5.8 (3.4)		
Peak velocity (°/s)		Pre-fatigue	21.3 (10.8)	19.5 (9.4)	$p = 0.41$	$p = 0.07$
		Post-fatigue	21.8 (10.8)	20.5 (7.1)		
Time to peak velocity (ms)		Pre-fatigue	238 (86)	217 (86)	$p \leq 0.001$	$p = 0.01$
		Post-fatigue	205 (67)	187 (79)		
Baseline (% MVC)	L	Pre-fatigue	8.2 (4.1)	7.6 (3.9)	$p = 0.03$	$p = 0.02$
		Post-fatigue	9.6 (5.1)	9.1 (4.6)		
	R	Pre-fatigue	9.9 (5.2)	9.6 (5.6)	$p = 0.18$	$p = 0.57$
		Post-fatigue	10.7 (6.1)	10.6 (5.7)		
Reflex latency (ms)	L	Pre-fatigue	94.3 (31.9)	89.3 (32.5)	$p = 0.19$	$p = 0.08$
		Post-fatigue	102.1 (39.2)	96.1 (42.4)		
	R	Pre-fatigue	93.8 (29.5)	98.2 (44.8)	$p = 0.75$	$p = 0.25$
		Post-fatigue	95.9 (39.1)	97.9 (36.7)		
Reflex peak (% MVC)	L	Pre-fatigue	60.1 (26.7)	49.5 (23.9)	$p = 0.38$	$p \leq 0.001$
		Post-fatigue	60.4 (26.9)	54.4 (24.4)		
	R	Pre-fatigue	66.7 (25.6)	52.5 (17.6)	$p = 0.02$	$p \leq 0.001$
		Post-fatigue	70.2 (27.9)	65.4 (25.1)		

*p based on the repeated measures ANOVA.

main effect of fatigue on both sides of the erector spinae (for the right side ($F_{(1,23)} = 0.11$, $p = 0.75$); for the left side ($F_{(1,23)} = 1.80$, $p = 0.19$). No significant adaptation effect was observed on either sides (for the right side ($F_{(1,23)} = 1.41$, $p = 0.25$); for the left side ($F_{(1,23)} = 3.34$, $p = 0.08$; see **Table 1** for mean and SD values). The ICC obtained for reflex latency values was moderate ($ICC_{3,1} = 0.63$, 95% CI = 0.31–082) and the SEM was small (SEM = 0.016).

Reflex Peak

Following the muscle fatigue task, erector spinae reflex peak value was increased, while adaptations over perturbation trials were altered. Results from the mixed model repeated measure ANOVA showed a main effect of fatigue for reflex peak with a higher peak value after the fatigue task on the right side ($F_{(1,23)} = 6.47$, $p = 0.02$), but not on the left side ($F_{(1,23)} = 0.80$, $p = 0.38$). Moreover, a significant main effect of adaptation, represented by a reduction of reflex peak amplitude through the perturbation trials, was observed on the right side ($F_{(1,23)} = 19.55$, $p \leq 0.001$), and on the left side ($F_{(1,23)} = 19.70$, $p \leq 0.001$). The analyses also showed a significant fatigue × adaptation interaction effect on the right side ($F_{(1,23)} = 7.68$, $p = 0.011$); a similar tendency, although not significant, was observed on the left side ($F_{(1,23)} = 3.16$, $p = 0.089$; see **Table 1** for mean and SD values). As illustrated in **Figure 4**, *post hoc* analyses revealed higher reflex peak values in the first perturbation trials vs. the last ones in the condition pre-fatigue, but not under the influence of muscle fatigue ($p \leq 0.001$). Moreover, a significant higher peak

reflex value was found in the last perturbation trials after vs. before fatigue protocol ($p \leq 0.001$).

Since the first trial reaction is known to have a higher impact on postural balance (Allum et al., 2011), all these analyses were performed a second time without taking into account the first trial before and after the fatigue protocol. This procedure was conducted to explore whether or not the reflex peak attenuation observed over perturbation trials was only due to the first trial. Once again, results from the repeated measure ANOVA showed a main effect of fatigue for reflex peak with a higher peak value after the fatigue task on the right side ($F_{(1,23)} = 8.35$, $p = 0.008$; **Figure 5**), but not on the left side ($F_{(1,23)} = 2.02$, $p = 0.17$). A significant main effect of adaptation was also observed on the right side ($F_{(1,23)} = 6.99$, $p = 0.015$), and on the left side ($F_{(1,23)} = 9.66$, $p = 0.005$). The analyses also showed a significant fatigue × adaptation interaction effect on the right side ($F_{(1,23)} = 12.09$, $p = 0.002$), but not on the left side ($F_{(1,23)} = 0.96$, $p = 0.33$). As illustrated in **Figure 4**, *post hoc* analyses showed higher reflex peak values in the first perturbation trials vs. the last ones in the condition pre-fatigue, but not under the influence of muscle fatigue ($p \leq 0.001$). *Post hoc* analyses also revealed that a significant higher peak reflex value was found in the last perturbation trials after the fatigue protocol vs. the last trials performed before muscle fatigue ($p \leq 0.001$).

Polynomial quadratic trend analyses yielded a significant adaptation (decreasing response) before the fatigue protocol on both sides (for the right side $p = 0.01$, contrast estimate of 0.99; for the left side $p = 0.007$, contrast estimate of 1.02), but not under the influence of muscle fatigue (for the right side $p = 0.45$, contrast

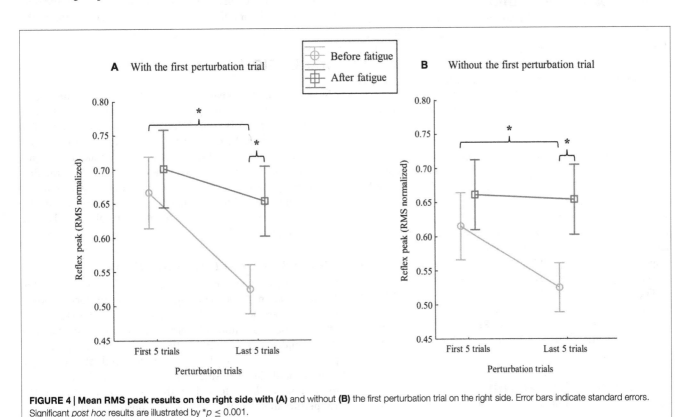

FIGURE 4 | Mean RMS peak results on the right side with (A) and without **(B)** the first perturbation trial on the right side. Error bars indicate standard errors. Significant *post hoc* results are illustrated by *$p \leq 0.001$.

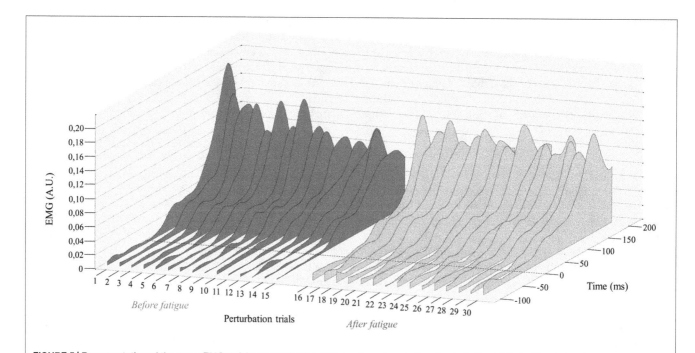

FIGURE 5 | Representation of the mean EMG activity traces for the right erector spinae before (perturbation trials 1–15) and after (perturbation trials 16–30) the fatigue task. The red dotted line represents the perturbation onset. (A.U. Arbitrary Unit).

estimate of 0.35; for the left side $p = 0.26$, contrast estimate of 0.46).

Reflex Spatial Distribution

A higher reflex spatial distribution was observed before the fatigue protocol. Dependent t-tests revealed a significant difference between the protocol before fatigue ($M = 1.13$, $SD = 0.25$) and after ($M = 0.95$, $SD = 0.29$) for the dispersion variable on the left side of the erector spinae ($p = 0.02$). A higher dispersion value, yet not significant ($p = 0.08$), was found on the right side before the fatigue ($M = 1.16$, $SD = 0.34$) when compared to trials performed following fatigue (mean = 1.03, $SD = 0.30$).

Dependent t-tests were repeated a second time without taking into account the first trial before and after the fatigue protocol. Results from the left side also revealed a significant higher value before the muscle fatigue ($M = 1.10$, $SD = 0.22$) compared to the trials following muscle fatigue ($M = 0.93$, $SD = 0.29$; $p = 0.02$). Once again, a higher dispersion value, yet not significant ($p = 0.07$), was found on the right side before the fatigue ($M = 1.12$, $SD = 0.35$) compared to the trials following muscle fatigue ($M = 0.99$, $SD = 0.29$).

Figure 6 provides an illustration of the complex and variable muscle activity distribution pattern during the perturbation trials before and after the fatigue task. Results showed a smaller centroid migration through the perturbation trials after the fatiguing task.

Abdominal Reflex Activity

Results from the repeated measures ANOVA showed a main effect of fatigue for abdominal reflex activity with a decrease

of reflex activity after the fatigue task for the rectus abdominis ($F_{(1,20)} = 8.82$, $p = 0.008$) and the external obliquus ($F_{(1,20)} = 9.50$, $p = 0.006$). Moreover, a significant main effect of adaptation, showing a reduction of abdominal reflex activity, was found only for the rectus abdominis ($F_{(1,20)} = 8.01$, $p = 0.01$), but not for the external obliquus ($F_{(1,20)} = 0.79$, $p = 0.39$).

DISCUSSION

Understanding the neuromuscular responses to unexpected loading of the trunk is highly relevant in view of everyday life and to the investigation of spinal stability and movement control. The present study assessed how erector spinae muscle adapts after a fatigue task fatigue following a series of repeated sudden external perturbations. Using high-density sEMG, this study is the first one showing variability in lower back muscle activity recruitment pattern strategies with a condition perturbing spinal stability. Moreover, this neuromuscular adaptation was altered following back muscle fatigue.

Methodological Considerations

Some fatigue recovery may have occurred over the 15 perturbation trials following the fatigue protocol. Several measures were taken to limit attenuation of muscle fatigue effects. The transition between the fatigue protocol and the second series of perturbation was made as quickly as possible. The time needed between the end of the fatigue protocol and the acquisition of the data ranged from 2 min to 4 min, while it took less than 8 min to conduct the 15 perturbation trials. A study demonstrated that recovery from back muscle fatigue occurs after approximately

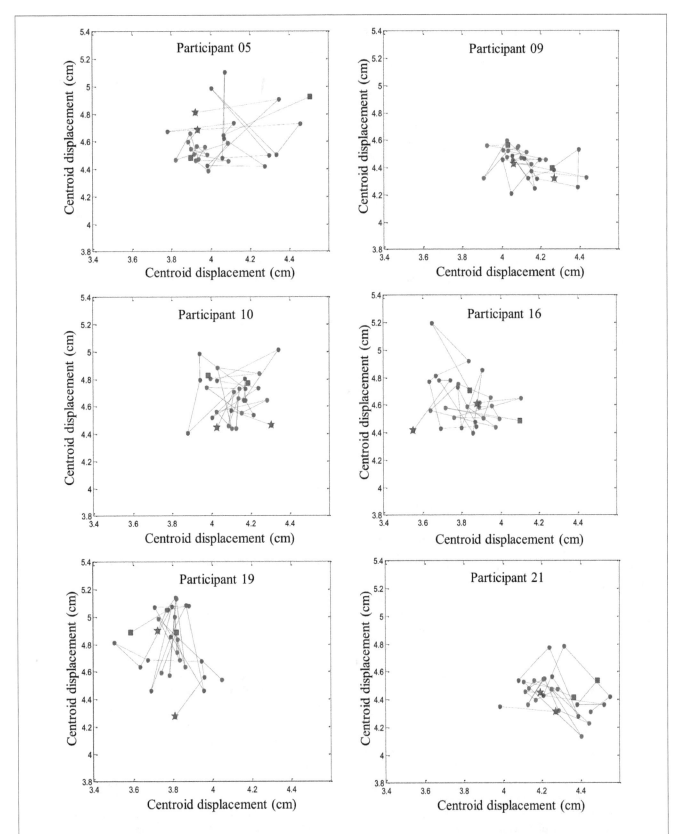

FIGURE 6 | Representation of six random participants' centroid displacement between perturbation trials on the right erector spinae muscles. Blue line represents centroid displacement before the fatigue task. Red line represents centroid displacement after the fatigue task. Stars represent the first trials and squares represent the last trials of each condition (pre- and post-fatigue).

10–15 min of rest (Larivière et al., 2003). However, in this study, participants had to perform a 30 s trunk extension at 75% of their MVC. In the present study, there was no time-limit for the fatigue task and participants were encouraged to maintain position until total exhaustion was reached.

The different acquisition frequencies used in EMG (2048 Hz) and kinematics (100 Hz) system can be considered as a methodological limitation of the study. The difference between acquisition frequencies could lead, under a worst case scenario, to a 10-ms margin of error, when identifying the onset of perturbations. However, the perturbation onset was only used to compute the reflex latencies and consequently did not affect other EMG variables.

Muscle Fatigue Effect

During the experiment, muscle fatigue manifestation in the erector spinae muscles was confirmed by a marked decreased in the MDF slope (De Luca, 1984; Mannion and Dolan, 1994). Moreover, participants perceived the fatigue task as a very hard exertion (Borg, 1982). Finally, a decrease in erector spinae EMG amplitude during post-fatigue MVC is also considered as a valid indicator of muscle fatigue (Enoka and Duchateau, 2008). These observations taken together suggest that the participant were in a fatigue state following the fatigue task. Regarding the impact of muscle fatigue on kinematic variables, results showed no difference between pre- and post-fatigue for trunk flexion angle following the perturbation. This observation is in accordance with previous studies that have also demonstrated that trunk flexion angle is not affected by acute back muscle fatigue following an unexpected perturbation (Granata et al., 2004; Mawston et al., 2007). Moreover, participant peak velocities remained unchanged with the presence of muscle fatigue. On the other hand, the present study is the first one showing that in the presence of muscle fatigue, participants decreased their time to peak velocity in response to the perturbation. These results suggest that fatigue did induce some changes in the neuromuscular control of postural balance, but the sensorimotor system remained partly efficient when the low back region was fatigued. This strategy could be explained by the trunk muscle system's redundancy which offers various adaptation possibilities to achieve a similar goal (Latash and Anson, 2006). Even if the trunk flexion angle were similar with or without fatigue, there were probably other neuromuscular strategies that prevented the effect of fatigue, such as variability in muscle activity recruitment pattern (see "New Insights into Motor Adaptation to Spinal Instability" Section for further explanation).

Using high-density sEMG, this study is the first one exploring EMG reflex variables with muscle fatigue. In the current study, baseline activity seemed to show a slight trend towards higher muscle activation after the fatigue protocol (only significant on one side of the erector spinae). Current evidence have not find a common understanding on baseline activity prior a perturbation under the influence of muscle fatigue (Granata et al., 2001, 2004; Herrmann et al., 2006; Mawston et al., 2007; Grondin and Potvin, 2009; Dupeyron et al., 2010). Baseline activity is

directly linked to EMG amplitude signals, which corresponds to the number of active motor units. Muscle fatigue is characterized by an increase of active motor units (De Luca, 1997), which is usually reflected by an increase in EMG amplitude signals in submaximal muscle contractions. A recent review has shown that muscle fatigue induced by a submaximal isometric contraction is associated with variable responses in motor units firing rates according to the intensity of the fatiguing task (Taylor et al., 2016). For example, motor unit behavior during submaximal isometric contraction at moderate intensity (50% MVC), which correspond to the Sorensen test (Demoulin et al., 2006), is first associated with a decrease in firing rate followed by an increased motor units recruitment (Heckman and Enoka, 2012). Since others studies have used different fatigue protocol, with effort intensity varying from approximately 20–60% of the MVC (Granata et al., 2001; Herrmann et al., 2006; Dupeyron et al., 2010), a variation in motor unit behavior could partly explain discrepancies across studies. In the current study, two methods were used to determine the exact time between the onset of the perturbation and the reflex response. Despite a moderate reliability between those detection methods (ICC 0.63), reflex latency values (≈95 ms) are similar to those observed in the studies (ranging from ≈60 ms to 125 ms) measuring the impact of muscle fatigue on reflex latency (Chow et al., 2004; Granata et al., 2004; Herrmann et al., 2006; Dupeyron et al., 2010; Sánchez-Zuriaga et al., 2010). Furthermore, no change was observed under the influence of muscle fatigue in the present study. This observation is consistent with most of the studies (Granata et al., 2004; Herrmann et al., 2006; Dupeyron et al., 2010; Sánchez-Zuriaga et al., 2010). In the literature, reflex amplitude of low back muscles was found not to be affected by muscle fatigue in several studies (Granata et al., 2004; Grondin and Potvin, 2009; Sánchez-Zuriaga et al., 2010), whereas two studies found a higher back reflex amplitude following a fatigue protocol (Herrmann et al., 2006; Dupeyron et al., 2010). In the present study, an increase in reflex peak values was observed after the fatiguing task. An interesting assumption to explain the discrepancy in reflex peak results could be the presence of an association between baseline activity responses, reflex peak and muscle fatigue. Indeed, studies who have reported an increase in baseline activity are the same that did not observe a change in reflex peak amplitude after muscle fatigue (Granata et al., 2004; Grondin and Potvin, 2009), and vice versa (Herrmann et al., 2006; Dupeyron et al., 2010). It could be hypothesized that increased muscle pre-activation is sufficient to counteract the fatigue effect in response to an external perturbation. On the other hand, with negligible change in pre-activation level, as observed in our study, neuromuscular adaptations are reflected in the variation of reflex peak amplitude.

In parallel to the observation of an increased reflex activity amplitude in the back muscle following fatigue, a decreased abdominal reflex activity was identified. This observation suggests that an increase in erector spinae activity would be sufficient to increase spinal stability in order to compensate for acute back fatigue effect (Cholewicki et al., 2000; Andersen et al., 2004). However, these results should be interpreted with caution since abdominal muscle EMG reflex amplitude remained higher than 50% of their activity during the MVC.

Trial-to-Trial Adaptation

In the current study, participants were submitted to a series of the exact same unexpected perturbation of the trunk. Kinematic variables including trunk flexion angles and velocity peaks remained constant through the perturbation trials. However, a decrease in time to peak velocity was observed across trials of the same unexpected perturbation. This suggest that participants adapted to the unexpected perturbation by taking less time to stop their trunk movement. A group of authors have also shown, across 10 trunk perturbation trials, a progressive reduction in the time interval between forward trunk movement initiation and complete cessation of trunk movement (Skotte et al., 2004). These observations suggest that, when first facing an unexpected perturbation, the sensorimotor systems allows irrelevant components of a motor task to fluctuate. According to the minimal intervention principle, the irrelevant aspects from the resulting behavior should be left uncorrected in order to maximize motor performance (Todorov and Jordan, 2002). Based on this principle and the findings of this study, one could argue that trunk movements triggered by the perturbations (6° on average) were not sufficient, and consequently no adaptation of the trunk flexion angle was needed to optimize spinal stabilization. In such context, trunk flexion angle and peak velocity would be considered irrelevant aspect of spinal stability while time to peak velocity would have more significant consequences on stability and potential tissue damage.

Across perturbation trials, a small attenuation of baseline activity was observed, while no adaptation was found for the reflex latency. The absence of reflex latency trial-to-trial adaptation was also observed in a previous study (Skotte et al., 2004). As for reflex peak amplitude, a clear reduction of amplitude values through the repetition of the unexpected trunk perturbation was found in the present study. It is known that the first trial reaction to an unexpected perturbation has a higher impact on postural balance in standing or seated positions (Allum et al., 2011). Results from the present study have shown that even without considering the first trial response, an attenuation of the reflex response still occurred. However, it is important to note that as we get closer to the last perturbation trial, the attenuation lessens. Similar observations were found following unexpected tilts of a surface platform, with authors showing a rapid adaptation of EMG amplitude between the first two trials, whereas adaptation was more gradual over the next trials (Oude Nijhuis et al., 2010). Again, based on this motor behavior, it could be suggested that, in the presence of an unknown movement or perturbation, the optimal strategy would be to first adopt a broader but less specific motor response (Todorov and Jordan, 2002). Following repetitions of the same unexpected perturbation, the trunk muscle system's redundancy could offer corrections by using the appropriate number of degrees of freedom (Latash and Anson, 2006). Such adaptations would also explain the

progressive time to peak velocity reduction across perturbation trials.

Interestingly, this progressive decrease continued throughout perturbation trials following the fatigue task. This suggests that even when muscle fatigue is present, participants continued their adaptation to perturbations by taking less time to stabilize their trunk. Since trunk flexion angle and velocity peak remained unchanged, it suggests that participants were able to stabilize trunk movement using alternative neuromuscular strategies. Indeed, following muscle fatigue, the trial-to-trial adaptation of the EMG reflex peak appeared to be limited. To our knowledge, the present study is the first one showing that adaptation of the reflex peak across perturbation trials is altered following muscle fatigue. The amplitude of the reflex peak remained almost constantly at the same level from the first to the last external perturbation. It could be hypothesized that muscle fatigue limited the possibility of using across-trial redundancy to adapt and optimize spinal stabilization using retroactive control. Moreover, since postural balance, expressed as a trunk angle, also remained constant throughout the perturbation trials with or without muscle fatigue, it could be suggested that alterations of the EMG reflex adaptation are an attempt to preserve a constant postural balance despite the presence of muscle fatigue.

As discussed in the methodological considerations section, some recovery may have been present throughout the last perturbation trials. In a previous study, the effect of recovery from muscle fatigue on adaptation to external perturbations was explored (Takahashi et al., 2006). Results showed that recovery affects recall of the internal model. The authors suggested that participants overestimated the muscle activity required to counteract the perturbation because their muscle force-generation capacity recovered during rest. Although fatigue and recovery effects cannot be teased out, results from the present study show that following a fatigue protocol, a modification of EMG reflex peak and trunk kinematics (time to peak velocity) occurred whereas trial-to-trial adaptation in EMG reflex peak was found to be limited following a protocol of fatigue.

Finally, the adaptation throughout the first perturbation trial following muscle fatigue was almost inexistent. Results from the present study showed that only time to peak velocity was affected when participants experienced, for the first time, an unexpected perturbation following a fatigue task. Similarly to the adaptation phenomenon observed across perturbation trials, participants took less time to stabilize their trunk following the fatigue protocol. These findings suggest that in most cases, the neuromuscular component of spinal stability is not significantly challenged in the presence of muscle fatigue, regardless of the number of exposure to a specific trunk perturbation.

New Insights into Motor Adaptation to Spinal Instability

Using high-density sEMG, dispersion of muscle activity, representing the area of reflex activity spatial distribution, was used to better understand trial-to-trial adaptation with and without muscle fatigue. A higher variability in muscle activity spatial distribution was observed before muscle fatigue was induced, while under the influence of fatigue, a reduction of the centroid migration was found. Changes in muscle activity distribution to different regions of the lumbar erector spinae could be associated with changes in variation in the control of motor units within this muscle. As mentioned earlier, adaptation of muscle reflex activity occurred through the repetition of similar sudden external perturbations. This observation suggests that the trial-to-trial adaptation was associated with higher levels of muscle activity spatial distribution. Conversely, such adaptation was not present when erector spinae muscles were in a state of fatigue. This suggests that changing spatial distribution of EMG activity, consistent with increased motor variability (Latash, 1998), may help face a series of unexpected perturbation. On the other hand, the reduced muscle activity spatial distribution observed in presence of muscle fatigue could be explained by the initiation of protective and restrictive neuromuscular strategies. This study suggests that under the influence of fatigue, the nervous system chooses to adopt a more stable muscle activity distribution when spinal stability is challenged. This observation are complementary with the work of Missenard et al., which showed that muscle fatigue increases the variance of motor commands during voluntary movements (Missenard et al., 2008, 2009). Motor variability can be measured using multiple parameters, such as muscle activity, kinetic or kinematic components of the movement pattern, or external force developed (Srinivasan and Mathiassen, 2012). In the present study, a more stable pattern of muscle activity distribution following fatigue, can be explained by the decreased number of motor unit available to generate muscle responses during perturbations. This reduced number of available motor unit may lead to more stable spatial distribution as illustrated by the reduced centroid migration in the presence of muscle fatigue (**Figure 6**). Moreover, muscle fatigue by reducing the number of available motor units may increase the variability in movement patterns (Missenard et al., 2008, 2009).

It is also important to note that the migration of muscle activity was highly variable between participants before and after the fatigue task. While spatial muscle activity distribution has been shown to shift laterally and caudally during a fatigue task in the low back region (Abboud et al., 2014), no distinctive muscle activity migration pattern was identified following a repeated unexpected perturbation. A recent study has provided similar results when a group of healthy participants were injected with a saline solution to induce acute low back pain (Hodges et al., 2013). After the injection, none of the participants activated their trunk muscles in the same manner in response to an external trunk perturbation (Hodges et al., 2013). These results reflect the complexity of the redundant trunk system, which offers various motor possibilities to achieve a similar goal. This raises the question whether these adaptations are maintained across various perturbation tasks or if the nervous system triggers individual similar adaptations for each person. Further research will be needed to verify if the alteration of trial-to-trial response is also present in a different external environment trunk perturbation such as chronic low back pain or spinal tissue creep.

In conclusion, the results of the present study suggest that participants adapt differently under the influence of muscle fatigue when they experience an unknown perturbation. While the EMG reflex amplitude remains constant over perturbation trials after the fatigue task, participants continue to habituate their trunk movements. Moreover, this study suggests that the nervous system chooses to adopt a more restrictive muscle activity recruitment pattern, when the unknown perturbation is repeated after a muscle fatigue task. Since this study is the first one describing such motor adaptations, it seems reasonable to propose that following muscle fatigue, the motor system can still generate proper stabilizing responses to spinal perturbations using alternative strategies. These strategies, however, may have detrimental long-term consequences that should also be considered in the context of spine rehabilitation.

AUTHOR CONTRIBUTIONS

JA, FN, AL, CD and MD: substantial contributions to the conception or design of the work, or acquisition, analysis, or interpretation of data for the work; drafting the work and revising it critically for important intellectual content; final approval of the version to be published; agreement to be accountable for all aspects of the work in ensuring that questions related to the accuracy or integrity of any part of the work are appropriately investigated and resolved.

FUNDING

This study was funded through the Natural Sciences and Engineering Research Council of Canada in the form of a scholarship.

ACKNOWLEDGMENTS

The authors wish to acknowledge the contribution of Frédéric Boivin, B.Sc., and Catherine Daneau, B.Sc., who assisted the authors during the experiment, and Louis Laurencelle, Ph.D. for his contribution and guidance in the statistical analyses.

REFERENCES

Abboud, J., Nougarou, F., Loranger, M., and Descarreaux, M. (2015). Test-retest reliability of trunk motor variability measured by large-array surface electromyography. *J. Manipulative Physiol. Ther.* 38, 359–364. doi: 10.1016/j.jmpt.2015.06.007

Abboud, J., Nougarou, F., Pagé, I., Cantin, V., Massicotte, D., and Descarreaux, M. (2014). Trunk motor variability in patients with non-specific chronic low back pain. *Eur. J. Appl. Physiol.* 114, 2645–2654. doi: 10.1007/s00421-014-2985-8

Allison, G. T., and Henry, S. M. (2001). Trunk muscle fatigue during a back extension task in standing. *Man. Ther.* 6, 221–228. doi: 10.1054/math.2001.0412

Allum, J. H. J., Tang, K.-S., Carpenter, M. G., Oude Nijhuis, L. B., and Bloem, B. R. (2011). Review of first trial responses in balance control: influence of vestibular loss and Parkinson's disease. *Hum. Mov. Sci.* 30, 279–295. doi: 10.1016/j.humov.2010.11.009

Andersen, T. B., Essendrop, M., and Schibye, B. (2004). Movement of the upper body and muscle activity patterns following a rapidly applied load: the influence of pre-load alterations. *Eur. J. Appl. Physiol.* 91, 488–492. doi: 10.1007/s00421-004-1040-6

Blouin, J. S., Descarreaux, M., Bélanger-Gravel, A., Simoneau, M., and Teasdale, N. (2003). Attenuation of human neck muscle activity following repeated imposed trunk-forward linear acceleration. *Exp. Brain Res.* 150, 458–464. doi: 10.1007/s00221-003-1466-9

Borg, G. A. V. (1982). Psychophysical bases of perceived exertion. *Med. Sci. Sports Exerc.* 14, 377–381. doi: 10.1249/00005768-198205000-00012

Boyas, S., and Guével, A. (2011). Neuromuscular fatigue in healthy muscle: underlying factors and adaptation mechanisms. *Ann. Phys. Rehabil. Med.* 54, 88–108. doi: 10.1016/j.rehab.2011.01.001

Champagne, A., Descarreaux, M., and Lafond, D. (2009). Comparison between elderly and young males' lumbopelvic extensor muscle endurance assessed during a clinical isometric back extension test. *J. Manipulative Physiol. Ther.* 32, 521–526. doi: 10.1016/j.jmpt.2009.08.008

Cholewicki, J., Simons, A. P., and Radebold, A. (2000). Effects of external trunk loads on lumbar spine stability. *J. Biomech.* 33, 1377–1385. doi: 10.1016/s0021-9290(00)00118-4

Chow, D. H. K., Man, J. W. K., Holmes, A. D., and Evans, J. H. (2004). Postural and trunk muscle response to sudden release during stoop lifting tasks before and after fatigue of the trunk erector muscles. *Ergonomics* 47, 607–624. doi: 10.1080/0014013031000151659

Côté, J. N., Mathieu, P. A., Levin, M. F., and Feldman, A. G. (2002). Movement reorganization to compensate for fatigue during sawing. *Exp. Brain Res.* 146, 394–398. doi: 10.1007/s00221-002-1186-6

Criswell, E., and Cram, J. R. (2011). *Cram's Introduction to Surface Electromyography*. Sudbury, MA: Jones and Bartlett.

De Luca, C. J. (1984). Myoelectrical manifestations of localized muscular fatigue in humans. *Crit. Rev. Biomed. Eng.* 11, 251–279.

De Luca, C. J. (1997). The use of surface electromyography in biomechanics. *J. Appl. Biomech.* 13, 135–163. doi: 10.1123/jab.13.2.135

Demoulin, C., Vanderthommen, M., Duysens, C., and Crielaard, J. M. (2006). Spinal muscle evaluation using the Sorensen test: a critical appraisal of the literature. *Joint Bone Spine* 73, 43–50. doi: 10.1016/j.jbspin.2004.08.002

Dupeyron, A., Perrey, S., Micallef, J. P., and Pélissier, J. (2010). Influence of back muscle fatigue on lumbar reflex adaptation during sudden external force perturbations. *J. Electromyogr. Kinesiol.* 20, 426–432. doi: 10.1016/j.jelekin.2009.05.004

Enoka, R. M., and Duchateau, J. (2008). Muscle fatigue: what, why and how it influences muscle function. *J. Physiol.* 586, 11–23. doi: 10.1113/jphysiol.2007.139477

Falla, D., Gizzi, L., Tschapek, M., Erlenwein, J., and Petzke, F. (2014). Reduced task-induced variations in the distribution of activity across back muscle regions in individuals with low back pain. *Pain* 155, 944–953. doi: 10.1016/j.pain.2014.01.027

Fuller, J. R., Fung, J., and Côté, J. N. (2011). Time-dependent adaptations to posture and movement characteristics during the development of repetitive reaching induced fatigue. *Exp. Brain Res.* 211, 133–143. doi: 10.1007/s00221-011-2661-8

Granata, K. P., Orishimo, K. F., and Sanford, A. H. (2001). Trunk muscle coactivation in preparation for sudden load. *J. Electromyogr. Kinesiol.* 11, 247–254. doi: 10.1016/s1050-6411(01)00003-7

Granata, K. P., Slota, G. P., and Wilson, S. E. (2004). Influence of fatigue in neuromuscular control of spinal stability. *Hum. Factors* 46, 81–91. doi: 10.1518/hfes.46.1.81.30391

Grondin, D. E., and Potvin, J. R. (2009). Effects of trunk muscle fatigue and load timing on spinal responses during sudden hand loading. *J. Electromyogr. Kinesiol.* 19, e237–e245. doi: 10.1016/j.jelekin.2008.05.006

Heckman, C. J., and Enoka, R. M. (2012). Motor unit. *Compr. Physiol.* 2, 2629–2682. doi: 10.1002/cphy.c100087

Herrmann, C. M., Madigan, M. L., Davidson, B. S., and Granata, K. P. (2006). Effect of lumbar extensor fatigue on paraspinal muscle reflexes. *J. Electromyogr. Kinesiol.* 16, 637–641. doi: 10.1016/j.jelekin.2005.11.004

Hodges, P. W., and Bui, B. H. (1996). A comparison of computer-based methods for the determination of onset of muscle contraction using electromyography. *Electroencephalogr. Clin. Neurophysiol.* 101, 511–519. doi: 10.1016/s0013-4694(96)95190-5

Hodges, P. W., Coppieters, M. W., MacDonald, D., and Cholewicki, J. (2013). New insight into motor adaptation to pain revealed by a combination of modelling and empirical approaches. *Eur. J. Pain* 17, 1138–1146. doi: 10.1002/j.1532-2149.2013.00286.x

Hodges, P. W., and Tucker, K. (2011). Moving differently in pain: a new theory to explain the adaptation to pain. *Pain* 152, S90–S98. doi: 10.1016/j.pain.2010.10.020

Holobar, A., Farina, D., Gazzoni, M., Merletti, R., and Zazula, D. (2009). Estimating motor unit discharge patterns from high-density surface electromyogram. *Clin. Neurophysiol.* 120, 551–562. doi: 10.1016/j.clinph.2008.10.160

Kennedy, A., Guevel, A., and Sveistrup, H. (2012). Impact of ankle muscle fatigue and recovery on the anticipatory postural adjustments to externally initiated perturbations in dynamic postural control. *Exp. Brain Res.* 223, 553–562. doi: 10.1007/s00221-012-3282-6

Larivière, C., Forget, R., Vadeboncoeur, R., Bilodeau, M., and Mecheri, H. (2010). The effect of sex and chronic low back pain on back muscle reflex responses. *Eur. J. Appl. Physiol.* 109, 577–590. doi: 10.1007/s00421-010-1389-7

Larivière, C., Gravel, D., Arsenault, A. B., Gagnon, D., and Loisel, P. (2003). Muscle recovery from a short fatigue test and consequence on the reliability of EMG indices of fatigue. *Eur. J. Appl. Physiol.* 89, 171–176. doi: 10.1007/s00421-002-0769-z

Latash, M. L. (1998). *Progress in Motor Control: Bernstein's Traditions in Movement Studies*. Champaign, IL: Human Kinetics.

Latash, M. L., and Anson, J. G. (2006). Synergies in health and disease: relations to adaptive changes in motor coordination. *Phys. Ther.* 86, 1151–1160.

Mannion, A. F., and Dolan, P. (1994). Electromyographic median frequency changes during isometric contraction of the back extensors to fatigue. *Spine (Phila Pa 1976)* 19, 1223–1229. doi: 10.1097/00007632-199405310-00006

Martinez-Valdes, E., Laine, C. M., Falla, D., Mayer, F., and Farina, D. (2016). High-density surface electromyography provides reliable estimates of motor unit behavior. *Clin. Neurophysiol.* 127, 2534–2541. doi: 10.1016/j.clinph.2015.10.065

Mawston, G. A., McNair, P. J., and Boocock, M. G. (2007). The effects of prior warning and lifting-induced fatigue on trunk muscle and postural responses to sudden loading during manual handling. *Ergonomics* 50, 2157–2170. doi: 10.1080/00140130701510139

Merletti, R., Holobar, A., and Farina, D. (2008). Analysis of motor units with high-density surface electromyography. *J. Electromyogr. Kinesiol.* 18, 879–890. doi: 10.1016/j.jelekin.2008.09.002

Missenard, O., Mottet, D., and Perrey, S. (2008). Muscular fatigue increases signal-dependent noise during isometric force production. *Neurosci. Lett.* 437, 154–157. doi: 10.1016/j.neulet.2008.03.090

Missenard, O., Mottet, D., and Perrey, S. (2009). Adaptation of motor behavior to preserve task success in the presence of muscle fatigue. *Neuroscience* 161, 773–786. doi: 10.1016/j.neuroscience.2009.03.062

Monjo, F., Terrier, R., and Forestier, N. (2015). Muscle fatigue as an investigative tool in motor control: a review with new insights on internal models and posture-movement coordination. *Hum. Mov. Sci.* 44, 225–233. doi: 10.1016/j.humov.2015.09.006

Nashner, L. M. (1976). Adapting reflexes controlling the human posture. *Exp. Brain Res.* 26, 59–72. doi: 10.1007/bf00235249

Oude Nijhuis, L. B., Allum, J. H., Valls-Sole, J., Overeem, S., and Bloem, B. R. (2010). First trial postural reactions to unexpected balance disturbances: a comparison with the acoustic startle reaction. *J. Neurophysiol.* 104, 2704–2712. doi: 10.1152/jn.01080.2009

Panjabi, M. M. (1992). The stabilizing system of the spine. Part I. Function, dysfunction, adaptation and enhancement. *J. Spinal Disord.* 5, 383–389; discussion 397. doi: 10.1097/00002517-199212000-00001

Radebold, A., Cholewicki, J., Panjabi, M. M., and Patel, T. C. (2000). Muscle response pattern to sudden trunk loading in healthy individuals and in patients with chronic low back pain. *Spine (Phila Pa 1976)* 25, 947–954. doi: 10. 1097/00007632-200004150-00009

Rantanen, J., Rissanen, A., and Kalimo, H. (1994). Lumbar muscle fiber size and type distribution in normal subjects. *Eur. Spine J.* 3, 331–335. doi: 10. 1007/bf02200146

Reeves, N. P., Cholewicki, J., and Milner, T. E. (2005). Muscle reflex classification of low-back pain. *J. Electromyogr. Kinesiol.* 15, 53–60. doi: 10.1016/j.jelekin. 2004.07.001

Sánchez-Zuriaga, D., Adams, M. A., and Dolan, P. (2010). Is activation of the back muscles impaired by creep or muscle fatigue? *Spine (Phila Pa 1976)* 35, 517–525. doi: 10.1097/BRS.0b013e3181b967ea

Shadmehr, R., and Mussa-Ivaldi, F. A. (1994). Adaptive representation of dynamics during learning of a motor task. *J. Neurosci.* 14, 3208–3224.

Siegmund, G. P., Sanderson, D. J., Myers, B. S., and Inglis, J. T. (2003). Rapid neck muscle adaptation alters the head kinematics of aware and unaware subjects undergoing multiple whiplash-like perturbations. *J. Biomech.* 36, 473–482. doi: 10.1016/s0021-9290(02)00458-x

Skotte, J. H., Fallentin, N., Pedersen, M. T., Essendrop, M., Strøyer, J., and Schibye, B. (2004). Adaptation to sudden unexpected loading of the low back–the effects of repeated trials. *J. Biomech.* 37, 1483–1489. doi: 10.1016/j. jbiomech.2004.01.018

Srinivasan, D., and Mathiassen, S. E. (2012). Motor variability in occupational health and performance. *Clin. Biomech. (Bristol, Avon)* 27, 979–993. doi: 10. 1016/j.clinbiomech.2012.08.007

Takahashi, C. D., Nemet, D., Rose-Gottron, C. M., Larson, J. K., Cooper, D. M., and Reinkensmeyer, D. J. (2006). Effect of muscle fatigue on internal model formation and retention during reaching with the arm. *J. Appl. Physiol. (1985)* 100, 695–706. doi: 10.1152/japplphysiol.00140.2005

Taylor, J. L., Amann, M., Duchateau, J., Meeusen, R., and Rice, C. L. (2016). Neural contributions to muscle fatigue: from the brain to the muscle and back again. *Med. Sci. Sports Exerc.* 48, 2294–2306. doi: 10.1249/mss.0000000000000923

Todorov, E., and Jordan, M. I. (2002). Optimal feedback control as a theory of motor coordination. *Nat. Neurosci.* 5, 1226–1235. doi: 10.1038/nn963

Tucker, K., Falla, D., Graven-Nielsen, T., and Farina, D. (2009). Electromyographic mapping of the erector spinae muscle with varying load and during sustained contraction. *J. Electromyogr. Kinesiol.* 19, 373–379. doi: 10.1016/j.jelekin.2007.10.003

Zwarts, M. J., and Stegeman, D. F. (2003). Multichannel surface EMG: basic aspects and clinical utility. *Muscle Nerve* 28, 1–17. doi: 10.1002/mus.10358

17

Elderly Fallers Enhance Dynamic Stability Through Anticipatory Postural Adjustments during a Choice Stepping Reaction Time

Romain Tisserand[1], Thomas Robert[1]*, Pascal Chabaud[2], Marc Bonnefoy[3] and Laurence Chèze[1]

[1] IFSTTAR, UMR_T9406, Laboratoire de Biomécanique et Mécanique des Chocs (LBMC), Université de Lyon, Université Claude Bernard Lyon 1, Lyon, France, [2] Laboratoire Interuniversitaire de Biologie de la Motricité (LIBM), Université de Lyon, Université Claude Bernard Lyon 1, Villeurbanne, France, [3] Service de Médecine Gériatrique, Centre Hospitalier Lyon Sud, Pierre-Bénite, France

*Correspondence:
Thomas Robert
thomas.robert@ifsttar.fr

In the case of disequilibrium, the capacity to step quickly is critical to avoid falling in elderly. This capacity can be simply assessed through the choice stepping reaction time test (CSRT), where elderly fallers (F) take longer to step than elderly non-fallers (NF). However, the reasons why elderly F elongate their stepping time remain unclear. The purpose of this study is to assess the characteristics of anticipated postural adjustments (APA) that elderly F develop in a stepping context and their consequences on the dynamic stability. Forty-four community-dwelling elderly subjects (20 F and 24 NF) performed a CSRT where kinematics and ground reaction forces were collected. Variables were analyzed using two-way repeated measures ANOVAs. Results for F compared to NF showed that stepping time is elongated, due to a longer APA phase. During APA, they seem to use two distinct balance strategies, depending on the axis: in the anteroposterior direction, we measured a smaller backward movement and slower peak velocity of the center of pressure (CoP); in the mediolateral direction, the CoP movement was similar in amplitude and peak velocity between groups but lasted longer. The biomechanical consequence of both strategies was an increased margin of stability (MoS) at foot-off, in the respective direction. By elongating their APA, elderly F use a safer balance strategy that prioritizes dynamic stability conditions instead of the objective of the task. Such a choice in balance strategy probably comes from muscular limitations and/or a higher fear of falling and paradoxically indicates an increased risk of fall.

Keywords: balance, fall, elderly, anticipatory postural adjustments, dynamic stability, step initiation

INTRODUCTION

Falling is a common and unexpected event that is a concerning health problem for the elderly population (World Health Organisation, 2008). Normal aging increases the risk of fall (Rubenstein, 2006), because of a reduced capacity to use the different resources involved in the control of balance (Horak, 2006). The physical consequences of a fall are more severe than for a young person (van Dieën and Pijnappels, 2008) and falls induce psychological issues, notably by increasing the fear of falling (FoF; Maki et al., 1991). As such, falls currently represent a large and increasing health cost for societies (Stevens et al., 2006; World Health Organisation, 2008). Early identification of community-dwelling elderly that are at risk of fall is a priority, in order to: (1) prevent them from the loss of different capacities leading to dependency and frailty; and (2) reduce the health costs of falls.

In community-dwelling elderly, "most falls occur as a result of an inability to react appropriately [to the imbalance] and produce an effective compensatory response" (Brauer et al., 2002). A natural, effective and privileged reaction to recover when balance is compromised is taking a step (Rogers et al., 1996; Maki and McIlroy, 1997). The choice stepping reaction time test (CSRT; Lord and Fitzpatrick, 2001) is a simple test to assess the capacity of a person to rapidly trigger and execute a step. The subject has to step as quickly as possible on one of several targets placed in front or around her/him. The time to reach the targets is an effective way to assess the risk of fall in elderly, as several studies showed that elderly fallers (F) have significantly longer performances compared to non-fallers (NF; Lord and Fitzpatrick, 2001; Melzer et al., 2007; St George et al., 2007; Ejupi et al., 2014). Moreover, the time to perform the CSRT appears to be a good predictor for the future risk of fall (Pijnappels et al., 2010). However, the reasons why the CSRT predicts this risk are not well established. In particular, it has been shown in simple (one leg, one target) stepping reaction time (RT) condition that elderly F are able to move their foot as fast as NF (White et al., 2002; Melzer et al., 2007). So the difference is probably made before, i.e., during the mechanisms that precede the step.

A voluntary step initiation is a self-perturbation of balance, with a modification of the base of support (BoS) and a transition from a static to a dynamic situation. To keep balance, coordinated muscular activations preceding the voluntary focal movement, namely anticipatory postural adjustments (APA), are performed (for a review see Bouisset and Do, 2008). They are part of the motor command elaborated by the central nervous system (CNS; Massion, 1992; Aruin and Latash, 1995; Brunt et al., 1999, 2005). In step (or gait) initiation, their functional role is to put the whole-body center of mass (CoM_{WB}) in motion: (1) in the desired direction; and (2) toward the future stance foot (Winter, 1995). This strategy reduces the subject's mediolateral instability during the forthcoming single support phase (Jian et al., 1993; Patla et al., 1993; Lyon and Day, 1997), where the BoS is reduced to only one foot. The motor program of this strategy has been well described, with coordinated ankle and hip muscles activations and inhibitions (Crenna and Frigo, 1991; Brunt et al., 1999). This coordination creates joint torques that move the center of pressure (CoP) backward and laterally (Brenière et al., 1987; Jian et al., 1993; Winter, 1995; Lyon and Day, 1997). Then, the movement of the subject's CoM_{WB} is principally driven by gravity effects during the swing phase (SP; Lepers and Brenière, 1995; Lyon and Day, 1997).

If APA are a very automatized postural control process, they are not invariant. They are adapted by the CNS to the external context, depending on the own resources of the subject (Patla et al., 1993; McIlroy and Maki, 1999; Luchies et al., 2002; Zettel et al., 2002; Yiou et al., 2012). In the context of a simple step initiation without a specific target, the studies that were interested in step preparation phases showed that elderly have APA elongated in time and reduced in amplitude compared to young adults (Halliday et al., 1998; Polcyn et al., 1998; Luchies et al., 2002). In the context of a CSRT, similar results have been found for elderly compared to young (Patla et al., 1993; Luchies et al., 2002) and for elderly F compared to NF, under normal (Lord and Fitzpatrick, 2001; St George et al., 2007) and dual-task conditions (Melzer et al., 2007; St George et al., 2007; Uemura et al., 2012a). Moreover, liftoff time is increased in CSRT compared to a simple RT test, increasing the landing time of the stepping foot (Luchies et al., 2002). So, the adaptable APA phase seems to be the major reason why the landing step timing is increased in elderly, and particularly in F, during a CSRT.

Why are APA elongated in time in elderly F? First, it is reported in the literature that a high FoF is associated to APA elongated in time and reduced in amplitude (Maki et al., 1991; Adkin et al., 2000; Yiou et al., 2011; Uemura et al., 2012b) and elderly F have an increased FoF compared to NF (Lajoie and Gallagher, 2004). The FoF has been shown to reduce the attentional resources available (Gage et al., 2003) and movement reinvestment (Huffman et al., 2009). So, elderly F probably have reduced attentional resources available. Moreover, normal aging reduces cognitive capacities. A reduced cognitive capacity is correlated to a longer stepping performance in elderly F during the CSRT (Lord and Fitzpatrick, 2001; Pijnappels et al., 2010; Schoene et al., 2015). The APA phase is also lengthened in elderly F during the CSRT, under dual-task paradigm (Melzer et al., 2007; St George et al., 2007; Sturnieks et al., 2008). This is probably because they need more attentional resources than NF during postural tasks under dual-task (Brauer et al., 2002; Woollacott and Shumway-Cook, 2002). Finally, elongated stepping performance is related to reduced proprioception (Pijnappels et al., 2010) and both sensorial and muscular capacity (Lord and Fitzpatrick, 2001). The muscular capacity of the lower limb is affected in elderly F, particularly around the hips (Johnson et al., 2004; Inacio et al., 2014; Morcelli et al., 2016).

Few studies have focused on the mechanics of the APA and its consequences on the stability, in a population of elderly F during a CSRT. We only found three studies talking about stability in the interpretation of their results in the conditions of step initiation. Patla et al. (1993) showed that elderly have a longer weight transfer time than young adults during CSRT, which resulted in a slower stepping response. Notably, in case of lateral steps, they found that elderly need more time because they choose to load their swing leg first, which is a sub-optimal strategy. They interpreted it as a "safer" strategy that helps elderly to increase their balance conditions. Later, Luchies et al. (2002) observed a slower weight transfer and a larger percentage of weight on the stance foot for elderly compared to young adults, in both simple step initiation and CSRT. They also used the term "safer" to describe the stepping strategy used by elderly. Unfortunately, the population of these two studies did not include elderly F. In the context of an induced step under dual-task condition the elderly—and even more for those who experienced a fall—reduce their secondary task performance (Brauer et al., 2002). They would do so to focus most of the available resources on the postural control, and by extension to increase the stability.

According to their results there could be a prioritization of a more "stable" balance strategy in elderly and particularly in elderly F. This would be observed because their CNS has better integrated than NF that falling engages the physical integrity. Nevertheless, there still is a lack in the literature of a precise biomechanical analysis of the dynamic stability for a group of elderly F during a CSRT.

To sum-up, elderly F are slower to step than NF under both normal and dual-task conditions of CSRT. As already observed in stepping tasks, a hypothesis would be that it comes from a lengthened APA phase, in an attempt to maximize their stability. The aim of this study is to investigate the characteristics of the APA for both F and NF community-dwelling elderly subjects, in normal CSRT conditions (i.e., without a secondary task). We expect that APA will be longer for F compared to NF, as a result of a strategy that elderly F use to increase their conditions for dynamic stability.

MATERIALS AND METHODS

Population

Forty-four healthy subjects participated in this study. They were divided in two groups: elderly F and elderly NF. Subjects were retrospectively categorized as F if they experienced at least a fall in the past year. A fall was defined as "an event, following an imbalance, which results in a person coming to rest inadvertently to a lower level, involving an impact, consecutive to the balance recovery actions failure and not a result of a major intrinsic event or overwhelming hazard". This definition was chosen based on previous literature (Tinetti et al., 1988; Hauer et al., 2006; Segev-Jacubovski et al., 2011). Headcounts and anthropometrical data of the two groups are summarized in **Table 1**.

All subjects were included if they: (1) were aged 70 or more; (2) performed at least 25 on the Mini Mental State Examination (MMSE); and (3) had no neurological, musculoskeletal or sensorial (vision and cutaneous sensation) disorders, after a medical inspection. Forty-four healthy elderly adults participated in the study. Their mean age, mass and height were 75 years (ranging from 70 to 82), 66 kg (45 to 95) and 1.62 m (1.50 to 1.95), respectively. All subjects provided written informed consent to

TABLE 1 | Mean (standard deviation) anthropometrical and MMSE data relative to the participants.

	Elderly F	Elderly NF
Number of subjects	20	24
Number of women	15	14
Right-shooters	16	20
Age [years]	76.0 (3.9)	74.2 (3.9)
Age range [years]	70–82	70–82
Height [m]	1.61 (0.10)	1.64 (0.09)
Weight [kg]	68.6 (12.2)	65.3 (11.9)
BMI [kg.m^{-2}]	26.5 (3.7)	24.2 (3.5)
MMSE [score]	28.7 (1.4)	28.9 (1.0)

No statistical difference (using a T-test) was seen between the two groups. BMI, Body Mass Index; MMSE, Mini Mental State Examination.

the experiment as conformed to the Declaration of Helsinki and was approved by the ethics committee Comité de Protection des Personnes Lyon Sud Est III.

Protocol

Each subject performed a CSRT. Subjects initially stood quietly, in a comfortable position, with arms along the body, eyes open and feet on two force platforms (60 cm × 40 cm, Bertec®, OH, USA). The positions of the feet was freely chosen by the subject and marked on the ground in order to repeat trials from the same initial posture. Four large targets (squared panels, 10 cm × 10 cm) were positioned on the ground at 40% of the subject's lower limb length (LLL; see **Figure 1**). This distance was comfortable for the subject. The LLL was measured vertically, between the femoral trochanter center (Van Sint Jan, 2007) and the ground. Two targets were placed strictly anterior to the right and left foot (Central). The two others were placed 30° on each lateral side (Lateral). A light-emitting diode (LED) was placed in front of each target. LEDs were initially turned off. Instructions given to the subjects were: "as soon as one of the LED gets illuminated, step with the ipsilateral foot (i.e., left foot for the two left targets, right foot for the two right targets) on the corresponding target, as quickly as possible". Each subject performed four trials on each target, randomly presented. To enhance the unpredictability of the imperative signal, the duration between the subjects said he/she was "ready" and the illumination of the LED was randomly chosen between 1 and 10 s.

Subjects were equipped with 39 reflective markers located on anatomical landmarks (Van Sint Jan, 2007) and recorded by eight cameras (Eagle 1.3 Mpx, Motion Analysis®, Santa Rosa, CA, USA) at 100 Hz sample frequency. Markers trajectories were filtered at 6 Hz with a Butterworth filter. The whole-body center of mass (CoM_{WB}) trajectory was calculated using these markers trajectories and a segmental method (Dumas et al., 2007, 2015). Ground reaction forces (GRFs) were recorded at a sampling frequency of 1000 Hz with four force platforms, to integrate both the starting and landing areas (see **Figure 1**). The CoP was then estimated from the GRF measured by the force platforms at the same frequency. The CoP was estimated only when the resultant vertical force was higher than a threshold fixed at 20 N. No additional filtering was performed.

Data Analysis

Step Phases Duration

All signals (markers' positions, GRFs and LEDs' voltage) were recorded on the same data acquisition card (National Instruments USB 6218) and synchronized. They were further time shifted so that the beginning of the trial (T0) corresponded to the LED's lightning (given by a raise in the LED's voltage). Three particular instants were then defined relative to T0, based on the vertical components of the GRFs (see **Figure 2**):

- *Beginning of loading* (BL) which corresponds to the beginning of APA is the instant where the force under the swing leg increases more than two standard deviations of a reference

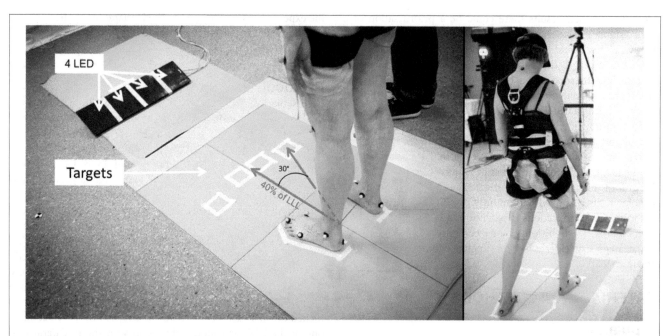

FIGURE 1 | Experimental set up for the choice stepping reaction time test (CSRT). Initial position of the subject, targets and board with light-emitting diode (LED) are shown on the left. Distance from the middle of the ankles and center of each target was 40% of the subject's lower limb length (LLL). On the right, the same subject in the final position, after the lightning of the "Lateral-Right" target.

period calculated between the beginning of the recording and T0;
- *Foot-Off* (FO) is the first instant where the swing leg force is inferior to 2.5% of the subject's body weight;
- *Foot Landing* (FL) is the first instant where the swing leg force is superior to 2.5% of the subject's body weight after FO.

Then, the three temporal phases were identified: the RT between T0 and BL, the anticipated postural adjustments (APA) between BL and FO and the SP between FO and FL.

APA and Swing Phases Analysis

Specific variables were extracted and analyzed during the APA and the SP phases. First, we measured the presence of an APA error. An APA error was considered when the lateral trajectory of the CoP first moved toward the stance foot side—instead of the swing foot side—more than two standard deviations of the reference period measured between 0 and T0. Then, we were interested in the two subphases of APA used during forward step initiation (see **Figure 3**): a "loading" subphase where the CoP moves backward and toward the swing foot, leading the CoM_{WB} to be put in motion forward and toward the stance foot; and an "unloading" subphase, during which the swing foot is unloaded, leading the CoP to move laterally under the stance foot (Jian et al., 1993). The beginning of the unloading subphase (BU)—corresponding the end of the loading subphase—was identified as the time when the vertical force under the swing leg was maximal (see **Figure 2**). The unloading subphase ended with the APA at FO. During the two APA subphases, the CoP displacements were characterized using the six following variables:

- CoP_B: the maximal excursion of the CoP backward along the AP axis during the loading subphase;
- CoP_L: the maximal excursion of the CoP along the ML axis toward the swing foot during the loading subphase;
- CoP_U: the amplitude of the CoP displacement along the ML axis during the unloading subphase;
- $VCoP_B$: the peak of the AP component of the velocity of the CoP during the loading subphase;
- $VCoP_L$: the peak of the ML component of the velocity of the CoP during the loading subphase;
- CoM_U: the peak of the ML component of the velocity of the CoP during the unloading subphase;

The CoP velocity was obtained by the first time derivative of the CoP trajectory, with a 2nd order lowpass digital Butterworth filter and a cutoff frequency of 20 Hz. Finally, during the SP, we analyzed the horizontal tangential velocity of the swing foot, using the first derivative of the ankle center trajectory given by the middle of the two malleolus markers. The horizontal distance traveled by the CoM_{WB} between T0 and FL was also calculated.

Dynamic Stability: XCoM and MoS Analysis

The position of the XCoM in the horizontal plane was computed with the following equation (Hof et al., 2005):

$$XCoM = \left(CoM_{WB} + \frac{1}{\omega_0}\dot{CoM}_{WB}\right) \cdot e_{proj} \quad \omega_0 = \sqrt{\frac{g}{h}} \quad (1)$$

$\dot{CoM}_{WB}$ is the vector of the CoM_{WB}'s velocity, obtained by numerical derivation and filtering. g is the gravitational constant and h the distance along the vertical axis between the ankle

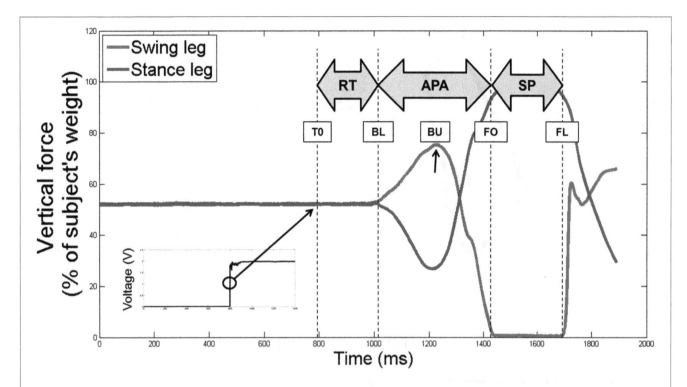

FIGURE 2 | An example of the raw vertical component of the ground reaction forces (GRFs) under the swing (in red) and stance (in blue) legs of a non-faller subject, before being time shifted. The four particular instants identified (T0, BL, FO and FL) are reported with dotted lines. The beginning of the unloading is also reported with a black arrow (BU). The black squared signal in the bottom left shows the voltage signal of the LED, used to determine the T0. Abbreviations used: T0, first instant lighting the LED; BL, beginning of loading; BU, beginning of unloading; FO, foot off; FL, foot landing; RT, reaction time phase; APA, anticipated postural adjustments; SP, swing phase.

and CoM_{WB}'s position in static initial posture. The vector e_{proj} projects the results in the horizontal plane of the laboratory coordinate system.

The dynamic stability was quantified at FO using the minimal distance between the positions of the XCoM and the edges of the stance foot, along both the AP and ML directions of the stance foot (see **Figure 3**). These variables, further referred as MoS_{AP} and MoS_{ML}, could be seen as the margin of stability (MoS; Hof et al., 2005) in these two directions. AP and ML directions of the stance foot were first defined as the lines passing through the markers positioned on calcaneus and 3rd toe and through the markers positioned on 1st and 5th metatarsal heads, respectively (dotted blue lines on **Figure 3**). The advantage of this method is that it takes into account the horizontal orientation of the foot. The anterior and medial edges of the BoS were then obtained by translating these lines to pass through the 1st metatarsal head marker and the 3rd toe marker, respectively (solid blue lines in **Figure 3**). Note that recent articles suggested the use of a functional BoS, i.e., a proportion of the initial BoS, instead of the mechanical BoS to correctly analyze the MoS values (Vallée et al., 2015; Hof and Curtze, 2016). However, the correct proportions to be used are still debated and using the mechanical or functional BoS will not change the meaning and interpretation of our results. At FO the BoS is the stance foot. MoS_{AP} and MoS_{ML} were calculated as the perpendicular distances between XCoM and the BoS edges (see **Figure 3**) and normalized by

the BoS length (distance between the calcaneus and 3rd toe markers) and width (distance between the 1st and 5th metatarsal markers of the stance foot), respectively. For interpretation, the higher (and positive) these values, the higher the stability. Note that the XCoM being most of the time medial to the ML BoS edge (as it is shown on **Figure 3**), MoS_{ML} is quasi-systematically negative. It means that the subject is in condition of instability and, not surprisingly, that a static stable standing posture can only be reached by placing the swing foot laterally to the stance foot.

Statistics and Graphic Representations

The steps on the left side were reflected about the laboratory AP axis to the steps on the right side. T-tests performed on the total duration comparing left and right target for both Central and Lateral conditions inside each group revealed probabilities to be different superior to 0.50 (for example in NF, $p = 0.85$ for Central and $p = 0.64$ for Lateral). So, right and left trials were combined in the two targets: Central and Lateral.

A first analysis on the frequency of APA error was performed with a χ^2 test. Next, the normality of the distribution in the other variables was evaluated with a Shapiro-Wilk test. All of them were reported normal, so we tested them with two-way repeated measures ANOVA. The factors tested are the independent factor "Group" (F or NF) and the repeated factor "Target" (Central or Lateral). When an interaction was found, *post hoc* T-tests with

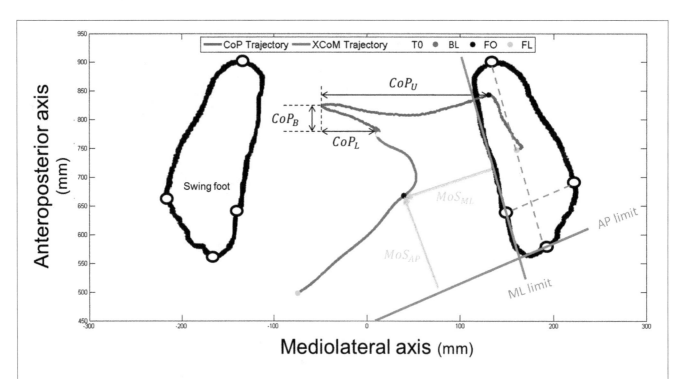

FIGURE 3 | An example of the horizontal center of pressure (CoP; in dark blue) and XCoM (in red) trajectories of a non-faller subject during the CSRT, seen from the top. Particular instants identified (T0, BL, FO and FL) are reported with colored points on CoP trajectory. Only FO and FL are reported on both trajectories. Foot markers are represented with white disks circled in black. Amplitudes of the CoP displacements are represented with black double arrows (CoP_B = backward; CoP_L = loading and CoP_U = unloading). The horizontal foot orientation is represented with dotted light blue lines that are then translated to the edges of the stance foot (solid light blue lines). Margin of stability (MoS) sizes at FO are represented with orange arrows. AP, anteroposterior; ML, mediolateral.

the Bonferroni correction were performed. We did all statistical tests using the $R^®$ software and a $p < 0.05$ was considered for a statistical difference.

For clarity, we choose to represent on the graphs the results for the two groups on each target even if an interaction was absent. In this case only the main factor effects of the ANOVA are reported. If an interaction was present, the results of the *post hoc* test are added to the main factor results coming from the ANOVA.

RESULTS

Seven hundred and four trials were collected. Twenty-Seven were instantly removed for the following reasons: subjects stepped with the wrong foot (19) or problems with forceplates data recordings appeared (signal partly or totally absent, 8). The 677 trials left were analyzed to detect the presence of APA errors. APA errors were observed in 21.6% (146) of the trials. Results of APA errors were 22.7% and 20.6% for F and 24.9% and 21.4% for NF in Central and Lateral targets, respectively. For both targets, there were no statistical difference between F and NF: $\chi^2 = 0.02$, $p = 0.89$ and $\chi^2 = 0.03$, $p = 0.87$ for Central and Lateral, respectively.

As no difference was seen between F and NF, we chose to analyze only the 78.4% left of the collected trials. So, the following results concern only the 531 "correct" trials of the initial 677.

In those trials, the results of the ANOVA tests have been summed up in **Table 2**.

A significant effect of the factor "Group" was found on the total step duration. F compared to NF needed 1131 ± 231 ms vs. 997 ± 175 ms in Central and 1019 ± 161 ms vs. 870 ± 117 ms in Lateral, to execute a quick step during the CSRT (see **Figure 4**, top). This observation was independent from the target, although no significant differences between F and NF were observed on the CoM_{WB} displacement (see **Figure 5**, top). Indeed, for F compared to NF, the CoM_{WB} horizontal displacement was 12.5 ± 4.0% vs. 13.3 ± 4.0% of the subject's height for Central and 10.2 ± 2.6% vs. 12.1 ± 3.0% of the subject's height for Lateral. We also found an effect of the factor "Target", indicating that the total step duration was significantly increased in Central compared to Lateral targets.

The analysis of each step phase duration (**Figure 4**, bottom) showed that APA was the only phase significantly elongated in elderly F compared to NF (534 ± 150 ms vs. 457 ± 139 ms in Central and 441 ± 98 ms vs. 357 ± 84 ms and in Lateral). As for the total step duration, this result was independent from the target and the mean values measured on Central targets were significantly higher than on Lateral targets.

The mean values measured on the RT phase duration for F compared to NF were 261 ± 61 ms vs. 272 ± 82 ms in Central and 249 ± 57 ms vs. 247 ± 55 ms in Lateral. Analysis of this phase reported neither effect of the factors "Group" nor "Target" (see **Table 2**).

For the SP duration and swing foot velocity, a significant effect of the factor "Target" was found, whereas the effect of the factor

TABLE 2 | Recapitulation of the results using two-way repeated measures ANOVA performed for all the variables in this study.

		Group		Target		Interaction	
		F	p	F	p	F	p
Durations							
	Total	9.86	**<0.01**	105.39	**<0.001**	<0.01	0.97
	Reaction time	2.34	0.13	0.25	0.62	2.01	0.16
	APA phase	13.01	**<0.001**	102.04	**<0.001**	0.10	0.75
	Swing phase	2.79	0.10	20.71	**<0.001**	0.49	0.49
	Loading subphase	5.98	**0.02**	54.80	**<0.001**	1.73	0.19
	Unloading subphase	6.84	**0.01**	34.59	**<0.001**	0.06	0.81
CoP amplitude							
	CoP_B	4.88	**0.03**	1.81	0.18	0.24	0.63
	CoP_L	0.49	0.49	37.57	**<0.001**	0.04	0.83
	CoP_U	1.60	0.31	26.84	**<0.001**	2.29	0.14
CoP velocity							
	$VCoP_B$	11.31	**0.02**	0.38	0.54	0.02	0.88
	$VCoP_L$	0.94	0.34	8.37	**<0.01**	0.44	0.51
	$VCoP_U$	2.17	0.15	3.52	0.07	2.80	0.10
MoS sizes							
	MoS_{AP}	4.64	**0.04**	7.93	**<0.01**	0.48	0.49
	MoS_{ML}	2.45	0.13	385.11	**<0.001**	5.48	**0.02**
Swing phase							
	Foot velocity	2.21	0.15	24.00	**<0.001**	0.01	0.94
CoM_{WB} displacement		0.31	0.58	75.09	**<0.001**	0.53	0.47

F and p from the ANOVA are provided. p inferior to 0.05 are indicated in bold.

"Group" revealed trends (see **Table 2, Figures 4, 5**). Those trends indicated that the mean values for SP duration are always longer for F compared to NF (336 ± 111 vs. 290 ± 87 ms in Central and 305 ± 79 vs. 265 ± 73 ms in Lateral), and that the mean values for swing foot velocity were always smaller in F than in NF (0.16 ± 0.04 vs. 0.18 ± 0.04 m.s^{-1} in Central and 0.15 ± 0.4 vs. 0.17 ± 0.4 m.s^{-1} in Lateral).

In order to illustrate the APA mechanisms and their consequences on stability, the CoP and XCoM trajectories were plotted between T0 and FO. Results for Lateral targets are provided in **Figure 6**. Similar patterns were observed for Central targets. For clarity, all trajectories have been normalized on zero. Only for the representation, the BL instant has been averaged between the two groups. This figure highlights the differences in APA between F and NF and their consequences on the stability. First, as previously mentioned, we observed that the APA duration was elongated in F. Indeed, FO arose around 100 ms later in F than in NF. Also, the plot of the CoP displacement along the ML axis illustrates well the two APA subphases (bottom left in **Figure 6**): the "loading" is when the CoP move to the swing-foot side while the "unloading" is when the CoP moves to the stance-foot side. The duration of these two subphases (see **Figure 7**) were significantly increased for F compared to NF: 254 ± 45 ms vs. 237 ± 45 ms in Central and 220 ± 30 ms vs. 183 ± 26 ms in Lateral to complete the loading subphase; 263 ± 47 ms vs. 217 ± 52 ms in Central and 227 ± 35 ms vs. 173 ± 24 ms in Lateral to complete the unloading subphase.

Two different CoP displacement strategies were observed in the AP and ML directions, respectively (see **Figure 6**, left panels). Both resulted in a similar effect on the stability (see **Figure 6**,

right panels): an increased stability in the AP direction and a less important instability (the XCoM is mostly external to the BoS at FO) in the ML direction, for the elderly F compared to NF (see **Figures 8, 9**).

• In the AP direction F moved their CoP less backward than NF: 9 ± 3.8% vs. 13.4 ± 5.5% of the BoS length in Central and 9.8 ± 3.9 vs. 14.7 ± 5.7% of the BoS length in Lateral. They also moved their CoP slower than NF: 0.21 ± 0.07 m.s^{-1} vs. 0.32 ± 0.12 m.s^{-1} in Central and 0.21 ± 0.07 m.s^{-1} vs. 0.34 ± 0.11 m.s^{-1} in Lateral. Consecutively, this strategy resulted in a smaller forward displacement of the XCoM (see **Figure 6**) and a significantly increased MoS_{AP} (23.2 ± 7.7% vs. 14.1 ± 11.5% of the BoS length in Central and 24.6 ± 6.6% vs. 16.6 ± 9.2% in Lateral).

• In the ML direction there were no significant differences between F and NF in the amplitude of CoP displacements. For F compared to NF, we measured mean CoP displacements of 16.0 ± 5.6% vs. 17.2 ± 5.7% of the initial BoS width in Central and of 14.4 ± 4.4% vs. 14.0 ± 5.0% of the initial BoS width in Lateral during the loading subphase. During the unloading subphase, the amplitude of this displacement was 32.7 ± 8.1% vs. 32.8 ± 7.5% of the initial BoS width in Central and 30.6 ± 6.7% vs. 29.6 ± 7.4% in Lateral. We also did not found any significant differences between F and NF for the CoP velocity peaks ($VCoP_L$ and $VCoP_U$). For F compared to NF, the mean $VCoP_L$ measured were 0.46 ± 0.21 m.s^{-1} vs. 0.50 ± 0.31 m.s^{-1} in Central and 0.39 ± 0.13 m.s^{-1} vs. 0.42 ± 0.16 m.s^{-1} in Lateral. We found however a significant effect of the factor "Target" ($p < 0.01$), with mean values measured on Central targets significantly higher than those on Lateral. $VCoP_U$ was 1.21 ± 0.37 m.s^{-1} vs. 1.45 ± 0.64 m.s^{-1} in

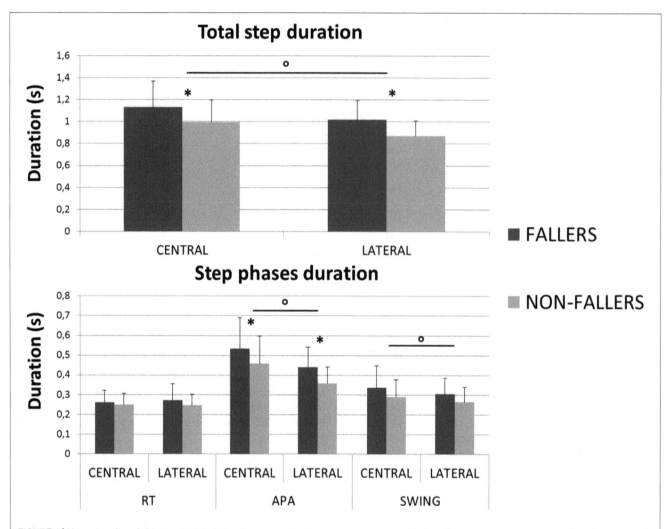

FIGURE 4 | Mean durations (with standard deviations) measured for both groups and targets during the CSRT. On top are presented results for the total step duration. On the bottom are presented results for the three steps phases (RT, APA and Swing). *Indicates a significant effect of the main factor "Group". °Indicates a significant effect of the main factor "Target".

Central and 1.31 ± 0.43 m.s^{-1} vs. 1.46 ± 0.50 m.s^{-1} in Lateral, for F compared to NF. Nonetheless, longer APA duration for F tended to induce a larger lateral displacement of the XCoM at FO (see **Figure 6**). Whether the MoS_{ML} was not significantly different between F and NF ($-9.6 \pm 19.8\%$ vs. $-24.2 \pm 27.1\%$ of the stance-foot BoS width in Central and -40.0 ± 20.6 vs. $-60.0 \pm 29.4\%$ of the stance-foot BoS width in Lateral), the significant interaction Group * Target (see **Table 2**) showed that this result depended on the Target. Independent analysis of each target revealed that F had a significantly larger MoS_{ML} than NF only for the Lateral targets ($p < 0.01$ after Bonferroni correction).

DISCUSSION

Step and Step Phases Durations

As previously in the literature (Lord and Fitzpatrick, 2001; St George et al., 2007), we found that elderly F need more time

to perform a CSRT under normal conditions (i.e., no secondary task). This result confirms that this test is relevant to identify community-dwelling elderly that are at risk of fall, with a simple measurement (the total duration of the step) conceivable outside of the laboratory (clinical environment, home, etc.) (Lord and Fitzpatrick, 2001; Schoene et al., 2011; Ejupi et al., 2014). The total mean durations obtained in our study are shorter than in Lord and Fitzpatrick (2001) study: 1075 ms vs. 1322 ms for F and 933 ms vs. 1168 ms for NF. This difference could be explained by the fact that we removed the trials with APA errors from analysis. Interestingly, the mean difference between the two groups is similar in both studies ($\sim$150 ms). So, the total step duration difference between F and NF does not seem to be influenced by the presence of APA errors. Despite the fact that they need more time to step, elderly F made similar steps (see results in **Figure 5**) and as many APA errors as NF. This last result may seem contradictory with those from the previous studies (St George et al., 2007; Sparto et al., 2014) who found that subjects who make more APA errors are mostly the subjects

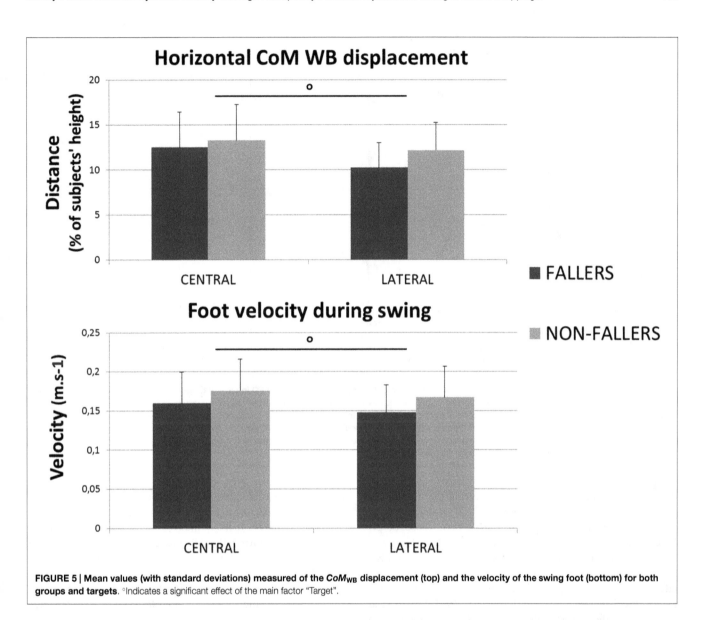

FIGURE 5 | Mean values (with standard deviations) measured of the CoM_WB displacement (top) and the velocity of the swing foot (bottom) for both groups and targets. °Indicates a significant effect of the main factor "Target".

with a history of fall and with a high risk of fall, respectively. It could be explained by the fact that Sparto et al. (2014) used purely lateral targets and reported an "error" when a loading subphase was observed, which is a very strict criterion (the presence of a loading subphase being more a sub-optimal response than an error). In St George et al. (2007) study subjects were under dual-task most of the time, which could have complicated the target identification for F. To sum-up, we found that elderly F are slower but able to execute the same step as NF during the CSRT and that the presence of an APA error is apparently not a reason to explain why they need more time to step during this test.

Regarding the step phases independently we found similar RT phase duration for F and NF. The mean value obtained for the RT is close to previous measurements in elderly (Luchies et al., 2002), but differs from the longer durations measured by Patla et al. (1993) (~400 ms vs. 280 ms in our study) and St George et al. (2007) in their condition without secondary task (~350 ms).

In Patla et al. (1993), targets also involved posterior steps. As the CoP has to move first forward in posterior steps, subjects may have taken more time to ensure the identification of the direction of the target before starting APA. In St George et al. (2007) study, this difference could be explained by the determination of the beginning of APA: they took the first activation of gastrocnemius that, as soleus, are ankle plantar flexors who are firstly turned off during the forward step initiation (Crenna and Frigo, 1991). Moreover, our results indicate that the F and the NF have similar SP durations and swing foot velocity (see **Figures 4, 5**).

So, an important result of this study is that the total duration of the step is elongated in elderly F compared to NF because their APA phase is elongated. This result is similar to what Patla et al. (1993) found for elderly compared to young adults, and the timing difference between F and NF related here is similar to St George et al.'s (2007) measurements in their condition without secondary task. It confirms the hypothesis that the

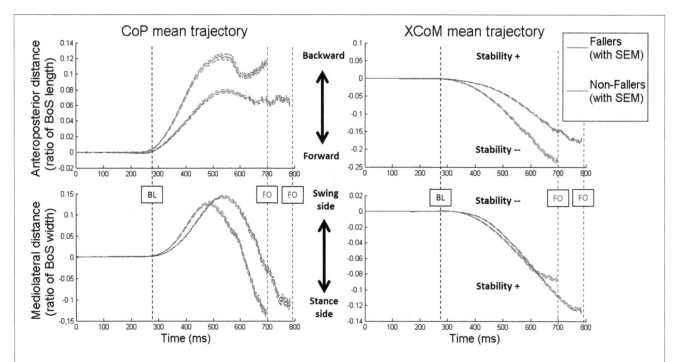

FIGURE 6 | Mean values of the CoP (on the left) and XCoM (on the right) trajectories from T0 to FO in Lateral targets. For both groups the two components of the movement are presented: anteroposterior (on top) and mediolateral (on the bottom). Blue lines are the results for Fallers (F) and red lines for Non-fallers (NF). The lines represent the mean value and the standard error to the mean (SEM). For clarity, the BL is the mean of the two groups. Note that for the anteroposterior displacement of the XCoM (top right) the less negative the XCoM indicates a better stability while for the mediolateral displacement of the XCoM (bottom right) the less negative XCoM indicate a worst the stability. For this representation, the base of support (BoS) width has been calculated between the positions of the two 5th metatarsal head markers, along the mediolateral axis.

difference between F and NF is made during the mechanisms preceding the step execution. Our result is reinforced by the fact that APA of elderly F last longer than those of NF, independently of the direction of the target (see **Figure 4**). Indeed, even for the Lateral targets, a situation that needs *a priori* reduced APA because of the advantages of the gravity effects on the frontal plane during the SP (Patla et al., 1993; Lepers and Brenière, 1995; Lyon and Day, 1997; Sparto et al., 2014), this difference is highly significant ($p < 0.001$). So, as Patla et al. (1993) observed for elderly in lateral steps, elderly F may chose not to take advantage of the gravity as much as elderly NF do during the execution of APA for lateral steps.

Two Different Balance Strategies, Depending on the Axis

Looking at the biomechanical mechanisms occurring during the APA, we showed that elderly F tend to keep their XCoM closer to the stance foot at FO than NF (see **Figure 6**). This situation allows them to increase their conditions for dynamic stability at this particular instant, i.e., when the BoS is reduced to only one foot (although this result was not significant in the ML direction for the Central targets). Moreover, as the body behaves almost as a passive mechanism during the SP (Lyon and Day, 1997) and as the swing characteristics observed here (foot location at FL and SP duration) are unchanged between F and NF, differences in dynamic stability at FL could be

expected from the differences in XCoM locations at FO. In particular, the XCoM is further from the stance foot at FO for NF (see **Figure 6**). It likely induces a larger ML displacement of the XCoM during the SP and could result in a smaller dynamic stability at FL for NF compared to F, similar to what was observed at FO. This should nevertheless be confirmed by proper estimations of the XCoM and of the BoS at FL. Interestingly, the increased conditions for stability were obtained

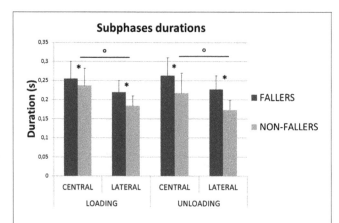

FIGURE 7 | Mean durations (with standard deviations) measured for the two subphases of APA for both groups and targets. *Indicates a significant effect of the main factor "Group". °Indicates a significant effect of the main factor "Target".

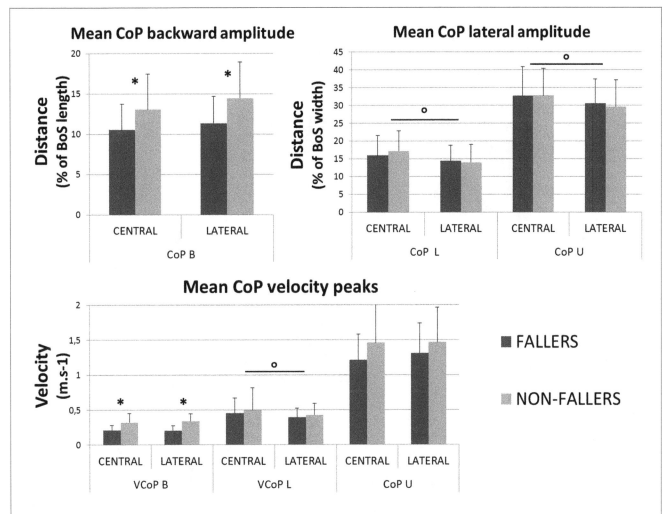

FIGURE 8 | Mean characteristics (with standard deviations) of CoP movement measured for both groups and targets during APA. Backward (top left) and mediolateral (top right) maximal amplitudes are presented with velocity peaks (bottom). *Indicates a significant effect of the main factor "Group". °Indicates a significant effect of the main factor "Target". Note that here the BoS width refers to the initial BoS width, which is calculated between the positions of the two 5th metatarsal head markers, along the mediolateral axis.

through two different strategies observed in the ML and AP directions.

In the ML direction, we did not find any statistical difference in the CoP trajectory between F and NF, both in amplitude and velocity variables (CoP_L, CoP_U, $VCoP_L$ and $VCoP_U$, respectively, see **Figures 6**, **8**). Longer durations of both loading and unloading subphases (see **Figure 7**) implied however that the CoP stayed lateral to the CoM_{WB} on the swing foot side for a longer time in F than in NF. Consequently, the torque that propels the CoM_{WB} toward the stance leg is more efficient in F and so the XCoM is more shifted toward the stance foot (see **Figure 6**). Thus, the ML instability at FO is reduced: MoS_{ML} is less negative (although it was only significant for Lateral targets, see **Figure 9**). This elongated duration implies a poorer performance in the CSRT task (Patla et al., 1993; Lord and Fitzpatrick, 2001). Interestingly, a similar result in terms of stability could be obtained without lengthening the APA phase duration. It would consist in increasing the

CoP peak velocity or excursion, i.e., in performing more efficient APA than NF. Why F do not to use this later strategy remains an open question. Two hypotheses could be proposed: (1) a physical limitation, in particular in the hip abductors/adductors that are primarily responsible for the CoP ML displacement (Winter, 1995); and (2) the FoF that would prevent the subjects to unbalance themselves more quickly. This study does not bring firm arguments for or against one of these hypotheses. By elongating their APA without modifying the amplitude, F subjects may have tried to minimize the muscular effort (Zettel et al., 2002). Indeed, a larger CoP displacement in the mediolateral direction (excursion and peak velocity) will require a high level of muscular strength at the hip abductors/adductors. It has been reported that elderly and particularly F have both weaker hip adductor/abductors capacity (Johnson et al., 2004; Inacio et al., 2014; Morcelli et al., 2016) and a reduced lateral stability (Rogers et al., 2001; Johnson-Hilliard et al., 2008). Elderly F also have a

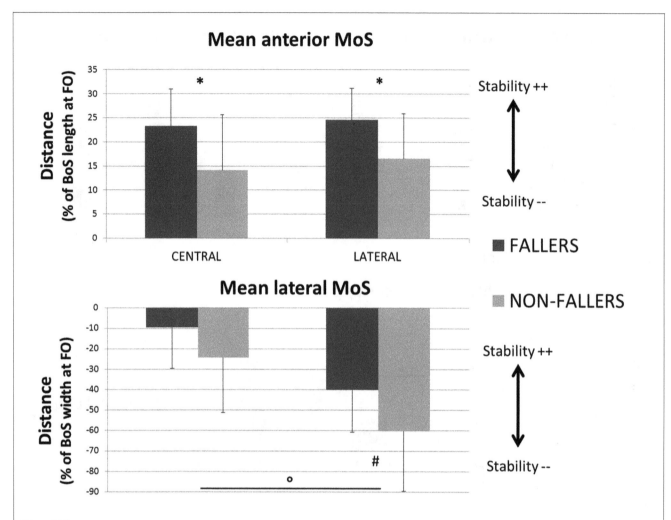

FIGURE 9 | Mean values (with standard deviations) of the MoS measured at FO for both the two groups and targets. Anteroposterior component is presented on the top and mediolateral component on the bottom. Indicators of the quality of stability are provided for each of them (Stability ++ = a higher stability, Stability -- = a smaller stability). *Indicates a significant effect of the main factor "Group". °Indicates a significant effect of the main factor "Target". #Indicates a significant difference between F and NF measured with the *post hoc* test. Note that here the BoS width is the width of the stance foot, the current BoS at FO.

higher FoF (Maki et al., 1991; Vellas et al., 1997; Lajoie and Gallagher, 2004). A high FoF affects the development of APA (Adkin et al., 2000; Yiou et al., 2011), and so F subjects may have tried to reduce the risk to fall on a particular side. Finally, it could be a combination of these two hypotheses. Nevertheless, it is remarkable that in the present study F performed at least as well as NF in terms of CoP excursion and peak velocity in the ML direction. As such, a lengthened APA phase measured during a CSRT test appears to be an earlier indicator of the risk of fall for community-dwelling elderly subjects than the capacity to move the CoP during the APA.

The situation is different in the AP direction: elderly F limited the CoP backward excursion (CoP_B) and peak velocity ($VCoP_B$) compared to NF (see **Figure 8**). According to Brenière and collaborators model (Brenière et al., 1987; Lepers and Brenière, 1995), it means that during APA the F reduced the distance between the CoP and the CoM_{WB} in the AP

direction. Consecutively, F did not create a forward propulsive torque as efficient as NF. This mechanism led to a smaller displacement of the XCoM in the forward direction and to an increased stability at FO. This is typically what we observed for F compared to NF (see **Figures 6, 9**). We could interpret these results in two different ways: (1) F cannot move their CoP further or faster backward, due to physical limitations or a higher FoF, and the APA last as long as the XCoM is forward enough to step; and (2) F chose to decrease the CoP excursion in order to enhance the stability at FO. In this case the decrease is even more pronounced that APA duration is increased, probably due to limitations in the ML direction (see paragraph above). Nonetheless, our results on elderly F show that they were as able as NF in: (1) moving their CoP in the ML direction inside the BoS; and (2) moving their foot during the SP (a part of the movement that also engages muscular capacity). Again, this study does not bring enough firm arguments pro or against any of these interpretations. According to our results the second interpretation seems however to correspond the best.

Different APA strategies in ML and AP directions are used by F compared to NF. Both resulted in an increase of the dynamic stability at FO. It seems that the increase in APA duration is primarily due to limitations of the ML direction. A lengthened APA phase measured during a CSRT appears to be an earlier indicator of the risk of fall than the capacity to move the CoP, in community-dwelling elderly subjects.

Two Strategies that Aim to Increase Stability Instead of Rapidity in Elderly F

As discussed previously, elderly F displays a higher stability at FO. One of the counterpart is that they take less advantage of the disequilibrium torque given by gravity to propel the body in the direction of the targets, at the beginning of the SP (Lepers and Brenière, 1995; Lyon and Day, 1997). Another negative consequence is that it necessitates longer APA duration that decreases performances at the CSRT (Lord and Fitzpatrick, 2001).

To interpret those results, we can see the CSRT as a test involving two "tasks" for the CNS: stepping on the target as fast as possible (rapidity) and maintaining balance (stability). The results we observed in this study resemble to a "safer" strategy—as previously suggested by Patla et al. (1993), Brauer et al. (2002) and Luchies et al. (2002)—where the elderly F seem to enhance stability to the detriment of rapidity. In a different context, Brauer et al. (2002) showed that elderly having balance troubles prioritize stability instead of a dual task, probably because they involve maximal attentional resources in the accomplishment of the primary "task" (i.e., maintain balance). Similarly to what they suggested, a hypothesis would be that elderly F may see stability as the "primary task" during the CSRT and choose to prioritize it. We suggest that F make a choice because they "go against" the instructions of the test which were clearly to give priority to the rapidity.

This choice could also be qualified as a "conservative" strategy (Nakano et al., 2016), because elderly F seems to use unnecessary large conditions of stability at FO—as elderly do regarding to young adults in lateral steps (Patla et al., 1993). This inability of F to limit, in reasonable proportions, their stability at FO could even be seen as a limited capacity to adapt their motor command to the external context. Elderly F may perform this "conservative" strategy during the CSRT because the initiation of a voluntary step can always be delayed. In a more demanding context, such as a protective step (Rogers et al., 1996; Maki and McIlroy, 1997), this strategy would probably induce balance issues and a higher risk of fall. During protective steps the APA are usually shortened in time and reduced in amplitude in the ML direction to adapt to the perturbation (McIlroy and Maki, 1999) and the lateral balance has been shown to be the most determinant capacity for F to prevent from falling (Rogers et al., 2001; Johnson-Hilliard et al., 2008). The results pointing out that elderly F prioritize a more stable strategy than NF at FO could be interpreted as a poorer control of balance and an increased risk of fall. It has recently been suggested that an increased MoS is an indicator of a decreased control of lateral balance and a higher risk of fall during gait (Vistamehr et al., 2016).

Why would elderly F prioritize a more stable strategy than NF at FO? As the postural control is complex and involve multiple capacities and processes (Horak, 2006), there is never only one reason. If elderly F are effectively choosing a more stable balance strategy, it is probably because of the use of different processes and the integration of their own capacities, which are different from one subject to another. Reasons could be found in numerous capacities and processes, as the literature has already shown in the past (sensorial, cognitive, muscular, psychological). It appears important to us to point out that all subjects of our group of elderly F have one characteristic in common: they fell in the past year. This has probably significantly increased their FoF (Maki et al., 1991; Lajoie and Gallagher, 2004). Then, as the FoF reduces attentional resources available (Gage et al., 2003) and movement reinvestment (Huffman et al., 2009), an interaction between FoF and cognitive processes that acts in APA elaboration may have influenced their choice. A higher FoF is probably the most important reason why we observed this balance strategy in elderly F.

Limitations

This study presents several limitations. The location of our "Lateral" targets may not have been enough lateral (see **Figure 1**). The main limitation for balance in elderly F seems to come from the ML control of the CoP and our results are the most significant for these targets. More pronounced effects may be obtained using, for instance, 45° targets rather than 30°.

Another limitation comes from the fact that there is no simple RT test in that study, such as in Luchies et al. (2002). Such data could have helped to determine if sensory processing was reduced in our group of F and/or if they needed more time than NF to program the correct APA during a CSRT.

We did not study our population under a secondary task during this test, making impossible to know if our F subjects suffered from reduced attentional or inhibition capacities. As the balance strategy observed may come from a choice of a more "safer" or stable strategy, it could have been interesting to see if FoF has an interaction with the decisional process. We cannot currently conclude on those processes, which need to be further investigated.

CONCLUSION AND PERSPECTIVES

The results presented here confirmed our hypothesis. Elderly F have an elongated performance in the CSRT due to longer APA phase. By lengthening the APA duration in the ML direction without increasing the CoP displacement performance (excursion and peak velocity), F increase the MoS at FO.

This strategy can be qualified as a "safer" strategy—as suggested previously by Patla et al. (1993), Brauer et al. (2002) and Luchies et al. (2002)—used to the detriment of the CSRT performance. This strategy probably comes from a choice due to a higher FoF, which changes the way posture and balance are controlled (Maki et al., 1991; Adkin et al., 2000; Brauer et al., 2002; Huffman et al., 2009; Yiou et al., 2011) and/or an attempt to minimize the muscular effort (Zettel et al., 2002). In a more demanding environment, this incapacity to adjust the stability to the task would probably induce balance issues and a higher risk of fall. Programs for the risk of fall prevention in community-dwelling elderly adults should focus on helping elderly F to get confidence back in their capacity to manage balance in different situations and, by so, improve balance performances.

In perspective of this study, we will look more specifically at the trials with APA errors. It would be indicative to know how elderly F correct these errors. Such information would particularly inform about their inhibition capacity, as Sparto et al.

(2014) showed. Further improvements of this test are also to consider, like for example use of 45° targets during a CSRT.

AUTHOR CONTRIBUTIONS

RT contributed with project creation, data collection, data analysis and drafted the manuscript. TR contributed with project creation and data analysis. PC contributed in data analysis. MB contributed with project creation and recruitment of the subjects. LC contributed with project creation, data collection and data analysis. All authors discussed the results and participated in the revision of the manuscript.

FUNDING

RT held a doctoral fellowship from La Région Rhône-Alpes.

REFERENCES

Adkin, A. L., Frank, J. S., Carpenter, M. G., and Peysar, G. W. (2000). Postural control is scaled to level of postural threat. *Gait Posture* 12, 87–93. doi: 10.1016/s0966-6362(00)00057-6

Aruin, A. S., and Latash, M. L. (1995). The role of motor action in anticipatory postural adjustments studied with self-induced and externally triggered perturbations. *Exp. Brain Res.* 106, 291–300. doi: 10.1007/BF00241125

Bouisset, S., and Do, M.-C. (2008). Posture, dynamic stability, and voluntary movement. *Neurophysiol. Clin.* 38, 345–362. doi: 10.1016/j.neucli.2008.10.001

Brauer, S. G., Woollacott, M., and Shumway-Cook, A. (2002). The influence of a concurrent cognitive task on the compensatory stepping response to a perturbation in balance-impaired and healthy elders. *Gait Posture* 15, 83–93. doi: 10.1016/s0966-6362(01)00163-1

Brenière, Y., Cuong Do, M., and Bouisset, S. (1987). Are dynamic phenomena prior to stepping essential to walking? *J. Mot. Behav.* 19, 62–76. doi: 10.1080/00222895.1987.10735400

Brunt, D., Liu, S. M., Trimble, M., Bauer, J., and Short, M. (1999). Principles underlying the organization of movement initiation from quiet stance. *Gait Posture* 10, 121–128. doi: 10.1016/s0966-6362(99)00020-x

Brunt, D., Santos, V., Kim, H. D., Light, K., and Levy, C. (2005). Initiation of movement from quiet stance: Comparison of gait and stepping in elderly subjects of different levels of functional ability. *Gait Posture* 21, 297–302. doi: 10.1016/j.gaitpost.2004.03.003

Crenna, P., and Frigo, C. (1991). A motor program for the initiation of forward oriented movements in humans. *J. Physiol.* 437, 635–653. doi: 10.1113/jphysiol.1991.sp018616

Dumas, R., Chèze, L., and Verriest, J.-P. (2007). Adjustments to McConville et al. and Young et al. body segment inertial parameters. *J. Biomech.* 40, 543–553. doi: 10.1016/j.jbiomech.2006.02.013

Dumas, R., Robert, T., Cheze, L., and Verriest, J.-P. (2015). Thorax and abdomen body segment inertial parameters adjusted from McConville et al. and Young et al. *Int. Biomech.* 2, 113–118. doi: 10.1080/23335432.2015.1112244

Ejupi, A., Brodie, M., Gschwind, Y. J., Schoene, D., Lord, S., and Delbaere, K. (2014). Choice stepping reaction time test using exergame technology for fall risk assessment in older people. *Conf. Proc. IEEE Eng. Med. Biol. Soc.* 2014, 6957–6960. doi: 10.1109/EMBC.2014.6945228

Gage, W. H., Sleik, R. J., Polych, M. A., McKenzie, N. C., and Brown, L. A. (2003). The allocation of attention during locomotion is altered by anxiety. *Exp. Brain Res.* 150, 385–394. doi: 10.1007/s00221-003-1468-7

Halliday, S. E., Winter, D. A., Frank, J. S., Patla, A. E., and Ontario, N. L. G. (1998). The initiation of gait in young, elderly, and Parkinson's disease subjects. *Gait Posture* 8, 8–14. doi: 10.1016/s0966-6362(98)00020-4

Hauer, K., Lamb, S. E., Jorstad, E. C., Todd, C., Becker, C., and PROFANE-Group. (2006). Systematic review of definitions and methods of measuring falls in randomised controlled fall prevention trials. *Age Ageing* 35, 5–10. doi: 10.1093/ageing/afi218

Hof, A. L., and Curtze, C. (2016). A stricter condition for standing balance after unexpected perturbations. *J. Biomech.* 49, 580–585. doi: 10.1016/j.jbiomech.2016.01.021

Hof, A. L., Gazendam, M. G. J., and Sinke, W. E. (2005). The condition for dynamic stability. *J. Biomech.* 38, 1–8. doi: 10.1016/j.jbiomech.2004.03.025

Horak, F. B. (2006). Postural orientation and equilibrium: what do we need to know about neural control of balance to prevent falls? *Age Ageing* 35, Suppl 2, ii7–ii11. doi: 10.1093/ageing/afl077

Huffman, J. L., Horslen, B. C., Carpenter, M. G., and Adkin, A. L. (2009). Does increased postural threat lead to more conscious control of posture? *Gait Posture* 30, 528–532. doi: 10.1016/j.gaitpost.2009.08.001

Inacio, M., Ryan, A. S., Bair, W.-N., Prettyman, M., Beamer, B. A., and Rogers, M. W. (2014). Gluteal muscle composition differentiates fallers from non-fallers in community dwelling older adults. *BMC Geriatr.* 14:37. doi: 10.1186/1471-2318-14-37

Jian, Y., Winter, D., Ishac, M., and Gilchrist, L. (1993). Trajectory of the body COG and COP during initiation and termination of gait. *Gait Posture* 1, 9–22. doi: 10.1016/0966-6362(93)90038-3

Johnson, M. E., Mille, M. L., Martinez, K. M., Crombie, G., and Rogers, M. W. (2004). Age-related changes in hip abductor and adductor joint torques. *Arch. Phys. Med. Rehabil.* 85, 593–597. doi: 10.1016/j.apmr.2003.07.022

Johnson-Hilliard, M., Martinez, K. M., Janssen, I., Edwards, B. J., Mille, M.-L., Zhang, Y., et al. (2008). Lateral balance factors predict future falls in community-living older adults. *Arch. Phys. Med. Rehabil.* 89, 1708–1713. doi: 10.1016/j.apmr.2008.01.023

Lajoie, Y., and Gallagher, S. P. (2004). Predicting falls within the elderly community: comparison of postural sway, reaction time, the Berg balance scale and the Activities-specific Balance Confidence (ABC) scale for comparing fallers and non-fallers. *Arch. Gerontol. Geriatr.* 38, 11–26. doi: 10.1016/s0167-4943(03)00082-7

Lepers, R., and Brenière, Y. (1995). The role of anticipatory postural adjustments and gravity in gait initiation. *Exp. Brain Res.* 107, 118–124. doi: 10.1007/bf00228023

Lord, S. R., and Fitzpatrick, R. C. (2001). Choice stepping reaction time: a composite measure of falls risk in older people. *J. Gerontol. A. Biol. Sci. Med. Sci.* 56, M627–M632. doi: 10.1093/gerona/56.10.m627

Luchies, C. W., Schiffman, J., Richards, L. G., Thompson, M. R., Bazuin, D., and DeYoung, A. J. (2002). Effects of age, step direction, and reaction condition on the ability to step quickly. *J. Gerontol. A. Biol. Sci. Med. Sci.* 57, M246–M249. doi: 10.1093/gerona/57.4.m246

Lyon, I. N., and Day, B. L. (1997). Control of frontal plane body motion in human stepping. *Exp. Brain Res.* 115, 345–356. doi: 10.1007/pl00005703

Maki, B. E., Holliday, P. J., and Topper, A. K. (1991). Fear of falling and postural performance in the elderly. *J. Gerontol.* 46, M123–M131. doi: 10.1093/geronj/46.4.m123

Maki, B. E., and McIlroy, W. E. (1997). The role of limb movements in maintaining upright stance: the "change-in-support" strategy. *Phys. Ther.* 77, 488–507.

Massion, J. (1992). Movement, posture and equilibrium: interaction and coordination. *Prog. Neurobiol.* 38, 35–56. doi: 10.1016/0301-0082(92)90034-c

McIlroy, W. E., and Maki, B. E. (1999). The control of lateral stability during rapid stepping reactions evoked by antero-posterior perturbation: does anticipatory control play a role? *Gait Posture* 9, 190–198. doi: 10.1016/s0966-6362(99)00013-2

Melzer, I., Kurz, I., Shahar, D., Levi, M., and Oddsson, L. (2007). Application of the voluntary step execution test to identify elderly fallers. *Age Ageing* 36, 532–537. doi: 10.1093/ageing/afm068

Morcelli, M. H., LaRoche, D. P., Crozara, L. F., Marques, N. R., Hallal, C. Z., Rossi, D. M., et al. (2016). Neuromuscular performance in the hip joint of elderly fallers and non-fallers. *Aging Clin. Exp. Res.* 28, 443–450. doi: 10. 1007/s40520-015-0448-7

Nakano, W., Fukaya, T., Kobayashi, S., and Ohashi, Y. (2016). Age effects on the control of dynamic balance during step adjustments under temporal constraints. *Hum. Mov. Sci.* 47, 29–37. doi: 10.1016/j.humov.2016. 01.015

Patla, A. E., Frank, J. S., Winter, D. A., Rietdyk, S., Prentice, S., and Prasad, S. (1993). Age-related changes in balance control system: initiation of stepping. *Clin. Biomech.* 8, 179–184. doi: 10.1016/0268-0033(93)90012-7

Pijnappels, M., Delbaere, K., Sturnieks, D. L., and Lord, S. R. (2010). The association between choice stepping reaction time and falls in older adults—a path analysis model. *Age Ageing* 39, 99–104. doi: 10.1093/ageing/afp200

Polcyn, A. F., Lipsitz, L. A., Kerrigan, D. C., and Collins, J. J. (1998). Age-related changes in the initiation of gait: degradation of central mechanisms for momentum generation. *Arch. Phys. Med. Rehabil.* 79, 1582–1589. doi: 10. 1016/s0003-9993(98)90425-7

Rogers, M. W., Hain, T. C., Hanke, T. A., and Janssen, I. (1996). Stimulus parameters and inertial load: effects on the incidence of protective stepping responses in healthy human subjects. *Arch. Phys. Med. Rehabil.* 77, 363–368. doi: 10.1016/s0003-9993(96)90085-4

Rogers, M. W., Hedman, L. D., Johnson, M. E., Cain, T. D., and Hanke, T. A. (2001). Lateral stability during forward-induced stepping for dynamic balance recovery in young and older adults. *J. Gerontol. A. Biol. Sci. Med. Sci.* 56, M589–M994. doi: 10.1093/gerona/56.9.m589

Rubenstein, L. Z. (2006). Falls in older people: epidemiology, risk factors and strategies for prevention. *Age Ageing* 35, Suppl 2, ii37–ii41. doi: 10. 1093/ageing/afl084

Schoene, D., Lord, S. R., Verhoef, P., and Smith, S. T. (2011). A novel video game–based device for measuring stepping performance and fall risk in older people. *Arch. Phys. Med. Rehabil.* 92, 947–953. doi: 10.1016/j.apmr.2011.01.012

Schoene, D., Valenzuela, T., Toson, B., Delbaere, K., Severino, C., Garcia, J., et al. (2015). Interactive cognitive-motor step training improves cognitive risk factors of falling in older adults–A randomized controlled trial. *PLoS One* 10:e0145161. doi: 10.1371/journal.pone.0145161

Segev-Jacubovski, O., Herman, T., Yogev-Seligmann, G., Mirelman, A., Giladi, N., and Haudsdorff, J. M. (2011). The interplay between gait, falls and cognition: can cognitive therapy reduce fall risk? *Expert Rev. Neurother.* 11, 1057–1075. doi: 10.1586/ern.11.69

Sparto, P. J., Jennings, J. R., Furman, J. M., and Redfern, M. S. (2014). Lateral step initiation behavior in older adults. *Gait Posture* 39, 799–803. doi: 10.1016/j. gaitpost.2013.10.021

Stevens, J., Corso, P., Finkelstein, E., and Miller, T. (2006). The costs of fatal and non-fatal falls among older adults. *InJ. Prev.* 12, 290–295. doi: 10.1136/ip.2005. 011015

St George, R. J., Fitzpatrick, R. C., Rogers, M. W., and Lord, S. R. (2007). Choice stepping response and transfer times: effects of age, fall risk, and secondary tasks. *J. Gerontol. A Biol. Sci. Med. Sci.* 62, 537–542. doi: 10.1093/gerona/62. 5.537

Sturnieks, D. L., St George, R., Fitzpatrick, R. C., and Lord, S. R. (2008). Effects of spatial and nonspatial memory tasks on choice stepping reaction time in older people. *J. Gerontol. A Biol. Sci. Med. Sci.* 63, 1063–1068. doi: 10.1093/gerona/63. 10.1063

Tinetti, M., Speechley, M., and Ginter, S. (1988). Risk factors for fall among elderly persons living in the community. *N. Engl. J. Med.* 319, 1701–1707. doi: 10. 1056/NEJM198812293192604

Uemura, K., Yamada, M., Nagai, K., Shinya, M., and Ichihashi, N. (2012a). Effect of dual-tasking on the center of pressure trajectory at a gait initiation in elderly fallers and non-fallers. *Aging Clin. Exp. Res.* 24, 152–156. doi: 10. 1007/bf03325161

Uemura, K., Yamada, M., Nagai, K., Tanaka, B., Mori, S., and Ichihashi, N. (2012b). Fear of falling is associated with prolonged anticipatory postural adjustment during gait initiation under dual-task conditions in older adults. *Gait Posture* 35, 282–286. doi: 10.1016/j.gaitpost.2011.09.100

Vallée, P., Tisserand, R., and Robert, T. (2015). Possible recovery or unavoidable fall? A model to predict the one step balance recovery threshold and its stepping characteristics. *J. Biomech.* 48, 3905–3911. doi: 10.1016/j.jbiomech.2015. 09.024

van Dieën, J. H., and Pijnappels, M. (2008). Falls in older people. *J. Electromyogr. Kinesiol.* 18, 169–171. doi: 10.1016/j.jelekin.2007.06.001

Van Sint Jan, S. (2007). *Color Atlas of Skeletal Landmark Definitions–Guidelines for Reproductible Manual and Virtual Palpations.* Edinburgh: Churchill Livingstone Elsevier.

Vellas, B. J., Wayne, S. J., Romero, L. J., Baumgartner, R. N., and Garry, P. J. (1997). Fear of falling and restriction of mobility in elderly fallers. *Age Ageing* 26, 189–193. doi: 10.1093/ageing/26.3.189

Vistamehr, A., Kautz, S. A., Bowden, M. G., and Neptune, R. R. (2016). Correlations between measures of dynamic balance in individuals with post-stroke hemiparesis. *J. Biomech.* 49, 396–400. doi: 10.1016/j.jbiomech.2015. 12.047

White, K. N., Gunter, K. B., Snow, C. M., and Hayes, W. C. (2002). The quick step: a new test for measuring reaction time and lateral stepping velocity. *J. Appl. Biomech.* 18, 271–277. doi: 10.1123/jab.18.3.271

Winter, D. A. (1995). Human balance and posture control during standing and walking. *Gait Posture* 3, 193–214. doi: 10.1016/0966-6362(96) 82849-9

Woollacott, M., and Shumway-Cook, A. (2002). Attention and the control of posture and gait: a review of an emerging area of research. *Gait Posture* 16, 1–14. doi: 10.1016/s0966-6362(01)00156-4

World Health Organisation. (2008). *Global Report on Falls: Prevention in Older Age.* Geneva: Ageing and Life Course Family and Community Health.

Yiou, E., Deroche, T., Do, M. C., and Woodman, T. (2011). Influence of fear of falling on anticipatory postural control of medio-lateral stability during rapid leg flexion. *Eur. J. Appl. Physiol.* 111, 611–620. doi: 10.1007/s00421-010-1680-7

Yiou, E., Hussein, T., and LaRue, J. (2012). Influence of temporal pressure on anticipatory postural control of medio-lateral stability during rapid leg flexion. *Gait Posture* 35, 494–499. doi: 10.1016/j.gaitpost.2011. 11.015

Zettel, J. L., McIlroy, W. E., and Maki, B. E. (2002). Environmental constraints on foot trajectory reveal the capacity for modulation of anticipatory postural adjustments during rapid triggered stepping reactions. *Exp. Brain Res.* 146, 38–47. doi: 10.1007/s00221-002-1150-5

18

Ehlers-Danlos Syndrome, Hypermobility Type: Impact of Somatosensory Orthoses on Postural Control

Emma G. Dupuy[1], Pascale Leconte[1], Elodie Vlamynck[1], Audrey Sultan[1,2], Christophe Chesneau[3], Pierre Denise[1], Stéphane Besnard[1], Boris Bienvenu[1,2] and Leslie M. Decker[1]*

[1]COMETE, INSERM, UNICAEN, Normandie Université, Caen, France, [2]Department of Internal Medicine, University Hospital Center of Caen, UNICAEN, Normandie Université, Caen, France, [3]LMNO, CNRS, UNICAEN, Normandie Université, Caen, France

*Correspondence:
Leslie M. Decker
leslie.decker@unicaen.fr

Elhers-Danlos syndrome (EDS) is the clinical manifestation of connective tissue disorders, and comprises several clinical forms with no specific symptoms and selective medical examinations which result in a delay in diagnosis of about 10 years. The EDS hypermobility type (hEDS) is characterized by generalized joint hypermobility, variable skin hyperextensibility and impaired proprioception. Since somatosensory processing and multisensory integration are crucial for both perception and action, we put forth the hypothesis that somatosensory deficits in hEDS patients may lead, among other clinical symptoms, to misperception of verticality and postural instability. Therefore, the purpose of this study was twofold: (i) to assess the impact of somatosensory deficit on subjective visual vertical (SVV) and postural stability; and (ii) to quantify the effect of wearing somatosensory orthoses (i.e., compressive garments and insoles) on postural stability. Six hEDS patients and six age- and gender-matched controls underwent a SVV (sitting, standing, lying on the right side) evaluation and a postural control evaluation on a force platform (Synapsys), with or without visual information (eyes open (EO)/eyes closed (EC)). These two latter conditions performed either without orthoses, or with compression garments (CG), or insoles, or both. Results showed that patients did not exhibit a substantial perceived tilt of the visual vertical in the direction of the body tilt (Aubert effect) as did the control subjects. Interestingly, such differential effects were only apparent when the rod was initially positioned to the left of the vertical axis (opposite the longitudinal body axis). In addition, patients showed greater postural instability (sway area) than the controls. The removal of vision exacerbated this instability, especially in the mediolateral (ML) direction. The wearing of orthoses improved postural stability, especially in the eyes-closed condition, with a particularly marked effect in the anteroposterior (AP) direction. Hence, this study suggests that hEDS is associated with changes in the relative contributions of somatosensory and vestibular inputs to verticality perception. Moreover, postural control impairment was offset, at least partially, by wearing somatosensory orthoses.

Keywords: subjective vertical, proprioception, compressive garments, proprioceptive insoles, postural sway

INTRODUCTION

The Ehlers-Danlos syndrome (EDS) is a heterogeneous group of hereditary connective tissue diseases, which are present in at least 1/5000 individuals with a majority of women (Sobey, 2014). Degradation of the composition and elasticity of connective tissue results in a broad, pronounced and unspecific symptomatology. Consequently, the revised Brighton criteria classified EDS in six subtypes, according to the predominance of their clinical manifestations (Beighton et al., 1998). The EDS hypermobility subtype (hEDS) is the most frequently encountered. Besides common symptoms with other subtypes such as fatigue and pain, hEDS is characterized by generalized joint hypermobility combined with variable cutaneous hyperelasticity and proprioceptive impairment (Beighton et al., 1998; Castori, 2012). Indeed, few studies that have investigated proprioceptive sensitivity (i.e., joint position sense) in hEDS, have demonstrated the existence of proprioceptive impairment in this population (Rombaut et al., 2010a; Clayton et al., 2015). A strong hypothesis to explain the neurophysiological basis of this impairment suggests that the generalized joint hypermobility specific to hEDS induces excessive and repeated extension of the ligaments, which damages the surrounding proprioceptive receptors (Ruffini's and Pacini's corpuscles; Golgi tendon organs). Additionally, changes in cutaneous elasticity probably affects pressure information transmitted by cutaneous tactile mechanoreceptors to cortical areas. Hence, it is likely that hEDS induces not only a proprioceptive deficit but, more broadly, a somatosensory deficit. Consequently, the major functional disabilities expressed by these patients, including clumsiness and falls, which sometimes lead to kinesiophobia, could be the result of this somatosensory impairment (Rombaut et al., 2012).

Indeed, somatosensory information, arising from muscles, skin, and joints, plays a key role in perception, balance and, more broadly in movement. Currently, there is growing evidence that balance and movement are both based on heteromodal integration of three types of sensory modality, visual, vestibular, and somatosensory, which carry redundant, specific and complementary information (Massion, 1992; Lacour et al., 1997). The integration of these sensory modalities by the central nervous system provides three spatial frames of reference—egocentric (i.e., body), geocentric (i.e., gravity) and allocentric (i.e., external cues)—which contribute to the development of internal models crucially involved in balance and movement (Gurfinkel et al., 1981; Massion, 1994; Mergner and Rosemeier, 1998). In the sensorimotor processes, internal models refer to a neural process responsible for synthesizing information from sensory modalities and combine efferent and afferent information to resolve sensory ambiguity (Merfeld et al., 1999). Furthermore, sensory processing is a flexible mechanism (Peterka, 2002). The central nervous system continually modulates weight assigned to each sensory modality to provide a dynamic internal representation, making it possible to always generate an appropriate muscle response to maintain and adapt balance to the continuously changing environment (Van der Kooij et al., 2001; Zupan et al., 2002; Peterka and Loughlin, 2004; Logan et al., 2014). Within

this process, the somatosensory system specifically provides information about the position of different parts of the body with respect to one another. Moreover, it allows characterization and localization of touch and pain (Dijkerman and De Haan, 2007). Thus, the somatosensory system mainly contributes to the sensorimotor map of body space in internal models, an unconscious process also called the "body schema" (De Vignemont, 2010).

Mittelstaedt (1983) reported that information provided by proprioception contributes considerably to the maintenance of body verticality. The perception of vertical is considered be the outcome of synthesizing visual, somatosensory and vestibular information (Brandt et al., 1994; Bisdorff et al., 1996; Merfeld et al., 1999; Van Beuzekom and Van Gisbergen, 2000; Bronstein et al., 2003; Barbieri et al., 2008; Pérennou et al., 2008; Tarnutzer et al., 2009). However, it is known that the contribution of each sensory modality in verticality perception varies between subjects and, to a greater extent, in populations presenting either vestibular impairments (e.g., patients with unilateral vestibular loss; Lopez et al., 2008) or somatosensory impairments (e.g., stroke patients with a hypoesthesia pressure and paraplegic patients; Barra et al., 2010). Interestingly, the Aubert effect, consisting in tilting of the visual vertical towards the body during lateral body tilt due to the resultant of the gravitational vector (i.e., perception of the otolith organ) and the idiotropic vector (i.e., perception of the main longitudinal axis of the body), is modified in favor of gravitational vector proportionally to the degree of somatosensory impairment (Barra et al., 2010). Hence, it seems reasonable to inquire whether somatosensory impairment in hEDS patients might modify the Aubert effect. At the same time, it has been previously shown that hEDS patients develop body schema disorders resulting in partial loss of movement control (Rombaut et al., 2010b) and postural instability (Galli et al., 2011). This deterioration in postural stability is manifested in both static (standing) and dynamic (walking) conditions (Rombaut et al., 2011; Rigoldi et al., 2013). Previous studies have already shown a strong connection between somatosensory impairments and balance disorders, especially in Parkinson's disease (Jacobs and Horak, 2006; Vaugoyeau et al., 2011). Typically, these patients, as in normal aging, compensate for their sensory deficit by an overreliance on visual information (Lord and Webster, 1990; Isableu et al., 1997; Azulay et al., 2002). Therefore, one can speculate that somatosensory impairment could be responsible to a large extent for this postural instability, and that it could be compensated for by using a high level of visual information.

Compression garments (CG) have been tested empirically in clinical practice in hEDS, resulting in beneficial effects on pain, fatigue and mobility. Speculatively, the CG, due to their mechanical effect, are thought to enhance joint coaptation and increase the pressure of the subcutaneous connective tissue to a normal range. Hence, CG may enhance somatosensory feedback to the brain and, thus, its contribution to postural control. Similarly, proprioceptive insoles (PI) may enhance plantar cutaneous afferents and postural stability. Therefore, somatosensory orthoses (i.e., CG and PI) offer a therapeutic solution to reduce somatosensory impairments, however weakly evaluated. Along with these observations, previous studies have demonstrated that CG induced an improvement in knee proprioception, and PI decreased the attentional demand for gait (Clark et al., 2014; Ghai et al., 2016). Conversely, these two ortheses showed no impact in healthy young subjects, and CG appeared to induce a deterioration of postural stability in elderly subjects (Hijmans et al., 2009; Dankerl et al., 2016). In the light of these conflicting observations, we aimed to quantify the impact of these somatosensory orthoses on postural stability in a population with a specific impairment of the somatosensory system. Indeed, it seems plausible that, although the wearing of CG has probably no immediate impact on the damaged joint proprioceptive receptors, its compressive effect applied to subcutaneous connective tissue could allow better somatosensory transmission from cutaneous tactile mechanoreceptors. Hence, somatosensory deficit could be partially reduced by CG, which would compensate for joint proprioception impairment. Similarly, enhanced plantar cutaneous afferents induced by PI could increase the available sensory information for postural control.

The goal of the present study was to assess: (i) the impact of somatosensory deficit on subjective visual vertical (SVV) and postural stability; and (ii) the effects of somatosensory orthoses (i.e., CG and PI) on static postural control. We hypothesized that: (i) somatosensory impairments would modify SVV, strongly impair postural stability and increase the use of visual information; and (ii) enhancing somatosensory feedback with the orthoses would restore the balance in the use of sensory modalities, thus reducing the use of visual information, and consequently enhance postural stability.

MATERIALS AND METHODS

Study Population

Six patients with hEDS (6 females; mean age ± SD: 37 ± 10.41 years) and six healthy, age- and gender-matched control subjects (6 females; mean age ± SD: 36 ± 11.52 years) participated in this study. Patient selection was carried out in the Internal Medicine Department of Caen University Hospital. Inclusion criteria were based on the revised Villefranche criteria, including the presence of generalized joint hypermobility, skin hyperelasticity, chronic musculoskeletal pain, and/or a positive family history (Beighton et al., 1998). Additionally, patients must have reported hypersensoriality (e.g., a low hearing threshold). Exclusion criteria were: (i) wearing of somatosensory orthoses (i.e., PI and CG); (ii) inability to maintain a minimum of postural stability in static conditions (i.e., holding an upright stance during 1 min); (iii) treatment by a physical therapist; and (iv) other pathologies that directly impact postural control (e.g., Ménière's disease). Finally, patients were checked for vestibular disorders by ENT examination with otolithic myogenic evoked potentials, and videonystagmography. Healthy controls subjects were recruited by local phone call. Control subjects were excluded if they had a neurologic (with

a special focus on vestibular disease using the Fukuda test; Fukuda, 1959) or orthopedic disorder (analysis of foot plantar pressure distributions using a podoscope) that could affect their postural stability, and a generalized disease affecting joints, or a Beighton score >4/9.

All subjects were treated in strict compliance with the Declaration of Helsinki. The protocol was approved by the CERSTAPS (Ethical Committee of Sport and Physical Activities Research), Notice Number: 2016-26-04-13, approved by the National Academic Commission (CNU) on April 26, 2016. Written informed consent was obtained from all participants.

Instrumentation

Somatosensory Orthoses

The CG and PI required in this study were customized based on the needs of each patient by orthotic and prosthetic practitioners (Novatex Medical). CG included pants, vest, and mittens, which covered the entire body of all participants (i.e., trunk, upper and lower limbs; **Figure 1**).

Postural Control

Postural sway was recorded using a motorized force platform (SYNAPSYS, France). Three strain gauges integrated into the force platform recorded the vertical ground reaction force component. The data were sampled at 100 Hz and transformed by computer-automated stability analysis software (i.e., Synapsys software) to obtain x-y coordinates of the center of pressure (COP).

Subjective Visual Vertical

Perception of the vertical was assessed by the SVV test using the Perspective System® (Framiral®, France).

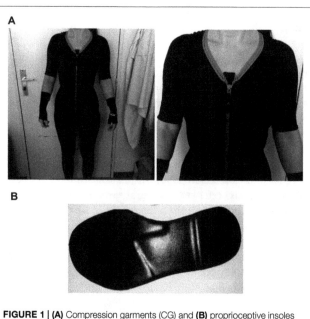

FIGURE 1 | (A) Compression garments (CG) and **(B)** proprioceptive insoles (PI) worn by an Ehlers-Danlos syndrome hypermobility type (hEDS) patient during the experiment.

Experimental Procedure

In the first part of the experiment, participants underwent postural control assessment (duration: 1 h 45 min for patients, and 20 min for controls) followed by SVV assessment (duration: 15 min for all participants).

Subjective Visual Vertical Assessment

To assess the SVV, each participant, in a completely darkened room, was shown, in front of them, the projection of a luminous rod (laser line 2 m in length placed 3 m in front of them). Participants could rotate the rod around its center in the clockwise or counterclockwise directions using a transmitter, and were instructed to place the rod vertically with respect to the true gravitational vertical. All subjects performed the SVV test in three conditions: standing, sitting and lying on their right side. In this latter condition, participants lay in a standard position on a stretcher with an adjustable head-rest, which was positioned identically initially for each participant (body and head were tilted, respectively, at 90° and 72°). Subjects were asked to minimize their movements during the tests. Each condition comprised four trials: two with the rod initially oriented to the right side (i.e., 30° to the right—clockwise) and two to the left side (i.e., −30° to the left—counterclockwise). The tests and conditions were randomly distributed within each participant.

Postural Control Assessment

Postural sway was measured for 52 s while participants stood on a force platform. Participants were asked to stand still, barefoot, arms hanging freely, feet positioned at an angle of 30°, and to focus on a visual reference mark fixed 1.5 m in front of them in their individual line of vision. The assessment comprised four conditions with two tests each lasting 52 s, with a 20 s rest between each test, and 5 min between each condition. The start and stop signals were given 3 s before and 3 s after each acquisition. The four conditions were: (1) control condition (CC; without orthoses); (2) CG; (3) PI; and (4) the combination of CG and PI (CG-PI). Each condition was performed with either eyes open (EO) or eyes closed (EC). Participants also underwent dual-task (combining postural control with a cognitive task) and dynamic (sinusoidal translation of support) trials under the four above-mentioned conditions (results are not included in the present article). To minimize any order effects during testing, such as fatigue effects, all conditions and trials (EO/EC) were randomized among subjects. A training test was performed before testing (**Figure 2**).

Data Analysis

Subjective Visual Vertical Analysis

SVV evaluation error was scored in degrees of deviation from the vertical. Mean errors were calculated across conditions, according to the initial orientation of the rod. Errors were scored negatively when the subjective vertical was oriented to the left, and positively when it was oriented to the right.

Postural Control Analysis

Postural sway parameters calculated from the COP recordings were as follows: the anteroposterior and mediolateral sway standard deviation (SD-AP/SD-ML; mm) and the sway area (AREA-CE; mm^2) corresponding to the 95% confidence elliptic area included within the COP path.

Statistical Analysis

The SVV (angle of deviation from the vertical) and postural (AREA-CE, SD-AP and SD-ML) dependent variables failed to display an acceptable normal distribution (Shapiro-Wilk test). Consequently, non-parametric tests were used for statistical analysis.

The Mann-Whitney U-test was used to compare healthy controls to hEDS patients on verticality perception and postural stability. A Friedman test was used to determine differences between the performances carried out in each postural condition (CC, CG, PI and CG/PI) and each SVV condition (standing, seated, lying: right and left initial orientation). When the result of the Friedman test was significant, we subsequently used a Wilcoxon test for matched samples to determine the effects of vision (EO and EC) and somatosensory orthoses on postural stability. We used the Bonferroni method to correct for multiple comparisons. Statistical significance was set at 0.05. Statistica (version 10, Statsoft, Inc., Tulsa, OK, USA) was used to perform all analyses.

RESULTS

Subjective Visual Vertical

We first analyzed perception of the visual vertical in each position (standing, seated, lying on the right side) using the Mann-Whitney U-test. In standing condition, hEDS patients oriented the vertical more in left side than controls, when the initial orientation of the rod was also on the left ($U = 4, p = 0.026$). Simultaneously, in lying on the right condition, when the initial orientation of the rod was on the left, patients did not exhibit the substantial perceived tilt of the visual vertical in the direction of the body tilt (Aubert effect), and oriented their vertical closer to the real vertical compared to controls, ($U = 0$, $p = 0.002$). Interestingly, in sitting condition, perception of visual vertical was similar in both groups (**Figure 3**).

The Friedman test revealed significant differences in verticality perception according to the initial orientation of the rod (right and left) and body position (sitting, standing and lying on the right) in hEDS patients ($p = 0.0001$) and controls ($p = 0.00034$). As 30 side-by-side comparisons were carried out for each *post hoc* analysis, the Bonferroni method was used to correct the significance level at 0.0016. Consequently, all the results from the Wilcoxon test reported below with a $p > 0.0016$ have been used because of our small sample size, and thus have a descriptive vocation.

Regardless of the position, the initial orientation of the rod seems to influence the verticality perception of hEDS patients (sitting: $Z = 2.20$, $p = 0.027$; standing: $Z = 2.20$, $p = 0.027$;

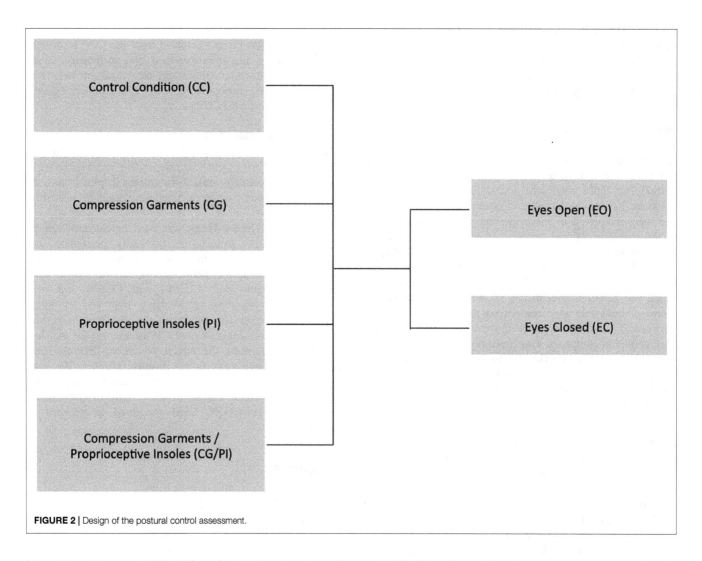

FIGURE 2 | Design of the postural control assessment.

lying: $Z = 2.20$, $p = 0.027$). When the initial orientation of the rod was to the right, patients showed a greater degree of deviation of verticality perception in standing compared to sitting ($Z = 2.20$, $p = 0.027$), and to a larger extent, when lying compared to sitting ($Z = 2.20$, $p = 0.027$) and standing ($Z = 2.20$, $p = 0.027$). In contrast, no difference was observed when the initial orientation of the rod was to the left. Likewise, in controls, the initial orientation of the rod did not influence verticality perception. In addition, controls presented a greater deviation of their verticality perception when lying as opposed to sitting and standing, regardless the initial orientation of the rod (right initial orientation: sitting vs. lying: $Z = 2.20$, $p = 0.027$, standing vs. lying: $Z = 2.20$, $p = 0.027$; left initial orientation: sitting vs. lying: $Z = 2.20$, $p = 0.027$, standing vs. lying: $Z = 2.20$, $p = 0.027$).

Postural Control without Somatosensory Orthoses

Compared with controls, hEDS patients showed impaired postural stability, as reflected by their increased sway area (EO, $U = 4$, $p = 0.052$) and increased AP sway SD (EO, $U = 3$,

$p = 0.015$). These latter effects became more pronounced in the absence of visual information (AREA-CE: EC, $U = 2$, $p = 0.017$; SD-AP: EC, $U = 0$, $p = 0.004$). Furthermore, postural stability also deteriorated in the ML direction without vision ($U = 4$, $p = 0.052$). Besides, the Wilcoxon test comparing EO and EC revealed an increased sway area ($Z = 2.022$, $p = 0.043$) and an increased ML sway SD in hEDS patients ($Z = 2.022$, $p = 0.043$). Removal of vision had no effect on postural stability in controls (**Figure 4**).

Postural Control with Somatosensory Orthoses

The Friedman test was conducted to assess the effects of somatosensory orthoses on postural stability in hEDS patients in four conditions (control, PI, CG, and PI-CG), with (EO) and without (EC) vision. Then, as six side-by-side comparisons were carried out within each *post hoc* analysis, the significance threshold was set at 0.00833, as indicated by Bonferroni correction. Similar to the SSV, all the results from the Wilcoxon test reported below with a $p > 0.00833$ have a descriptive vocation.

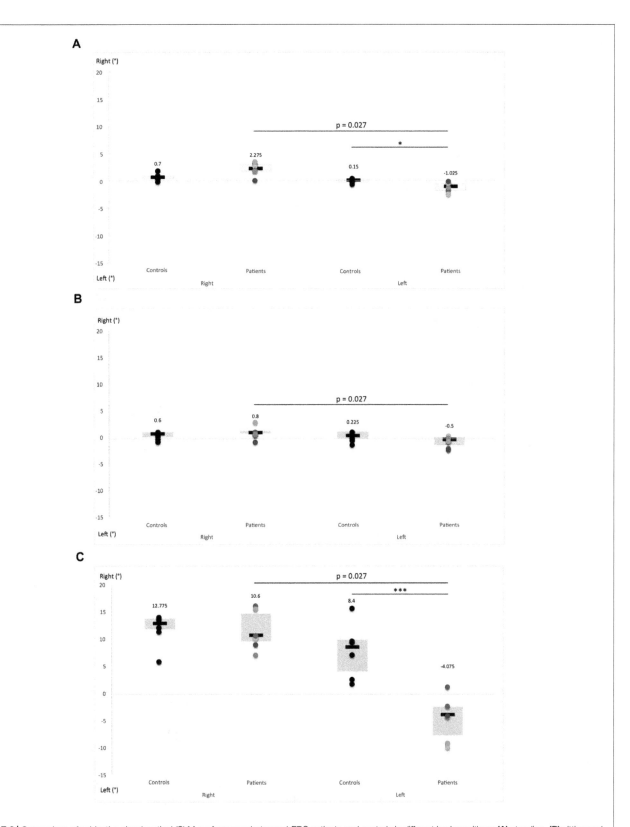

FIGURE 3 | Comparison of subjective visual vertical (SVV) performance between hEDS patients and controls in different body positions: **(A)** standing, **(B)** sitting and **(C)** lying on the right side. SVV was measured by presenting a laser rod 12 times in total darkness with a 30-degree deviation from the vertical alternately on the right and the left. Subjects were asked to reposition the rod vertically using a remote control. Box plots represent median and quartiles, and dots represent performance of each participant as follows: controls: black; patient 1: red; patient 2: green; patient 3: purple; patient 4: light blue; patient 5: orange; patient 6: dark blue. $*p < 0.05$, $***p < 0.005$.

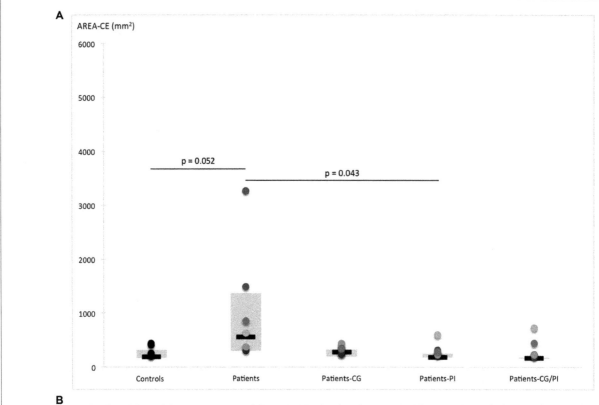

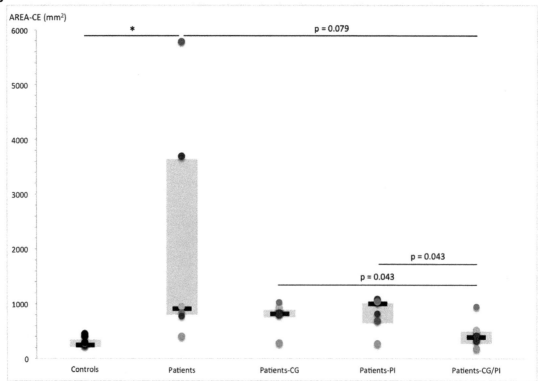

FIGURE 4 | Comparison of AREA-CE (area of 95% confidence circumference, mm²) obtained by hEDS patients and controls, with and without somatosensory orthoses (CG, compression garments; PI, proprioceptive insoles; CG-PI, both somatosensory orthoses): in **(A)** eyes-open, and **(B)** eyes-closed conditions. Box plots represent median and quartiles, and dots represent performance of each participant as follows: controls: black; patient 1: red; patient 2: green; patient 3: purple; patient 4: light blue; patient 5: orange; patient 6: dark blue. *$p < 0.05$.

With Vision

The Friedman test revealed that somatosensory orthoses tended to have a significant effect on sway area ($p = 0.069$), with an improvement in postural stability (decreased sway area) in the presence of PI compared to the CC ($Z = 2.022$, $p = 0.043$; **Figure 4A**). However, the patients' performance distribution within each orthosis condition indicates that this result may be due to a lower inter-individual heterogeneity than in CG/PI condition, and a median slightly lower than in CG condition (**Figure 4A**). Consequently, there is little evidence that the PI condition induced an improvement of postural stability greater than the other conditions (CG, CG/PI), which all seem to induce a beneficial but similar effect on postural stability. This effect appeared to be even more pronounced when the patient was unstable in the CC. On the other hand, somatosensory orthoses had no significant effect on AP and ML sway SD (**Figures 5A, 6**).

Without Vision

The Friedman test revealed that somatosensory orthoses significantly impacted AP sway SD ($p = 0.040$), and tended to have a significant effect on sway area ($p = 0.06$). Importantly, the simultaneous wearing of the two orthoses seems to have induced further improvement on AP sway SD ($Z = 2.022$, $p = 0.043$; **Figure 5B**), compared to control, as opposed to the wearing of each orthosis separately. Indeed, the observed effects were more pronounced when the two orthoses were worn together rather than separately (AREA-CE: CG vs. CG/PI: $Z = 2.022$, $p = 0.043$; PI vs. CG/PI: $Z = 2.022$, $p = 0.043$; **Figure 4B**; SD-AP: CG vs. CG/PI: $Z = 1.75$, $p = 0.079$; PI vs. CG/PI: $Z = 2.022$, $p = 0.043$; **Figure 5B**). Also, the decreased AP sway SD induced by CG ($Z = 2.022$, $p = 0.043$) tended to be greater than that induced by PI ($Z = 1.75$, $p = 0.079$; **Figure 5B**). However, in light of patients' performance distribution under these two conditions, it is difficult to identify an additional effect of CG as compared to PI. In the ML direction, somatosensory orthoses did not show any significant impact on postural stability.

With vs. Without Vision

The increased sway area found in hEDS patients without vision and somatosensory orthoses ($Z = 2.022$, $p = 0.043$) persisted when they wore orthoses, alone (PI: $Z = 2.022$, $p = 0.043$; CG: $Z = 1.75$, $p = 0.079$) or in combination ($Z = 2.022$, $p = 0.043$). A similar result was observed for ML sway SD (PI: $Z = 2.022$, $p = 0.043$; CG: $Z = 1.75$, $p = 0.079$, PI/CG: $Z = 1.75$ $p = 0.079$; **Figure 6**). In contrast, visual removal did not appear to affect AP sway SD, regardless of the presence of somatosensory orthoses.

DISCUSSION

Subjective Visual Vertical in hEDS

In the standing condition, the results obtained by hEDS patients suggest a greater deviation from true gravitational vertical than controls. This effect seems to be less apparent in the sitting condition. These findings suggest that hEDS is associated with changes in the neural processing of somatosensory inputs,

which could in turn alter judgment of the SVV (Trousselard et al., 2003). Moreover, one can speculate that, as previously observed in stroke patients, this specific alteration of verticality perception in the standing condition could be associated with postural instability in hEDS patients, and especially with lower limb asymmetry (Bonan et al., 2006, 2007). However, correlational analyses did not strongly confirm a direct link between these two factors. The small number of subjects included in this pilot study makes these analyses irrelevant due to pronounced heterogeneity between patients in both postural stability and verticality perception performances. In addition, certain technical limitations prevented us from computing parameters able to quantify postural asymmetry. Nevertheless, these observations provide preliminary data that should be explored further. More relevantly, when lying in the right condition, the Aubert or A-effect (i.e., SVV deviation from the true vertical in the same direction as the body tilt; Aubert, 1861) was found when the rod was tilted to the right in both groups, but absent when the rod was initially left-oriented in hEDS patients. In healthy controls, the A-effect is considered to result from the subject's tendency to shift the SVV toward the longitudinal body axis, independently of the initial orientation of the rod (Mittelstaedt and Glasauer, 1993). More specifically, it may result from changes in vestibular (i.e., otolithic organs; *gravitational vector*) and somatosensory (i.e., muscular and articulatory endocaptors, cutaneous exocaptors; interception *idiotropic vector*) inputs related to a body tilt in the dark (Bronstein, 1999). In their study, Bronstein et al. (1996) demonstrated that when patients with bilateral peripheral labyrinthine lesion are lying at approximately 90° on their right side, they presented an A-effect twice as large as controls. The authors suggested that tilt-mediated effect on the visual vertical is more likely to be of somatosensory rather than vestibular origin. The implication of the somatosensory system in verticality perception was confirmed by studies on SVV in somatosensory deficient populations (Yardley, 1990; Anastasopoulos and Bronstein, 1999). In these studies, the authors found a unilateral loss of A-effect when hemianesthetic patients were lying on the same side as their lesion, and a bilateral loss in patients with severe polyneuropathy. Thus, our results are consistent with those reported in the literature for healthy controls. A striking finding is that the perceived vertical of hEDS patients was not far from the true vertical when the rod was initially oriented to the left side. This finding is also consistent with earlier studies (Yardley, 1990; Anastasopoulos and Bronstein, 1999), and another study conducted by Barra et al. (2010), who found that the A-effect was markedly reduced in patients with somatosensory deficit (i.e., hemiplegia and paraplegia). The explanation advanced is that these patients cannot integrate somatosensory inputs. Hence, their SVV relies mainly on gravitational (vestibular) input. Another interesting finding is that this phenomenon did not appear when the rod was initially right-oriented. A plausible explanation is that, in this condition, the initial orientation of the rod was directly congruent with the joint combination of the idiotropic and gravitational vectors (internal representation of the vertical). This was not the case when

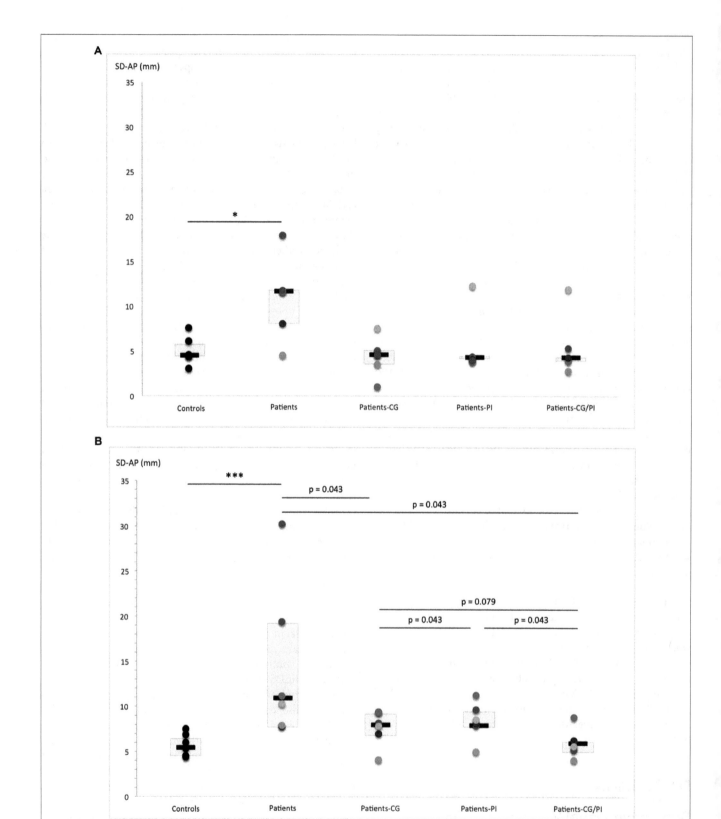

FIGURE 5 | Comparison of SD-AP (standard deviation of anteroposterior center-of-pressure (COP) displacement: mm) obtained by hEDS patients and controls, with and without somatosensory orthoses (CG, compression garments; PI, proprioceptive insoles; CG-PI, both somatosensory orthoses): in **(A)** eyes-open, and **(B)** eyes-closed conditions. Box plots represent median and quartiles, and dots represent performance of each participant as follows: controls: black; patient 1: red; patient 2: green; patient 3: purple; patient 4: light blue; patient 5: orange; patient 6: dark blue. *$p < 0.05$, ***$p < 0.005$.

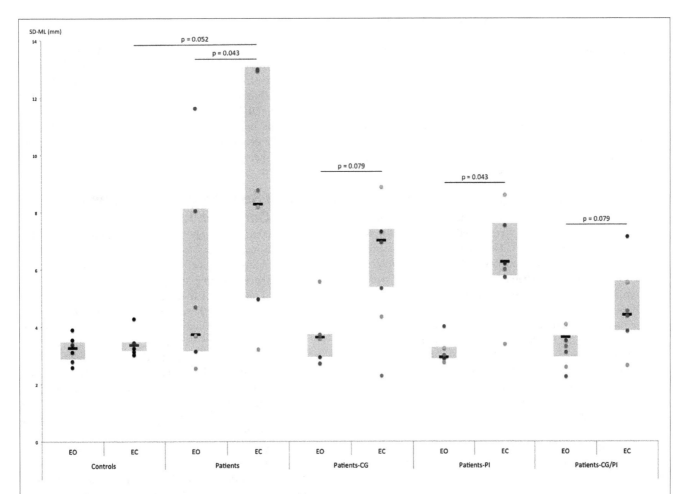

FIGURE 6 | Comparison of SD-ML (standard deviation of mediolateral COP displacement: mm) obtained by hEDS patients and controls, with eyes open (EO) and eyes closed (EC) depending on the somatosensory orthoses worn (CG, compression garments; PI, proprioceptive insoles; CG-PI, both somatosensory orthoses). Box plots represent median and quartiles, and dots represent performance of each participant as follows: controls: black; patient 1: red; patient 2: green; patient 3: purple; patient 4: light blue; patient 5: orange; patient 6: dark blue.

the rod was initially left-oriented (i.e., rotated in a direction opposite to the longitudinal body axis). This may be due to the greater complexity of the task that led patients to preferentially rely on gravitational (vestibular) input. Indeed, to adjust the rod with their verticality perception when it was initially left-oriented, the rod systematically passed through the true vertical. Consequently, one can postulate that the predominance of vestibular input relative to somatosensory input led patients to perceive as vertical the position where the rod converged with gravitational vector. This finding is consistent with the fact that somatosensory input is not absent, but is compromised by damage to its receptors and the poor pressure transmission induced by degraded connective tissue. Hence, we could suggest that somatosensory input is also present, but its contribution to perception could be inhibited or reduced due to its lack of reliability. Finally, taken together, these findings highlight changes in the relative contributions of somatosensory and vestibular inputs to verticality perception in hEDS patients (i.e., central adaptation in somato-vestibular perceptual systems).

Baseline Characteristics of Postural Control in hEDS

In line with previous studies, hEDS patients showed significant difficulties in controlling COP displacements (i.e., increased sway area—confidence ellipse area), especially when visual information was absent (Galli et al., 2011; Rigoldi et al., 2013). Interestingly, controls did not show any difference in their postural stability between EO and EC conditions as observed in other studies (e.g., Lacour et al., 1997; Błaszczyk et al., 2014). This result is not surprising given the fact that the healthy controls included in this study were fairly young (approximately 37 years old) and presented no orthopedic and sensory disorders. In addition, it is also possible that postural parameters used in this study were not the most sensitive to assess the effect of visual removal in healthy young subjects (Prieto et al., 1996). However, our result suggests that hEDS patients (especially the most unstable cases) relied on vision for postural stability. Marigold and Eng (2006) found that the removal of vision in stroke patients increased postural instability, particularly in the ML direction, and all the more so in presence of postural asymmetry. To explain this observation, the authors suggested that, in stroke patients, the body schema formed by the CNS may lack appropriate somatosensory information due to altered supraspinal centers (Niam et al., 1999). In hEDS patients, impairment of somatosensory receptors would induce a down-weighting of this sensory modality, compensated by an up-weighting of visual modality (slow dynamic; Chiba et al., 2015). The balance between the contributions of each sensory modality is essential in continuous sensory reweighting (fast dynamic), which permits the maintenance of efficient and adaptable postural control (Nashner, 1976; Asslander and Peterka, 2014; Chiba et al., 2015). Furthermore, hEDS patients also had great difficulty in maintaining their ML postural stability when vision was withdrawn. Therefore, ML stability appears to depend upon two factors: reliance on vision and asymmetry in postural control. Our results tend to confirm an overreliance on visual information, but suggest only the presence of postural asymmetry in hEDS patients. It would be interesting to investigate this question in future studies. Regardless of visual condition, the intergroup difference in sway SD was more pronounced in the AP direction. Increased AP sway was also found in stroke patients when somatosensory information was altered (Marigold et al., 2004). To interpret these results, the authors hypothesized that the ability to integrate information from cutaneous sensation can reduce the contribution of ankle proprioception in controlling postural sway. Consequently, the increased AP sway observed in stroke patients in whom ankle proprioception was compromised would be due to their inability to compensate by using cutaneous plantar information (Marigold et al., 2004; Marigold and Eng, 2006). However, the authors found no correlation between cutaneous plantar foot sensation and postural sway. Thus, it is still unclear how somatosensory information affects AP postural sway in stroke patients. This finding, also observed in hEDS patients with specific somatosensory impairment, suggests that AP stability results, at least in part, from accurate somatosensory information. Moreover, a previous study conducted in healthy young subjects showed that the neuromuscular system must allocate 50 percent more effort to control AP stability in the upright stance (Błaszczyk et al., 2014). Thus, the greater AP sway SD in hEDS patients suggests that they may have difficulty generating sufficient neuromuscular effort to maintain their postural stability. However, this hypothesis needs to be confirmed as Błaszczyk et al. (2014) used COP velocity (sway ratio and sway directional index) to quantify postural stability. Technological limitations prevented us from computing this parameter. Hence, we posit that the greater neuromuscular effort allocated for controlling AP stability may produce higher recruitment of the somatosensory system. Therefore, somatosensory impairment could prevent hEDS patients from producing sufficient neuromuscular effort to stabilize their balance in the AP direction. To summarize, specificities of postural control in hEDS patients appear to result from both their somatosensory impairment and the adoption of postural compensatory strategies. This imbalance in multisensory integration complicates control of the upright stance and, therefore, is at least partly responsible for their

postural instability. Finally, this process seems to be relatively variable between participants. This finding was not surprising given that considerable variability in clinical expression is commonly observed in hEDS patients. Consequently, it has recently been proposed to consider hEDS as a spectrum of pathogenetically-related manifestations of joint hypermobility (Malfait et al., 2017). Hence, it would be interesting to further investigate the link between severity of clinical expression of hEDS and the evolution of the sensori-motor strategy adopted by these patients.

Effects of Somatosensory Orthoses on Postural Control in hEDS

In hEDS patients (notably the most unstable cases), the wearing of somatosensory orthoses seems to reduce their postural instability (i.e., sway area) to such an extent that their performances became comparable to those of controls in eyes-open condition. However, further investigations will be required to confirm these preliminary observations with a larger sample. Interestingly, this effect turned out to be even more pronounced in the absence of visual information. Wearing the two orthoses in combination seems to help patients stabilize their balance and minimize their AP sway SD. Thus, the combined wearing of orthoses could induce a synergetic effect. Indeed, it seems to improve postural stability more than the wearing of the CG or PI separately in the eyes-closed condition for both sway area and AP sway SD. Therefore, one can reasonably hypothesize that the increased cutaneous plantar sensation applied by pressure on sole receptors from PI could be concurrent with the increased cutaneous sensation and joint position sense promoted by CG. Hence, the combination of CG and PI could possibly enhance the available somatosensory information and, consequently, balance, even without vision. In addition, it is noteworthy that removal of visual information increases the impact of somatosensory orthoses on postural stability, especially in the AP direction. We thus suggest that, in the EO condition, visual information compensates for the lack of somatosensory information. Consequently, the removal of vision obliges patients to rebalance their use of sensory modalities in favor of somatosensory information, thus reinforcing the somatosensory input provided by orthoses. In contrast, ML stability appears to be scarcely affected by the somatosensory orthoses and remained sensitive to visual input. This result supports our previous hypothesis, which assumed that visual information was, at least in part, responsible for ML stability. Besides, our results showed no effect of somatosensory orthoses on overreliance on visual input in hEDS patients. Also, their postural strategy, which consists in compensating their lack of somatosensory information by ample use of visual information, appears to have persisted although the somatosensory input was enhanced. It is thus legitimate to assume that, in order to modify the strategy adopted by these patients, prolonged wearing of somatosensory orthoses would be necessary. The long-term use of somatosensory orthoses would both stimulate and preserve somatosensory receptors and thus develop and consolidate the neural network, supporting a more balanced sensory-motor strategy. Lastly, unlike previous studies which found no effect for PI and CG, our study suggested their efficacy on postural stability in hEDS patients (Hijmans et al., 2009; Dankerl et al., 2016). Indeed, in healthy controls, it is possible that the improved somatosensory input provided by CG actuate more information than needed to control their posture. Hence, the wearing of CG may induce noise in the somatosensory input in healthy subjects, whereas it helps adjust the somatosensory threshold in hEDS patients (Hijmans et al., 2009). Likewise, PI did not induce any effect on postural stability in healthy subjects, probably because no proprioceptive enhancement was required (Dankerl et al., 2016).

Study Limitations

This pilot study presents a number of limitations. First, the study was conducted on a small sample. Second, the methodology used to investigate SVV could be improved in several respects: (i) the number of trials performed (Piscicelli et al., 2015: a minimum of six trials are required); (ii) the subject's head should be fixed to their support to prevent any speculative movements; (iii) the head could be placed in the same alignment as the body; and (iv) the lying position could also be performed on the left side.

Conclusions

Collectively, the functional explorations performed on hEDS patients, using posturography and SVV, suggest an imbalance in the integration of sensory inputs. The results tended to show that somatosensory impairment modifies both verticality perception (Aubert effect) and postural instability. More specifically, results from postural assessment suggest a re-weighting of multisensory integration in favor of visual input. This compensatory strategy, adopted by the patients in order to maintain their balance, may

diminish their adaptability, which could, at least in part, account for their postural instability. In contrast, our findings suggest an enhancement of somatosensory feedback induced by the orthoses, thus facilitating postural control, which in turn tends to become more stable. Lastly, this is the first investigation assessing the effect of somatosensory orthoses in hEDS patients, providing new perspectives for improving medical care. However, the observations in this pilot study need to be confirmed by further investigations with a larger number of subjects. Yet, they strongly suggest that postural and SVV assessments are potentially useful tools for the diagnosis and monitoring of this pathology.

AUTHOR CONTRIBUTIONS

LMD and EGD designed the study. LMD, EGD and PL carried out the experiment. EGD, LMD and CC analyzed the data. EGD and LMD conceived the figures. EGD, LMD, SB, BB and PD interpreted the results and drafted the manuscript. BB, AS and EV screened potential participants to determine their eligibility for the study. All authors revised the manuscript and approved its final version.

ACKNOWLEDGMENTS

This research was funded by the Normandy Integrative Biology, Health, Environment Doctoral School (EGD), the Regional Council of Basse-Normandie (equipment funding), and the "Association des Patients Normands Ehlers Danlos" (APNED, President: Dr. Claire El Moudden). We sincerely thank the company NOVATEX Medical® for providing customized compression garments and proprioceptive insoles for the patients, and all the participants in our study.

REFERENCES

Anastasopoulos, D., and Bronstein, A. M. (1999). A case of thalamic syndrome: somatosensory influences on visual orientation. J. Neurol. Neurosurg. Psychiatry 67, 390–394. doi: 10.1136/jnnp.67.3.390

Asslander, L., and Peterka, R. J. (2014). Sensory reweighting dynamics in human postural control. J. Neurophysiol. 111, 1852–1864. doi: 10.1152/jn.00669.2013

Aubert, H. (1861). Eine scheinbare bedeutende Drehung von Objecten bei Neigung des Kopfes nach rechts oder links. Archiv f. Pathol. Anat. 20, 381–393. doi: 10.1007/bf02355256

Azulay, J. P., Mesure, S., Amblard, B., and Pouget, J. (2002). Increased visual dependence in Parkinson's disease. Percept. Mot. Skills 95, 1106–1114. doi: 10.2466/pms.2002.95.3f.1106

Barbieri, G., Gissot, A. S., Fouque, F., Casillas, J. M., Pozzo, T., and Pérennou, D. (2008). Does proprioception contribute to the sense of verticality? Exp. Brain Res. 185, 545–552. doi: 10.1007/s00221-007-1177-8

Barra, J., Marquer, A., Joassin, R., Reymond, C., Metge, L., Chauvineau, V., et al. (2010). Humans use internal models to construct and update a sense of verticality. Brain 133, 3552–3563. doi: 10.1093/brain/awq311

Beighton, P., De Paepe, A., Steinmann, B., Tsipouras, P., and Wenstrup, R. J. (1998). Ehlers-Danlos syndromes: revised nosology, Villefranche, 1997. Am. J. Med. Genet. 77, 31–37. doi: 10.1002/(SICI)1096-8628(19980428)77:131::AID-AJMG8>3.3.CO;2-P

Bisdorff, A., Wolsley, C., Anastasopoulos, D., Bronstein, A., and Gresty, M. A. (1996). The perception of body verticality (subjective postural vertical)

in peripheral and central vestibular disorders. Brain 119, 1523–1534. doi: 10.1093/brain/119.5.1523

Błaszczyk, J. W., Beck, M., and Sadowska, D. (2014). Assessment of postural stability in young healthy subjects based on directional features of posturographic data: vision and gender effects. Acta. Neurobiol. Exp. 74, 433–442.

Bonan, I. V., Guettard, E., Leman, M. C., Colle, F. M., and Yelnik, A. P. (2006). Subjective visual vertical perception relates to balance in acute stroke. Arch. Phys. Med. Rehabil. 87, 642–646. doi: 10.1016/j.apmr.2006.01.019

Bonan, I. V., Hubeaux, K., Gellez-Leman, M. C., Guichard, J. P., Vicaut, E., and Yelnik, A. P. (2007). Influence of subjective visual vertical misperception on balance recovery after stroke. J. Neurol. Neurosurg. Psychiatry 20, 49–55. doi: 10.1136/jnnp.2006.087791

Brandt, T., Dieterich, M., and Danek, A. (1994). Vestibular cortex lesions affect the perception of verticality. Ann. Neurol. 35, 403–412. doi: 10.1002/ana.410350406

Bronstein, A. M. (1999). The interaction of otolith and proprioceptive information in the perception of verticality. The effects of labyrinthine and CNS disease. Ann. N Y Acad. Sci. 871, 324–333. doi: 10.1111/j.1749-6632.1999.tb09195.x

Bronstein, A. M., Pérennou, D. A., Guerraz, M., Playford, D., and Rudge, P. (2003). Dissociation of visual and haptic vertical in two patients with vestibular nuclear lesions. Neurology 61, 1260–1262. doi: 10.1212/01.wnl.0000086815.22816.dc

Bronstein, A. M., Yardley, L., Moore, A. P., and Cleeves, L. (1996). Visually and posturally mediated tilt illusion in Parkinson's disease and in labyrinthine defective subjects. Neurology 47, 651–656. doi: 10.1212/wnl.47.3.651

Castori, M. (2012). Ehlers-Danlos syndrome, hypermobility type: an underdiagnosed hereditary connective tissue disorder with mucocutaneous, articular and systemic manifestations. *ISRN Dermatol.* 2012, 1–22. doi: 10.5402/2012/751768

Chiba, R., Takakusaki, K., Ota, J., Yozu, A., and Haga, N. (2015). Human upright posture control models based on multisensory inputs; in fast and slow dynamics. *Neurosci. Res.* 104, 96–104. doi: 10.1016/j.neures.2015.12.002

Clark, D. J., Christou, E. A., Ring, S. A., Williamson, J. B., and Doty, L. (2014). Enhanced somatosensory feedback reduces prefrontal cortical activity during walking in older adults. *J. Gerontol. A Biol. Sci. Med. Sci.* 69, 1422–1428. doi: 10.1093/gerona/glu125

Clayton, H. A., Jones, S. A., and Henriques, D. Y. (2015). Proprioceptive precision is impaired in Ehlers-Danlos syndrome. *Springerplus* 4:323. doi: 10.1186/s40064-015-1089-1

Dankerl, P., Keller, A. K., Häberle, L., Stumptner, T., Pfaff, G., Uder, M., et al. (2016). Effects on posture by different neuromuscular afferent stimulations and proprioceptive insoles: rasterstereographic evaluation. *Prosthet. Orthot. Int.* 40, 369–376. doi: 10.1177/0309364614554031

De Vignemont, F. (2010). Body schema and body image-pros and cons. *Neuropsychologia* 48, 669–680. doi: 10.1016/j.neuropsychologia.2009.09.022

Dijkerman, H. C., and De Haan, E. H. (2007). Somatosensory processes subserving perception and action. *Behav. Brain. Sci.* 30, 189–201. doi: 10.1017/S0140525X07001392

Fukuda, T. (1959). Vertical writing with eyes covered; a new test of vestibulo-spinal reaction. *Acta. Otolaryngol.* 50, 26–36. doi: 10.3109/00016485909129150

Galli, M., Rigoldi, C., Celletti, C., Mainardi, L., Tenore, N., Albertini, G., et al. (2011). Postural analysis in time and frequency domains in patients with Ehlers-Danlos syndrome. *Res. Dev. Disabil.* 32, 322–325. doi: 10.1016/j.ridd.2010.09.009

Ghai, S., Driller, M. W., and Masters, R. S. (2016). The influence of below-knee compression garments on knee-joint proprioception. *Gait Posture* doi: 10.1016/j.gaitpost.2016.08.008 [Epub ahead of print].

Gurfinkel, V. S., Lipshits, M. I., Mori, S., and Popov, K. E. (1981). Stabilization of body position as the main task of postural regulation. *Hum. Physiol.* 7, 155–165.

Hijmans, J. M., Zijlstra, W., Geertzen, J. H., Hof, A. L., and Postema, K. (2009). Foot and ankle compression improves joint position sense but not bipedal stance in older people. *Gait Posture* 29, 322–325. doi: 10.1016/j.gaitpost.2008.10.051

Isableu, B., Ohlmann, T., Cremieux, J., and Amblard, B. (1997). Selection of spatial frame of reference and postural control variability. *Exp. Brain Res.* 114, 584–589. doi: 10.1007/pl00005667

Jacobs, J. V., and Horak, F. B. (2006). Abnormal proprioceptive-motor integration contributes to hypometric postural responses of subjects with Parkinson's disease. *Neuroscience* 141, 999–1009. doi: 10.1016/j.neuroscience.2006.04.014

Lacour, M., Barthelemy, J., Borel, L., Magnan, J., Xerri, C., Chays, A., et al. (1997). Sensory strategies in human postural control before and after unilateral vestibular neurotomy. *Exp. Brain Res.* 115, 300–310. doi: 10.1007/pl00005698

Logan, D., Kiemel, T., and Jeka, J. J. (2014). Asymmetric sensory reweighting in human upright stance. *PLoS One* 9:e100418. doi: 10.1371/journal.pone.0100418

Lopez, C., Lacour, M., Léonard, J., Magnan, J., and Borel, L. (2008). How body position changes visual vertical perception after unilateral vestibular loss. *Neuropsychologia* 46, 2435–2440. doi: 10.1016/j.neuropsychologia.2008.03.017

Lord, S. R., and Webster, I. W. (1990). Visual field dependence in elderly fallers and non-fallers. *Int. J. Aging. Hum. Dev.* 31, 267–277. doi: 10.2190/38mh-2ef1-e36q-75t2

Malfait, F., Francomano, C., Byers, P., Belmont, J., Berglund, B., Black, J., et al. (2017). The 2017 international classification of the Ehlers-Danlos syndromes. *Am. J. Med. Genet. C Semin. Med. Genet.* 175, 8–26. doi: 10.1002/ajmg.c.31552

Marigold, D. S., and Eng, J. J. (2006). The relationship of asymmetric weight-bearing with postural sway and visual reliance in stroke. *Gait Posture* 23, 249–255. doi: 10.1016/j.gaitpost.2005.03.001

Marigold, D. S., Eng, J. J., Tokuno, C. D., and Donnelly, C. A. (2004). Contribution of muscle strength and integration of afferent input to postural instability in persons with stroke. *Neurorehabil. Neural Repair* 18, 222–229. doi: 10.1177/1545968304271171

Massion, J. (1992). Movement, posture and equilibrium: interaction and coordination. *Prog. Neurobiol.* 38, 35–56. doi: 10.1016/0301-0082(92)90034-c

Massion, J. (1994). Postural control system. *Curr. Opin. Neurobiol.* 4, 877–887. doi: 10.1016/0959-4388(94)90137-6

Merfeld, D. M., Zupan, L., and Peterka, R. J. (1999). Humans use internal models to estimate gravity and linear acceleration. *Nature* 15, 615–618.

Mergner, T., and Rosemeier, T. (1998). Interaction of vestibular, somatosensory and visual signals for postural control and motion perception under terrestrial and microgravity conditions—a conceptual model. *Brain. Res. Rev.* 28, 118–135. doi: 10.1016/s0165-0173(98)00032-0

Mittelstaedt, H. (1983). A new solution to the problem of the subjective vertical. *Naturwissenschaften* 70, 272–281. doi: 10.1007/bf00404833

Mittelstaedt, H., and Glasauer, S. (1993). Illusions of verticality in weightlessness. *Clin. Investig.* 71, 732–739. doi: 10.1007/bf00209728

Nashner, L. M. (1976). Adapting reflexes controlling the human posture. *Exp. Brain Res.* 26, 59–72. doi: 10.1007/bf00235249

Niam, S., Cheung, W., Sullivan, P. E., Kent, S., and Gu, X. (1999). Balance and physical impairments after stroke. *Arch. Phys. Med. Rehabil.* 80, 1227–1233. doi: 10.1016/s0003-9993(99)90020-5

Pérennou, D. A., Mazibrada, G., Chauvineau, V., Greenwood, R., Rothwell, J., Gresty, M. A., et al. (2008). Lateropulsion, pushing and verticality perception in hemisphere stroke: a causal relationship? *Brain* 131, 2401–2413. doi: 10.1093/brain/awn170

Peterka, R. J. (2002). Sensorimotor integration in human postural control. *J. Neurophysiol.* 883, 1097–1118. doi: 10.1152/jn.00605.2001

Peterka, R. J., and Loughlin, P. J. (2004). Dynamic regulation of sensorimotor integration in human postural control. *J. Neurophysiol.* 91, 410–423. doi: 10.1152/jn.00516.2003

Piscicelli, C., Nadeau, S., Barra, J., and Pérennou, D. (2015). Assessing the visual vertical: how many trials are required? *BMC Neurol.* 15:215. doi: 10.1186/s12883-015-0462-6

Prieto, T. E., Myklebust, J. B., Hoffmann, R. G., Lovett, E. G., and Myklebust, B. M. (1996). Measures of postural steadiness: differences between healthy young and elderly adults. *EEE. Trans. Biomed. Eng* 4, 956–966. doi: 10.1109/10.532130

Rigoldi, C., Cimolin, V., Camerota, F., Celletti, C., Albertini, G., Mainardi, L., et al. (2013). Measuring regularity of human postural sway using approximate entropy and sample entropy in patients with Ehlers-Danlos syndrome hypermobility type. *Res. Dev. Disabil.* 34, 840–846. doi: 10.1016/j.ridd.2012.11.007

Rombaut, L., De Paepe, A., Malfait, F., Cools, A., and Calders, P. (2010a). Joint position sense and vibratory perception sense in patients with Ehlers-Danlos syndrome type III (hypermobility type) . *Clin. Rheumatol.* 29, 289–295. doi: 10.1007/s10067-009-1320-y

Rombaut, L., Malfait, F., Cools, A., De Paepe, A., and Calders, P. (2010b). Musculoskeletal complaints, physical activity and health-related quality of life among patients with the Ehlers-Danlos syndrome hypermobility type. *Disabil. Rehabil.* 32, 1339–1345. doi: 10.3109/09638280903514739

Rombaut, L., Malfait, F., De Wandele, I., Taes, Y., Thijs, Y., De Paepe, A., et al. (2012). Muscle mass, muscle strength, functional performance and physical impairment in women with the hypermobility type of Ehlers-Danlos syndrome. *Arthritis Care Res. (Hoboken)* 63, 1584–1592. doi: 10.1002/acr.21726

Rombaut, L., Malfait, F., De Wandele, I., Thijs, Y., De Paepe, A., and Calders, P. (2011). Balance, gait, falls and fear of falling in women with the hypermobility type of Ehlers-Danlos Syndrome. *Arthritis Care Res. (Hoboken)* 63, 1432–1439. doi: 10.1002/acr.20557

Sobey, G. (2014). Ehlers-Danlos syndrome - a commonly misunderstood group of conditions. *Clin. Med.* 14, 432–436. doi: 10.7861/clinmedicine.14-4-432

Tarnutzer, A. A., Bockisch, C., Straumann, D., and Olasagasti, I. (2009). Gravity dependence of subjective visual vertical variability. *J. Neurophysiol.* 102, 1657–1671. doi: 10.1152/jn.00007.2008

Trousselard, M., Cian, C., Nougier, V., Pla, S., and Raphel, C. (2003). Contribution of somesthetic cues to the perception of body orientation and subjective visual vertical. *Percept. Psychophys.* 65, ,1179–1187. doi: 10.3758/bf03194843

Van Beuzekom, A. D., and Van Gisbergen, J. A. (2000). Properties of the internal representation of gravity inferred from spatial-direction and body-tilt estimates. *J. Neurophysiol.* 84, 11–27.

Van der Kooij, H., Jacobs, R., Koopman, B., and Van der Helm, F. (2001). An adaptive model of sensory integration in a dynamic environment applied to human stance control. *Biol. Cybern.* 84, 103–115. doi: 10.1007/s004220 000196

Vaugoyeau, M., Hakam, H., and Azulay, J. P. (2011). Proprioceptive impairment and postural orientation control in Parkinson's disease. *Hum. Mov. Sci.* 30, 405–414. doi: 10.1016/j.humov.2010.10.006

Yardley, L. (1990). Contribution of somatosensory information to perception of the visual vertical with body tilt and rotating visual field. *Percept. Psychophys.* 48, 131–134. doi: 10.3758/bf03207079

Zupan, L. H., Merfeld, D. M., and Darlot, C. (2002). Using sensory weighting to model the influence of canal, otolith and visual cues on spatial orientation and eye movements. *Biol. Cybern.* 86, 209–230. doi: 10.1007/s00422-001-0290-1

19

Specific Posture-Stabilising Effects of Vision and Touch Are Revealed by Distinct Changes of Body Oscillation Frequencies

Stefania Sozzi[1], Antonio Nardone[2] and Marco Schieppati[3]*

[1] Centro Studi Attività Motorie (CSAM), Istituti Clinici Scientifici Maugeri SB (Istituto di Ricovero e Cura a Carattere Scientifico, IRCCS), Pavia, Italy, [2] Neurorehabilitation and Spinal Unit, Department of Clinical-Surgical, Diagnostic and Pediatric Sciences, Istituti Clinici Scientifici Maugeri SB (Istituto di Ricovero e Cura a Carattere Scientifico, IRCCS), University of Pavia, Pavia, Italy, [3] Istituti Clinici Scientifici Maugeri SB, Istituto di Ricovero e Cura a Carattere Scientifico (IRCCS), Pavia, Italy

*Correspondence:
Marco Schieppati
marco.schieppati@icsmaugeri.it

We addressed postural instability during stance with eyes closed (EC) on a compliant surface in healthy young people. Spectral analysis of the centre of foot pressure oscillations was used to identify the effects of haptic information (light-touch, EC-LT), or vision (eyes open, EO), or both (EO-LT). Spectral median frequency was strongly reduced by EO and EO-LT, while spectral amplitude was reduced by all "stabilising" sensory conditions. Reduction in spectrum level by EO mainly appeared in the high-frequency range. Reduction by LT was much larger than that induced by the vision in the low-frequency range, less so in the high-frequency range. Touch and vision together produced a fall in spectral amplitude across all windows, more so in anteroposterior (AP) direction. Lowermost frequencies contributed poorly to geometric measures (sway path and area) for all sensory conditions. The same subjects participated in control experiments on a solid base of support. Median frequency and amplitude of the spectrum and geometric measures were largely smaller when standing on solid than on foam base but poorly affected by the sensory conditions. Frequency analysis but not geometric measures allowed to disclose unique tuning of the postural control mode by haptic and visual information. During standing on foam, the vision did not reduce low-frequency oscillations, while touch diminished the entire spectrum, except for the medium-high frequencies, as if sway reduction by touch would rely on rapid balance corrections. The combination of frequency analysis with sensory conditions is a promising approach to explore altered postural mechanisms and prospective interventions in subjects with central or peripheral nervous system disorders.

Keywords: stance, critical conditions, body oscillation, spectral analysis, centre of foot pressure, length and area of sway path, vision, haptic

INTRODUCTION

The sensory control of bipedal human stance has been a matter of investigation for many years (1–3). A plethora of studies has been published on this topic, including some from our group (4, 5). Body sway when standing upright on a solid base of support is normally almost negligible in healthy subjects, witnessing accurate and precise neural control (6, 7) based on the internal model of gravitational and inertial forces (8) and on multiple inputs from the receptors detecting the body state. The excursions of the centre of foot pressure (CoP) of subjects standing quietly on the firm ground are approximately contained within the size of a dime, even if there is a large variability in sway across different healthy subjects (9). In several conditions, though, sway area can significantly increase, such as standing on sloped surfaces or when leaning forward or backward (4, 10), or decrease when subjects stand on elevated platforms (11). Standing on viscoelastic, compliant support like a foam pad produces larger sway and obvious body unsteadiness (12–14). This can in some cases lead to falls (15, 16), especially when vision is not available (17) or when sensory deficits are present (18–20).

Vision is important for body stabilisation during standing (21, 22). Sway may increase without vision compared to eyes open during quiet stance on a firm platform (23) with the effects depending on the distance between the feet (22, 24–26). Vision is also able to gate the effects of vibration (activating the primary receptors of the muscle spindles) of the neck muscles, consisting of a large forward sway when the eyes are closed (27). Vision also moderates the postural effects of the Achilles tendon vibration (28) and plays a more important role in postural stability under challenging conditions compared to quiet stances, such as on a mobile platform or on a foam surface (13, 29–31). When vision is available, subjects reduce reliance on proprioception and increase reliance on visual information (25).

Proprioception is crucial in the control of body stability and orientation in space (32–35), and various manoeuvres have been put in place to clarify its role, including muscle vibration as a tool for activating the spindles (36) or leg ischemia by compression to attenuate the transmission of their firing (37, 38). However, the contribution of the spindles to standing posture may not have been completely elucidated, not to speak of the role of the information from the foot sole and from the intrinsic foot muscles (39–41). These inputs under a quiet stance on the firm ground would play a limited function because the information originating in the primary spindle terminations, which are mainly sensitive to the velocity of muscle stretch (42), may not be crucial in the absence of rapid changes in muscle length. Under a quiet stance, the small-diameter fibres originating in the secondary spindle terminations may play a predominant role (43). Further, reweighting of the proprioceptive information normally occurs, as attested by the reduction in the amplitude of the soleus muscle H-reflex during unperturbed stance (44). Moreover, the reflex excitability of the motor neurons of the leg muscles is decreased when the stance is stabilised by holding onto a solid frame (45, 46) or by lightly touching fixed support (47). The role of proprioception can be more important when the balance is challenged (48) without vision. Under perturbed conditions or with a major reduction of the support surface (49, 50), when the postural muscle activity plays a major stabilising role, the role of proprioception is amplified and that of vision becomes of minor importance (51, 52). Moreover, velocity information would be crucial to stabilise posture during standing on foam support, where the task difficulty is increased and balance is controlled by many muscles acting at several joints (49, 53–57).

Haptic information is effective in reducing postural sway. The effect of a light fingertip touch is comparable to that obtained by opening the eyes (58–63). It can selectively originate from touch receptors (64) and occurs with contact forces below those necessary to mechanically stabilise the body (65–67). Touch-induced stabilisation occurs both when standing on firm ground and when standing on foam (68, 69) or after a balance perturbation (70, 71). With eyes closed, a light touch of an object next to the body, or a touch of the ground by the cane (66, 72), modifies the control of posture, because finger or cane can be appropriately moved to get the information they are searching for (73). The integration of visual and haptic cues in the control of stance has received much less attention than for the identification of object features (74, 75), but the same operating principles might underpin the effects of either or both inflows. For that matter, reaching and grasping (76) are in fact coordinated with postural adjustments (46, 77).

It is easy to measure sway. The force platform upon which subjects stand captures the path of the wandering centre of foot pressure in a given time period, and its length can be measured along with the surface covered by its journey. The geometric and statistical measures of sway (length of sway path and ellipses containing 95% of the acquired points) show a reasonable reproducibility (78) but bear large inter subject variability (79). Further, although sway path and sway area often co-vary, the correspondence between the former and the latter measure may not be consistent across subjects or patients (27, 80), because the same length of the oscillation skein may not occupy the same surface all the time (81). These measures can also overlap between eyes-open and eyes-closed conditions or between young and elderly (82, 83). In turn, the stabilising effect of vision is indistinguishable from that of touch (62). A different analytical approach might more consistently disclose unique attributes of the visual and haptic stabilising effects (21, 84).

When vision and touch are available, sway can further decrease compared to either information alone (63, 74). On the other hand, removal of peripheral sensation, as by anaesthesia or cooling of the skin of the foot sole, increases body oscillations (40). It might be supposed that integration of multiple inputs, as from the eye, the skin, the proprioceptors, or the graviceptors, can afford excellent body stabilisation (reduction of CoP sway) in accordance with the assumption that "more is better." This view would implicitly assume the existence of one posture-controlling centre able to integrate the sensory inputs and produce the adequate motor commands, which are evidently optimally designed when the centre receives the best possible amount of information. Body oscillations during quiet stance should then diminish monotonically as a function of the number and competence of the sensory inputs.

The assumption of the present study is that potential differences in the effect of vision or touch on stance control cannot be clearly evinced from the geometric analysis of the standard sway variables such as sway path length or area. Sway metrics more closely connected to the muscle synergies and to the presumably responsible supra-spinal and spinal control modes, expressed by the rambling and trembling behaviour (85, 86), would be more telling. Other methods, like indexing postural dynamics, have been exploited with attention to the multiple time scales of control that subserve standing postures (87, 88), such as the stabilogram-diffusion analysis (89, 90), the wavelet-based spectral analysis (91–93), and the sample entropy (94, 95), which provides measures advising automaticity of postural behaviour.

The purpose of this study has been to increase our knowledge on the role of the sensory control of stance by leveraging the tool of spectral frequency analysis (96–99) rather than through the sole use of geometric sway measures, such as the amplitude of sway area and length of sway path (23). Since oscillations frequencies have a strong relationship to leg and foot muscle activity (100), we hypothesised that the frequencies prevalent under certain conditions may offer a straightforward way of identifying whether the control of stance selects distinct balancing modes under a given sensory condition.

Different laboratories have identified a few frequency windows within the frequency spectrum and have connected these windows to the contribution of vestibular or visual or somatosensory information (99, 101–105). Occasionally, criteria for choosing the width of the frequency windows (106) have been provided. Further, the opinion that proprioception would be disrupted when standing on foam is at variance with the plain consideration that proprioception may be modest and downweighed in a quiet stance (see above), while a massive proprioceptive input must reach the central nervous system during the complex adjustments (often unconsciously produced) carried out when standing on foam (107).

Hence, we addressed the sensory modulation (visual, haptic) of postural behaviour in healthy young people through the use of spectral analysis of the CoP displacement. We have hypothesised that vision and touch stabilise body sway through at least partially different modes of action detectable by the spectral analysis. We first critically examined the use of this tool since there is a wide divergence in the way frequency spectra and frequency windows are defined by different laboratories. We then considered the distribution of the frequency spectrum oscillations when stabilisation was achieved through the use of haptic information (light touch, EC-LT) or vision (EO) or both (EO-LT). In addition, we compared the data obtained by the frequency analysis to those based on geometric sway measures. Finally, we compared the results obtained on the foam to those obtained on a solid base of support (BoS). Consistent modulations of the median frequency of the spectrum and of specific frequency windows thereof emerged, suggesting different neural mechanisms of sway-minimisation strategy for vision and haptic sense.

MATERIALS AND METHODS

Participants
Nineteen healthy young adults (9 men and 10 women) participated in the study. Their average age was 29 ± 4.2 years (mean ± SD), height 172.6 ± 7.2 cm, and weight 68.9 ± 13.5 kg. All subjects were free of neurological and musculoskeletal disorders and either had no sight problems or if so, had their visual acuity corrected during the procedure. All gave written informed consent to participate in the experiments that were performed in accordance with the Declaration of Helsinki and approved by the institutional Ethics Committee (Istituti Clinici Scientifici Maugeri, approval number #2564CE).

Procedures
Subjects stood barefoot for at least 100 s on a force platform (Kistler 9286BA, Switzerland). The outer profiles of the parallel feet were set at hip width. The head was facing forward. Balance was measured under two Base of Support (BoS) conditions, solid and foam, two visual conditions, eyes open (EO) and eyes closed (EC), and two touch conditions, no-touch and light-touch (LT), resulting in eight experimental conditions. The foot position was marked on a paper sheet placed on top of the platform or of the foam pad (Airex-Balance Pad 50 cm L × 41 cm W × 6 cm H) for consistency across trials.

Subjects were asked to stand at ease (108), not to stare at a fixed point (109) but to look at the visual scene of the laboratory wall at 6 m distance, featuring the horizontal and vertical profiles of a bookcase. They were asked to avoid the head pitch, roll, and yaw movements, and if possible, ample gaze deviations. In the EC condition, subjects were asked to close their eyes before the start of the acquisition epoch and to keep their eyes closed throughout the trial. In the LT condition, the index finger of the dominant hand was kept on the surface of a haptic device made by a flat horizontal wooden square (10 × 10 cm) fixed on top of a strain gauge (**Figure 1**). The instruction was to maintain a constant "light touch" on this smooth plane. The output of the strain gauge was recorded by a device that beeped when the vertical force passed the threshold of 1 N. The haptic device was located in front of the subject at about the height of the belly button and distant about 15 cm from it in the sagittal plane. There was no instruction to keep the finger immobile on the force pad and hence, small fluctuations in the hand and finger position were allowed. The finger never slipped off the force pad. The device seldom beeped, mostly in the time period before the acquisition.

The data presented here originate from an investigation that required each volunteer to come to the laboratory eight times on separate days. Each day, the subject completed eight equal-duration (100 s) consecutive standing trials in one of the conditions of interest (EC, EO, EC-LT, and EO-LT). In the following analysis, only the first of the eight trials for each sensory condition has been considered and analysed because an adaptation process proved to take place in the successive trials (manuscript in preparation).

Data Acquisition and Processing
The last 90 s epoch of each 100 s stance trial was acquired in order to avoid the accustoming phase occurring immediately after mounting on the platform (with/without foam). This duration of the trials had been selected in order to be the longest possible to avoid exhaustion while at the same time allowing a good resolution of the oscillation frequencies. Critical parameters to obtain a reliable power spectrum were the duration of the acquired epoch (that defines the lowest detectable frequency) and the sampling rate (that defines the highest detectable frequency) (110–112).

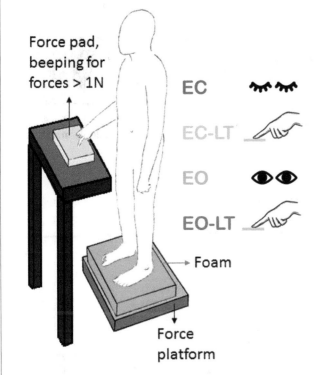

FIGURE 1 | Sketch of the test situation showing a standing subject in front of the force pad (yellow) during the light-touch (LT) trials. The force pad device beeped when the force exceeded 1 N. Subjects rarely reached this force level during the trials. In the sketch, the foam is shown (blue). In the absence of touch, both arms were along the trunk. The same position(s) were assumed with the eyes closed (EC) or open (EO).

All platform data and the data from the haptic device were captured at the sampling frequency of 140 Hz by a PC on which the dedicated software was running (Smart-D, BTS, Italy). All data were moved to another PC for *post-hoc* analysis, and calculations were done using the Excel software and customised LabVIEW programs (National Instrument, USA). The force platform signals of the CoP displacements along both the anteroposterior (AP) and mediolateral (ML) directions were high-pass filtered at 0.01 Hz with a 4th order Butterworth philtre after removing the respective mean values. The length of the sway path was the total length of the wandering CoP during the 90 s epoch, calculated using a software compiled on LabVIEW, and sway area was the surface of the 95% ellipse fitted to the dispersion of the time-series of the AP data plotted against those of the ML recorded in the same epoch (113).

The frequency analysis was performed by applying the fast Fourier transform to the ML and AP CoP time-series data of each trial, subject, sensory, and BoS conditions. This was done by means of the Auto power spectrum VI algorithms of the LabVIEW functions. The frequency resolution, i.e., the sampling frequency (140 Hz) divided by the number of samples acquired by the platform (12,600 samples), was 0.011 Hz. The power spectrum signal was expressed as cm^2_{rms} since the root mean square (rms) of a signal is defined by $u_{rms} = \sqrt{\frac{1}{T}\int_0^T u(t)^2 * t}$. For

example, in the case of a sinusoidal waveform like u (t) = A sin $(2\pi/T^*t)$, where A is the peak amplitude, T = 1/f, and f is the waveform frequency, the rms of this waveform is $u_{rms} = A/\sqrt{2}$ = 0.707*A. In the case of a sinusoidal peak to peak displacement of 10 cm amplitude, the amplitude of the power spectrum signal would be about 18 cm^2_{rms}.

An example of this analysis is shown in **Figure 2**. The analysis has been applied to the data of a pilot test made under dynamic EO foam condition consisting of continuous deliberate mediolateral oscillations around 0.5 Hz (left panels) performed by one experimenter following the rhythm of a metronome for a 90 s period. The amplitude of the rhythmic ML displacement was set by the distance between the feet. The computed oscillation frequency in the ML direction (**Figure 2A**, red) has a peak around 0.5 Hz, and the amplitude of this peak is about 21 cm^2_{rms}. In the AP direction (green), the oscillations are smaller and less regular than in the ML direction with a peak frequency of about 1 Hz (**Figure 2G**). In the right panels of the Figure, the results of the same analysis are reported and applied to a performance during which the same subject was asked to deliberately shake like a raving lunatic on the foam for 90 s (**Figures 2C,D**). In this case, the spectral analysis shows oscillations at frequencies >2 Hz, and the amplitude of the spectrum is negligible above 5 Hz (**Figures 2F,H**).

In the analysis of our experimental trials performed under quiet stance, the frequency range of interest was not predefined. However, we decided to limit the analysis to the part of the frequency spectrum below 2 Hz owing to the negligible amplitude of the power spectrum from 2 Hz onwards. In the EC foam condition, the area under the profile (calculated as the sum of the amplitude of the values of every sample) of the spectrum from 0.01 to 2 Hz corresponded to the 98.8 and 99.0% of the area of the entire spectrum from 0.01 to 70 Hz, for ML and AP, respectively (114).

The amplitude of the body sway (area of the 95% confidence ellipse fitted to the CoP path in the horizontal plane) was hardly affected by oscillation frequencies beyond 2 Hz. **Figure 3** shows that the ellipse fitted onto the CoP of the ML and AP traces plotted after high-pass filtering at 2 Hz (**Figure 3B**) contains a very small percentage (0.7%) of the original unfiltered signal (**Figure 3A**). The CoP path length diminishes to a much smaller extent (52%).

Median frequency and mean level of the spectrum were calculated for each sensory and BoS condition between 0.01 and 2 Hz for the AP and the ML CoP displacements. Median frequency (at which the power spectrum is divided into two parts of equal area) was calculated by means of Matlab software. Then, specific frequency windows (Ws) were identified for further analysis of the effects of the manipulation of conditions on the power spectrum. The Ws identification was made based on the "default" condition (the EC foam trial), which featured the maximum overall amplitude of the entire power spectrum profile compared to all other conditions tested. Then, the boundaries of the Ws were selected based on the profile of the mean power spectrum obtained by averaging the profiles of the EC foam trial of all the subjects (**Figure 4**). In detail, the Ws have been operationally identified by the superimposition of the mean EC

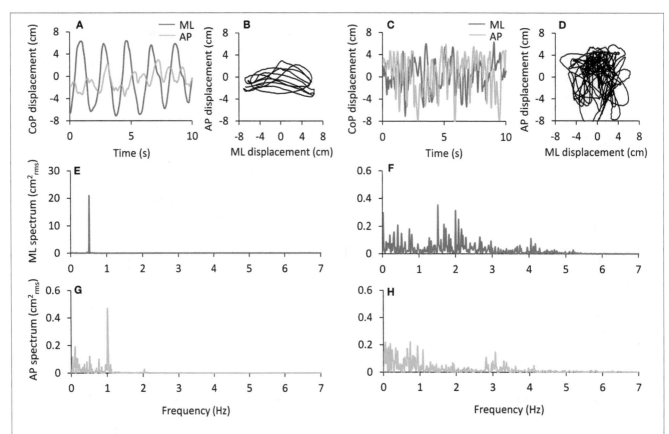

FIGURE 2 | Examples of deliberate sway of the body are performed in order to test the recording and analysis procedures. Voluntary, wide, and rhythmic predominantly mediolateral oscillations were performed in response to 0.5 Hz beeps of a metronome **(A,B)**. The relevant power spectrum profiles in the frontal (ML, with a large peak at 0.5 Hz) and sagittal (AP) planes are reported in **(E,G)**. Note the difference in the ordinates of **(E,G)**. The same subject deliberately performed large body movements at the highest frequency possible **(C,D)**. The relevant power spectrum profiles are shown in **(F,H)**. Now the oscillation frequencies have a wider range and smaller peak amplitudes. Under both circumstances, the deliberate oscillations were performed with the eyes open and lasted 90 s. In **(A–D)**, only 10 s are depicted for easily identifying the CoP oscillations. The traces are dispersed around zero because their mean value has been removed. The power spectra are computed over the 90 s trial.

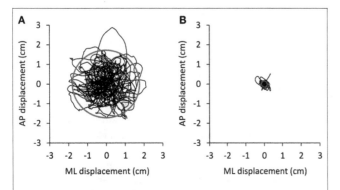

FIGURE 3 | Effect of high-pass filtering. Body oscillations during a 90 s trial were performed with EC on the foam base of support by a representative subject. The oscillations normally ranged about 3–4 cm in both mediolateral (ML) and anteroposterior (AP) directions **(A)**. **(B)** The shrink of the oscillation pattern of the same trial as in A when the AP and ML time series were computed on the 2 Hz high-pass filtered signals.

power spectra separately for the frontal (ML) and the sagittal (AP) planes. The local *minima* were identified in successive epochs of 0.05 Hz of the traces. The same procedure was repeated for the local *minima* of the profile of the SD trace of the mean power spectrum as a companion criterion. It turned out that the local *minima* in the successive epochs of the mean power spectrum trace and of its SD trace almost coincided in most cases. These points would correspond to oscillation frequencies poorly represented in our population. They were arbitrarily considered critical discriminating points for the identification of the boundaries of the Ws. Further, in order to simplify the interpretation, some of the *minima* were disregarded and a few adjacent Ws merged. Hence, the analysis was restricted to six windows only.

Moreover, based on the visual comparison of the profiles of the mean power spectra obtained for the ML and AP directions of CoP oscillations and of their SD, which were similar and almost superimposable across the entire frequency range, we decided to utilise the same Ws identified for the ML direction for the AP direction. This procedure allowed to identify the following frequency Ws, which were equal for both the ML and the AP directions: W1 (the lowest frequency), from 0.01 to 0.055 Hz; W2, 0.055 to 0.2 Hz; W3, 0.2 to 0.44 Hz; W4, 0.44 to 0.8 Hz; W5, 0.8 to

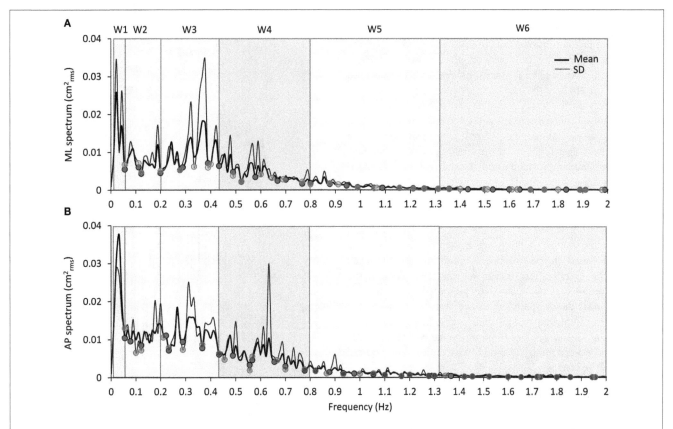

FIGURE 4 | Frequency windows identification. The graphs show the mean profile of the power spectrum (average of the profiles obtained in all the subjects, the thick black line) in the ML and AP directions [**(A,B)**, respectively]. The thin dark grey lines are the corresponding profiles of the SD of the means. A similar pattern for the ML and AP spectra is obvious. The superimposed SD traces largely reproduce the up and downs of the mean spectra and show minimum values close to the relative minimum values of the mean spectra. The blue and red dots correspond to the local minima of the mean and SD traces, respectively, computed in the consecutive 0.05 Hz windows. The pale-coloured rectangles indicate the frequency windows used in the analysis.

1.31 Hz; and W6, 1.31 to 2 Hz. For each W, the mean level of the spectrum was calculated and compared across the sensory and BoS conditions.

Data Treatment and Statistics

The mean power spectra profiles (mean + SD) obtained for the CoP oscillations were point-by-point compared by Student's t-test according to a procedure used in this laboratory (115). The oscillation frequencies at which the Student's t-test value bypassed the probability of 0.05 (two-tailed pairwise test) were taken as the frequencies at which ML and AP oscillations became different. This procedure was used to compare the ML and AP power spectra in the EC condition and the spectra under both EC-LT and EO conditions on foam in order to investigate the differences in the contribution to the stabilisation process of touch and vision.

The data pertaining to the mean profile of the AP power spectrum were plotted against those of the mean profile of the ML power spectrum for the EC foam condition. This relationship was studied by a linear regression model and the coefficient of determination (R^2) was calculated. Also, the relationships between the mean level of the ML and AP spectrum in each

frequency window and the CoP path length and sway area were studied by a linear regression model and the R^2 was calculated.

Assumptions for parametric statistics were met for all variables of interest as assessed by the Kolmogorov-Smirnov and Levene's test. The following analyses were performed separately for the two BoS conditions (solid and foam). A 2 (ML and AP directions) × 4 (vision and touch conditions) repeated measure (rm) ANOVA was used to compare the median frequency and the mean level of the spectrum between 0.01 and 2 Hz. A 2 (ML and AP directions) × 4 (vision and touch conditions) × 6 (frequency windows) rm ANOVA was used to compare the mean level of the spectrum calculated in each frequency window. In order to highlight the difference between sensory conditions in each window, a 2 (ML and AP directions) × 4 (vision and touch conditions) rm ANOVA was applied to the mean level, separately for each window. The effects of the different sensory conditions on path length and sway area of the CoP were compared by a 1-way rm ANOVA. A two-tailed paired t-test was used to compare the force exerted by the subjects on the touch pad between EC-LT and EO-LT conditions.

The main effects of BoS (foam and solid) on the median frequency and on the mean level of the spectrum between 0.01 Hz and 2 Hz were compared by a 2 (BoS) × 2 (ML and AP directions) ×4 (vision and touch conditions) rm ANOVA. A 2 (BoS) × 4 (vision and touch conditions) rm ANOVA was used to test the effect of the two BoS on CoP path length and sway area. A 2 (BoS) × 2 (EC-LT and EO-LT conditions) rm ANOVA was used to compare the effect of the base of support on the force exerted by the subjects on the touch pad. The *post-hoc* was the Fisher's LSD test. The significance level was set at 0.05. The value of η_p^2 was reported as well. Where the differences were significant, the Cohen's d effect sizes highlighted the strength of the difference. Statistical tests were performed using Statistica (Statsoft, USA).

RESULTS

The findings are itemised for the sake of clarity. The CoP data collected in the foam condition are presented first, followed by those recorded in the solid BoS condition. Within each branch of the investigation, the power spectrum data in the different experimental conditions are presented first, followed by the geometric data of path length and sway area and by the comparisons of frequency and geometric data. In both cases, the data regarding the ML precede those of the AP oscillations. The comparisons between foam and solid BoS conditions are reported at the end of the section.

Foam Base of Support
Power Spectrum
ML and AP Oscillations (EC) Have Similar Profiles
The analysed range of the power spectrum reached from 0.01 to 2 Hz. The area under the curve of this range corresponded to more than 98% of that of the entire spectrum (along both the ML and the AP directions). In particular, no frequency peak however small was obvious in the profile of the power spectrum beyond 2 Hz.

Figure 5 shows the mean power spectra superimposed for the ML and AP oscillations (**Figure 5A**) in the EC condition and the result of applying the *t*-test to each of the frequency values (**Figure 5C**). The profiles were similar. However, differences between the two spectra were detected by the Student's *t*-test between 0.1 and 0.3 Hz and in scattered positions for higher frequencies. In inset **Figure 5B**, the data pertaining to the mean profile of the AP power spectrum were plotted against those of the mean ML power spectrum for the EC condition. Each sampled frequency point is considered ($n = 180$ data points corresponding to the frequency units). Clearly, there is a good regression line, indicating that when the value of the power spectrum profile at a certain sampled frequency was low in ML, the corresponding AP value was also low and vice versa.

Sensory Conditions
The mean profiles of the power spectra in the four tested conditions (EC, EC-LT, EO, EO-LT) when standing on foam are shown in **Figures 6A,B**. For each condition and each subject, the median frequency and the mean level of the spectrum was calculated (**Figures 6C–F**). All conditions included, the median frequency was not different between ML and AP [$F_{(1, 18)} = 0.86, p = 0.36$]. However, there was a significant difference in the

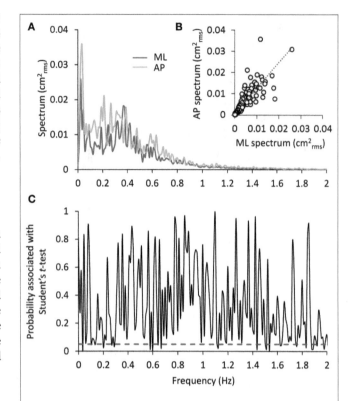

FIGURE 5 | Comparison between the ML and AP spectra. In **(A)**, the superimposed power spectra in the ML and AP directions (EC) appear similar, except for a slightly higher amplitude of the AP (green) compared to the ML spectrum (red). The regression line fitted to the data points of AP vs. ML **(B)** has a slope slightly higher than 1 and the intercept close to origin of the axes ($y = 1.15 \times + 0.0008, R^2 = 0.72, p < 0.001$). The plot in **(C)** shows the probability values associated with the *t*-test of the point-to-point differences between the two spectra. The red dashed line indicates the significance of the differences at $p < 0.05$. Consistent but limited differences between the two spectra were observed at low frequencies.

median frequency between sensory conditions [$F_{(3, 54)} = 64.5, p < 0.001, d = 3.76, \eta_p^2 = 0.78$] and a significant interaction between ML and AP directions and sensory conditions [$F_{(3, 54)} = 3.16, p = 0.03, d = 0.84, \eta_p^2 = 0.15$]. For both ML and AP, the median frequency was higher with EC (EC and EC-LT) than with EO (EO and EO-LT) (*post-hoc*, $p < 0.05$ for all comparisons). In the ML direction, there was no difference in the median frequency between EC and EC-LT ($p = 0.76$) and between EO and EO-LT ($p = 0.73$). In the AP direction, instead, the median frequency was higher with EC-LT than with EC ($p < 0.001$), but there was no significant difference between EO and EO-LT ($p = 0.14$). All conditions included, there was a significant difference in the mean level of the spectrum between ML and AP directions [$F_{(1, 18)} = 5.53, p = 0.03, d = 1.1, \eta_p^2 = 0.23$], a significant difference between sensory conditions [$F_{(3, 54)} = 88.35, p < 0.001, d = 4.43, \eta_p^2 = 0.83$] and a significant interaction between ML and AP directions and sensory conditions [$F_{(3, 54)} = 27.11, p < 0.001, d = 2.45, \eta_p^2 = 0.6$]. In the ML direction, the mean level of the spectrum under EC condition was the highest (*post-hoc*, $p < 0.001$ for all comparisons) and became the smallest

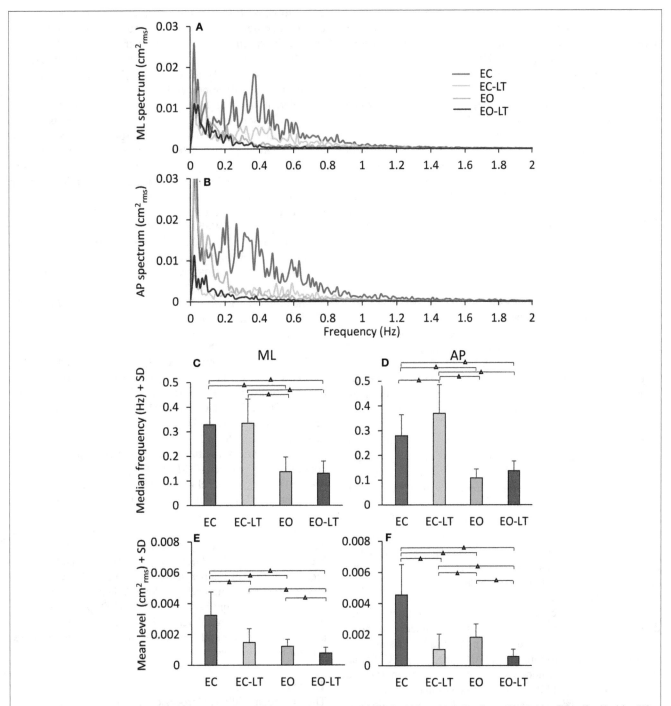

FIGURE 6 | Power spectra under different sensory conditions. This contrasts the spectra during the trials performed on foam without vision (EC, red), with vision (EO, green), and with the addition of touch (EC-LT, yellow; EO-LT, blue). Obviously, the level of the spectrum for all the "stabilised" conditions is smaller than with EC **(A,B)**. The median frequency of the spectrum **(C,D)** is definitely smaller with vision (EO and EO-LT) than without vision (EC and EC-LT), both in the frontal and sagittal plane. Conversely, the mean level **(E,F)** is small in the three "stabilised" conditions. In this case, the reduction in the mean level also applies to EC-LT. Triangles indicate significant differences ($^{\Delta}p < 0.001$).

in the EO-LT condition ($p < 0.01$ for all comparisons). In the EC-LT condition, the mean level was not different to the mean level under EO ($p = 0.1$). Also, in the AP direction, the mean level of the spectrum under EC condition was the highest (*post-hoc, $p <$*

0.001 for all comparisons) and became the smallest in the EO-LT condition ($p < 0.01$ for all comparisons). Moreover, in the EC-LT condition, the mean level of the AP spectrum was smaller than in the EO condition ($p < 0.001$).

In **Figure 7**, the median frequency of the spectrum is plotted against its mean level for ML and AP directions in the four sensory conditions for each subject. A large variability across subjects is obvious in the plots. However, it is clear that the red and yellow circles (no vision, EC and EC-LT, respectively), have high median-frequency values, while the green and blue circles (vision, EO and EO-LT, respectively) mostly include low frequencies values. Conversely, touch (EC-LT and EO-LT, the clusters of the yellow and blue symbols, respectively), produced the largest reduction in the mean level, regardless of the visual condition. This consideration applies to both ML and AP directions. In the plots, the large circles correspond to the mean values of the clusters. As expected, the conditions EO and EO-LT feature small values for both variables. The median frequencies with touch were just larger (even not significantly so for the ML direction) than under the corresponding EC and EO conditions (without touch) for both the ML and the AP directions.

Distinct Effects Are Elicited by the Sensory Conditions in the Different Frequency Windows

Figure 8 shows the mean level of the spectrum calculated for the ML (**Figure 8A**) and AP directions (**Figure 8B**) across all the subjects in each of the identified frequency windows. In the bottom panels (**Figures 8C,D**), the percent changes with respect to the EC condition are reported for the 'stabilised' conditions. There was a difference between the mean level of the spectra of the ML and AP directions, all conditions included [$F_{(1, 18)} = 13.1, p < 0.01, d = 1.7, \eta_p^2 = 0.42$], a difference between sensory conditions [$F_{(3, 54)} = 96.6, p < 0.001, d = 4.62, \eta_p^2 = 0.84$] and between frequency windows [$F_{(5, 90)} = 115.6, p < 0.001, d = 5.06, \eta_p^2 = 0.86$]. There was a significant interaction between ML and AP directions and sensory conditions [$F_{(3, 54)} = 22.2, p < 0.001, d = 2.23, \eta_p^2 = 0.55$], ML and AP directions and frequency windows [$F_{(5, 90)} = 3.4, p < 0.01, d = 0.87, \eta_p^2 = 0.16$], between sensory conditions and frequency windows [$F_{(15, 270)} = 15.4, p < 0.001, d = 1.83, \eta_p^2 = 0.45$], and between ML and AP directions, sensory conditions and frequency windows [$F_{(15, 270)} = 5.26, p < 0.001, d = 1.08, \eta_p^2 = 0.23$].

Figures 8C,D give an easy view of the similarities and differences in the mean levels of the distinct frequency windows in the three "stabilised" conditions. In W1 and W2, vision (EO, green) had a small effect in ML and AP compared to EC. For all remaining frequency windows, vision reduced the mean level to a large extent in AP and ML. Touch without vision (EC-LT, yellow) moderately reduced the mean level in all frequency windows in ML, more so in AP. Touch and vision (EO-LT, blue) reduced the mean level of the entire spectrum in ML, particularly for the W3–W6, more so in AP.

ML Direction. In detail, in W1, the mean levels in the EC and EO conditions were not much different (*post-hoc*, $p = 0.09$). The mean level with EC was >2 conditions with touch (EC-LT and EO-LT, $p < 0.05$ for both comparisons). When touch was added (EC-LT condition), the mean level of the spectrum was not different from the mean level of the EO and of the EO-LT conditions ($p > 0.4$ for both comparisons). When touch was

added to vision (EO-LT), there was no difference compared to the EO condition ($p = 0.67$). In W2, touch diminished the mean level of the spectrum with respect to the corresponding visual condition without touch (*post-hoc*, EC-LT vs. EC: $p < 0.001$; EO-LT vs. EO: $p < 0.05$). Touch under the EC condition diminished the mean level with respect to EO ($p < 0.01$). EC and EO were not different ($p = 0.6$). In W3, EC had the largest spectrum than the other sensory conditions ($p < 0.001$ for all comparisons). When touch was added (EC-LT), the spectrum diminished to less than half of EC ($p < 0.001$) but remained greater than EO ($p < 0.05$) and EO-LT ($p < 0.01$). When touch was added to vision, there was no difference in the amplitude of the spectrum compared to EO ($p = 0.33$). In W4, the EC had the largest spectrum compared to the other sensory conditions ($p < 0.001$ for all comparisons). With EC-LT, the mean level was greater than with EO and EO-LT ($p < 0.05$ for both comparisons). There was no difference between EO and EO-LT ($p = 0.51$). In W5, EC was greater than EO ($p < 0.05$). When touch was added (EC-LT), the mean level was smaller with respect to EC ($p < 0.001$). There was no difference between EO and EO-LT ($p = 0.14$). In W6, the mean level in the EC condition was the greatest ($p < 0.05$ for all comparisons).

AP Direction. In W1, touch with respect to no-touch diminished the mean level of the spectrum both with EC and EO (*post-hoc*, $p < 0.001$ for all comparisons). There was no difference between EC and EO either with (EC-LT vs. EO-LT, $p = 0.62$) or without touch (EC vs. EO, $p = 0.39$). The mean level in W2 behaved similarly to W1. Again, touch diminished the mean level of the spectrum with respect to the corresponding visual condition without touch (EC-LT vs. EC, $p < 0.001$; EO-LT vs. EO: $p < 0.01$). The mean level without vision (EC) was reduced by a touch more than by vision ($p < 0.001$). There was a significant difference in this window between EC and EO ($p < 0.01$), but there was no difference between EC-LT and EO-LT ($p = 0.18$). The pattern of the spectrum in the four sensory conditions was broadly reproduced in W3, W4, W5, and W6. EC had the largest mean level than the other sensory conditions ($p < 0.001$ for all comparisons within each window). When touch was added (EC-LT), the spectrum became similar to EO ($p > 0.08$ in each window). There was a difference between EO and EO-LT in W3 and W5 ($p < 0.05$ for both windows) but not in W4 and W6 ($p > 0.14$ for both windows).

Touch and Vision

The potentially different processes subserving the "stabilising" effects of touch without vision (EC-LT) and of vision without touch (EO) have been the object of additional analysis. In **Figure 9**, the spectrum of the EC-LT condition is superimposed to that of the EO condition for the ML (**Figure 9A**) and AP (**Figure 9B**) directions, and the result of applying the point-by-point *t*-test analysis (**Figures 9C,D**) is shown. For the ML direction, touch (EC-LT) significantly decreased the amplitude of the spectrum between 0.07 and 0.15 Hz (approximately corresponding to the frequency window W2) with respect to the EO (no-touch), while the amplitude of the spectrum was greater for EC-LT with respect to EO between 0.3 and 0.8 Hz

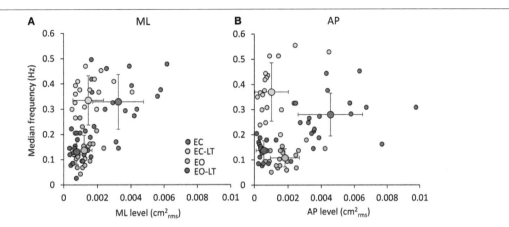

FIGURE 7 | Relationship between median frequency and mean level of the spectrum. There is a weak relationship between the value of the median frequency and the mean value of the entire spectra in each subject ($n = 19$), in both the frontal **(A)** and the sagittal planes **(B)**. The relatively large variability across subjects is underscored by the plots. However, when the mean values of each of the coloured clusters are considered (the large circles with their SDs), it appears that vision (EO, green) and vision and touch (EO-LT, blue) feature small oscillation frequencies with small oscillation amplitudes. Without vision, however, touch clearly reduces the mean level (EC-LT, yellow) compared to no-vision (EC, red), while the oscillation frequencies are hardly changed, particularly along the ML direction.

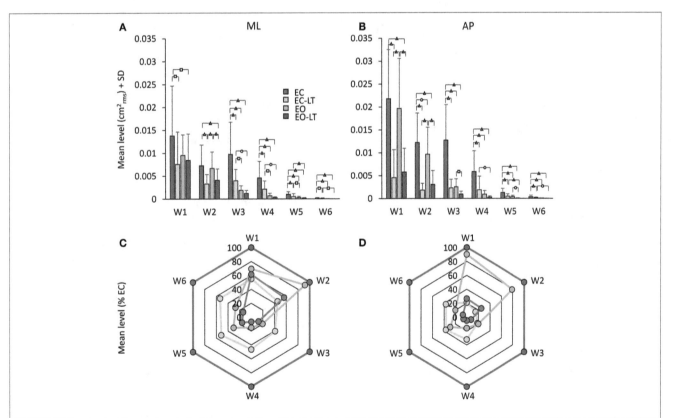

FIGURE 8 | Mean levels of the spectrum in the frequency windows (Ws) standing on foam. The mean level of the spectrum is irregularly distributed across the distinct Ws **(A,B)**. The EC condition (red bars) features a large mean level compared to the other sensory conditions in all the Ws, regardless of the ML or AP direction and of the progressive decrease in amplitude at the higher frequencies. The "stabilised" conditions show a non-uniform pattern depending on Ws and sensory conditions. EC-LT reduces the mean level in all the Ws in ML and more so in AP. Whereas, in ML and AP, EO (green) shows large mean levels at the low frequencies. Overall, the mean level at the highest frequencies is broadly reduced in all "stabilised" conditions. Distinct symbols indicate significant differences ($^{\square}p < 0.05$; $^{\circ}p < 0.01$; $^{\Delta}p < 0.001$). A compact compendium of the percent reduction compared to EC (red outermost trace) in the mean level of the distinct frequency Ws under the EC-LT, EO, EO-LT conditions is given by the radar plots in **(C)** (ML) and **(D)** (AP).

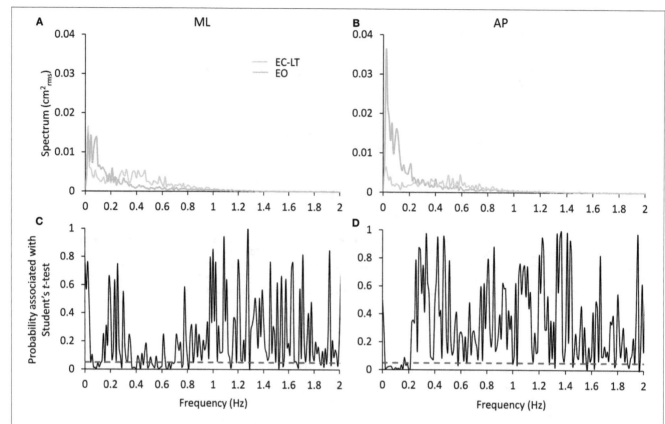

FIGURE 9 | Comparison of the effects of the "stabilising" touch and vision conditions. EC-LT (yellow) and EO (green) are compared in **(A,B)** for the ML and AP directions, respectively. Touch compared to vision remarkably decreases the spectrum in the very low frequency range (~0.01–0.2 Hz) but increases its level in the range 0.3–0.8 Hz. Graphs **(C,D)** (reporting the p-values of the point-to-point differences between the mean values of the entire spectra) show that the mean levels are significantly different in these ranges. The differences are less strong in the higher frequency range for the AP direction. The red dashed lines indicate the level at which the differences are significant at p < 0.05.

(approximately corresponding to W4). For the AP direction, the amplitude of the spectrum was smaller with EC-LT than EO only at low frequency, while there was an increased amplitude for frequencies in W4 (EC-LT > EO). This analysis confirms the emergence of a relatively large high-frequency component of the spectrum, for both ML and AP, selective for touch. However, this component did not raise the spectrum up to its EC values and disappeared when vision was available (EO-LT, see **Figures 5, 7**).

Geometric Sway Measures

The statokinesigrams of a representative subject under the four different conditions while standing on the foam BoS are shown in **Figures 10A–D**. Sway area diminished with touch and with vision with respect to EC. The bottom panels show the mean CoP path length (**Figure 10E**) and the mean sway area (**Figure 10F**) calculated across all subjects. The CoP path length was different between conditions [$F_{(3, 54)} = 18.4$, $p < 0.001$, $d = 4.76$, $\eta_p^2 = 0.85$] and there was a difference between each condition (EC > EC-LT > EO > EO-LT, *post-hoc*, $p < 0.01$, for all paired comparisons). When vision and touch were combined (EO-LT), the CoP path length became the smallest ($p < 0.001$ for all paired comparisons). Of note, the force applied by the fingertip to the

force pad (**Figure 10G**) was virtually the same regardless of the vision condition (EC-LT and EO-LT, paired t-test, $p = 0.63$).

Similar but not identical results were obtained considering the sway area. There was a significant difference between conditions [$F_{(3, 54)} = 83.4$, $p < 0.001$, $d = 4.3$, $\eta_p^2 = 0.82$]. With EC, the sway area was the largest with respect to the other sensory conditions (*post-hoc*, $p < 0.0001$ for all comparisons) and became the smallest with EO-LT ($p < 0.0001$ for all comparisons). When touch was added to EC, the sway area become not different from EO (EC-LT vs. EO, $p = 0.23$) but remained greater than with EO-LT ($p < 0.001$).

The relationship between the mean level of the spectrum in the ML (**Figures 11A–F**) and AP directions (**Figures 11G–L**) vs. the CoP path length and sway area in the different frequency windows are shown in **Figure 11**. W1 and W2 are shown in the first two columns. In the panels of the right column, the frequency windows from W3 to W6 (containing the highest frequencies) and their levels are merged. There was no relationship between the mean level of the ML or AP spectrum and the CoP path length or sway area in the first frequency window (W1). The relationship improved from the W2 to the higher frequency windows, especially for the CoP sway area ($p < 0.001$ for all regression lines) for both ML and AP directions. The

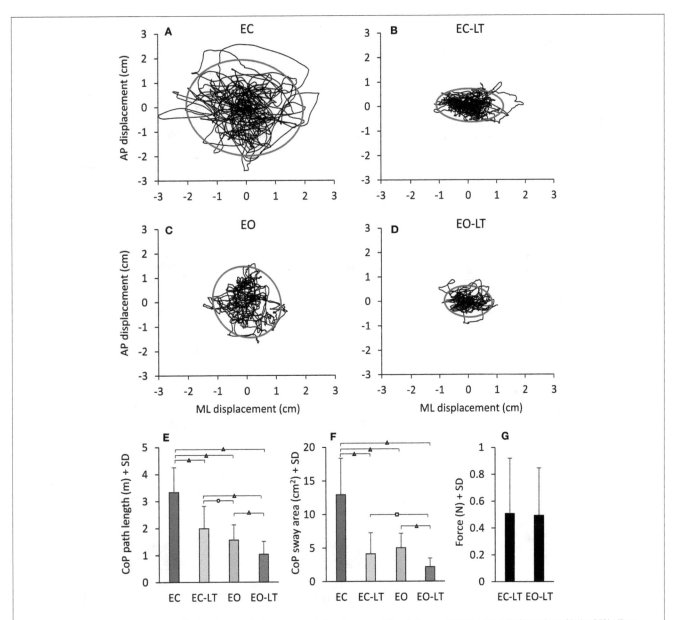

FIGURE 10 | Geometric sway measures. The four top panels show representative diagrams of the CoP sway trajectory (black line) together with the 95% ellipse profile (red) in one subject in the four sensory conditions tested on foam (A–D). The diagrams broadly match the mean values of path length (E) and sway area (F) of the entire cohort of subjects. There is a discordance in the two metrics (length and area), whereby the path length diminishes with EC-LT and EO-LT, but the sway area decreases proportionally more. (G) The fingertip forces applied to the force pad during the touch conditions (both EC-LT and EO-LT) were similar. Distinct symbols indicate significant differences ($^{\square}p < 0.05$; $^{\circ}p < 0.01$; $^{\triangle}p < 0.001$).

equation of the regression lines fitted to the data is reported in **Table 1** for the ML and AP directions.

Solid Base of Support
Power Spectrum
The mean power spectra profiles computed for the four tested conditions (EC, EC-LT, EO, EO-LT) when standing on the solid BoS are shown in **Figures 12A,B**. For each condition and for each subject, the median frequency and the mean level of the spectrum were calculated between 0.01 and 2 Hz (**Figures 12C–F**).

Sensory Conditions
All conditions included, the median frequency was not different between ML and AP [$F_{(1, 18)} = 0.2, p = 0.65$]. There was a difference between conditions [$F_{(3, 54)} = 4.1, p < 0.05, d = 4.25, \eta_p^2 = 0.18$] and an interaction between median frequency of ML and AP directions and sensory conditions [$F_{(3, 54)} = 4.01, p < 0.05, d = 4.14, \eta_p^2 = 0.18$]. For the ML direction, the median frequency was much higher with EC than with all other sensory conditions (*post-hoc*, $p < 0.05$ for all comparisons). There was no difference between EC-LT and the two conditions with eyes open (EO and EO-LT) ($p > 0.4$ for both comparisons) and between EO

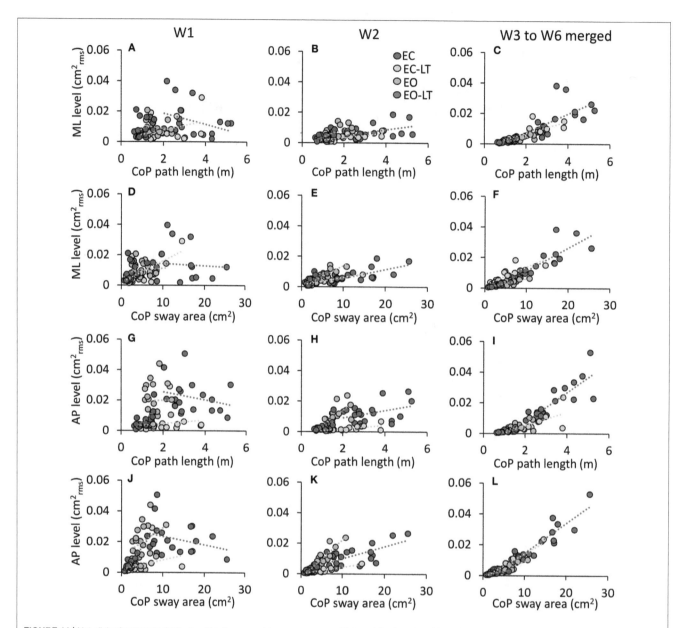

FIGURE 11 | Not all the frequency windows match the geometric sway measures. The contribution of the ML **(A–F)** and AP **(G–L)** sway frequencies to the geometric sway measures is limited to high frequency windows (EC, red; EC-LT, yellow; EO, green; EO-LT, blue). The columns refer to W1 **(A,D,G,J)**, W2 **(B,E,H,K)**, and from W3–W6 **(C,F,I,L)**. Each symbol refers to one subject. **(A–C,G–I)** The spectrum amplitudes vs. the CoP path length, and **(D–F,J–L)** the spectrum amplitudes vs. the sway area. For both sway area and path length, the slope of the regression lines increases with frequency under all sensory conditions but only for W2 onwards.

and EO-LT ($p = 0.22$). For the AP direction, EC was not different from the other sensory conditions ($p > 0.1$ for all comparisons). EC-LT was larger with respect to EO ($p < 0.05$) and EO-LT ($p < 0.05$). There was no difference between EO and EO-LT conditions ($p = 0.44$).

The mean level of the spectrum between 0.01 and 2 Hz was different between ML and AP [$F_{(1, 18)} = 16.45$, $p < 0.001$, $d = 1.91$, $\eta_p^2 = 0.48$]. There was a difference between conditions [$F_{(3, 54)} = 11.4, p < 0.001, d = 1.59, \eta_p^2 = 0.39$] and an interaction between ML and AP directions and sensory conditions [$F_{(3, 54)} = 12.6, p < 0.001, d = 1.67, \eta_p^2 = 0.41$]. For ML, the mean level

was not different between sensory conditions (*post-hoc*, $p > 0.2$ for all comparisons). For AP, the mean level with EC was higher than with EC-LT and EO-LT ($p < 0.001$), but was not different from EO ($p = 0.35$). The mean level with EC-LT was smaller than EO ($p < 0.001$) and similar to EO-LT ($p = 0.57$). Compared to the foam condition, the median frequency was lower for the solid BoS [$F_{(1, 18)} = 60.7$, $p < 0.001$, $d = 3.66$, $\eta_p^2 = 0.77$] when all sensory conditions were included. The mean level of the spectrum between 0.01 and 2 Hz was also different between foam and solid BoS [foam > solid, $F_{(1, 18)} = 108.19$, $p < 0.001$, $d = 4.89$, $\eta_p^2 = 0.86$].

TABLE 1 | Relationship between level of mediolateral (ML, left part) and anteroposterior (AP, right part) spectrum and CoP path length and sway area.

FW	Condition	ML spectrum vs. CoP path length			ML spectrum vs. sway area			AP spectrum vs. CoP path length			AP spectrum vs. sway area		
		Equation	R^2	p-value	Equation	R^2	p-value	Equation	R^2	p-value	Equation	R^2	p-value
Entire spectrum (from 0.01 to 2 Hz)	EC	$y = -0.001x - 0.00006$	0.41	<0.01	$y = 0.0003x - 0.0001$	0.85	<0.001	$y = 0.0016x - 0.0009$	0.7	<0.001	$y = 0.0003x + 0.0003$	0.8	<0.001
	EC LT	$y = 0.0009x - 0.0003$	0.68	<0.001	$y = 0.0003x + 0.0003$	0.89	<0.001	$y = 0.0009x - 0.0007$	0.58	<0.001	$y = 0.0003x - 0.0002$	0.94	<0.001
	EO	$y = 0.0009x - 0.0002$	0.54	<0.001	$y = 0.0002x + 0.0001$	0.94	<0.001	$y = 0.0013x - 0.0003$	0.4	<0.01	$y = 0.0004x - 0.0002$	0.96	<0.001
	EO LT	$y = 0.0009x - 0.0002$	0.56	<0.01	$y = 0.0003x + 0.0002$	0.74	<0.001	$y = 0.0012x - 0.0007$	0.57	<0.001	$y = 0.0004x - 0.0002$	0.9	<0.001
FW 1	EC	$y = -0.0036x + 0.026$	0.1	0.2	$y = -0.0001x + 0.016$	0.005	0.77	$y = -0.0026x + 0.03$	0.06	0.32	$y = -0.0005x + 0.03$	0.08	0.25
	EC LT	$y = 0.003x + 0.0016$	0.13	0.13	$y = 0.0014x + 0.002$	0.4	<0.01	$y = 0.0012x + 0.002$	0.03	0.5	$y = 0.0006x + 0.002$	0.1	0.19
	EO	$y = -0.002x + 0.013$	0.035	0.44	$y = 0.0003x + 0.008$	0.02	0.54	$y = 0.0005x + 0.02$	0.0003	0.95	$y = 0.002x + 0.01$	0.13	0.12
	EO LT	$y = -0.0055x + 0.003$	0.08	0.18	$y = 0.0021x + 0.004$	0.2	0.05	$y = 0.012x - 0.007$	0.5	<0.001	$y = 0.004x - 0.002$	0.85	<0.001
FW 2	EC	$y = 0.002x + 0.0008$	0.18	0.07	$y = 0.0006x - 0.0002$	0.5	<0.001	$y = 0.0025x + 0.004$	0.14	0.11	$y = 0.0006x - 0.0002$	0.5	<0.001
	EC LT	$y = 0.0015x + 0.0002$	0.41	<0.01	$y = 0.0005x + 0.001$	0.55	<0.001	$y = 0.0011x - 0.0004$	0.43	<0.01	$y = 0.0005x + 0.001$	0.55	<0.001
	EO	$y = 0.0054x - 0.0017$	0.35	<0.01	$y = 0.0014x - 0.0003$	0.7	<0.001	$y = 0.0099x - 0.006$	0.43	<0.01	$y = 0.0014x - 0.0003$	0.7	<0.001
	EO LT	$y = 0.06x - 0.0021$	0.5	0.07	$y = 0.0014x + 0.001$	0.54	<0.001	$y = 0.0067x - 0.004$	0.42	<0.01	$y = 0.0014x + 0.001$	0.54	<0.001
FW 3	EC	$y = 0.0036x - 0.0024$	0.26	<0.05	$y = 0.001x - 0.003$	0.57	<0.001	$y = 0.0053x - 0.005$	0.45	<0.01	$y = 0.001x - 0.003$	0.57	<0.001
	EC LT	$y = 0.0016x + 0.0008$	0.3	<0.05	$y = 0.0005x + 0.002$	0.38	<0.01	$y = 0.0015x - 0.0006$	0.44	<0.01	$y = 0.0005x + 0.002$	0.38	<0.01
	EO	$y = 0.0015x - 0.0005$	0.35	<0.01	$y = 0.0003x + 0.0003$	0.46	<0.01	$y = 0.0017x - 0.0001$	0.15	0.1	$y = 0.0003x + 0.0003$	0.46	<0.01
	EO LT	$y = 0.0016x - 0.0004$	0.5	<0.05	$y = 0.0004x + 0.0003$	0.63	<0.001	$y = 0.0014x - 0.0005$	0.41	<0.01	$y = 0.0004x + 0.0003$	0.63	<0.001
FW 4	EC	$y = 0.002x - 0.002$	0.3	<0.05	$y = 0.0005x - 0.001$	0.46	<0.01	$y = 0.0036x - 0.006$	0.6	<0.001	$y = 0.0005x - 0.001$	0.46	<0.01
	EC LT	$y = 0.0018x - 0.0014$	0.72	<0.001	$y = 0.0005x + 0.001$	0.74	<0.001	$y = 0.0025x - 0.003$	0.5	<0.001	$y = 0.0005x + 0.001$	0.74	<0.001
	EO	$y = 0.0009x - 0.0006$	0.38	<0.01	$y = 0.0002x - 0.0003$	0.65	<0.001	$y = 0.0012x - 0.001$	0.4	<0.01	$y = 0.0002x - 0.0003$	0.65	<0.001
	EO LT	$y = 0.0005x - 0.0002$	0.85	<0.05	$y = 0.0001x + 5 \times 10^{-5}$	0.78	<0.001	$y = 0.0006x - 0.0004$	0.6	<0.001	$y = 0.0001x + 5 \times 10^{-5}$	0.78	<0.001
FW 5	EC	$y = 0.0004x - 4 \times 10^{-4}$	0.5	<0.001	$y = 0.00006x + 0.0002$	0.37	<0.01	$y = 0.0006x - 0.0006$	0.43	<0.01	$y = 0.00006x + 0.0002$	0.37	<0.01
	EC LT	$y = 0.0005x - 0.0006$	0.58	<0.001	$y = 0.0002x - 0.0002$	0.76	<0.001	$y = 0.0005x - 0.0004$	0.6	<0.001	$y = 0.0002x - 0.0002$	0.76	<0.001
	EO	$y = 0.0006x - 0.0006$	0.92	<0.001	$y = 0.000007x - 4 \times 10^{-5}$	0.4	<0.01	$y = 0.0005x - 0.0004$	0.45	<0.01	$y = 0.000007x - 4 \times 10^{-5}$	0.4	<0.01
	EO LT	$y = 0.0004x - 2 \times 10^{-4}$	0.75	<0.001	$y = 0.00009x - 4 \times 10^{-5}$	0.77	<0.001	$y = 0.0001x - 7 \times 10^{-5}$	0.63	<0.001	$y = 0.00009x - 4 \times 10^{-5}$	0.77	<0.001
FW 6	EC	$y = 0.00009x - 0.0001$	0.64	<0.001	$y = 0.00001x + 2 \times 10^{-5}$	0.43	<0.01	$y = 0.0003x - 0.0005$	0.56	<0.001	$y = 0.00001x + 2 \times 10^{-5}$	0.43	<0.01
	EC LT	$y = 0.0001x - 9 \times 10^{-5}$	0.7	<0.001	$y = 0.00003x - 1 \times 10^{-5}$	0.75	<0.001	$y = 0.0001x - 0.0001$	0.76	<0.001	$y = 0.00003x - 1 \times 10^{-5}$	0.75	<0.001
	EO	$y = 0.00005x - 3 \times 10^{-5}$	0.7	<0.001	$y = 0.000007x + 1 \times 10^{-5}$	0.78	<0.001	$y = -0.00009x - 7 \times 10^{-5}$	0.62	<0.001	$y = 0.000007x + 1 \times 10^{-5}$	0.78	<0.001
	EO LT	$y = 0.00005x - 3 \times 10^{-5}$	0.74	<0.001	$y = 0.00001x + 4 \times 10^{-6}$	0.54	<0.001	$y = 0.00005x - 3 \times 10^{-5}$	0.4	<0.01	$y = 0.00001x + 4 \times 10^{-6}$	0.54	<0.001

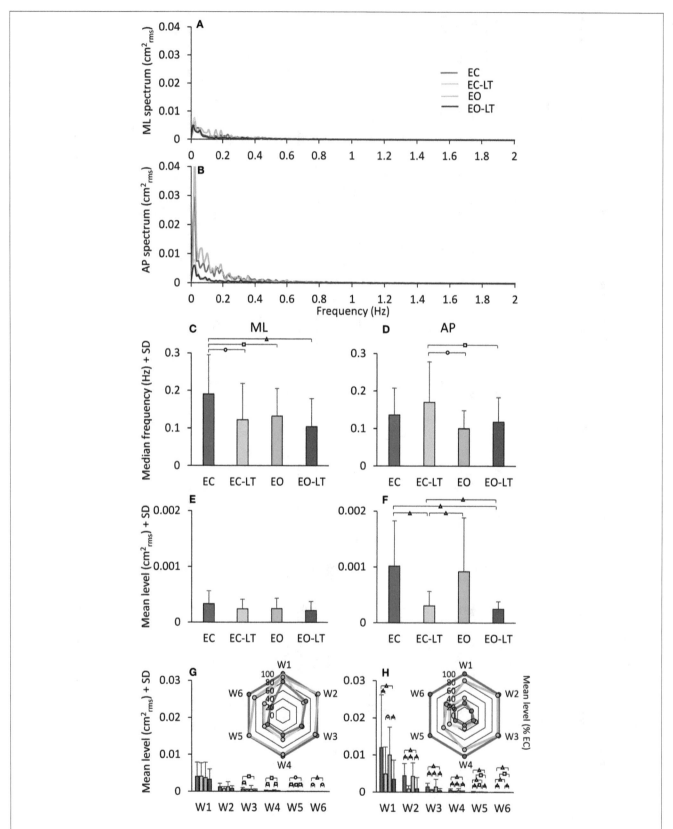

FIGURE 12 | Power spectrum on solid BoS. **(A,B)** compare the power spectra during quiet stance EC (red), EO (green), EC-LT (yellow), and EO-LT (blue). For the low-frequency range, the mean level with EO was not smaller than with EC (for both ML and AP directions). Touch (EC-LT) and vision (EO) produced the smallest

(Continued)

FIGURE 12 | amplitudes of the spectrum. The median frequency of the entire spectrum was not much different across conditions (C,D). However, the mean level was larger in AP than ML (both EC and EO), and much larger without touch (E,F). Overall, median frequencies were about half, and the mean level was about half to a quarter of those with foam (compare to **Figure 5**). The changes with respect to EC of the distinct frequency windows are shown in the radar plots (G,H) for both ML and AP directions. Compared to the foam conditions (see **Figure 8**), the mean levels are less than half. Distinct symbols indicate significant differences ($^{\square}p < 0.05$; $^{\circ}p < 0.01$; $^{\triangle}p < 0.001$).

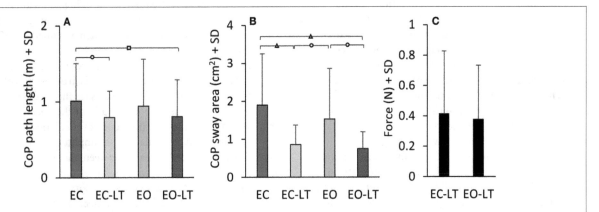

FIGURE 13 | CoP path length and sway area on solid BoS. The path length and 95% ellipse area with the solid BoS are much smaller than in the foam condition. While the path length is not very different across sensory conditions (A), sway area shows larger differences across conditions, the minimal excursions of the CoP being present when touch is available (B). In the solid BoS condition, the touch forces (C) are similar, with and without vision. Distinct symbols indicate significant differences ($^{\square}p < 0.05$; $^{\circ}p < 0.01$; $^{\triangle}p < 0.001$).

Frequency Windows

In **Figures 12G,H**, the mean level of the spectrum in the different frequency windows and their percent reduction with respect to EC condition is reported for each sensory condition.

There was a difference in the spectrum mean level between the ML and AP directions when all conditions included [$F_{(1, 18)} = 17.4, p < 0.001, d = 1.97, \eta_p^2 = 0.49$]. There was also a difference between conditions [$F_{(3, 54)} = 9.08, p < 0.001, d = 1.42, \eta_p^2 = 0.33$] and between frequency windows [$F_{(5, 90)} = 38.1, p < 0.001, d = 2.91, \eta_p^2 = 0.68$]. There was an interaction between ML and AP directions and sensory conditions [$F_{(3, 54)} = 10.3, p < 0.001, d = 1.51, \eta_p^2 = 0.36$], ML and AP directions and frequency windows [$F_{(5, 90)} = 8.6, p < 0.001, d = 1.38, \eta_p^2 = 0.32$], between sensory conditions and frequency windows [$F_{(15, 270)} = 4.8, p < 0.001, d = 1.03, \eta_p^2 = 0.21$], and between ML and AP directions, sensory conditions and frequency windows [$F_{(15, 270)} = 4.5, p < 0.001, d = 0.99, \eta_p^2 = 0.20$]. For the ML direction, there was no significant difference between sensory conditions for W1 and W2 (*post-hoc*, $p > 0.2$ for all comparisons). In W3 to W6 there was no difference in the mean levels between EC-LT and EO-LT ($p > 0.6$ for all comparisons) and between EC and EO ($p > 0.3$). Touch reduced the level under both EC-LT and EO-LT conditions ($p < 0.05$). The level of the EC-LT condition was not much different to EO ($p > 0.07$), and that of EO-LT was smaller than EO ($p < 0.05$). For the AP direction, touch reduced the mean levels in all the frequency windows (EC-LT vs. EC and EO-LT vs. EO, $p < 0.001$). There was no difference between EC and EO ($p > 0.07$). Similarly, EC-LT and EO-LT were not different across the windows ($p > 0.3$).

Geometric Sway Measures

The mean CoP path length and the mean sway area calculated across subjects standing on solid BoS are shown in **Figures 13A,B**. ANOVA on the CoP path length showed a difference between sensory conditions [$F_{(3, 54)} = 3.46, p = 0.02, d = 0.88, \eta_p^2 = 0.16$]. With EC, the path length was greater than EC-LT and EO-LT (*post-hoc*, $p < 0.05$ for both comparisons), but not different from EO ($p = 0.4$). There was no difference between the two conditions with touch (EC-LT vs. EO-LT, $p = 0.92$). ANOVA, on the sway area, showed a significant difference between sensory conditions [$F_{(3, 54)} = 11, p < 0.001, d = 1.56, \eta_p^2 = 0.38$]. Sway area with EC and EO was greater than EC-LT (*post-hoc*, $p < 0.01$ for both comparisons) and EO-LT ($p < 0.01$ for both comparisons). There was no difference in sway area between EC and EO ($p = 0.17$) and between EC-LT and EO-LT ($p = 0.68$). Path length [$F_{(1, 18)} = 90.5, p < 0.001, d = 4.48, \eta_p^2 = 0.83$] and sway area [$F_{(1, 18)} = 93.97, p < 0.001, d = 4.56, \eta_p^2 = 0.84$] were greater with foam than solid BoS when all sensory conditions are included. Much as with foam, during the trials performed on the solid BoS vision did not affect the force applied by the subjects onto the force pad (**Figure 13C**) (paired t-test, $p = 0.29$). In turn, the touch forces exerted on solid BoS were not different from those recorded when standing on foam [$F_{(1, 18)} = 2.6, p = 0.12$].

DISCUSSION

Our hypothesis was that vision and light touch stabilise body sway through at least partially different actions (31). To this objective, we have computed and analysed both the usual stabilometric indices (sway path and sway area) and the power spectra of the oscillation frequency along with both the frontal and the sagittal planes in healthy young subjects standing on a compliant and on a solid surface.

Spectral analysis of body oscillations during stance has been repeatedly exploited in order to understand the processes underpinning the control of equilibrium in the absence of external perturbations (35–39, 116–120). Singh et al. (98) had a contiguous research question and emphasised open issues in attributing specific frequencies to the effect of different sensory modalities on standing posture. Inconsistencies in the methodological approach across the literature might have detracted researchers and clinicians from the use of standardised approaches. The span of considered frequencies varies across laboratories, and one wonders whether frequencies as high or higher than, say, 2 Hz can have a practical counterpart for the interpretation of the sway of healthy, non-trembling subjects (121, 122). Moreover, the value of the ordinate in the power spectrum is sometimes of difficult interpretation, also because of dissimilar modes in the signal processing (e.g., filtered/non-filtered) and the metrics used in different studies, so that attention seems to have been devoted more to the frequencies themselves than to the effective amplitude of their power spectrum. We have leveraged this approach in order to test the possibility that the effects of different sensory conditions and support bases on the body sway can be easily detected by the frequency analysis compared to the commonly used metrics and can yield details not granted by the simple analysis of the CoP path length or sway area.

We have tried to identify ranges and amplitudes of oscillation frequencies presumably having an actual physical counterpart in the wandering of the CoP of the standing body, and to detect spectrum windows which could be questioned for elucidating the effects of adding haptic and visual sensory information on the CoP oscillations identified in the most unstable condition (eyes closed, EC). As a consequence, we have limited our analysis to the region of the power spectrum (below 2 Hz) encompassing about 99% of the total available spectrum (i.e., containing the frequencies up to 70 Hz, which depend on the frequency of sampling of the CoP signal). We have also checked that the oscillations beyond 2 Hz represent a tiny proportion of the geometric metrics, the sway area, and the path length. The oscillations beyond 2 Hz do indeed represent a minor part of the sway area (<1%) (see **Figure 3B**). They contribute to the path length by about 50%, though. The incongruous length of the sway path compared to its area is due to the long period of acquisition, when the filtered signal does negligibly oscillate but may show minimal displacements, the sum of which gives rise to sizeable total lengths over the 90 s epoch. Perhaps, for this reason, frequencies from 2 to 20 Hz have been considered in some studies on dizzy patients (123, 124).

With EC foam, the frequency spectra and their amplitudes were broadly similar in both ML and AP directions, but larger in AP for frequencies in the W1 and W2. This was not unexpected because the spontaneously oscillating body during quiet stance does not really care about the space directions along which to move, and the balancing strategies of a double-inverted

pendulum are not really functionally separated (56, 125) unless imposed by the feet distance (24, 126, 127). In our subjects, this distance (the outer profile of the feet was about the hip distance) was appropriate for promoting omni-directional sway, as obvious in the shape of the wandering of the CoP on the horizontal plane (see **Figures 3A, 10A,C**).

The median frequencies are higher without vision (EC). The median frequencies remain high (or get relatively higher in the AP direction) when touch is added to EC. Hence, the median frequency is not a good predictor of the effect of the haptic information. Conversely, vision is associated with low median frequency values. This is true both with and without touch. In general, vision diminishes the median frequency, while touch diminishes the amplitude of the spectrum. It seems that vision prescribes the frequency of oscillation, upon which touch quantitatively modulates the amplitude. As expected, there is a broad correspondence between the amplitude of the spectra and the geometric sway measures (compare **Figures 6E,F** with **Figures 10E,F**). Across the sensory conditions, the length of the sway path is broadly reflected in the amplitude of the mean level of the spectrum along the ML direction, and the sway area is rather reflected in the mean level along the AP direction.

Vision and Touch Stabilise the Standing Body on the Foam
Vision

The power spectrum of the oscillation frequencies with EC foam has been considered here the default condition, against which to compare the stabilising effects of vision and touch and both together. Compared to EC, vision (EO) reduced the area of the ellipse by about 61% and the CoP path length by about 53% (see **Figure 10**). In the spectral analysis, the addition of vision remarkably lowered the median frequency of the entire spectrum. This diminution affected the entire spectrum both in the ML (63%) and in the AP (60%) directions (see **Figure 5**). This was consistent with a decrease in the amplitude of the medium-high frequencies with sparing of the low frequencies. While the amplitude of each of the oscillation frequency windows was smaller with EO than with EC, the vision had no effect on the spectral mean level of the low-frequency windows in the ML and AP directions. This is in keeping with the findings by Yamagata et al. (86), who showed that slow oscillations, or drifts, appear to be poorly sensitive to vision. Conversely, the reduction was conspicuous for the subsequent windows (between 0.2 and 0.8 Hz), i.e., for oscillation cycles lasting from 5 to nearly 1 s. The highest-frequency windows (beyond 0.8 Hz) were scarcely influenced by vision, much as had been previously shown (56, 117). Under unstable conditions (as standing on an inclined surface or on a balance trainer ball), the slow components of the postural sway appear to depend on vision compared to more stable conditions (128–130). No significant vision effects on the oscillation frequency were noted by Šarabon et al. (82), probably because they measured the average frequency. In our hands, the reduction was clear in the median frequency, just because of the preserved low-frequency and reduced high-frequency oscillations. The frequency window W3 (from 0.2 to 0.44 Hz) should contain frequencies related to ventilation (131), i.e., broadly between 0.2 and 0.3 Hz for ventilation cycles from 12 to 18 per minute, which are probably blunted in the mean spectrum by inter-subject variability. In our hands, the amplitude of the postulated ventilation component diminishes with the general decay of the mean level of the spectrum in the stabilised conditions, making it difficult to draw strong deductions. Interestingly, stabilisation by vision (EO vs. EC) reduced both length and area of the CoP wandering without decreasing the level of the lowest part of the spectrum (the frequency Ws 1 and 2, spanning 0.01–0.2 Hz). The absence of influence of this part of the spectrum on the geometric sway measures is "compensated" by the strong relationships between the level of the higher-frequency windows with CoP path length and sway area (see **Figure 11**).

Touch

A light touch is a potent stabilising stimulus, able to replace vision in subjects with impaired vestibular system (132–134). In the present study, like in several others [(7), see Lackner (47) for a recent review], the haptic information arose from the index fingertip lightly touching the force pad and from the muscles active in this task. In many studies, the vertical force of the fingertip on the force pad representing the earth-fixed reference was generally well-below 1 N and was considered to be inadequate for mechanical stabilisation (60, 135, 136). Importantly, during our experimental trials, the force did not change across the different sensory or BoS conditions.

Compared to EC, the light touch without vision (EC-LT) reduced the sway area (by about 68%) and the path length (40%). In the frequency domain, EC-LT had minimal effects on the median frequencies of the ML and AP spectra (see **Figures 6–9**). However, EC-LT reduced the level of the spectrum, along with the ML (by 55%) and more so along with the AP (77%) direction (137–139). It is not unlikely that the haptic reference helped diminish the "slow" sway oscillations more in the sagittal than in the frontal plane (140, 141). This would depend on the haptic task, whereby the reference (the fingertip onto the force pad) was located just in front of the subjects, almost coinciding with the sagittal plane, and broadly congruent with the direction of the gaze (142, 143). However, we would not exclude that, when standing on foam, a minor but non-negligible additional advantage might have been furnished by the contact of the finger with the force pad. We have no information on the amplitude or direction of the friction forces on the force pad, though. Although minimal, these cannot be disregarded (144). Since the body oscillations reduction along the ML direction was similar for touch and vision, we suppose that the added reduction in the AP direction was due to the anterior position of the force pad. Qualitative changes occur, however, even when the haptic stimulus is applied to diverse body sites and has no definite direction of action (145). As to the location of the haptic device, we would remind that similar stabilising effects are obtained by using a cane touching the ground (146). The use of a tool

is as helpful as the fingertip input and does not produce a different stabilisation.

Touch and Vision Stabilise Balance Through Distinct Actions

The stabilising effects of touch (EC-LT) and vision (EO) have been directly compared. While both conditions resulted in a similar reduction of path length and sway area (147), their modulation of the spectrum frequencies was definitely divergent. This was clear in the superimposition of the frequency spectra obtained in the two conditions on foam. While the addition of vision (EO) had no effect on the very low frequencies of the spectrum, the same frequencies abated with touch (EC-LT). Conversely, while the higher frequencies were reduced with vision, a broad peak intruded with touch between 0.3 and 0.8 Hz (148), as if the former frequency window drop and the increase of the latter were a necessary quality of the touch effect. It has been known for decades that touching or even aiming to a stable structure diminishes the amplitude of the leg muscle long-latency reflex responses to stretch (46, 149, 150), whereas the short-latency responses are hardly affected. Touch would not be powerful enough for cancelling the medium-high frequencies, likely sustained by continuous operation of short-chain reflexes that represent a major share of the oscillations EC. Further, a new inter-foot coordination pattern (26) would emerge when a midline reference (the LT in front of the subject) is available and attenuate slow omnidirectional oscillations in favour of fast, short displacements. The sway area reflects this effect, as shown by the major shrinkage of the ellipses fitted to the EC-LT (but not EO) data, with a minor reduction in path length. One might speculate that touch *without* vision sustains the elevated level of excitability of the proprioceptive circuits operating with EC as if this would serve prompt postural corrections when an obstacle challenges the equilibrium in the frontal plane. We would add that, while the spectrum profiles of EC-LT and EO (i.e., during stabilisation by vision or touch) clearly intersected on foam (**Figure 8**), this pattern disappeared when standing on solid BoS. On the other hand, even the differences between EC and EO disappear with solid BoS, where the sensory information is less crucial for stabilisation.

The Combination of Touch and Vision Produces the Maximal Stabilisation

The integration of touch and vision has been often studied in the context of studies on space perception (151). The interaction of both inputs would take place in cortical areas that are related, among other things, with the control of equilibrium (152–155). In our hands, the condition touch and vision together (EO-LT) clearly proved to be able to further reduce the sway area and the path length (more so the area than the path length) compared to EC (area and path length were reduced by 83 and 69%, respectively). Sway area and path length were also reduced compared to touch (EC-LT) (by 47 and 48%) (see **Figure 10**) and to EO when separately considered (by 57 and 34%), confirming the findings of Honeine et al. (63). Regarding the frequency spectrum, EO-LT was superior in attenuating the oscillations on foam compared to vision alone (EO). However, EO-LT was not superior to touch without vision (EC-LT) in the low-frequency windows (W1 and W2). In this vein, we would mention that, while the integration of haptic and visual inputs in cortical regions likely plays a role, other probably concurrent processes cannot be overlooked. Effectiveness in visuo-haptic integration is enhanced by object-selective brain regions with increased salience of the stimulus (156). Salience can be attributed to our light touch here because attention was devoted to keeping the force within the required range, even if subjects did not look at the force pad with EO. The level of attention would be most likely different in the foam than in the solid BoS condition. In the former case, a precision task would be implicit (141), even if not expressly required. In the latter case, the task can be more easily carried out and provide a simple haptic reference in the absence of accidental displacement (73).

Foam and Solid BoS

The solid BoS, compared to foam, diminished the median frequency of the spectra almost selectively for the EC condition (both EC and EC-LT), whereas the median frequencies with vision (both EO and EO-LT) were similar in the two BoS conditions. However, the oscillations in the 0.3–0.8 Hz and higher frequency windows (W3–W6) under EC-LT conditions appear only when standing on foam, as if this frequency range were a distinctive feature of standing on a compliant surface. Instead, the mean level of the spectrum was much reduced for all sensory conditions on solid BoS in both ML and AP directions. The effect of touch on the mean level seems to be proportionally stronger on foam in keeping with the observation that unstable balance enhances the haptic sensitivity (157). Generally speaking, it seems that the distinct qualitative contributions to the stabilisation process by vision, touch, or both are hard-wired. These contributions are modulated in amplitude. When the body is in a stable condition (solid BoS), it would continue to operate but are adaptively scaled (or "downweighed") to the new state.

The balancing behaviour standing on a compliant surface must adapt to the spring-like properties of the foam that influence sway by its own mechanical compliance. This would favour higher activity in the muscles controlling mediolateral oscillations (49, 98). For example, the mean levels of the AP and ML spectra were less different on foam than on solid BoS, suggesting proportionally larger mediolateral adjustments on foam. The inverted pendulum model does not apply to this condition, and movements at several joints contribute to the equilibrium control (13, 158). Analogously, it seems simplistic to posit that the proprioceptive system is disturbed, or its contribution attenuated or invalidated when standing on foam (43, 159, 160). Sway while on foam compared to solid BoS may be less useful for "exploration" of the support base (161) and for "resetting" of the input from the adapting receptors of the foot sole (40). Whereas, pelvis and trunk movements may be more important in getting information about body segments' orientation in space when task difficulty increases (134, 162). The continuous corrections of the body segment displacements on the foam are likely dependent on proprioceptive volleys, which send a continuous (meaningful) input to various regions of the brain

and produce appropriate short- and long-latency reflexes (163). Conversely, the vibration of the leg muscles, producing a non-meaningful proprioceptive input, has a smaller effect on body sway while standing on foam (164) or on an unstable support (165, 166). If anything, these findings support the notion that proprioception continues to operate (and likely much more) on a compliant (foam) than solid BoS. The vibration of trunk muscles has, instead, a larger effect compared to the vibration of the leg muscles (164), a finding that we interpret as a shift in excitability of different circuits rather than mere disruption of proprioceptive information by vibration. Of note, touch increases the postural tone in trunk muscles (167). It is not clear, though, whether the new trunk postural activity can be responsible for the relative increase in medium-high frequencies seen while standing on foam in EC-LT condition (168, 169).

With EC, our subjects were actually unstable on foam (but never made a step during these trials) and became stable with touch (EC-LT). Touch devoid of mechanical action (always < 1 N) could have had such effect just because proprioception was properly working. In a sense, the ampler the joint movements on foam, the more substantial the proprioceptive input from multiple muscles, not excluding those of the forearm muscles enabling and contributing to a significant haptic input (64, 170). Mastering a complex proprioceptive input can be difficult and lead to instability. However, there must be a large safety margin compensating for unpredictable alteration in proprioceptive input. Young subjects, healthy except for the Marfan syndrome, a disorder targeting the connective tissue, show impaired balance control under critical conditions (unstable BoS, eyes closed) (171). However, just a few of them had to be supported during the trials despite presumably altered reflex patterns due to their unique joint hypermobility.

Frontal and Sagittal Planes

Control of balance in the mediolateral direction is critical (52, 172) and is often impaired in older adults and when the asymmetry of stance is present, like for instance in stroke patients (173, 174). There were considerable differences in the mean level of the spectrum of all the frequency windows between ML and AP directions, and the overall pattern of the effects of touch and vision were distinct along the frontal and sagittal planes and both on foam and solid BoS (compare **Figures 8, 12**). On the other hand, the median frequency was not different between the frontal and the sagittal planes for both foam and solid BoS. Touch compared to no-touch, regardless of vision availability, exerted a larger stabilising effect in the AP than in the ML direction. Such a stabilised condition (EC-LT and EO-LT) may have reduced the "rambling" component of the control while favouring the "trembling" omponent (86, 175), thanks to the haptic reference in the AP direction. With vision, a difference also emerged between ML and AP directions in the mean level of the spectrum because spectrum amplitude relatively prevailed in the AP direction on solid BoS.

Limitations

The sample size was not determined prior to the study. However, the effect size of the significant differences indicates always large effects. Given our sample size of 19 participants, the study proved to have a sufficient power (>80%) to detect an effect in median frequency larger than 0.12 Hz between the EC-LT and EO conditions. The data have been collected here and analysed on the basis of one single trial per subject per condition (i.e., the first trial of a series of eight trials), administered in order to investigate the effect of the sensory conditions in the adaptation to repeated stance performances. Given the inter-individual variability in the stance performance (9, 176), particularly when standing on foam, this procedure is certainly a limitation however hardly avoidable because repetition of stance trials produces significant adaptation in the balancing pattern (8, 127, 177–180). Alsubaie et al. (181) have recently shown that different measures of postural sway are reliable when recorded at two visits 1 week apart, including measures with unstable BoS and sensory conditions. We do not know whether the frequencies might change as a function of the viewing scene (the characteristics of the patterned environment or the visual target being close or far) or of the position, texture, and orientation with respect to the body of the force pad, or of the force exerted by the finger. Further, the effect of the inner mechanical spring-like properties of the foam on the recorded signal has not been addressed, thereby preventing quantitative considerations on the role of proprioception standing on foam (or on solid BoS as well) and its potential interaction with vision and touch. Moreover, the feet position has not been manipulated, contrary to Šarabon et al. (82), who however found no major difference in the oscillation frequencies across different positions.

No estimation of the role of the vestibular information is provided here (182, 183), and no measure of the displacement in space of body segments such as the head and the pelvis. The information from the plantar foot sole, certainly different between foam and solid BoS, must have played a role. It has been proposed that our perception of verticality on a compliant surface, dependent in part on the plantar foot mechanoreceptor input, decreases when vision is not available (39, 184). We made no attempt to assess the contribution of these receptors. Electrical activity of the muscles involved in the control of equilibrium under the tested conditions has not been recorded, either. This information would help define the coordination properties underpinning the changes in oscillation frequency prescribed by the sensory conditions and the factors leading to the specific power spectrum features of postural sway. Moreover, this preliminary investigation is limited to young adult healthy subjects, and no information on the behaviour of aged healthy persons

(185–187) or of patients with equilibrium disorders has been collected and analysed in these conditions according to this methodology (188).

CONCLUSION

The data suggest that the oscillation frequency analysis, in spite of its relative complexity, gives information on the control mode of critical stance exerted by different sensory inputs, not supplied by common and simpler geometric sway measures. The use of foam highlighted a significant increase in medium-high frequencies with touch in the absence of vision compared to vision alone. In perspective, the approach based on the analysis of distinct windows in the frequency spectrum of the body oscillations would help postulate the existence, and define the respective mechanisms, of the specific process through which different sensory information contributes to body stabilisation under critical conditions (31). Differences in balance control between young and older subjects would also be easily defined and exploited as a measure of balance alterations in patients due to impairments of various origins (189–192).

AUTHOR CONTRIBUTIONS

MS conceived the idea for the manuscript. SS performed the recruitment of participants and the collection of data. SS and MS performed the data analysis and drafted the article. AN revised it critically for important intellectual content. All authors approved the submitted version.

FUNDING

The funding for this study was provided by the Ricerca Corrente of the Italian Ministry of Health.

ACKNOWLEDGMENTS

The authors would like to thank the ICS Maugeri SB, Pavia, Italy, that helped make this work possible.

REFERENCES

Honeine JL, Schieppati M. Time-interval for integration of stabilizing haptic and visual information in subjects balancing under static and dynamic conditions. *Front Syst Neurosci.* (2014) 8:190. doi: 10.3389/fnsys.2014.00190

Forbes PA, Chen A, Blouin JS. Sensorimotor control of standing balance. *Handb Clin Neurol.* (2018) 159:61–83. doi: 10.1016/B978-0-444-63916-5.00004-5

Peterka RJ. Sensory integration for human balance control. *Handb Clin Neurol.* (2018) 159:27–42. doi: 10.1016/B978-0-444-63916-5.00002-1

Schieppati M, Hugon M, Grasso M, Nardone A, Galante M. The limits of equilibrium in young and elderly normal subjects and in parkinsonians. *Electroencephalogr Clin Neurophysiol.* (1994) 93:286–98. doi: 10.1016/0168-5597(94)90031-0

Nardone A, Tarantola J, Giordano A, Schieppati M. Fatigue effects on body balance. *Electroencephalogr Clin Neurophysiol.* (1997) 105:309– 20. doi: 10.1016/S0924-980X(97)00040-4

Masani K, Popovic MR, Nakazawa K, Kouzaki M, Nozaki D. Importance of body sway velocity information in controlling ankle extensor activities during quiet stance. *J Neurophysiol.* (2003) 90:3774–82. doi: 10.1152/jn.00730.2002

Morasso P. Centre of pressure versus centre of mass stabilization strategies: the tightrope balancing case. *R Soc Open Sci.* (2020) 7:200111. doi: 10.1098/rsos.200111

Lhomond O, Juan B, Fornerone T, Cossin M, Paleressompoulle D, Prince F, et al. Learned overweight internal model can be activated to maintain equilibrium when tactile cues are uncertain: evidence from cortical and behavioral approaches. *Front Hum Neurosci.* (2021) 15:635611. doi: 10.3389/fnhum.2021.635611

Sakanaka TE, Lakie M, Reynolds RF. idiosyncratic characteristics of postural sway in normal and perturbed standing. *Front Hum Neurosci.* (2021) 15:660470. doi: 10.3389/fnhum.2021.660470

Svensson I, Gao C, Halder A, Gard G, Magnusson M. Standing balance on inclined surfaces with different friction. *Ind Health.* (2018) 56:292– 99. doi: 10.2486/indhealth.2018-0005

Cleworth TW, Carpenter MG. Postural threat influences conscious perception of postural sway. *Neurosci Lett.* (2016) 620:127–31. doi: 10.1016/j.neulet.2016.03.032

Teasdale N, Stelmach GE, Breunig A. Postural sway characteristics of the elderly under normal and altered visual and support surface conditions. *J Gerontol.* (1991) 46:B238–44. doi: 10.1093/geronj/46.6.B238

Patel M, Fransson PA, Johansson R, Magnusson M. Foam posturography: standing on foam is not equivalent to standing with decreased rapidly adapting mechanoreceptive sensation. *Exp Brain Res.* (2011) 208:519– 27. doi: 10.1007/s00221-010-2498-6

Hsiao D, Belur P, Myers PS, Earhart GM, Rawson KS. The impact of age, surface characteristics, and dual-tasking on postural sway. *Arch Gerontol Geriatr.* (2020) 87:103973. doi: 10.1016/j.archger.2019.103973

Johansson J, Nordström A, Gustafson Y, Westling G, Nordström P. Increased postural sway during quiet stance as a risk factor for prospective falls in community-dwelling elderly individuals. *Age Ageing.* (2017) 46:964– 70. doi: 10.1093/ageing/afx083

Anson E, Bigelow RT, Studenski S, Deshpande N, Agrawal Y. Failure on the foam eyes closed test of standing balance associated with reduced semicircular canal function in healthy older adults. *Ear Hear.* (2019) 40:340– 44. doi: 10.1097/AUD.0000000000000619

Kapoula Z, Lê TT. Effects of distance and gaze position on postural stability in young and old subjects. *Exp Brain Res.* (2006) 173:438– 45. doi: 10.1007/s00221-006-0382-1

Horlings CG, Küng UM, Bloem BR, Honegger F, Van Alfen N, Van Engelen BG, et al. Identifying deficits in balance control following vestibular or proprioceptive loss using posturographic analysis of stance tasks. *Clin Neurophysiol.* (2008) 119:2338–46. doi: 10.1016/j.clinph.2008.07.221

Morrison S, Rynders CA, Sosnoff JJ. Deficits in medio-lateral balance control and the implications for falls in individuals with multiple sclerosis. *Gait Posture.* (2016) 49:148–54. doi: 10.1016/j.gaitpost.2016.06.036

Allum JH, Carpenter MG. A speedy solution for balance and gait analysis: angular velocity measured at the centre of body mass. *Curr Opin Neurol.* (2005) 18:15–21. doi: 10.1097/00019052-200502000-00005

Amblard B, Crémieux J, Marchand AR, Carblanc A. Lateral orientation and stabilization of human stance: static versus dynamic visual cues. *Exp Brain Res.* (1985) 61:21–37. doi: 10.1007/BF00235617

Day BL, Steiger MJ, Thompson PD, Marsden CD. Effect of vision and stance width on human body motion when standing: implications for afferent control of lateral sway. *J Physiol.* (1993) 469:479–99. doi: 10.1113/jphysiol.1993.sp019824

Nardone A, Schieppati M. The role of instrumental assessment of balance in clinical decision making. *Eur J Phys Rehabil Med.* (2010) 46:221–37.

Šarabon N, Rosker J, Loefler S, Kern H. Sensitivity of body sway parameters during quiet standing to manipulation of support surface size. *J Sports Sci Med.* (2010) 9:431–8.

Goodworth AD, Mellodge P, Peterka RJ. Stance width changes how sensory feedback is used for multisegmental balance control. *J Neurophysiol.* (2014) 112:525–42. doi: 10.1152/jn.00490.2013

Wang Z, Newell KM. Inter-foot coordination dynamics of quiet standing postures. *Neurosci Biobehav Rev.* (2014) 47:194– 202. doi: 10.1016/j.neubiorev.2014.08.007

Bove M, Bonzano L, Trompetto C, Abbruzzese G, Schieppati M. The postural disorientation induced by neck muscle vibration subsides on lightly touching a stationary surface or aiming at it. *Neuroscience.* (2006) 143:1095– 103. doi: 10.1016/j.neuroscience.2006.08.038

Kabbaligere R, Lee BC, Layne CS. Balancing sensory inputs: sensory reweighting of ankle proprioception and vision during a bipedal posture task. *Gait Posture.* (2017) 52:244–50. doi: 10.1016/j.gaitpost.2016.12.009

Lord SR, Menz HB. Visual contributions to postural stability in older adults. *Gerontology.* (2000) 46:306–10. doi: 10.1159/000022182

De Nunzio AM, Schieppati M. Time to reconfigure balancing behaviour in man: changing visual condition while riding a continuously moving platform. *Exp Brain Res.* (2007) 178:18–36. doi: 10.1007/s00221-006-0708-z

Lee IC, Pacheco MM, Newell KM. Constraints specific influences of vision, touch and surface compliance in postural dynamics. *Gait Posture.* (2018) 59:117–21. doi: 10.1016/j.gaitpost.2017.09.014

Fitzpatrick R, Rogers DK, McCloskey DI. Stable human standing with lower-limb muscle afferents providing the only sensory input. *J Physiol.* (1994) 480:395–403. doi: 10.1113/jphysiol.1994.sp020369

Fitzpatrick RC, Gorman RB, Burke D, Gandevia SC. Postural proprioceptive reflexes in standing human subjects: bandwidth of response and transmission characteristics. *J Physiol.* (1992) 458:69–83. doi: 10.1113/jphysiol.1992.sp019406

Gatev P, Thomas S, Kepple T, Hallett M. Feedforward ankle strategy of balance during quiet stance in adults. *J Physiol.* (1999) 514:915– 28. doi: 10.1111/j.1469-7793.1999.915ad.x

Courtine G, De Nunzio AM, Schmid M, Beretta MV, Schieppati M. Stance- and locomotion-dependent processing of vibration-induced proprioceptive inflow from multiple muscles in humans. *J Neurophysiol.* (2007) 97:772– 9. doi: 10.1152/jn.00764.2006

Gritti I, Schieppati M. Short-latency inhibition of soleus motoneurones by impulses in Ia afferents from the gastrocnemius muscle in humans. *J Physiol.* (1989) 416:469–84. doi: 10.1113/jphysiol.1989.sp017772

Bussel B, Morin C, Pierrot-Deseilligny E. Mechanism of monosynaptic reflex reinforcement during jendrassik manoeuvre in man. *J Neurol Neurosurg Psychiatry.* (1978) 41:40–4. doi: 10.1136/jnnp.41.1.40

Leukel C, Lundbye-Jensen J, Gruber M, Zuur AT, Gollhofer A, Taube W. Short-term pressure induced suppression of the short-latency response: a new methodology for investigating stretch reflexes. *J Appl Physiol.* (2009) 107:1051–8. doi: 10.1152/japplphysiol.00301.2009

Nedelkou A, Hatzitaki V, Chatzinikolaou K, Grouios G. Does somatosensory feedback from the plantar foot sole contribute to verticality perception? *Somatosens Mot Res.* (2021) 38:1–9. doi: 10.1080/08990220.2021.1949977

Felicetti G, Thoumie P, Do MC, Schieppati M. Cutaneous and muscular afferents from the foot and sensory fusion processing: physiology and pathology in neuropathies. *J Peripher Nerv Syst.* (2021) 26:17– 34. doi: 10.1111/jns.12429

Schieppati M, Nardone A, Siliotto R, Grasso M. Early and late stretch responses of human foot muscles induced by perturbation of stance. *Exp Brain Res.* (1995) 105:411–22. doi: 10.1007/BF00233041

Roll JP, Vedel JP, Ribot E. Alteration of proprioceptive messages induced by tendon vibration in man: a microneurographic study. *Exp Brain Res.* (1989) 76:213–22. doi: 10.1007/BF00253639

Nardone A, Schieppati M. Group II spindle fibres and afferent control of stance. Clues from diabetic neuropathy. *Clin Neurophysiol.* (2004) 115:779– 89. doi: 10.1016/j.clinph.2003.11.007

Bove M, Trompetto C, Abbruzzese G, Schieppati M. The posture- related interaction between Ia-afferent and descending input on the spinal reflex excitability in humans. *Neurosci Lett.* (2006) 397:301– 6. doi: 10.1016/j.neulet.2005.12.049

Nardone A, Giordano A, Corrà T, Schieppati M. Responses of leg muscles in humans displaced while standing. Effects of types of perturbation and of postural set. *Brain.* (1990) 113 (Pt. 1):65–84. doi: 10.1093/brain/113.1.65

Schieppati M, Nardone A. Free and supported stance in Parkinson's disease. The effect of posture and 'postural set' on leg muscle responses to perturbation, and its relation to the severity of the disease. *Brain.* (1991) 114 (Pt. 3):1227–44. doi: 10.1093/brain/114.3.1227

Lackner JR. The importance of being in touch. *Front Neurol.* (2021) 12:646640. doi: 10.3389/fneur.2021.646640

De Nunzio AM, Nardone A, Schieppati M. Head stabilization on a continuously oscillating platform: the effect of a proprioceptive disturbance on the balancing strategy. *Exp Brain Res.* (2005) 165:261– 72. doi: 10.1007/s00221-005-2297-7

Fransson PA, Gomez S, Patel M, Johansson L. Changes in multi- segmented body movements and EMG activity while standing on firm and foam support surfaces. *Eur J Appl Physiol.* (2007) 101:81– 9. doi: 10.1007/s00421-007-0476-x

Mademli L, Mavridi D, Bohm S, Patikas DA, Santuz A, Arampatzis A. Standing on unstable surface challenges postural control of tracking tasks and modulates neuromuscular adjustments specific to task complexity. *Sci Rep.* (2021) 11:6122. doi: 10.1038/s41598-021-84899-y

Allum JH, Pfaltz CR. Visual and vestibular contributions to pitch sway stabilization in the ankle muscles of normals and patients with bilateral peripheral vestibular deficits. *Exp Brain Res.* (1985) 58:82– 94. doi: 10.1007/BF00238956

Sozzi S, Honeine JL, Do MC, Schieppati M. Leg muscle activity during tandem stance and the control of body balance in the frontal plane. *Clin Neurophysiol.* (2013) 124:1175–86. doi: 10.1016/j.clinph.2012.12.001

Jeka J, Kiemel T, Creath R, Horak F, Peterka R. Controlling human upright posture: velocity information is more accurate than position or acceleration. *J Neurophysiol.* (2004) 92:2368–79. doi: 10.1152/jn.00983.2003

Horlings CG, Küng UM, Honegger F, Van Engelen BG, Van Alfen N, Bloem BR, et al. Vestibular and proprioceptive influences on trunk movements during quiet standing. *Neuroscience.* (2009) 161:904– 14. doi: 10.1016/j.neuroscience.2009.04.005

Hsu WL, Scholz JP, Schöner G, Jeka JJ, Kiemel T. Control and estimation of posture during quiet stance depends on multijoint coordination. *J Neurophysiol.* (2007) 97:3024–35. doi: 10.1152/jn.01142.2006

Zhang Y, Kiemel T, Jeka J. The influence of sensory information on two-component coordination during quiet stance. *Gait Posture.* (2007) 26:263–71. doi: 10.1016/j.gaitpost.2006.09.007

Kelly LA, Kuitunen S, Racinais S, Cresswell AG. Recruitment of the plantar intrinsic foot muscles with increasing postural demand. *Clin Biomech.* (2012) 27:46–51. doi: 10.1016/j.clinbiomech.2011.07.013

Holden M, Ventura J, Lackner JR. Stabilization of posture by precision contact of the index finger. *J Vestib Res.* (1994) 4:285–301.

Jeka JJ, Lackner JR. Fingertip contact influences human postural control. *Exp Brain Res.* (1994) 100:495–502. doi: 10.1007/BF02738408

Jeka JJ, Lackner JR. The role of haptic cues from rough and slippery surfaces in human postural control. *Exp Brain Res.* (1995) 103:267– 76. doi: 10.1007/BF00231713

Wing AM, Johannsen L, Endo S. Light touch for balance: influence of a time-varying external driving signal. *Philos Trans R Soc Lond B Biol Sci.* (2011) 366:3133–41. doi: 10.1098/rstb.2011.0169

Sozzi S, Do MC, Monti A, Schieppati M. Sensorimotor integration during stance: processing time of active or passive addition or withdrawal of visual or haptic information. *Neuroscience.* (2012) 212:59–76. doi: 10.1016/j.neuroscience.2012.03.044

Honeine JL, Crisafulli O, Sozzi S, Schieppati M. Processing time of addition or withdrawal of single or combined balance- stabilizing haptic and visual information. *J Neurophysiol.* (2015) 114:3097–110. doi: 10.1152/jn.00618.2015

Rocha-Silva C, Magalhães FH, Kohn AF. Fingertip-Coupled spindle signaling does not contribute to reduce postural sway under light touch. *Front Physiol.* (2019) 10:1072. doi: 10.3389/fphys.2019.01072

Kouzaki M, Masani K. Reduced postural sway during quiet standing by light touch is due to finger tactile feedback but not mechanical support. *Exp Brain Res.* (2008) 188:153–8. doi: 10.1007/s00221-008-1426-5

Sozzi S, Crisafulli O, Schieppati M. Haptic cues for balance: use of a cane provides immediate body stabilization. *Front Neurosci.* (2017) 11:705. doi: 10.3389/fnins.2017.00705

Prado-Rico JM, Alouche SR, Sodré AC, Garbus RBSC, Freitas SMSF. Effect of force magnitude of touch on the components of postural sway. *Gait Posture.* (2018) 65:15–19. doi: 10.1016/j.gaitpost.2018.06.164

Dickstein R. Stance stability with unilateral and bilateral light touch of an external stationary object. *Somatosens Mot Res.* (2005) 22:319– 25. doi: 10.1080/08990220500420640

Afzal MR, Byun HY, Oh MK, Yoon J. Effects of kinesthetic haptic feedback on standing stability of young healthy subjects and stroke patients. *J Neuroeng Rehabil.* (2015) 12:27. doi: 10.1186/s12984-015-0020-x

Kaulmann D, Saveriano M, Lee D, Hermsdörfer J, Johannsen L. Stabilization of body balance with light touch following a mechanical perturbation: adaption of sway and disruption of right posterior parietal cortex by cTBS. *PLoS ONE.* (2020) 15:e0233988. doi: 10.1371/journal.pone.0233988

Shiva T, Misiaszek JE. Activation of ankle muscles following rapid displacement of a light touch contact during treadmill walking. *Exp Brain Res.* (2018) 236:563–576. doi: 10.1007/s00221-017-5151-9

Albertsen IM, Temprado JJ, Berton E. Effect of haptic supplementation provided by a fixed or mobile stick on postural stabilization in elderly people. *Gerontology.* (2012) 58:419–29. doi: 10.1159/000337495

Bolton DA, McIlroy WE, Staines WR. The impact of light fingertip touch on haptic cortical processing during a standing balance task. *Exp Brain Res.* (2011) 212:279–91. doi: 10.1007/s00221-011-2728-6

Ernst MO, Banks MS. Humans integrate visual and haptic information in a statistically optimal fashion. *Nature.* (2002) 415:429–33. doi: 10.1038/415429a

Lacey S, Sathian K. Crossmodal and multisensory interactions between vision and touch. *Scholarpedia.* (2015) 10:7957. doi: 10.4249/scholarpedia.7957

Camponogara I, Volcic R. Integration of haptics and vision in human multisensory grasping. *Cortex.* (2021) 135:173– 85. doi: 10.1016/j.cortex.2020.11.012

Jeannerod M. Intersegmental coordination during reaching at natural visual objects. In: Long J, Baddeley A, editors. *Attention Performance IX.* Hillsdale, MI: Erlbaum (1981). p. 153–68.

Ruhe A, Fejer R, Walker B. The test-retest reliability of centre of pressure measures in bipedal static task conditions - a systematic review of the literature. *Gait Posture.* (2010) 32:436–45. doi: 10.1016/j.gaitpost.2010.09.012

Yamamoto T, Smith CE, Suzuki Y, Kiyono K, Tanahashi T, Sakoda S, et al. Universal and individual characteristics of postural sway during quiet standing in healthy young adults. *Physiol Rep.* (2015) 3:e12329. doi: 10.14814/phy2.12329

Marchese R, Bove M, Abbruzzese G. Effect of cognitive and motor tasks on postural stability in Parkinson's disease: a posturographic study. *Mov Disord.* (2003) 18:652–8. doi: 10.1002/mds.10418

Fitzgerald JE, Murray A, Elliott C, Birchall JP. Comparison of body sway analysis techniques. Assessment with subjects standing on a stable surface. *Acta Otolaryngol.* (1994) 114:115–9. doi: 10.3109/00016489409126028

Šarabon N, Rosker J, Loefler S, Kern H. The effect of vision elimination during quiet stance tasks with different feet positions. *Gait Posture.* (2013) 38:708–11. doi: 10.1016/j.gaitpost.2013.03.005

Bergamin M, Gobbo S, Zanotto T, Sieverdes JC, Alberton CL, Zaccaria M, et al. Influence of age on postural sway during different dual-task conditions. *Front Aging Neurosci.* (2014) 6:271. doi: 10.3389/fnagi.2014.00271

Schmid M, Nardone A, De Nunzio AM, Schmid M, Schieppati M. Equilibrium during static and dynamic tasks in blind subjects: no evidence of cross-modal plasticity. *Brain.* (2007) 130 (Pt. 8):2097– 107. doi: 10.1093/brain/awm157

Zatsiorsky VM, Duarte M. Rambling and trembling in quiet standing. *Motor Control.* (2000) 4:185–200. doi: 10.1123/mcj.4.2.185

Yamagata M, Popow M, Latash ML. Beyond rambling and trembling: effects of visual feedback on slow postural drift. *Exp Brain Res.* (2019) 237:865– 71. doi: 10.1007/s00221-019-05470-w

Bottaro A, Casadio M, Morasso PG, Sanguineti V. Body sway during quiet standing: is it the residual chattering of an intermittent stabilization process? *Hum Mov Sci.* (2005) 24:588–615. doi: 10.1016/j.humov.2005.07.006

Duarte M, Freitas MSF, Zatsiorsky V. Control of equilibrium in humans. Sway over sway. In: Danion F, Latash M, editors. *Motor Control: Theories, Experiments, and Applications.* Oxford: Oxford University Press (2011). p. 219–42. doi: 10.1093/acprof:oso/9780195395273.003.0010

Collins JJ, De Luca CJ. Open-loop and closed-loop control of posture: a random-walk analysis of center-of-pressure trajectories. *Exp Brain Res.* (1993) 95:308–18. doi: 10.1007/BF00229788

Rougier PR. What insights can be gained when analysing the resultant centre of pressure trajectory? *Neurophysiol Clin.* (2008) 38:363–73. doi: 10.1016/j.neucli.2008.09.006

Lacour M, Bernard-Demanze L, Dumitrescu M. Posture control, aging, and attention resources: models and posture-analysis methods. *Neurophysiol Clin.* (2008) 38:411–21. doi: 10.1016/j.neucli.2008.09.005

Potvin-Desrochers A, Richer N, Lajoie Y. Cognitive tasks promote automatization of postural control in young and older adults. *Gait Posture.* (2017) 57:40–5. doi: 10.1016/j.gaitpost.2017.05.019

St-Amant G, Rahman T, Polskaia N, Fraser S, Lajoie Y. Unveilling the cerebral and sensory contributions to automatic postural control during dual-task standing. *Hum Mov Sci.* (2020) 70:102587. doi: 10.1016/j.humov.2020.102587

Roerdink M, De Haart M, Daffertshofer A, Donker SF, Geurts AC, Beek PJ. Dynamical structure of center-of-pressure trajectories in patients recovering from stroke. *Exp Brain Res.* (2006) 174:256–69. doi: 10.1007/s00221-006-0441-7

King AC, Patton J, Dutt-Mazumder A, Newell KM. Center-of-pressure dynamics of upright standing as a function of sloped surfaces and vision. *Neurosci Lett.* (2020) 737:135334. doi: 10.1016/j.neulet.2020.135334

Schumann T, Redfern MS, Furman JM, El-Jaroudi A, Chaparro LF. Time-frequency analysis of postural sway. *J Biomech.* (1995) 28:603– 7. doi: 10.1016/0021-9290(94)00113-I

Hufschmidt A, Dichgans J, Mauritz KH, Hufschmidt M. Some methods and parameters of body sway quantification and their neurological applications. *Arch Psychiatr Nervenkr.* (1980) 228:135–50. doi: 10.1007/BF00365601

Singh NB, Taylor WR, Madigan ML, Nussbaum MA. The spectral content of postural sway during quiet stance: influences of age, vision and somatosensory inputs. *J Electromyogr Kinesiol.* (2012) 22:131– 6. doi: 10.1016/j.jelekin.2011.10.007

Kanekar N, Lee YJ, Aruin AS. Frequency analysis approach to study balance control in individuals with multiple sclerosis. *J Neurosci Methods.* (2014) 222:91–6. doi: 10.1016/j.jneumeth.2013.10.020

Tanabe H, Fujii K, Kouzaki M. Large postural fluctuations but unchanged postural sway dynamics during tiptoe standing compared to quiet standing. *J Electromyogr Kinesiol.* (2012) 22:975–82. doi: 10.1016/j.jelekin.2012.05.006

Golomer E, Dupui P, Bessou P. Spectral frequency analysis of dynamic balance in healthy and injured athletes. *Arch Int Physiol Biochim Biophys.* (1994) 102:225–9. doi: 10.3109/13813459409007543

Paillard T, Noé F, Rivière T, Marion V, Montoya R, Dupui P. Postural performance and strategy in the unipedal stance of soccer players at different levels of competition. *J Athl Train.* (2006) 41:172–6.

Tanaka S, Ando K, Kobayashi K, Nakashima H, Seki T, Ishizuka S, et al. Locomotive syndrome and the power spectral characteristics of body sway. *Geriatr Gerontol Int.* (2020) 20:691–6. doi: 10.1111/ggi.13937

Nagy E, Toth K, Janositz G, Kovacs G, Feher-Kiss A, Angyan L, et al. Postural control in athletes participating in an ironman triathlon. *Eur J Appl Physiol.* (2004) 92:407–13. doi: 10.1007/s00421-004-1157-7

Diaz-Artiles A, Karmali F. Vestibular precision at the level of perception, eye movements, posture, and neurons. *Neuroscience.* (2021) 468:282– 320. doi: 10.1016/j.neuroscience.2021.05.028

Mezzarane RA, Kohn AF. Postural control during kneeling. *Exp Brain Res.* (2008) 187:395–405. doi: 10.1007/s00221-008-1308-x

Hlavacˇka F, Njiokiktjien C. Sinusoidal galvanic stimulation of the labyrinths and postural responses. *Physiol Bohemoslov.* (1986) 35:63–70.

Bonnet CT. Advantages and disadvantages of stiffness instructions when studying postural control. *Gait Posture.* (2016) 46:208– 10. doi: 10.1016/j.gaitpost.2015.12.026

Stoffregen TA, Smart LJ, Bardy BG, Pagulayan RJ. Postural stabilization of looking. *J. Exp. Psychol. Hum. Percept. Performa.* (1999) 25:1641– 58. doi: 10.1037/0096-1523.25.6.1641

Michalak K, Ja´skowski P. Dimensional complexity of posturographic signals: I. Optimization of frequency sampling and recording time. *Curr Topics Biophys.* (2002) 26:235–44.

Vieira TM, Oliveira LF, Nadal J. Estimation procedures affect the center of pressure frequency analysis. *Braz J Med Biol Res.* (2009) 42:665– 73. doi: 10.1590/S0100-879X2009000700012

Scoppa F, Capra R, Gallamini M, Shiffer R. Clinical stabilometry standardization: basic definitions–acquisition interval–sampling frequency. *Gait Posture.* (2013) 37:290–2. doi: 10.1016/j.gaitpost.2012.07.009

Schubert P, Kirchner M. Ellipse area calculations and their applicability in posturography. *Gait Posture.* (2014) 39:518– 22. doi: 10.1016/j.gaitpost.2013.09.001

Jurkojc´ J. Balance disturbances coefficient as a new value to assess ability to maintain balance on the basis of FFT curves. *Acta Bioeng Biomech.* (2018) 20:143–51.

Sozzi S, Monti A, De Nunzio AM, Do MC, Schieppati M. Sensori- motor integration during stance: time adaptation of control mechanisms on adding or removing vision. *Hum Mov Sci.* (2011) 30:172–89. doi: 10.1016/j.humov.2010.06.002

Taguchi K. Spectral analysis of body sway. *ORL J Otorhinolaryngol Relat Spec.* (1977) 39:330–7. doi: 10.1159/000275375

Krizková M, Hlavacˇka F, Gatev P. Visual control of human stance on a narrow and soft support surface. *Physiol Res.* (1993) 42:267–72.

Nakagawa H, Ohashi N, Watanabe Y, Mizukoshi K. The contribution of proprioception to posture control in normal subjects. *Acta Otolaryngol. Suppl.* (1993) 504:112–6. doi: 10.3109/00016489309128134

Demura S, Kitabayashi T. Comparison of power spectrum characteristics of body sway during a static upright standing posture in healthy elderly people and young adults. *Percept Mot Skills.* (2006) 102:467– 76. doi: 10.2466/pms.102.2.467-476

Demura S, Kitabayashi T, Noda M. Power spectrum characteristics of sway position and velocity of the center of pressure during static upright posture for healthy people. *Percept Mot Skills.* (2008) 106:307– 16. doi: 10.2466/pms.106.1.307-316

Morrison S, Kerr G, Newell KM, Silburn PA. Differential time- and frequency-dependent structure of postural sway and finger tremor in Parkinson's disease. *Neurosci Lett.* (2008) 443:123–8. doi: 10.1016/j.neulet.2008.07.071

Schinkel-Ivy A, Singer JC, Inness EL, Mansfield A. Do quiet standing centre of pressure measures within specific frequencies differ based on ability to recover balance in individuals with stroke? *Clin Neurophysiol.* (2016) 127:2463–71. doi: 10.1016/j.clinph.2016.02.021

Krafczyk S, Schlamp V, Dieterich M, Haberhauer P, Brandt T. Increased body sway at 3.5-8 Hz in patients with phobic postural vertigo. *Neurosci Lett.* (1999) 259:149–52. doi: 10.1016/S0304-3940(98)00917-3

Anagnostou E, Stavropoulou G, Zachou A, Kararizou E. Spectral composition of body sway in persistent postural-perceptual dizziness. *Otol Neurotol.* (2021) 42:e1318–26. doi: 10.1097/MAO.000000000 0003252

Creath R, Kiemel T, Horak F, Peterka R, Jeka JJ. A unified view of quiet and perturbed stance: simultaneous co-existing ankle and hip strategies. *Neurosci Lett.* (2005) 377:75–80. doi: 10.1016/j.neulet.2004.11.071

Winter DA, Prince F, Frank JS, Powell C, Zabjek KF. Unified theory regarding A/P and M/L balance in quiet stance. *J Neurophysiol.* (1996) 75:2334– 43. doi: 10.1152/jn.1996.75.6.2334

Tarantola J, Nardone A, Tacchini E, Schieppati M. Human stance stability improves with the repetition of the task: effect of foot position and visual condition. *Neurosci Lett.* (1997) 228:75–8. doi: 10.1016/S0304-3940(97)00370-4

Mezzarane RA, Kohn AF. Control of upright stance over inclined surfaces. *Exp Brain Res.* (2007) 180:377–88. doi: 10.1007/s00221-007- 0865-8

Cawsey RP, Chua R, Carpenter MG, Sanderson DJ. To what extent can increasing the magnification of visual feedback of the centre of pressure position change the control of quiet standing balance? *Gait Posture.* (2009) 29:280–4. doi: 10.1016/j.gaitpost.2008.09.007

Lubetzky-Vilnai A, McCoy SW, Price R, Ciol MA. Young adults largely depend on vision for postural control when standing on a BOSU ball but not on foam. *J Strength Cond Res.* (2015) 29:2907– 18. doi: 10.1519/JSC.0000000000000935

Thurrell A, Jáuregui-Renaud K, Gresty MA, Bronstein AM. Vestibular influence on the cardiorespiratory responses to whole-body oscillation after standing. *Exp Brain Res.* (2003) 150:325–31. doi: 10.1007/s00221-003- 1422-8

Lackner JR, DiZio P, Jeka J, Horak F, Krebs D, Rabin E. Precision contact of the fingertip reduces postural sway of individuals with bilateral vestibular loss. *Exp Brain Res.* (1999) 126:459–66. doi: 10.1007/s0022100 50753

Creath R, Kiemel T, Horak F, Jeka JJ. The role of vestibular and somatosensory systems in intersegmental control of upright stance. *J Vestib Res.* (2008) 18:39–49. doi: 10.3233/VES-2008-18104

Honegger F, Tielkens RJ, Allum JH. Movement strategies and sensory reweighting in tandem stance: differences between trained tightrope walkers and untrained subjects. *Neuroscience.* (2013) 254:285–300. doi: 10.1016/j.neuroscience.2013.09.041

Chen FC, Tsai CL. The mechanisms of the effect of light finger touch on postural control. *Neurosci Lett.* (2015) 605:69– 73. doi: 10.1016/j.neulet.2015.08.016

Johannsen L, Coward SRL, Martin GR, Wing AM, Casteren AV, Sellers WI, et al. Human bipedal instability in tree canopy environments is reduced by "light touch" fingertip support. *Sci Rep.* (2017) 7:1135. doi: 10.1038/s41598-017-01265-7

Clapp S, Wing AM. Light touch contribution to balance in normal bipedal stance. *Exp Brain Res.* (1999) 125:521–4. doi: 10.1007/s0022100 50711

Huang CY, Cherng RJ, Yang ZR, Chen YT, Hwang IS. Modulation of soleus H reflex due to stance pattern and haptic stabilization of posture. *J Electromyogr Kinesiol.* (2009) 19:492–9. doi: 10.1016/j.jelekin.2007. 07.014

Bryanton MA, Chodan SDC, Vander Meulen J, Fenrich KK, Misiaszek JE. The effect of light touch on standing sway when the stability of the external touch reference becomes unreliable. *Exp Brain Res.* (2019) 237:663– 72. doi: 10.1007/s00221-018-5455-4

Rabin E, Bortolami SB, DiZio P, Lackner JR. Haptic stabilization of posture: changes in arm proprioception and cutaneous feedback for different arm orientations. *J Neurophysiol.* (1999) 82:3541–9. doi: 10.1152/jn.1999.82.6.3541

Lee IC, Pacheco MM, Newell KM. Postural coordination and control to the precision demands of light finger touch. *Exp Brain Res.* (2019) 237:1339– 46. doi: 10.1007/s00221-019-05513-2

Krishnamoorthy V, Slijper H, Latash ML. Effects of different types of light touch on postural sway. *Exp Brain Res.* (2002) 147:71– 9. doi: 10.1007/s00221-002-1206-6

Conrad V, Vitello MP, Noppeney U. Interactions between apparent motion rivalry in vision and touch. *Psychol Sci.* (2012) 23:940–8. doi: 10.1177/0956797612438735

Janko M, Primerano R, Visell Y. On frictional forces between the finger and a textured surface during active touch. *IEEE Trans Haptics.* (2016) 9:221–32. doi: 10.1109/TOH.2015.2507583

Rogers MW, Wardman DL, Lord SR, Fitzpatrick RC. Passive tactile sensory input improves stability during standing. *Exp Brain Res.* (2001) 136:514– 22. doi: 10.1007/s002210000615

Sozzi S, Decortes F, Schmid M, Crisafulli O, Schieppati M. Balance in blind subjects: cane and fingertip touch induce similar extent and promptness of stance stabilization. *Front Neurosci.* (2018) 12:639. doi: 10.3389/fnins.2018.00639

Goyal N, Lee Y, Luna G, Aruin AS. Individual and combined effects of a cognitive task, light finger touch, and vision on standing balance in older adults with mild cognitive impairment. *Aging Clin Exp Res.* (2020) 32:797–807. doi: 10.1007/s40520-019-01262-y

Andreopoulou G, Maaswinkel E, Cofré Lizama LE, van Dieën JH. Effects of support surface stability on feedback control of trunk posture. *Exp Brain Res.* (2015) 233:1079–87. doi: 10.1007/s00221-014-4185-5

Jergelová M, Podivinský F. Some conceptual remarks about supraspinal mechanisms in the control of voluntary and reflex motor activities. *Electromyogr Clin Neurophysiol.* (1992) 32:537–46.

Nardone A, Pasetti C, Schieppati M. Spinal and supraspinal stretch responses of postural muscles in early parkinsonian patients. *Exp Neurol.* (2012) 237:407–17. doi: 10.1016/j.expneurol.2012.07.003

Macaluso E, Maravita A. The representation of space near the body through touch and vision. *Neuropsychologia.* (2010) 48:782–95. doi: 10.1016/j.neuropsychologia.2009.10.010

Taube W, Schubert M, Gruber M, Beck S, Faist M, Gollhofer A. Direct corticospinal pathways contribute to neuromuscular control of perturbed stance. *J Appl Physiol.* (2006) 101:420– 9. doi: 10.1152/japplphysiol.01447.2005

Bolton DA, Brown KE, McIlroy WE, Staines WR. Transient inhibition of the dorsolateral prefrontal cortex disrupts somatosensory modulation during standing balance as measured by electroencephalography. *Neuroreport.* (2012) 23:369–72. doi: 10.1097/WNR.0b013e328352027c

Mierau A, Pester B, Hülsdünker T, Schiecke K, Strüder HK, Witte H. Cortical correlates of human balance control. *Brain Topogr.* (2017) 30:434– 46. doi: 10.1007/s10548-017-0567-x

Malcolm BR, Foxe JJ, Joshi S, Verghese J, Mahoney JR, Molholm S, et al. Aging-related changes in cortical mechanisms supporting postural control during base of support and optic flow manipulations. *Eur J Neurosci.* (2020). 1–19. doi: 10.1111/ejn.15004

Kim S, James TW. Enhanced effectiveness in visuo-haptic object-selective brain regions with increasing stimulus salience. *Hum Brain Mapp.* (2010) 31:678–93. doi: 10.1002/hbm.20897

Magre FL, Costa TDAD, Paiva ACS, Moraes R, Mauerberg-deCastro E. Does the level of difficulty in balancing tasks affect haptic sensitivity via light touch? *J Mot Behav.* (2020) 52:1–12. doi: 10.1080/00222895.2019.1565529

Kilby MC, Molenaar PC, Newell KM. Models of postural control: shared variance in joint and COM motions. *PLoS ONE.* (2015) 10:e0126379. doi: 10.1371/journal.pone.0126379

Sprenger A, Wojak JF, Jandl NM, Helmchen C. Postural control in bilateral vestibular failure: its relation to visual, proprioceptive, vestibular, and cognitive input. *Front Neurol.* (2017) 8:444. doi: 10.3389/fneur.2017.00444

Bacsi AM, Colebatch JG. Evidence for reflex and perceptual vestibular contributions to postural control. *Exp Brain Res.* (2005) 160:22–8. doi: 10.1007/s00221-004-1982-2

Carpenter MG, Murnaghan CD, Inglis JT. Shifting the balance: evidence of an exploratory role for postural sway. *Neuroscience.* (2010) 171:196– 204. doi: 10.1016/j.neuroscience.2010.08.030

Reynard F, Christe D, Terrier P. Postural control in healthy adults: determinants of trunk sway assessed with a chest-worn accelerometer in 12 quiet standing tasks. *PLoS ONE.* (2019) 14:e0211051. doi: 10.1371/journal.pone.0211051

Knikou M, Rymer Z. Effects of changes in hip joint angle on H-reflex excitability in humans. *Exp Brain Res.* (2002) 43:149–59. doi: 10.1007/s00221-001-0978-4

Kiers H, Brumagne S, van Dieën J, van der Wees P, Vanhees L. Ankle proprioception is not targeted by exercises on an unstable surface. *Eur J Appl Physiol.* (2012) 112:1577–85. doi: 10.1007/s00421-011-2124-8

Ivanenko YP, Talis VL, Kazennikov OV. Support stability influences postural responses to muscle vibration in humans. *Eur J Neurosci.* (1999) 11:647– 54. doi: 10.1046/j.1460-9568.1999.00471.x

Hatzitaki V, Pavlou M, Bronstein AM. The integration of multiple proprioceptive information: effect of ankle tendon vibration on postural responses to platform tilt. *Exp Brain Res.* (2004) 154:345–54. doi: 10.1007/s00221-003-1661-8

Franzén E, Gurfinkel VS, Wright WG, Cordo PJ, Horak FB. Haptic touch reduces sway by increasing axial tone. *Neuroscience.* (2011) 174:216– 23. doi: 10.1016/j.neuroscience.2010.11.017

Warnica MJ, Weaver TB, Prentice SD, Laing AC. The influence of ankle muscle activation on postural sway during quiet stance. *Gait Posture.* (2014) 39:1115–21. doi: 10.1016/j.gaitpost.2014.01.019

van Dieën JH, van Drunen P, Happee R. Sensory contributions to stabilization of trunk posture in the sagittal plane. *J Biomech.* (2018) 70:219– 27. doi: 10.1016/j.jbiomech.2017.07.016

Gandevia SC, Hall LA, McCloskey DI, Potter EK. Proprioceptive sensation at the terminal joint of the middle finger. *J Physiol.* (1983) 335:507– 17. doi: 10.1113/jphysiol.1983.sp014547

Monteleone S, Feltroni L, Arbustini E, Bernardi E, Carenzio G, Dalla Toffola E Schieppati M. Balance in patients with Marfan syndrome. *Transl Sci Rare Dis.* (2018) 3:145–56. doi: 10.3233/TRD-180029

Yiou E, Hussein T, Larue J. Influence of temporal pressure on anticipatory postural control of medio-lateral stability during rapid leg flexion. *Gait Posture.* (2012) 35:494–9. doi: 10.1016/j.gaitpost.2011. 11.015

Osoba MY, Rao AK, Agrawal SK, Lalwani AK. Balance and gait in the elderly: A contemporary review. *Laryngoscope Investig Otolaryngol.* (2019) 4:143–53. doi: 10.1002/lio2.252

Embrechts E, Van Criekinge T, Schröder J, Nijboer T, Lafosse C, Truijen S, et al. The association between visuospatial neglect and balance and mobility post-stroke onset: a systematic review. *Ann Phys Rehabil Med.* (2021) 64:101449. doi: 10.1016/j.rehab.2020.10.003

Shin S, Milosevic M, Chung CM, Lee Y. Contractile properties of superficial skeletal muscle affect postural control in healthy young adults: a test of the rambling and trembling hypothesis. *PLoS ONE.* (2019) 14:e0223850. doi: 10.1371/journal.pone.0223850

Michaud L, Richer N, Lajoie Y. Number of trials needed to assess postural control of young adults in single and dual-task. *J Mot Behav.* (2021) 53:30– 9. doi: 10.1080/00222895.2020.1723479

Sozzi S, Nardone A, Schieppati M. Adaptation of balancing behaviour during continuous perturbations of stance. Supra-postural visual tasks and platform translation frequency modulate adaptation rate. *PLoS ONE.* (2020) 15:e0236702. doi: 10.1371/journal.pone.0236702

Keller M, Pfusterschmied J, Buchecker M, Müller E, Taube W. Improved postural control after slackline training is accompanied by reduced H-reflexes. *Scand J Med Sci Sports.* (2012) 22:471– 7. doi: 10.1111/j.1600-0838.2010.01268.x

Kiss R, Brueckner D, Muehlbauer T. Effects of single compared to dual task practice on learning a dynamic balance task in young adults. *Front Psychol.* (2018) 9:311. doi: 10.3389/fpsyg.2018.00311

Beurskens R, Brueckner D, Muehlbauer T. Effects of motor versus cognitive task prioritization during dual-task practice on dual-task performance in young adults. *Front Psychol.* (2020) 11:581225. doi: 10.3389/fpsyg.2020.581225

Alsubaie SF, Whitney SL, Furman JM, Marchetti GF, Sienko KH, Sparto PJ. Reliability of postural sway measures of standing balance tasks. *J Appl Biomech.* (2018) 10:1–23. doi: 10.1123/jab.2017-0322

Fujimoto C, Kamogashira T, Kinoshita M, Egami N, Sugasawa K, Demura S, et al. Power spectral analysis of postural sway during foam posturography in patients with peripheral vestibular dysfunction. *Otol Neurotol.* (2014) 35:e317–23. doi: 10.1097/MAO.000000000 0000554

Rasman BG, Forbes PA, Tisserand R, Blouin JS. Sensorimotor manipulations of the balance control loop-beyond imposed external perturbations. *Front Neurol.* (2018) 9:899. doi: 10.3389/fneur.2018.00899

Viseux F, Lemaire A, Barbier F, Charpentier P, Leteneur S, Villeneuve P. How can the stimulation of plantar cutaneous receptors improve postural control? Review and clinical commentary. *Neurophysiol Clin.* (2019) 49:263– 8. doi: 10.1016/j.neucli.2018.12.006

Tremblay F, Mireault AC, Dessureault L, Manning H, Sveistrup H. Postural stabilization from fingertip contact: I. Variations in sway attenuation, perceived stability and contact forces with aging. *Exp Brain Res.* (2004) 157:275–85. doi: 10.1007/s00221-004-1830-4

Tremblay F, Mireault AC, Dessureault L, Manning H, Sveistrup H. Postural stabilization from fingertip contact II. Relationships between age, tactile sensibility and magnitude of contact forces. *Exp Brain Res.* (2005) 164:155– 64. doi: 10.1007/s00221-005-2238-5

Fujimoto C, Egami N, Demura S, Yamasoba T, Iwasaki S. The effect of aging on the center-of-pressure power spectrum in foam posturography. *Neurosci Lett.* (2015) 585:92–7. doi: 10.1016/j.neulet.2014.11.033

Pauelsen M, Jafari H, Strandkvist V, Nyberg L, Gustafsson T, Vikman I, et al. Frequency domain shows: fall-related concerns and sensorimotor decline explain inability to adjust postural control strategy in older adults. *PLoS One.* (2020) 15:e0242608. doi: 10.1371/journal.pone.0242608

Yoneda S, Tokumasu K. Frequency analysis of body sway in the upright posture. Statistical study in cases of peripheral vestibular disease. *Acta Otolaryngol.* (1986) 102:87–92. doi: 10.3109/00016488609108650

Baloh RW, Jacobson KM, Beykirch K, Honrubia V. Static and dynamic posturography in patients with vestibular and cerebellar lesions. *Arch Neurol.* (1998) 55:649–54. doi: 10.1001/archneur.55.5.649

Fino PC, Horak FB, El-Gohary M, Guidarelli C, Medysky ME, Nagle SJ, et al. Postural sway, falls, and self-reported neuropathy in aging female cancer survivors. *Gait Posture.* (2019) 69:136–42. doi: 10.1016/j. gaitpost.2019.01.025

Nagy E, Feher-Kiss A, Barnai M, Domján-Preszner A, Angyan L, Horvath G. Postural control in elderly subjects participating in balance training. *Eur J Appl Physiol.* (2007) 100:97–104. doi: 10.1007/s00421-007-0407-x

20

Tai Chi Training as a Primary Daily Care Plan for Better Balance Ability in People With Parkinson's Disease: An Opinion and Positioning Article

Ting Zhang [1,2], Zhenyu Lv [3] and Song Gao [1]*

[1] College of Physical Education and Health Sciences, Zhejiang Normal University, Jinhua, China, [2] University Hospital, Zhejiang Normal University, Jinhua, China, [3] Department of Chinese Medicine, Naval Special Medical Center, Naval Medical University, Shanghai, China

*Correspondence:
Song Gao
1811516014@sus.edu.cn

Keywords: Parkinson's disease, fall, tai chi, balance ability, limitations

INTRODUCTION

Parkinson's disease (PD) is a common degenerative disease of the central nervous system. Clinically, its incidence is second only to Alzheimer's disease, which seriously harms the health of middle-aged and elderly people (1). Main clinical manifestations of this disease include balance disorder, resting tremor, bradykinesia, and muscle stiffness, and this disease has a high incidence and disability rate. However, initial symptoms of PD are different, and the early symptoms are often ignored by people, which delays the optimal time to manage the disease. PD is closely related to age. Epidemiological surveys showed that the global prevalence of PD is 0.3%, among which the population over 65 years old accounts for 1–2%, and the prevalence rate over 85 years old increases to 3–5% (2, 3). A meta-analysis of people, both genders, with PD showed that men are at higher risk of PD than women (4). The progression of PD is unpredictable and may suddenly worsen. People with PD often complain that their symptoms clearly worsen within one year.

Fall is a balance disorder that often occurs in the late stage of PD. However, some studies have found that abnormal body swings occur in the early stages of PD, that is, mild balance dysfunction, which gradually worsens as the course of the disease progresses (5). Some researchers have found that people with Hoehn-Yahr stageII PD have balance adjustment disorders when they turn around (6). Newly diagnosed unmedicated people with PD have abnormal balance (7). Ultrasound of abnormal brain substantia nigra shows mild balance wobble in high-risk people with PD (8). Therefore, people with PD can have mild balance dysfunction in the early stage (9). As the course of the disease progresses, people with PD will inevitably show signs of abnormal dynamic balance, and even fall, leading to fractures and disability.

Although the apoptosis of dopaminergic cells in the substantia nigra striatum is the main cause of motor symptoms of PD, the balance disorder cannot be explained by lack of dopamine alone. Application of PET-CT found that apoptosis of the substantia nigra is closely related to motor retardation, but it has little to do with postural balance. It is well known that Medoba cannot alleviate or partially alleviate the symptoms of balance disorders in people with PD. Levodopa is the first-line drug for the treatment of PD. It has a good therapeutic effect on muscle stiffness and motor retardation, but there is no consensus on whether it can improve the symptoms of instability in PD (10, 11). In addition, long-term use of drugs can cause adverse drug reactions, such as nausea, vomiting, and orthostatic hypotension. Deep brain stimulation (DBS) is a surgical treatment for movement disorders such as PD (12). A study found that DBS stimulation of bilateral pontine nuclei can provide an effective treatment for alleviating gait and balance abnormalities in people with PD (13). In other studies, the effect of DBS on gait and balance disorders has been less successful and may even lead to freezing and increased gait imbalance (14). For the symptoms of PD, management rather than treatment is considered a more realistic strategy. Therefore, it is particularly important to actively seek safe and effective complementary and alternative therapies to improve the balance disorder in PD. Since 2002, Complementary and alternative therapy has been widely used in the United States and has attracted the attention of patients with neurological diseases (15). Short-term muscle stretching and functional electrical stimulation have also been shown to be effective in improving the gait of patients with PD (16, 17). Exercise therapy is considered to be an adjunct to medical and surgical treatments designed to maximize function, improve quality of life, and minimize or reduce complications (18). Although exercise therapy is recommended as an effective treatment for persons with PD, there is no uniform standard for specific exercise patterns (19, 20).

Fear of falling, decreased muscle strength, and decreased proprioception are the main factors that cause falls. A study reported that the elderly showed lower muscle use efficiency and greater postural swings in standing balance tasks, which means that the elderly has a greater risk of falls (21). Lelard et al. (22) considered that any form of physical activities can increase confidence in maintaining balance, and that strength and proprioception training is the most suitable balance exercises for healthy elderly people. However, due to practical considerations, the elderly, especially elderly people with PD, have a low chance of participating in special strength training.

Tai chi, a popular traditional Chinese martial art, has gradually developed into an exercise therapy. As we all know, tai chi is a form of exercise that requires long-term practice and continuous improvement, and Yang tai chi is the most popular (23). Tai chi can increase muscle strength and improve body coordination. Unlike other complementary and alternative therapies, tai chi training is very economical, and there is no need to consider whether the state can provide subsidies. According to a report, each tai chi class in the United States is worth USD 3.5, which is acceptable to most practitioners (24). Practitioners can choose actions that improve balance and flexibility rather than the entire set of actions. In recent years, tai chi has been proven to improve many diseases, such as chronic obstructive pulmonary disease, heart failure, and knee osteoarthritis (25). In the tai chi training process, participants continuously adjust their center of gravity while moving slowly in multiple directions to maintain their body balance. A meta-analysis showed that tai chi has a promoting effect on balance, and it is believed that it has a good effect on the strengthening of proprioception (26, 27). A study by Guo et al. (28) found that compared with a control group who had not practiced tai chi, the elderly who had practiced tai chi for an average of 9 years or more had a great advantage in proprioception of the knee and ankle joints. This shows that long-term tai chi exercise helps maintain or strengthen the proprioception of the elderly.

The balance and stability of people with PD are seriously threatened, and tai chi training has potential healing effects. Therefore, this article aims to outline the key role of tai chi training in enhancing balance ability and preventing falls in people with PD. Moreover, the authors emphasize the limitations and challenges of this research on tai chi to improve balance ability in PD.

TAI CHI PROMOTES THE BALANCE ABILITY OF PEOPLE WITH PD

Human daily activities cannot be performed without balance ability. Studies have shown that elderly people with PD are more likely to be admitted to a hospital for fractures due to falls (29). Therefore, seeking active and effective exercise methods to enhance the balance ability of elderly people with PD is particularly important for improving their quality of life. Tai chi has slow rhythm and continuous movements. It enhances the balance ability of people with PD by constantly shifting the center of gravity. The decreased balance ability of people with PD is closely related to loss of posture control. Tai chi training finely controls joints through muscle coordination. In addition, tai chi training can strengthen the sensory stimulation of the limbs and lower limb muscles, which is very important for the improvement of the movement and balance ability of people with PD.

In order to investigate how tai chi reduces the risk of falls, Rahal et al. (30) compared the balance ability between healthy elderly people who practiced Tai Chi and ballroom dancers. They found that the tai chi group had faster walking speed and shorter transfer time, and that in the sit-to-stand test the tai chi group had better balance performance in the final standing posture. Besides, Zhou et al. (31) reported the influence of tai chi training on posture control of elderly women. When the tai chi group shifted the center of gravity as quickly as possible to complete the special orientation posture, and remain stable without falling, the overall, lateral, and anteroposterior diameter swing paths of the center of gravity were smaller than those of the control group. The study by Holmes et al. (32) found that tai chi can reduce the swing of the body's center of gravity caused by respiratory disturbance, thereby reducing the instability of the body. Zhou et al. (33) found that Tai Chi can effectively increase muscle strength of the lower limbs for elderly people. Furthermore, crossing obstacles is a behavior that occurs in daily life, which requires better dynamic balance ability. Chang et al. (34) reported that when crossing obstacles, the flexion angle of the hip joint in a tai chi group was significantly greater when raising the leg, and that the tai chi group had a larger stride, faster stepping speed, and shorter time required to cross an obstacle. Therefore, tai chi training has a positive effect on maintaining balance when crossing obstacles. Another research by Zou et al. (35) showed that both the 24-style tai chi and the modified Chen-style tai chi can effectively enhance the balance function and adaptability of body posture control in elderly people with PD. Recent studies have shown that tai chi exercise can better promote balance function, and that it is significantly better than stretching exercises and multi-modal exercises in reducing the incidence of moderate injury falls and severe injury falls (36, 37). However, the results of this study cannot determine whether

Tai Chi is suitable for elderly PD patients since the participants were not PD patients though over 65 years old.

Tai Chi can effectively improve the static balance ability of middle-aged and elderly people, but there is no direct evidence to improve PD patients' static balance ability (38). In tai chi movements, such as "brushing keen and twisting step" and "parting the wild horse's mane," the legs should be open to a larger and suitable angle, and the maximum swing should be emphasized when doing the movements (39, 40). The knees should be bent and squat with the knee joints on the frontal axis. The angle between the sagittal axis and the sagittal axis is increased, and this posture can improve the control ability of the practitioner's lower limbs. This may be the key reason for long-term tai chi training to improve posture control ability and reduce the ellipse area that represents the static balance ability.

The significance of tai chi for the treatment of PD is mainly to improve gait and strengthen neuromuscular control to reduce the risk of falls. Characteristics of the included studies are shown in **Table 1**. A research study by Li et al. (39) found that tai chi can maintain and improve various body functions of elderly people with PD and that it is a very effective exercise therapy. In its follow-up study (41), 195 patients with PD, Hoehn-Yahr stages 1 to 4, were randomly divided into tai chi group, resistance training group, and stretching training group, each for 60 min/time, 2 times/week, for a total of 24 weeks of intervention. The results showed that the tai chi group performed better than the resistance group in terms of maximum excursion, with a difference of 5.55 percentage points (95% confidence interval [CI], 1.12–9.97, $P = 0.01$). In terms of directional control, the difference between groups was 10.45 percentage points (95% CI, 3.89–17, $P = 0.002$). Compared with the stretching group, the tai chi group had more obvious differences between the groups in maximum excursion and direction control. This showed that tai chi has significant effects on improving postural stability and functional ability of people with mild to moderate PD. Liu (42) et al. showed that tai chi exercise-assisted balance and gait training can reduce the occurrence of falls in people with PD, and that the improvement of traction in the tai chi training group was significantly better than that of the control group. A study by Gao et al. (43) found that the 12-week Yang Style tai chi was better than the control group in improving the Berg balance scale ($p < 0.05$), and that the number of falls in the Tai Chi group during the 6-month follow-up period was significantly less than that in the control group. The number of falls in the tai chi group was 0.3 ± 0.62 times, and in the control group it was $= 0.64 \pm 0.74$ times ($p < 0.05$). In a preliminary experiment conducted by Hackney et al. (44), 30 people with PD were randomly divided into a tai chi group and a control group. The tai chi group intervened for 1 h a day twice a week, for a total of 10 weeks. The control group did not intervene. The results showed that before and after exercise, the tai chi group had significant changes in the Berg Balance Scale, Unified Parkinson's Disease Rating Scale (UPDRS), Timed Up and Go, tandem stance test, 6-minute walk, and backward walking compared with the control group.

However, there are only few studies that believe tai chi has no significant effect on reducing falls in people with PD (45, 46). Amano et al. (47) found that tai chi training had no effect on the gait and posture control of people with PD, and that no improvement in people's balance ability was observed. It was speculated that the reason could be the short duration of training, which was only 16 weeks and only 2 to 3 practice sessions per week.

LIMITATIONS OF CURRENT TAI CHI RESEARCH

There are some limitations in the research on Tai Chi improving the balance ability of people with PD. This may be attributed to the following reasons: at present, most clinical control studies recruit subjects who have no foundation in tai chi training. After randomization, the trial group will be given tai chi training and practice for not more than 6 months to evaluate the difference with the control group (46, 47). Therefore, the reason for the diverse conclusions is the difference in the standard degree of tai chi movement and length of training. Moreover, when formulating tai chi to improve the balance ability of people with PD, the characteristics of different tai chi categories should be considered, and unified Tai Chi training movements should be performed. The selection and modification of Tai Chi actions for PD needs to focus on the severity of the disease of people with PD to enhance the reproducibility and generalization of the research results.

Tai Chi, as a medium-intensity aerobic exercise, with frequency of training of three times a week, can meet the recommended standards of American College of Sports Medicine (ACSM). Furthermore, tai chi is a kind of physical and mental exercise. During exercise, breathing and soothing music should be used to effectively improve the mood of people with PD, and it is beneficial to overcome the fear of falling. Compared with the rehabilitation training content of modern medicine, tai chi training improves the abnormal gait and balance disorders of elderly people with PD. It does not require special equipment and venues, and the exercise intensity and difficulty are not challenging, which is convenient for people with PD to practice. Tai chi improves the movement and balance abilities of people with PD, effectively reducing physical and psychological burdens of caregivers, and it has high social and economic benefits.

CONCLUSION

The authors of this article point out that tai chi can improve balance ability and reduce the risk of falls in people with mild to moderate PD. It is an effective non-drug intervention. In addition, in view of the differences in research results, the existing problems of Tai Chi intervention in PD should be deeply analyzed. This is also a key issue that needs attention and

TABLE 1 | Characteristics of the included studies.

Study	Participants	Interventions	Outcomes
Li et al. (39)	$n = 17$ Age: 71.51 (± 5.4) y HY scale1–3 stage ability to walk with/without aids	Yang style Tai Chi-based stepping exercises vs. no intervention 90min, 5 times/week, 5 weeks	50-ft walk, TUGT, FRT
Li et al. (41)	$n = 195$ Age: 40–85y HY scale scale1–4 stage ability to walk with/without aids	Tai Chi vs. resistance training vs. stretching 60 min, 2 times/week, 24 weeks	Falls, TUG, UPDRS-III, limit-of stability, FRT, gait, strength
Gao et al. (43)	$n = 76$ Age>40 y Independent walking≥1 fall during past 1 y	Yang style Tai Chi vs. no intervention 60 min, 3 times/week, 12 weeks	Occurrences of falls, BBS, TUGT, UPDRS-III
Amano et al. (47)	$n = 45$ Age: 50–7 0y HY scale 2–3 stage ability to walk with/without aids	Tai Chi vs. Qigong vs. no intervention 60 min, 2 times/week, 16 weeks	GI, gait, UPDRS-III
Hackney et al. (44)	$n = 26$ Age > 40 y HY scale 1.5–3 stageindependent walking with/without aids for 3 m	Yang short style Tai Chi vs. no intervention 60 min, 2 times/week, 20 sessions	BBS, TUG, TS, UPDRS-III,OLS, GAITRite, 6MWT

HY scale, Hoehn and Yahr scale; TUGT, timed up and go test; FRT, functional reach test; UPDRS, Unified Parkinson's Disease Rating Scale; BBS, Berg Balance Scale; GI, gait initiation; TS, tandem stance; OLS, one-leg stance; 6MWT, 6-min walk test.

consideration in the future research. However, more evidence-based research is needed to prove the effectiveness of tai chi in improving balance ability and preventing falls of people with PD. Researchers designing tai chi movements should take into full consideration the special physical conditions of people with PD, movements that are simple and easy to learn while having good effects on improving balance ability. Based on a good mass foundation, tai chi movement will be more widely used and promoted as a daily care plan for people with PD.

AUTHOR CONTRIBUTIONS

TZ and ZL conceived the manuscript and revised the drafts. SG wrote the first draft. All authors contributed to the article and approved the submitted version.

FUNDING

This study was supported by the College of Physical Education and Health Sciences, Zhejiang Normal University, Jinhua, China.

REFERENCES

Arii Y, Sawada Y, Kawamura K, Miyake S, Taichi Y, Izumi Y, et al. Immediate effect of spinal magnetic stimulation on camptocormia in Parkinson's disease. *J Neurol Neurosurg Psychiatry.* (2014) 85:1221–6. doi: 10.1136/jnnp-2014-30 7651

de Lau LML, Breteler MMB. Epidemiology of Parkinson's disease. *Lancet Neurol.* (2006) 5:525–35 doi: 10.1016/S1474-4422(06)70471-9

Elbaz A, Carcaillon L, Kab S, Moisan F. Epidemiology of Parkinson's disease. *Rev Neurol (Paris).* (2016) 172:14–26. doi: 10.1016/j.neurol.2015.09.012

Taylor KSM, Cook JA, Counsell CE. Heterogeneity in male to female risk for Parkinson's disease. *J Neurol Neurosurg Psychiatry.* (2007) 78:905– 6 doi: 10.1136/jnnp.2006.104695

Kim SD, Allen NE, Canning CG, Fung VSC. Postural instability in patients with Parkinson's disease. epidemiology, pathophysiology and management. *CNS Drugs.* (2013) 27:97–112. doi: 10.1007/s40263-012-0012-3

Song J, Sigward S, Fisher B, Salem GJ. Altered dynamic postural control during step turning in persons with early-stage parkinson's disease. *Parkinsons Dis.* (2012) 2012:386962. doi: 10.1155/2012/386962

Mancini M, Horak FB, Zampieri C, Carlson-Kuhta P, Nutt JG, Chiari L. Trunk accelerometry reveals postural instability in untreated Parkinson's disease. *Parkinsonism Relat Disord.* (2011) 17:557–62. doi: 10.1016/j.parkreldis.2011.05.010

Maetzler W, Mancini M, Liepelt-Scarfone I, Müller K, Becker C, van Lummel RC, et al. Impaired trunk stability in individuals at high risk for Parkinson's disease. *PLoS ONE.* (2012) 7:e32240. doi: 10.1371/journal.pone.0032240

Delafontaine A, Hansen C, Marolleau I, Kratzenstein S, Gouelle A. Effect of a concurrent cognitive task, with stabilizing visual information and withdrawal, on body sway adaptation of Parkinsonian's patients in an off-medication state: a controlled study. *Sensors (Basel).* (2020) 20:18. doi: 10.3390/s20185059

Nova IC, Perracini MR, Ferraz HB. Levodopa effect upon functional balance of Parkinson's disease patients. *Parkinsonism Relat Disord.* (2004) 10:411– 5 doi: 10.1016/j.parkreldis.2004.04.004

Rocchi L, Chiari L, Horak FB. Effects of deep brain stimulation and levodopa on postural sway in Parkinson's disease. *J Neurol Neurosurg Psychiatry.* (2002) 73:267–74 doi: 10.1136/jnnp.73.3.267

Fukaya C, Yamamoto T. Deep brain stimulation for Parkinson's disease: recent trends and future direction. *Neurol Med Chir.* (2015) 55:422–31. doi: 10.2176/nmc.ra.2014-0446

Stefani A, Lozano AM, Peppe A, Stanzione P, Galati S, Tropepi D, et al. Bilateral deep brain stimulation of the pedunculopontine and subthalamic nuclei in severe Parkinson's disease. *Brain.* (2007) 130(Pt 6):1596–607 doi: 10.1093/brain/awl346

Collomb-Clerc A, Welter ML. Effects of deep brain stimulation on balance and gait in patients with Parkinson's disease: A systematic neurophysiological review. *Neurophysiol Clin.* (2015) 45:371–88. doi: 10.1016/j.neucli.2015.07.001

Du S, Dong J, Zhang H, Jin S, Xu G, Liu Z, et al. Taichi exercise for self-rated sleep quality in older people: a systematic review and meta-analysis. *Int J Nurs Stud.* (2015) 52:368–79. doi: 10.1016/j.ijnurstu.2014.05.009

Delafontaine A, Fourcade P, Zemouri A, Diakhaté DG, Saiydoun G, Yiou E. In patients with parkinson's disease in an off-medication state, does bilateral electrostimulation of tibialis anterior improve anticipatory postural adjustments during gait initiation? *Front Hum Neurosci.* (2021) 15:692651. doi: 10.3389/fnhum.2021.692651

Vialleron T, Delafontaine A, Millerioux I, Memari S, Fourcade P, Yiou E. Acute effects of short-term stretching of the triceps surae on ankle mobility and gait initiation in patients with Parkinson's disease. *Clin Biomech.* (2021) 89:105449. doi: 10.1016/j.clinbiomech.2021.105449

Abbruzzese G, Marchese R, Avanzino L, Pelosin E. Rehabilitation for Parkinson's disease: Current outlook and future challenges. *Parkinsonism Relat Disord.* (2016) 22 Suppl 1:S60–S4. doi: 10.1016/j.parkreldis.2015.09.005

Luan X, Tian X, Zhang H, Huang R, Li N, Chen P, et al. Exercise as a prescription for patients with various diseases. *J Sport Health Sci.* (2019) 8:422–1. doi: 10.1016/j.jshs.2019.04.002

Guo S, Huang Y, Zhang Y, Huang H, Hong S, Liu T. Impacts of exercise interventions on different diseases and organ functions in mice. *J Sport Health Sci.* (2020) 9:53–73. doi: 10.1016/j.jshs.2019.07.004

Donath L, Kurz E, Roth R, Zahner L, Faude O. Leg and trunk muscle coordination and postural sway during increasingly difficult standing balance tasks in young and older adults. *Maturitas.* (2016) 91:60–8. doi: 10.1016/j.maturitas.2016.05.010

Lelard T, Ahmaidi S. Effects of physical training on age-related balance and postural control. *Neurophysiol Clin.* (2015) 45:357–69. doi: 10.1016/j.neucli.2015.09.008

Huang Z-G, Feng Y-H, Li Y-H, Lv C-S. Systematic review and meta-analysis: Tai Chi for preventing falls in older adults. *BMJ Open.* (2017) 7:e013661. doi: 10.1136/bmjopen-2016-013661

Li F, Harmer P, McAuley E, Duncan TE, Duncan SC, Chaumeton N, et al. An evaluation of the effects of Tai Chi exercise on physical function among older persons: a randomized contolled trial. *Ann Behav Med.* (2001) 23:139–46 doi: 10.1207/S15324796ABM2302_9

Lan C, Lai J-S, Chen S-Y. Tai Chi Chuan: an ancient wisdom on exercise and health promotion. *Sports Med.* (2002) 32:217–24 doi: 10.2165/00007256-200232040-00001

Winser SJ, Tsang WW, Krishnamurthy K, Kannan P. Does Tai Chi improve balance and reduce falls incidence in neurological disorders? a systematic review and meta-analysis. *Clin Rehabil.* (2018) 32:1157–68. doi: 10.1177/0269215518773442

Zou L, Han J, Li C, Yeung AS, Hui SS-C, Tsang WWN, et al. Effects of tai chi on lower limb proprioception in adults aged over 55: a systematic review and meta-analysis. *Arch Phys Med Rehabil.* (2019) 100:1102–13. doi: 10.1016/j.apmr.2018.07.425

Guo L-y, Yang C-p, You Y-l, Chen S-k, Yang C-h, Hou Y-y, et al. Underlying mechanisms of Tai-Chi-Chuan training for improving balance ability in the elders. *Chin J Integr Med.* (2014) 20:409–15. doi: 10.1007/s11655-013-1533-4

Lan C, Chen S-Y, Lai J-S, Wong AM-K. Tai chi chuan in medicine and health promotion. *Evid Based Complement Alternat Med.* (2013) 2013:502131. doi: 10.1155/2013/502131

Rahal MA, Alonso AC, Andrusaitis FR, Rodrigues TS, Speciali DS, Greve JMDA, et al. Analysis of static and dynamic balance in healthy elderly practitioners of Tai Chi Chuan versus ballroom dancing. *Clinics (São Paulo).* (2015) 70:157–61. doi: 10.6061/clinics/2015(03)01

Zhou J, Chang S, Cong Y, Qin M, Sun W, Lian J, et al. Effects of 24 weeks of Tai Chi Exercise on postural control among elderly women. *Res Sports Med.* (2015) 23:302–14. doi: 10.1080/15438627.2015.1040918

Holmes ML, Manor B, Hsieh W-h, Hu K, Lipsitz LA, Li L. Tai Chi training reduced coupling between respiration and postural control. *Neurosci Lett.* (2016) 610:60–5. doi: 10.1016/j.neulet.2015.10.053

Zhou M, Peng N, Dai Q, Li H-W, Shi R-G, Huang W. Effect of Tai Chi on muscle strength of the lower extremities in the elderly. *Chin J Integr Med.* (2016) 22:861–6 doi: 10.1007/s11655-015-2104-7

Chang Y-T, Huang C-F, Chang J-H. The effect of tai chi chuan on obstacle crossing strategy in older adults. *Res Sports Med.* (2015) 23:315–29. doi: 10.1080/15438627.2015.1040920

Zou L, Loprinzi PD, Yu JJ, Yang L, Li C, Yeung AS, et al. Superior effects of modified chen-style tai chi versus 24-style tai chi on cognitive function, fitness, and balance performance in adults over 55. *Brain Sci.* (2019) 9:5. doi: 10.3390/brainsci9050102

Moreland B, Kakara R, Henry A. Trends in nonfatal falls and fall-related injuries among adults aged ≥65 Years - United States, 2012-2018. *MMWR Morb Mortal Wkly Rep.* (2020) 69:875–81. doi: 10.15585/mmwr.mm6927a5

Li F, Harmer P, Eckstrom E, Fitzgerald K, Chou L-S, Liu Y. Effectiveness of tai ji quan vs multimodal and stretching exercise interventions for reducing injurious falls in older adults at high risk of falling: follow-up analysis of a randomized clinical trial. *JAMA Netw Open.* (2019) 2:e188280. doi: 10.1001/jamanetworkopen.2018.8280

Li Y, Devault CN, Van Oteghen S. Effects of extended Tai Chi intervention on balance and selected motor functions of the elderly. *Am J Chin Med.* (2007) 35:383–91 doi: 10.1142/S0192415X07004904

Li F, Harmer P, Fisher KJ, Xu J, Fitzgerald K, Vongjaturapat N. Tai Chi-based exercise for older adults with Parkinson's disease: a pilot-program evaluation. *J Aging Phys Act.* (2007) 15:139–51 doi: 10.1123/japa.15.2.139

Schleicher MM, Wedam L, Wu G. Review of Tai Chi as an effective exercise on falls prevention in elderly. *Res Sports Med.* (2012) 20:37–58. doi: 10.1080/15438627.2012.634697

Li F, Harmer P, Fitzgerald K, Eckstrom E, Stock R, Galver J, et al. Tai chi and postural stability in patients with Parkinson's disease. *N Engl J Med.* (2012) 366:511–9. doi: 10.1056/NEJMoa1107911

Liu H-H, Yeh N-C, Wu Y-F, Yang Y-R, Wang R-Y, Cheng F-Y. Effects of Tai Chi exercise on reducing falls and improving balance performance in parkinson's disease: a meta-analysis. *Parkinsons Dis.* (2019) 2019:9626934. doi: 10.1155/2019/9626934

Gao Q, Leung A, Yang Y, Wei Q, Guan M, Jia C, et al. Effects of Tai Chi on balance and fall prevention in Parkinson's disease: a randomized controlled trial. *Clin Rehabil.* (2014) 28:748–53 doi: 10.1177/0269215514521044

Hackney ME, Earhart GM. Tai Chi improves balance and mobility in people with Parkinson disease. *Gait Posture.* (2008) 28:456–60. doi: 10.1016/j.gaitpost.2008.02.005

Taylor-Piliae RE, Hoke TM, Hepworth JT, Latt LD, Najafi B, Coull BM. Effect of Tai Chi on physical function, fall rates and quality of life among older stroke survivors. *Arch Phys Med Rehabil.* (2014) 95:816–24. doi: 10.1016/j.apmr.2014.01.001

Kurlan R, Evans R, Wrigley S, McPartland S, Bustami R, Cotter A. Tai Chi in Parkinson!s Disease: a preliminary randomized, controlled, and rater-blinded study. *Adv Parkinson's Dis.* (2015) :9-12. doi: 10.4236/apd.2015.41002

Amano S, Nocera JR, Vallabhajosula S, Juncos JL, Gregor RJ, Waddell DE, et al. The effect of Tai Chi exercise on gait initiation and gait performance in persons with Parkinson's disease. *Parkinsonism Relat Disord.* (2013) 19:955–60. doi: 10.1016/j.parkreldis.2013.06.007

Permissions

The contributors of this book come from diverse backgrounds, making this book a truly international effort. This book will bring forth new frontiers with its revolutionizing research information and detailed analysis of the nascent developments around the world.

We would like to thank all the contributing authors for lending their expertise to make the book truly unique. They have played a crucial role in the development of this book. Without their invaluable contributions this book wouldn't have been possible. They have made vital efforts to compile up to date information on the varied aspects of this subject to make this book a valuable addition to the collection of many professionals and students.

This book was conceptualized with the vision of imparting up-to-date information and advanced data in this field. To ensure the same, a matchless editorial board was set up. Every individual on the board went through rigorous rounds of assessment to prove their worth. After which they invested a large part of their time researching and compiling the most relevant data for our readers.

The editorial board has been involved in producing this book since its inception. They have spent rigorous hours researching and exploring the diverse topics which have resulted in the successful publishing of this book. They have passed on their knowledge of decades through this book. To expedite this challenging task, the publisher supported the team at every step. A small team of assistant editors was also appointed to further simplify the editing procedure and attain best results for the readers.

Apart from the editorial board, the designing team has also invested a significant amount of their time in understanding the subject and creating the most relevant covers. They scrutinized every image to scout for the most suitable representation of the subject and create an appropriate cover for the book.

The publishing team has been an ardent support to the editorial, designing and production team. Their endless efforts to recruit the best for this project, has resulted in the accomplishment of this book. They are a veteran in the field of academics and their pool of knowledge is as vast as their experience in printing. Their expertise and guidance has proved useful at every step. Their uncompromising quality standards have made this book an exceptional effort. Their encouragement from time to time has been an inspiration for everyone.

The publisher and the editorial board hope that this book will prove to be a valuable piece of knowledge for researchers, students, practitioners and scholars across the globe.

List of Contributors

Olivier Beauchet
Department of Medicine, Division of Geriatric Medicine, Sir Mortimer B. Davis—Jewish General Hospital and Lady Davis Institute for Medical Research, McGill University, Montreal, QC, Canada
Dr. Joseph Kaufmann Chair in Geriatric Medicine, Faculty of Medicine, McGill University, Montreal, QC, Canada
Centre of Excellence on Aging and Chronic Diseases of McGill Integrated University Health Network, QC, Canada

Gilles Allali
Department of Neurology, Geneva University Hospital and University of Geneva, Geneva, Switzerland
Division of Cognitive & Motor Aging, Department of Neurology, Albert Einstein College of Medicine, Yeshiva University, Bronx, NY, United States

Harmehr Sekhon
Department of Medicine, Division of Geriatric Medicine, Sir Mortimer B. Davis—Jewish General Hospital and Lady Davis Institute for Medical Research, McGill University, Montreal, QC, Canada

Joe Verghese
Division of Cognitive & Motor Aging, Department of Neurology, Albert Einstein College of Medicine, Yeshiva University, Bronx, NY, United States

Sylvie Guilain
Geriatric Department, Liège University Hospital, Liege, Belgium
Laboratory of Human Motion Analysis, Liège University, Liege, Belgium

Jean-Paul Steinmetz
Centre for Memory and Mobility, Luxembourg City, Luxembourg

Reto W. Kressig
Basel University Center for Medicine of Aging, Felix Platter Hospital and University of Basel, Basel, Switzerland

John M. Barden
Faculty of Kinesiology and Health Studies, Neuromechanical Research Centre, University of Regina, Regina, SK, Canada

Tony Szturm
Department of Physical Therapy, College of Rehabilitation Sciences, University of Manitoba, Winnipeg, MB, Canada

Cyrille P. Launay
Division of Geriatrics, Angers University Hospital, Angers, France

Sébastien Grenier
Centre de Recherche, Institut Universitaire de Gériatrie de Montréal, Montreal, QC, Canada

Louis Bherer
Centre de Recherche, Institut Universitaire de Gériatrie de Montréal, Montreal, QC, Canada
Department of Medicine and Montreal Heart Institute, University of Montreal, Montreal, Canada

Teresa Liu-Ambrose
Aging, Mobility and Cognitive Neuroscience Laboratory, University of British Columbia, Vancouver, BC, Canada

Vicky L. Chester
Andrew and Marjorie McCain Human Performance Laboratory, Richard J. Currie Center, Faculty of Kinesiology, University of New Brunswick, Fredericton, NB, Canada

Michele L. Callisaya
Menzies Institute of Medical Research, University of Tasmania, Hobart, TAS, Australia
Stroke and Ageing Research Group, Department of Medicine, Southern Clinical School, Monash University, Melbourne, VIC, Australia

Velandai Srikanth
Stroke and Ageing Research Group, Department of Medicine, Southern Clinical School, Monash University, Melbourne, VIC, Australia

Guillaume Léonard
Research Center on Aging, CIUSSS de l'Estrie-CHUS, Sherbrooke, QC, Canada

Anne-Marie De Cock
Department of Geriatrics and Department of Primary and Interdisciplinary Care (ELIZA), University of Antwerp and AZ St. Maarten Mechelen, Antwerp, Belgium

Ryuichi Sawa
Department of Physical Therapy, School of Health Sciences at Narita, International University of Health and Welfare, Narita, Japan

Richard Camicioli
Division of Neurology, Department of Medicine, University of Alberta, Edmonton, AB, Canada

Gustavo Duque
Australian Institute for Musculoskeletal Science, University of Melbourne and Western Health, St. Albans, VIC, Australia

Jorunn L. Helbostad
Department of Neuro-Medicine and Movement Science, Faculty of Medicine and Health Sciences, Norwegian University of Science and Technology, Trondheim, Norway
Clinic for Clinical Services, St. Olav University Hospital, Trondheim, Norway

Hortense Chatard
UMR 1141, Institut National de la Santé et de la Recherche Médicale — Université Paris 7, Robert Debré University Hospital, Paris, France
Vestibular and Oculomotor Evaluation Unit, ENT Department, Robert Debré University Hospital, Paris, France
Centre Ophtalmologique du Val-d'Oise (OPH95), Osny, France

Laure Tepenier, Talal Beydoun and Sawsen Salah
Groupe Hospitalier Cochin-Hôtel-Dieu, Department of Ophthalmology, Assistance Publique-Hôpitaux de Paris, Paris Descartes University, Paris, France

Olivier Jankowski, Antoine Aussems and Alain Allieta
Centre Ophtalmologique du Val-d'Oise (OPH95), Osny, France

Maria P. Bucci
UMR 1141, Institut National de la Santé et de la Recherche Médicale — Université Paris 7, Robert Debré University Hospital, Paris, France
Vestibular and Oculomotor Evaluation Unit, ENT Department, Robert Debré University Hospital, Paris, France

Robert T. Thibault
Integrated Program in Neuroscience, Department of Neurology and Neurosurgery, McGill University, Montreal, QC, Canada

Amir Raz
Integrated Program in Neuroscience, Department of Neurology and Neurosurgery, McGill University, Montreal, QC, Canada
The Lady Davis Institute for Medical Research at the Jewish General Hospital, Montreal, QC, Canada
Department of Psychiatry, Institute for Community and Family Psychiatry, McGill University, Montreal, QC, Canada

Brice Isableu
Aix Marseille Univ, PSYCLE, Aix-en-Provence, France

Petra Hlavackova
Équipe d'Accueil Autonomy, Gerontology, E-health, Imaging & Society, Université Grenoble-Alpes, Grenoble, France
Grenoble Alpes University Hospital, Grenoble, France

Bruno Diot
Équipe d'Accueil Autonomy, Gerontology, E-health, Imaging & Society, Université Grenoble-Alpes, Grenoble, France
Informatique de Sécurité, Montceau-les-Mines, France

Nicolas Vuillerme
Équipe d'Accueil Autonomy, Gerontology, E-health, Imaging & Society, Université Grenoble-Alpes, Grenoble, France
Institut Universitaire de France, Paris, France

Eric Yiou, Romain Artico, Claudine A. Teyssedre, Ombeline Labaune and Paul Fourcade
CIAMS, Université Paris Sud, Université Paris-Saclay, Orsay, France
CIAMS, Université d'Orléans, Orléans, France

Carlo Bruttini, Roberto Esposti, Francesco Bolzoni and Paolo Cavallari
Human Motor Control and Posture Laboratory, Human Physiology Section of the DePT, Università degli Studi di Milano, Milan, Italy

Manh-Cuong Do
CIAMS, Université Paris-Sud Université Paris-Saclay, Orsay, France; CIAMS, Université d'Orléans, Orléans, France

Olivier Gagey
CIAMS, Université Paris-Sud Université Paris-Saclay, Orsay, France; CIAMS, Université d'Orléans, Orléans, France
Service de Chirurgie Orthopédique, C.H.U Kremlin Bicêtre, Kremlin Bicêtre, France

Silvia Colnaghi and Jean-Louis Honeine
CSAM Laboratory, Department of Public Health, University of Pavia, Pavia, Italy

Sébastien Ditcharles and Arnaud Delafontaine
CIAMS, Université Paris-Sud, Université Paris-Saclay, Orsay, France
CIAMS, Université d'Orléans, Orléans, France
Ecole Nationale de Kinésithérapie et Rééducation (ENKRE), Saint-Maurice, France

Thierry Lelard and Said Ahmaidi
EA-3300: Adaptations Physiologiques à l'Exercice et Réadaptation à l'Effort, Faculté des Sciences du Sport, Université de Picardie Jules Verne, Amiens, France

Alain Hamaoui
Laboratoire de Physiologie de la Posture et du Mouvement (PoM Lab), Université JF Champollion, Albi, France
Laboratoire Activité Physique, Performance et Santé (MEPS), Université de Pau et des Pays de l'Adour (UPPA), Tarbes, France

Christian A. Clermont and Dylan Kobsar
Faculty of Kinesiology, University of Calgary, Calgary, AB, Canada

Agnès Olivier
CIAMS, Univ Paris-Sud, Université Paris-Saclay, Orsay, France
CIAMS, Université d'Orléans, Orléans, France
Normandie Univ, UNICAEN, CESAMS, Caen, France

Elise Faugloire and Laure Lejeune
Normandie Univ, UNICAEN, CESAMS, Caen, France

Sophie Biau
ENE, Institut Français du Cheval et de l'Equitation, Saumur, France

Pierre-Louis Doutrellot
EA-3300: Adaptations Physiologiques à l'Exercice et Réadaptation à l'Effort, Faculté des Sciences du Sport, Université de Picardie Jules Verne, Amiens, France
Service Medecine Physique et Rééducation, Centre Hospitalier Universitaire, Amiens, France

Abdou Temfemo
EA-3300: Adaptations Physiologiques à l'Exercice et Réadaptation à l'Effort, Faculté des Sciences du Sport, Université de Picardie Jules Verne, Amiens, France
Department of Biological Sciences, Faculty of Medicine and Pharmaceutical Sciences, University of Douala, Douala, Cameroon

Julien Maitre and Thierry P. Paillard
Laboratoire Mouvement Equilibre, Performance et Santé, EA 4445, Département Sciences et Techniques des Activités Physiques et Sportives (STAPS), Université de Pau et des Pays de l'Adour, Tarbes, France

Cheng-Ya Huang
School and Graduate Institute of Physical Therapy, College of Medicine, National Taiwan University, Taipei City, Taiwan
Physical Therapy Center, National Taiwan University Hospital, Taipei, Taiwan

Clément Morant
Aix-Marseille Université, CNRS, Laboratoire de Neurosciences Cognitives, FR 3C, Marseille, France
Aix-Marseille Université, CNRS, Institut des Sciences du Mouvement, Marseille, France

Gwo-Ching Chang
Department of Information Engineering, I-Shou University, Kaohsiung City, Taiwan

Yi-Ying Tsai
Institute of Allied Health Sciences, College of Medicine, National Cheng Kung University, Tainan City, Taiwan

Ing-Shiou Hwang
Institute of Allied Health Sciences, College of Medicine, National Cheng Kung University, Tainan City, Taiwan
Department of Physical Therapy, College of Medicine, National Cheng Kung University, Tainan City, Taiwan

Jernej Čamernik
Department for Automation, Biocybernetics and Robotics, Jožef Stefan Institute, Ljubljana, Slovenia
Jožef Stefan International Postgraduate School, Ljubljana, Slovenia

Zrinka Potocanac and Jan Babič
Department for Automation, Biocybernetics and Robotics, Jožef Stefan Institute, Ljubljana, Slovenia

Luka Peternel
Department for Automation, Biocybernetics and Robotics, Jožef Stefan Institute, Ljubljana, Slovenia
HRI2 Laboratory, Department of Advanced Robotics, Istituto Italiano di Tecnologia, Genoa, Italy

Laurence Mouchnino and Olivia Lhomond
Aix-Marseille Université, CNRS, Laboratoire de Neurosciences Cognitives, FR 3C, Marseille, France

Pascale Chavet
Aix-Marseille Université, CNRS, Institut des Sciences du Mouvement, Marseille, France

Jacques Abboud
Département d'Anatomie, Université du Québec à Trois-Rivières, Trois-Rivières, QC, Canada

François Nougarou
Département de Génie Électrique, Université du Québec à Trois-Rivières, Trois-Rivières, QC, Canada

Arnaud Lardon
Institut Franco-Européen de Chiropraxie, Ivry-Sur-Seine, France
Département des Sciences de l'Activité Physique, Université du Québec à Trois-Rivières, Trois-Rivières, QC, Canada

Claude Dugas and Martin Descarreaux
Département des Sciences de l'Activité Physique, Université du Québec à Trois-Rivières, Trois-Rivières, QC, Canada

Romain Tisserand, Thomas Robert and Laurence Chèze
IFSTTAR, UMR_T9406, Laboratoire de Biomécanique et Mécanique des Chocs (LBMC), Université de Lyon, Université Claude Bernard Lyon 1, Lyon, France

Pascal Chabaud
Laboratoire Interuniversitaire de Biologie de la Motricité (LIBM), Université de Lyon, Université Claude Bernard Lyon 1, Villeurbanne, France

Marc Bonnefoy
Service de Médecine Gériatrique, Centre Hospitalier Lyon Sud, Pierre-Bénite, France

Emma G. Dupuy, Pascale Leconte, Elodie Vlamynck, Pierre Denise, Stéphane Besnard and Leslie M. Decker
COMETE, INSERM, UNICAEN, Normandie Université, Caen, France

Audrey Sultan and Boris Bienvenu
COMETE, INSERM, UNICAEN, Normandie Université, Caen, France
Department of Internal Medicine, University Hospital Center of Caen, UNICAEN, Normandie Université, Caen, France

Christophe Chesneau
LMNO, CNRS, UNICAEN, Normandie Université, Caen, France

Stefania Sozzi
Centro Studi Attività Motorie (CSAM), Istituti Clinici Scientifici Maugeri SB (Istituto di Ricovero e Cura a Carattere Scientifico, IRCCS), Pavia, Italy

Antonio Nardone
Neurorehabilitation and Spinal Unit, Department of Clinical-Surgical, Diagnostic and Pediatric Sciences, Istituti Clinici Scientifici Maugeri SB (Istituto di Ricovero e Cura a Carattere Scientifico, IRCCS), University of Pavia, Pavia, Italy

Marco Schieppati
Istituti Clinici Scientifici Maugeri SB, Istituto di Ricovero e Cura a Carattere Scientifico (IRCCS), Pavia, Italy

Ting Zhang
College of Physical Education and Health Sciences, Zhejiang Normal University, Jinhua, China
University Hospital, Zhejiang Normal University, Jinhua, China

Zhenyu Lv
Department of Chinese Medicine, Naval Special Medical Center, Naval Medical University, Shanghai, China

Song Gao
College of Physical Education and Health Sciences, Zhejiang Normal University, Jinhua, China

Index